W9-CSJ-602

Essentials of Health Care Finance
Sixth Edition

William O. Cleverley, PhD, CPA
President
Cleverley & Associates
Professor Emeritus
The Ohio State University
Columbus, OH

Andrew E. Cameron, PhD, MBA
Principal
Managing Director, Columbus, Ohio Office
Kurron Shares of America, Inc.
New York, NY

JONES AND BARTLETT PUBLISHERS
Sudbury, Massachusetts
BOSTON   TORONTO   LONDON   SINGAPORE

World Headquarters
Jones and Bartlett Publishers
40 Tall Pine Drive
Sudbury, MA 01776
978-443-5000
info@jbpub.com
www.jbpub.com

Jones and Bartlett Publishers
Canada
6339 Ormindale Way
Mississauga, Ontario L5V 1J2
CANADA

Jones and Bartlett Publishers
International
Barb House, Barb Mews
London W6 7PA
UK

Jones and Bartlett's books and products are available through most bookstores and online booksellers. To contact Jones and Bartlett Publishers directly, call 800-832-0034, fax 978-443-8000, or visit our website, www.jbpub.com.

Substantial discounts on bulk quantities of Jones and Bartlett's publications are available to corporations, professional associations, and other qualified organizations. For details and specific discount information, contact the special sales department at Jones and Bartlett via the above contact information or send an email to special-sales@jbpub.com.

Production Credits
Publisher: Michael Brown
Associate Editor: Kylah Goodfellow McNeill
Production Director: Amy Rose
Production Editor: Tracey Chapman
Marketing Manager: Sophie Fleck
Manufacturing Buyer: Therese Connell
Composition: Auburn Associates, Inc.
Cover Design: Kristin E. Ohlin
Cover Image: © Photos.com
Printing and Binding: Transcontinental
Cover Printing: Transcontinental

Library of Congress Cataloging-in-Publication Data
Cleverley, William O.
    Essentials of health care finance / William O. Cleverley, Andrew E. Cameron.—6th ed.
        p. cm.
    Includes bibliographical references.
    ISBN-13: 978-0-7637-4236-2 (casebound)
    ISBN-10: 0-7637-4236-8 (casebound)
    1. Hospitals—Finance. 2. Hospitals—Accounting. 3. Health facilities—Finance. 4. Health facilities—Accounting.
I. Cameron, Andrew E. II. Title.
    RA971.3.C528 2007
    362.11068'1—dc22
                                                                                    2006025213

6048

Printed in the United States of America
12 11 10 09 08   10 9 8 7 6 5 4 3

Dedication

Dr. Cleverley dedicates this book to his four grandchildren—Joshua, Riley, Mikaela, and Ainsley.

Dr. Cameron dedicates this book to his mentor and friend, Corbett A. Price, Chairman of Kurron, a visionary health care executive and strategic thinker.

Table of Contents

Preface

This book represents the sixth edition of a book published originally in 1978, entitled *Essentials of Hospital Finance*. The text has evolved from being a book containing seven chapters that dealt largely with understanding and interpreting hospital financial statements, to being a comprehensive financial text. The sixth edition has 22 chapters that cover most of the major areas of financial decision making that health care executives deal with on a daily basis.

There are many reasons why this book has been so widely used over the years. No other textbook so fully melds the best of current finance theory with the tools needed for day-to-day practice by health care managers. The textbook also encompasses virtually the whole spectrum of the health care industry, including hospitals, pharmaceutical companies, health maintenance organizations, home health agencies, skilled nursing facilities, surgical centers, physician practices, hospital departments, and integrated health care systems.

Building on the strong foundation of the previous editions, the sixth edition introduces a number of enhancements. We have continued the inclusion of learning objectives at the beginning of each chapter. The learning objectives orient the students to the material in the chapter and highlight some particular concepts and skills they should acquire by studying the chapter. A new feature of this edition is the repetition of each learning objective in the text preceding the discussion specific to that objective. This will allow students to easily locate topics of interest. As in previous editions, each chapter also has a real-world scenario, which illustrates how the chapter concepts and tools are used in practice. As with previous editions, each chapter

concludes with a summary, followed by a large number of assignments with related solutions.

Before discussing the coverage of this book, it is important to understand the objective, which has not changed in more than 20 years. This text is intended to provide a relevant and readable text for health care management students and executives. This is important to understand because *Essentials of Health Care Finance* is neither a traditional finance textbook, nor is it a traditional management or financial accounting textbook. It attempts to blend the topics of both accounting and finance that have become part of the everyday life of most health care executives. This textbook does not provide as much coverage of cost of capital, capital structure, and capital budgeting topics as is present in most financial management textbooks. *Essentials of Health Care Finance* likewise does not provide significant discussion on management control and budgeting systems, which are typically present in most cost accounting and management accounting textbooks. This book attempts to cover the types of financial decisions that health care executives are most likely to be involved with; it provides material that will help them understand the conceptual basis and mechanics of financial analysis and decision making, as they pertain to the health care industry sector.

CONTENT OF THE BOOK

The general basis of financial decision making in any business is almost always built upon understanding three critical elements. First, most financial decisions are based upon the use of accounting information. It is difficult to make intelligent decisions without having at least a basic understanding of accounting information. The user does not need to be a CPA, but it is essential to have a little understanding of what accounting is and is not. Second, all business units operate within an industry. The health care industry is a huge, complex industry that is unlike any other industry in many ways. Unless the student has an understanding and appreciation for these critical differences, major mistakes can be made. Finally, both accounting and finance are, in many ways, subsets of economics. The principles of economics form the conceptual basis upon which many types of business decisions are made.

Chapter 1 provides some introductory linkages to the role of information in decision making. Chapter 2, "Billing and Coding for Health Services," is a new chapter that recognizes the increasingly important role that billing and coding play in financial decision making. Chapter 3, "Financial Environment of Health Care Organizations," provides detailed information about the economic environment of health care firms. Specific coverage of payment methods for all types of providers, from hospitals to physicians, is included. Much of Chapter 3 was rewritten for this edition. For example, this edition incorporates information about current Medicare prospective payment systems for outpatient, home health, and skilled nursing facilities. Chapter 4 provides coverage of the numerous legal and regulatory provisions that affect today's health care manager. Chapter 5, "Revenue Determination: Pricing and Contracting," is the second new chapter in the sixth edition and devotes specific attention to pricing and managed care contract negotiations. Extensive coverage of managed care, its definition, concepts, organizational

structures, and its financial implications are included in Chapter 6 and woven throughout the remainder of the text. Managed care contracting is covered far more extensively in this edition.

Chapters 7, 8, and 9 discuss financial reporting for health care firms, while incorporating accounting jargon. Perhaps of more importance, these chapters refer to accounting terms specifically related to health care issues, such as self insurance of professional liability.

Chapters 10, 11, and 12 cover financial analysis and financial planning. Chapter 10 has been thoroughly revised to reflect the best analytical tools and techniques available for financial statement analysis. Chapter 11 provides specific coverage of health care firms other than hospitals. Comparative financial and operating benchmark values are included for hospitals, health maintenance organizations, nursing homes, and medical groups; these values are used later to evaluate the financial position of a number of different kinds of health care firms.

Topics discussed in Chapters 13 through 15 are cost finding, pricing, break-even analysis, budgeting, and other managerial care examples and concepts. This section of the book also features more extensive coverage of relative value units

Chapters 17 through 20 include coverage of capital budgeting, consolidations, valuation, and capital formation, as they pertain to health care firms. Special attention is given to capital formation in both taxable and voluntary nonprofit situations. Consolidations, mergers, and acquisitions are increasingly important topics in the health care industry and they are covered in Chapter 19. Detailed coverage of several valuation techniques are included. Chapters 21 and 22 cover the topics of working capital management and cash budgeting.

Acknowledgments

We have received the support and assistance of many people in the preparation of this sixth edition. Professor Cleverley was extremely fortunate to have taught health care finance for more than 20 years to a large number of very bright and very positive students both at Ohio State University (OSU) and in countless adult education seminars around the country. Much of the material that is presented in this book is a direct result of his teaching experiences. Although Professor Cleverley has recently retired from Ohio State University to focus on his firm, Cleverley & Associates, he is joined in this edition, as on the previous edition, by a colleague in health care finance, Andrew Cameron. Formerly at OSU, Dr. Cameron is now a principal with Kurron Shares of America. In prepar-ing this edition, Dr. Cameron drew on both his management consulting experience with Kurron and his teaching experiences at OSU, the University of Michigan, the University of North Carolina, and else-where.

We thank Jones and Bartlett Publishers for its ongo-ing support of this text and for its suggestions about how to improve it.

Professor Cleverley would like to thank his wife and three children for their understanding, love, and sup-port. His wife and children have constantly reminded him to say things as simply as possible. He hopes that this text is clearly spoken.

Finally, Dr. Cameron thanks Corbett Price, Chairman of Kurron, for his tremendous mentorship on health care management and strategy. Mr. Price's support and advice have been invaluable. Dr. Cameron also thanks his family for its love, patience and support.

We have tried our best to create a text that is relevant and readable for health care students. However, this book will evolve as the health care industry evolves.

About the Authors

William O. Cleverley, PhD, has been the President of Cleverley & Associates since its formation in January 2000. Prior to forming the company, Dr. Cleverley established the Center for Healthcare Industry Performance Studies (CHIPS) in 1992, which was acquired by United Healthcare in March 1998. In addition to his professional responsibilities, Dr. Cleverley is also Professor Emeritus at The Ohio State University where he has taught courses in healthcare finance since 1973.

Dr. Cleverley is the author of 47 books dealing with the application and use of financial management principles and data in healthcare organizations. In addition, he has authored over 170 articles on healthcare financial issues in a wide variety of both academic and professional journals.

Andrew E. Cameron, PhD, MBA, is director of the Midwest Division and principal with Kurron Shares of America, a health care management, consulting and strategic advisory company. Dr. Cameron brings 15 years of results-oriented corporate finance, academic, research, and consulting experience to Kurron and its clients. He specializes in financial analysis, performance measurement and improvement, capital investment decision-making, corporate valuation, financial modeling, financial engineering and strategic decision support analysis.

Prior to joining Kurron, Dr. Cameron was on the faculty of The Ohio State University. Previously, he was on the faculty at the University of North Carolina at Chapel Hill. He has also lectured at numerous other universities, including Duke University's Fuqua School of Business. During the time in academia, Dr. Cameron was the principal investigator for several applied health care finance research projects. Prior to academia, he gained corporate finance expertise in the Controller's Office of Ford Motor Credit Company. He also was a management consultant with the firm now known as Accenture, one of the world's largest management consulting firms.

Chapter 1

Financial Information and the Decision-Making Process

LEARNING OBJECTIVES

After studying this chapter, you should be able to do the following:

1. Describe the importance of financial information in health care organizations.
2. Discuss the uses of financial information.
3. List the users of financial information.
4. Describe the financial functions within an organization.
5. Discuss the common ownership forms of health care organizations, along with their advantages and disadvantages.

REAL-WORLD SCENARIO

In 1946, a small band of hospital accountants formed the American Association of Hospital Accountants (AAHA). They were interested in sharing information and experiences in their industry, which was beginning to show signs of growth. A small educational journal was put together, which was first published in 1947 in an attempt to disseminate information of interest to their members. About ten years later in 1956, the AAHA's membership had grown to over 2600 members. The real growth, however, was still to come with the advent of Medicare financing in 1965.

With the dramatic growth of hospital revenues came an escalation in both the number and functions delegated to the hospital accountant. Hospital finance had become much more than just billing patients and paying invoices. Hospitals were becoming big businesses with complex and varied financial functions. They had to arrange funding of major capital programs, which could no longer be supported through charitable campaigns. Cost accounting and management control were important functions that ensured the continued financial viability of their firms. Hospital accountants soon evolved into hospital financial managers and so the AAHA changed its name in 1968 to the Hospital Financial Management Association (HFMA).

The hospital industry continued to boom through the late 1960s and 1970s. Third-party insurance became the norm for most of the American population. Patients either received it through governmental programs such as Medicare and Medicaid, or obtained it as part of the fringe benefit program at their place of employment. Hospitals were clearly no longer quite as charitable as they once were. There was money, and plenty of it, to finance the growth required by increased demand and the new evolving medical technology. By 1980, HFMA was a large association with 19,000 members. Primary offices were located in Chicago, but an important office opened in Washington, DC, to provide critical input to both the executive and legislative branches of government. On many issues that affected either government payment or capital financing, HFMA became the credible voice that policy makers sought.

The industry adapted and evolved even more in the '80s as fiscal pressure hit the federal government. Hospital payments were increasing so fast that new systems were sought that would curtail the growth rate. Prospective payment systems were introduced in 1983 and alternative payment systems were developed, which provided incentives for treating patients in an ambulatory setting. Growth in the hospital industry was still rapid, but other sectors of health care began to experience colossal growth rates, such as ambulatory surgery centers. More and more health care was being transferred to the outpatient setting. The hospital industry was no longer the only large corporate player in health care. To recognize this trend, the HFMA changed its name in 1982 to the Healthcare Financial Management Association to reflect the more diverse elements of the industry and to better meet the needs of members in other sectors.

In 2000, HFMA had over 33,000 members in a wide variety of health care organizations. The daily activities of their members still involve basic accounting issues; patient bills must still be created and collected, payroll still needs to be met, but strategic decision making is much more critical in today's environment. It would be impossible to imagine any organization planning its future without financial projections and input. Many health care organizations may still be charitable from a taxation perspective, but they are too large to depend upon charitable giving to finance their future. Financial managers of health care firms are involved in a wide array of critical and complex decisions that will ultimately determine the destiny of their firms.

This book is intended to improve decision makers' understanding and use of financial information in the health care industry. It is not an advanced treatise in accounting or finance, but an elementary discussion of how financial information, in general, and health care industry financial information in particular are interpreted and used. It is written for individuals who are not experienced health care financial executives. Its aim is to make the language of health care finance readable and relevant for decision makers in the health care industry.

Three interdependent factors created the need for this book:

1. Rapid expansion and evolution of the health care industry
2. Health care decision makers' general lack of business and financial background
3. Financial and cost criteria's increasing importance in health care decisions

The health care industry's expansion is a trend visible even to individuals outside the health care system.

The hospital industry, the major component of the health care industry, consumes about five percent of the gross domestic product; other types of health care systems, although smaller than the hospital industry, are expanding at even faster rates. Table 1–1 lists the types of major health care institutions and indexes their relative size.

LEARNING OBJECTIVE 1

Describe the importance of financial information in health care organizations.

The rapid growth of health care facilities providing direct medical services has substantially increased the numbers of decision makers who need to be familiar with financial information. Effective decision making in their jobs depends on an accurate interpretation of financial information. Many health care decision makers involved directly in health care delivery—doctors,

Table 1–1 Health Care Expenditures 1998–2010 ($ in Billions)

	(Projected) 2010	2004	1998	Annual Growth Rate, 2004– 2010 (%)
Total health expenditures	$2,753.9	$1,804.7	$1,150.9	7.3
Percentage of gross domestic product (%)	17.3	15.4	13.2	
Health services and supplies	$2,648.6	$1,735.5	$1,112.6	7.3
Personal health care	2,353.1	1,549.0	1,009.8	7.2
Hospital care	795.4	551.8	378.5	6.3
Physician and clinical	599.0	397.2	256.8	7.1
Dental services	116.4	79.1	53.2	6.7
Home health	73.6	45.2	33.6	8.3
Other professional and personal health	171.0	104.9	65.7	8.5
Prescription Drugs	368.8	200.5	87.3	10.8
Other Medical Products	71.6	54.8	45.3	4.5
Nursing home care	157.3	115.4	89.5	5.3
Expenses for prepayment and administration	199.0	128.2	64.9	7.7
Government public health	96.5	58.3	37.9	8.7
Research and construction	105.4	69.2	38.2	7.3

Source: Centers for Medicare and Medicaid Services, Office of the Actuary.

nurses, dietitians, pharmacists, radiation technologists, physical therapists, inhalation therapists—are medically or scientifically trained, but lack education and experience in business and finance. Their specialized education, in most cases, did not include such courses as accounting. However, advancement and promotion within health care organizations increasingly entails assumption of administrative duties, requiring almost an instant, knowledgeable understanding of financial information. Communication with the organization's financial executives is not always helpful. As a result, executives without a strong knowledge of finance often end up ignoring financial information.

Governing boards of health care facilities, which are significant users of financial information, are expanding in size, in some cases to accommodate consumer demands for more representation. This trend can be healthy for both the community and the facilities. However, many board members, even those with backgrounds in business, are being overwhelmed by financial reports and statements. There are important distinctions between the financial reports and statements of business organizations and those of health care facilities, the latter of which only some board members are familiar. Governing board members must recognize these differences if they are to carry out their governing missions satisfactorily.

The increasing importance of financial and cost criteria in health care decision making is the third factor creating a need for more knowledge of financial information. For many years, accountants and others involved with financial matters have been caricatured as individuals with narrow visions, incapable of seeing the forest for the trees. In many respects, this may have been an accurate portrayal. However, few individuals in the health care industry today would deny the importance of financial concerns, especially cost. Payment pressures from payers, as described in the preceding real world scenario, underscore the need for attention to costs. Careful attention to these concerns requires knowledgeable consumption of financial information by a variety of decision makers. It is not an overstatement to say that inattention to financial criteria can lead to excessive costs and eventually to insolvency.

INFORMATION AND DECISION MAKING

The major function of information in general and financial information in particular is to oil the decision-making process. Decision making is basically the selection of a course of action from a defined list of possible or feasible actions. In many cases, the actual course of action followed may essentially be no action; decision makers may decide to make no change from their present policies. It should be recognized, however, that both action and inaction represent policy decisions.

Figure 1–1 shows how information is related to the decision-making process and gives an example to illustrate the sequence. Generating information is the key to decision making. The quality and effectiveness of decision making depend on accurate, timely, and relevant information. The difference between data and information is more than semantic: data become information only when they are useful and appropriate for the decision. Many financial data never become information because they are not viewed as relevant or intelligible.

For the illustrative purposes of the ambulatory surgery center (ASC) example in Figure 1–1, only two possible courses of action are assumed: to build or not to build an ASC. In most situations, there may be a continuum of alternative courses of action. For example, an ASC might vary by size or by number of facilities included in the unit. In this case, prior decision making seems to have reduced the feasible set of alternatives to a more manageable and limited number of analyses.

Once a course of action is selected in the decision-making phase, it must be accomplished. Implementing a decision may be extremely complex. In the ASC example, carrying out the decision to build the unit would require enormous management efforts to ensure that the projected results are actually obtained. Periodic measurement of results in a feedback loop, as in Figure 1–1, is a method commonly used to make sure that decisions are actually implemented according to plan.

As previously stated, forecasted results are not always guaranteed. Controllable factors, such as failure to adhere to prescribed plans, and uncontrollable circumstances, such as a change in reimbursement, may obstruct planned results.

Decision making is usually surrounded by uncertainty. No anticipated result of a decision is guaranteed. Events may occur that were analyzed but not anticipated. A results matrix concisely portrays the possible results of various courses of action, given the occurrence of possible events. Table 1–2 provides a results matrix for the sample ASC; it shows that approximately 50 percent utilization will enable this unit to operate in the black (or make a positive level of profit) and not drain resources from other areas. If forecasting shows that utilization below 50 percent is unlikely, decision makers may very well elect to build.

A good information system enables decision makers to choose those courses of action that have the highest expectation of favorable results. Based on the results matrix of Table 1–2, a good information system should specifically:

* list possible courses of action.
* list events that might affect the expected results.
* indicate the probability that those events will occur.

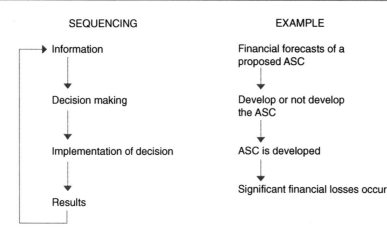

Figure 1–1 Information in the Decision-Making Process

Table 1–2 Results Matrix for the ASC

	Event		
Alternative Actions	*25% Utilization*	*50% Utilization*	*75% Utilization*
Build unit	$400,000 Loss	$10,000 Profit	$200,000 Profit
Do not build unit	0	0	0

• estimate the results accurately, given an action/event combination (e.g., profit in Table 1–2).

One thing an information system does not do is evaluate the desirability of results. Decision makers must evaluate results in terms of their organizations' preferences or their own. For example, construction of an ASC may be expected to lose $200,000 a year, but it could provide a needed community service. Weighing these results and determining criteria is purely a decision maker's responsibility—not an easy task, but one that can be improved with accurate and relevant information.

LEARNING OBJECTIVE 2

Discuss the uses of financial information.

USES OF FINANCIAL INFORMATION

As a subset of information in general, financial information is important for decision-making. For our purposes, we identify five uses of financial information that may be important in decision making:

1. Evaluating the *financial condition* of an entity
2. Evaluating *stewardship* within an entity
3. Assessing the *efficiency* of operations
4. Assessing the *effectiveness* of operations
5. Determining the *compliance* of operations with directives

Financial Condition

Evaluation of an entity's financial condition is probably the most common use of financial information. Usually, an organization's financial condition is equated with its viability or capacity to continue pursuing its stated goals at a consistent level of activity. Viability is a far more restrictive term than solvency; some health care organizations may be solvent but not viable. For example, a hospital may have its level of funds restricted so that it must reduce its scope of activity, but still remain solvent. A reduction in payment rates by a major payer may be the vehicle for this change in viability.

Assessment of the financial condition of business enterprises is essential to our economy's smooth and efficient operation. Most business decisions in our economy are directly or indirectly based on perceptions of financial condition. This includes the largely non-profit health care industry. Although attention is usually directed at organizations as whole units, assessment of the financial condition of organizational divisions is equally important. In the ASC example, information on the future financial condition of the unit is valuable. If continued losses from this operation are projected, impairment of the financial condition of other divisions in the organization could be in the offing.

Assessment of financial condition also includes consideration of short-run versus long-run effects. The relevant time frame may change, depending on the decision under consideration. For example, suppliers typically are interested only in an organization's short-run financial condition because that is the period in which they expect payment. However, investment bankers, as long-term creditors, are interested in the organization's financial condition over a much greater time period.

Stewardship

Historically, evaluation of stewardship was the most important use of accounting and financial information systems. These systems were originally designed to prevent the loss of assets or resources through employees' malfeasance. This use is still very important. In fact, the relatively infrequent occurrence of employee fraud and embezzlement may be due in part to the deterrence of well-designed accounting systems.

Efficiency

Efficiency in health care operations is becoming an increasingly important objective for many decision makers. Efficiency is simply the ratio of outputs to inputs, not the quality of outputs (good or not good), but the lowest possible cost of production. Adequate assessment of efficiency requires the availability of standards against which actual costs may be compared. In many health care organizations, these standards may be formally introduced into the budgetary process. Thus, a given nursing unit may have an efficiency standard of 4.3 nursing hours per patient day of care delivered. This standard may then be used as a benchmark by which to evaluate the relative efficiency of the unit. If actual employment were 6.0 nursing hours per patient day, management would be likely to reassess staffing patterns.

Effectiveness

Assessment of the effectiveness of operations is concerned with the attainment of objectives through production of outputs, not the relationship of outputs to cost. Measuring effectiveness is much more difficult than measuring efficiency because most organizations' objectives or goals are typically not stated quantitatively. Because measurement of effectiveness is difficult, there is a tendency to place less emphasis on effectiveness and more on efficiency. This may result in the delivery of unnecessary services at an efficient cost. For example, development of outpatient surgical centers may reduce costs per surgical procedure and thus create an efficient means of delivery. However, the necessity of those surgical procedures may still be questionable.

Compliance

Finally, financial information may be used to determine whether compliance with directives has taken place. The best example of an organization's internal directives is its budget, an agreement between two management levels regarding use of resources for a defined time period. External parties may also impose directives, many of them financial in nature, for the organization's adherence. For example, rate-setting or regulatory agencies may set limits on rates determined within an organization. Financial reporting by the organization is required to ensure compliance.

LEARNING OBJECTIVE 3

List the users of financial information and their uses for it.

Table 1–3 presents a matrix of users and uses of financial information in the health care industry. It identifies areas or uses that may interest particular decision-making groups. It does not consider relative importance.

Not every use of financial information is important in every decision. For example, in approving a health care organization's rates, a governing board may be interested in only two uses of financial information: (1) evaluation of financial condition and (2) assessment of operational efficiency. Other uses may be irrelevant. The board wants to ensure that services are being provided efficiently and that the rates being established are sufficient to guarantee a stable or improved financial condition. As Table 1–3 illustrates, most health care decision-making groups use financial information to assess financial condition and efficiency.

FINANCIAL ORGANIZATION

It is important to understand the management structure of businesses in general and health care organizations in particular. Figure 1–2 outlines the financial management structure of a typical hospital.

LEARNING OBJECTIVE 4

Describe the financial functions within an organization.

Financial Executives International has categorized financial management functions as either controllership or treasurership. Although few health care organizations have specifically identified treasurers and controllers at this time, the separation of duties is important to the understanding of financial management. The following describes functions in the two categories designated by Financial Executives International, along with an example of the type of activities conducted within each of these functions:

1. Controllership
   (a) Planning for control: Establishing budgetary systems (Chapters 12 and 15)
   (b) Reporting and interpreting: Preparing financial statements (Chapter 8)
   (c) Evaluating and consulting: Conducting cost analyses (Chapter 13)
   (d) Administrating taxes: Calculating payroll taxes owed
   (e) Reporting to government: Submitting Medicare bills and cost reports (Chapters 2 & 4)
   (f) Protecting assets: Developing internal control procedures
   (g) Appraising economic health: Analyzing financial statements (Chapters 10 and 11)
2. Treasurership
   (a) Providing capital: Arranging for bond issuance (Chapter 20)
   (b) Maintaining investor relations: Assisting in analysis of appropriate dividend payment policy (for-profit firms): (Chapters 19 and 20)
   (c) Providing short-term financing: Arranging lines of credit (Chapters 21 and 22)
   (d) Providing banking and custody: Managing overnight and short-term funds transfers (Chapters 21 and 22)

   (e) Overseeing credits and collections: Establishing billing, credit, and collection policies (Chapters 2 and 21)
   (f) Choosing investments: Analyzing capital investment projects (Chapter 18)
   (g) Providing insurance: Managing funds related to self-insurance program

The effectiveness of financial management in any business is the product of many factors, such as environmental conditions, personnel capabilities, and information quality. A major portion of the total financial management task is the provision of accurate, timely, and relevant information. Much of this activity is carried out through the accounting process. An adequate understanding of the accounting process and the data generated by it are thus critical to successful decision making.

LEARNING OBJECTIVE 5

Discuss the common ownership forms of health care organizations, along with their advantages and disadvantages.

Table 1–3 Users and Uses of Financial Information

Users	Uses				
	Financial Condition	Stewardship	Efficiency	Effectiveness	Compliance
External					
Health care coalitions	X		X	X	
Unions	X		X		
Rate-setting organizations	X		X	X	X
Creditors	X		X	X	
Third-party payers			X		X
Suppliers	X				
Public	X		X	X	
Internal					
Governing board	X	X	X	X	X
Top management	X	X	X	X	X
Departmental management			X		X

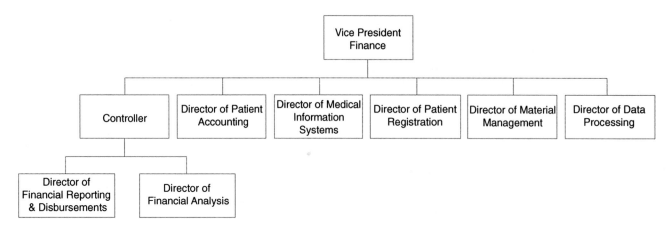

Figure 1–2 Financial Organization Chart of a Typical Hospital

FORMS OF BUSINESS ORGANIZATION

More so than in most other industries, firms in the health care industry consist of a wide array of ownership and organizational structures. In health care, there are four main types organizations (adapted from the American Institute of Certified Public Accountants Audit and Accounting Guide *Health Care Organizations,* 2006):

- Not-for-profit, Business-Oriented Organizations
- Investor-Owned Health Care Enterprises
  –Investor-Owned
  –Professional corporations/Professional associations
  –Sole proprietorships
  –Limited partnerships
  –Limited liability partnerships/Limited liability companies
- Governmental Health Care Organizations
- Not-for-Profit, Non-business-Oriented Organizations

These four main types of firms differ in terms of ownership structure. Additionally, different health care organizations require slightly different sets of financial statements.

Not-for-Profit, Business-Oriented Organizations

Not-for-profit health care organizations (HCOs) are owned by the entire community rather than by investor–owners. Unlike its for-profit counterpart, the primary goal of a not-for-profit organization is not to maximize profits, but to serve the community in which it operates through the health care services it provides. Not-for-profit HCOs must be run as a business, however, in order to ensure their long-term financial viability. With an annual budget of more than $10 billion, Ascension Healthcare is an example of one of the largest nonprofit HCOs.

Nonprofit organizations (described in Sec. 501(c)(3) of the Internal Revenue Code) usually are exempt from federal income taxes and property taxes. In return for this favorable tax treatment, nonprofit organizations are expected to provide a public benefit, which often comes in the form of providing more uncompensated care (vis-à-vis for-profit firms), setting lower prices, or by offering services that, from a financial perspective, might not be viable for for-profit firms. In addition to patient revenue in excess of expenses, nonprofits can additionally be funded by tax-exempt debt, grants, donations, and investments by other nonprofit firms.

The primary advantage of the nonprofit form of organization is its tax advantage. It also typically enjoys a lower cost of equity capital compared with for-profit firms. The main disadvantage of this form of organization is that nonprofits have limited access to capital. Nonprofits cannot raise capital in the equity markets.

While for-profit firms are becoming increasingly prevalent in many sectors of health care, nonprofits still dominate the hospital sector. About 80 percent of hospitals are nonprofit. In the future, however, this sector may witness the growth of investor-owned organizations, which will be owed mainly to their easier access to capital that will be necessary for adapting to the rapid changes in the health care system.

Investor-Owned Health Care Organizations

The main objective of most Investor-Owned Health Care Organizations is to earn profits that are distributed to the investor–owners of the firms or reinvested in the firm for the long-term benefit of these owners. For example, HCA, Inc. is an investor-owned health care organization headquartered in Nashville, Tennessee. It owns or operates 189 hospitals and related businesses in 23 states. In its fiscal year ending December 31, 2004, the company had after-tax income of $1.25 billion. For-profit hospital management must strike a balance between their fiduciary responsibilities to the owners of the company and with their other mission of providing acceptable-quality health care services to the community. Investor-Owned Health Care Organizations have a wide variety of organization and ownership structures, as discussed below.

Investor-owned firms are owned by risk-based equity investors who expect the managers of the corporation to maximize shareholder wealth. Most large for-profit firms use this legal form. Investor-owned firms have a relative advantage in terms of financing. In addition to debt, for-profit firms can raise funding through risk-based equity capital. They enjoy limited liability, but their earnings are taxed at both the corporate level and the shareholder level (so-called double taxation). The company pays corporate income tax and the shareholder pays both tax on dividends paid by the company and gains made on the sale of the company's stock.

A professional corporation (PC), also called a professional association (PA), is a corporate form for professionals who wanted to have the advantages of incorporation. A PC does not, however, shield its owners from professional liability. PCs and PAs have been widely used by physicians and other health care professionals.

Sole proprietorships are unincorporated businesses owned by a single individual. They do not necessarily have to be small businesses. Solo practitioner physicians often are sole proprietors. The main advantages are: easy and inexpensive to set up; no sharing of profits; total control; few government regulations; no special income taxes; easy and inexpensive to dissolve. Its two main disadvantages are unlimited liability and limited access to capital.

Partnerships are unincorporated businesses with two or more owners. Group practices of physicians sometimes were set up with this form. There are now a wide variety of partnership forms. They are easy to form, are subject to few government regulations, and are not subject to double-taxation. On the down side, partnerships have unlimited liability, are difficult to dissolve, and create potential for conflict among the partners.

In a limited partnership (LP) there is at least one general partner who has unlimited liability for the LP's debts and obligations. LPs offer limited liability to the limited partners along with tax flow-through treatment. The disadvantage to LPs is that they require a general partner who remains fully liable for the LP's debts and obligations.

A limited liability company (LLC), also called a *limited liability partnership* (LLP), is a business entity that combines the tax flow-through treatment characteristics of a partnership (i.e., no double taxation) with the liability protection of a corporation. In an LLC, the liability of the general partner is limited. LLCs are flexible in the sense that they permit owners to structure allocations of income and losses any way they desire, so long as the partnership tax allocation rules are followed.

Governmental Health Care Organizations

Governmental health care organizations are public corporations, typically owned by a state or local government. They are operated for the benefit of the communities they serve. A variation on this type of ownership is the public benefit organization. Assets (and accumulated earnings) of a nonprofit public benefit corporation belong to the public or to the charitable beneficiaries the trust was organized to serve. In 1999, for example, the Nassau County Medical Center (NCMC), a 1,500-bed health care system on Long Island, New York, converted from county ownership to a public benefit corporation. The purpose of the conversion was to give NCMC greater autonomy in its governing board and decision making, so that it could compete more effectively with the area's large private hospitals and networks.

Governmental HCOs have an additional revenue source not usually available to other HCOs. They often have the authority to raise funds by levying taxes. As with nonprofits, though, they are not able to raise funds through equity investments. Governmental HCOs, like nonprofits, are exempt from income taxes and property taxes.

Governmental HCOs can face political pressures if their earnings become too great. Rather than reinvesting their surplus in productive assets, the hospital might be pressured to return some of the surplus to the community, to reduce prices, or to initiate programs that are not financially advisable.

Not-for-Profit, Non-business Oriented Organizations

Not-for-Profit, Non-business Oriented Organizations perform voluntary services in their communities; accordingly, they are often called voluntary health and welfare organizations. They are tax-exempt and rely primarily on public donations for their funds. Examples include the American Red Cross and the American Cancer Society. Although these types of organizations provide invaluable services, the financial statements and financial management of these organizations are somewhat different from that of business-oriented firms. While many of the topics covered in this book would be applicable to these firms, these firms are not explicitly covered in this book.

SUMMARY

The health care sector of our economy is growing rapidly in both size and complexity. Understanding the financial and economic implications of decision making has become one of the most critical areas encountered by health care decision makers. Successful decision making can lead to a viable operation capable of providing needed health care services. Unsuccessful decision making can and often does lead to financial failure. The role of financial information in the decision-making process cannot be overstated. It is incumbent on all health care decision makers to become accounting-literate in our financially changing health care environment.

REFERENCES

American Institute of Certified Public Accountants Audit and Accounting Guide *Health Care Organizations,* 2006.

ASSIGNMENTS

1. Only in recent years have hospitals begun to develop meaningful systems of cost accounting. Why did they not begin such development sooner?

2. Your hospital has been approached by a major employer in your market area to negotiate a preferred provider arrangement. The employer is seeking a 25 percent discount from your current charges. Describe a structure that you might use to summarize the financial implications of this decision. Describe the factors that would be critical in this decision.

3. What type of financial information should be routinely provided to board members?

SOLUTIONS AND ANSWERS

1. Prior to 1983, most hospitals were paid actual costs for delivering hospital services. With the introduction of Medicare's prospective payment system in 1983, hospitals now receive prices based on diagnosis-related groupings that are fixed in advance. Cost control and, therefore, cost accounting are critical in a fixed-price environment. The expansion of managed care has further restricted revenue and fostered greater interest in costing.

2. This problem could be set up in a results matrix (see Table 1–2). The two actions to be charted are to accept or to reject the preferred provider arrangement opportunity. Possible events would center on the magnitude of volume changes, for example, to lose 1,000 patient days or to gain 500 patient days. A key concern in estimating the financial impact would be the hospital's incremental revenue and incremental cost positions. In short, how large would the revenue reduction and cost reduction be if significant volume were lost? Actuarial gains or losses of business would be functions of the hospital's market position.

3. Board members do not need to see detailed financial information that relates to their established plans to ensure that the plans are being met. If significant deviations have occurred, more details may be necessary to take corrective action or to modify established plans. High level financial reporting is usually recommended with summary financial values and ratios.

Chapter 2

Billing and Coding for Health Services

LEARNING OBJECTIVES

After studying this chapter, you should be able to do the following:

1. Describe the revenue cycle for health care firms.
2. Understand the role of coding information in health care organizations in claim generation.
3. Define the two major bill types used in health care firms.
4. Define the basic characteristics of chargemasters.
5. Appreciate the role of claims editing in the bill submission process.

REAL-WORLD SCENARIO

Riley Ilene, the Chief Financial Officer of Campbell Hospital, was concerned by the reduction in revenue during the last three months. The revenue reduction was most pronounced in the outpatient arena and represented a 15 percent reduction from prior year levels. Loss of this revenue had eroded Campbell's already thin operating margins and the hospital was now operating with losses.

Riley's first thought was that volume may be down from prior year levels. She asked her controller, Michael Dean, to report on comparative volumes for last year and this year. Michael's report showed that total numbers of outpatient visits were actually above last year. Furthermore, the increases in volumes appeared relatively uniform across all product line groupings. Riley then directed Michael to review "Revenue and Usage" summaries for the current and prior year. A revenue and usage summary would show the quantity of items billed by charge code and payer. The summaries would also break out the volumes by inpatient and outpatient areas.

After reviewing this data, Michael reported back to Riley with some startling news. Volumes for several procedures in the hospital's "Chargemaster" were well below prior year levels. Specifically, the numbers of drug administration codes that are reported when an injectable or infusible drug is administered were well below prior year levels. This was surprising because the number of injectable and infusible drugs had actually increased.

Riley Ilene thought she had discovered the problem and reported back to her CEO, Meredith Lynn. Meredith, however, asked Riley whether this could have caused the revenue reduction.

Meredith believed that a heavy percentage of the hospital's payment was related to either case payment for inpatients or APC (Ambulatory Patient Classification) groups for outpatients. Meredith believed that these bundled payments would not be impacted by a failure to document the drug administration procedures.

Riley said that this was a good point and she would do some additional research and report back to Meredith. Riley found that Medicare provides separate payments for the drug administration procedure when performed in outpatient visits. The average loss for the undocumented procedure codes appeared to average about $120 per occurrence. Riley also found that many of their commercial payers paid on a discount from a billed charge basis. Failure to report these procedures for these payers would result in lost revenue. The only remaining task was to discover why charges for drug administration procedures for outpatient procedures were not being recorded.

Health care firms are for the most part business-oriented organizations. Their ultimate financial survival is dependent upon a consistent and recurring flow of funds from the services that they provide to patients. Without an adequate stream of revenue these firms would be forced to cease operations. In this regard, health care firms are similar to most business entities that sell products or services in our economy. Figure 2–1 depicts the stages involved in the revenue cycle for a health care firm. The critical stages in the revenue cycle for health care firms are the provision of services to the patient, the generation of charges for those services, the preparation of a bill or claim, the submission of the bill or claim to the respective payer, and the collection of payment.

LEARNING OBJECTIVE 1

Describe the revenue cycle for health care firms.

A simple review of the five stages of the revenue cycle in Figure 2–1 hides the significant degree of complexity involved in revenue generation for health care providers. There is no other industry in our nation's economy that experiences the same level of billing complexity that most health care firms face. Part of this complexity is related to the nature and importance of the services provided. Regulation is also a factor that further complicates documentation and billing for health care services. Finally, the existence of different payment methods and rates for multiple payers further complicates the revenue cycle for most health care firms. Payment complexity is a topic that will be addressed in Chapter 3.

GENERATING HEALTH CARE CLAIMS

Figure 2–2 provides more detail on the steps and processes involved in the actual generation of a health care bill or claim. The process and steps mirror those in Figure 2–1, except additional detail unique to health care firms is included. The process often begins with the collection of information about the patient in the patient registration function, prior to the delivery of services. Information about the patient including address, date of birth, and insurance data is collected to facilitate bill preparation after services are provided. Once services have been provided, data from that encounter(s) flow into two areas: medical documentation and charge capture.

While the primary purpose of the data accumulated in the medical record may relate to clinical decision-making, a substantial proportion of the information may also be linked to billing. For example, the assignment of diagnosis and procedure codes within the medical record by physicians plays a key role in DRG (Diagnosis Related Group) assignment. Many health care payers provide payment for inpatient care based upon DRG assignment. Data in the medical record is also the primary source for documenting the provision of services. For example, if a patient's bill listed a series of drugs used by the patient, but the medical record did not show those drugs as being used, the claim would not be supported. The primary linkage between the claim and the medical record is related to the

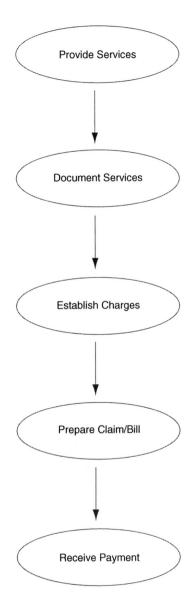

Figure 2–1 Revenue Cycle

documentation of specific services provided and their reporting in a series of clinical codes. We will explore the categories of coding and their importance to billing shortly.

Data from the provision of services also flow directly to billing indirectly through the capture of charges. The posting of charges to a patient's account is usually accomplished through the issuance and collection of "charge slips" in a manual mode, or through direct order entry or bar code readers in an automated system. The critical link here is the firm's price list, often referred to as its "chargemaster." The chargemaster is simply a list of all the items that the firm has

established specific prices for. In a hospital setting it is not unusual to find more than 20,000 items on a chargemaster.

Information from the medical record and the chargemaster then flow into the actual claim. For most health care firms, there are two basic categories of claims: the Uniform Bill(UB)–92 and the Center for Medicare and Medicaid Services(CMS)–1500. The UB–92 is the claim form that is used for most hospitals to report claims for both inpatient and outpatient services. The CMS–1500 is used primarily for physician and professional claims. Samples of these two claim forms are included in the Appendix to this chapter.

The final step before actual claim submission is claims editing. While this step may not be performed by all health care firms, it is a critical step for many. In this editing process, several key areas are reviewed. First, does the claim have enough information to trigger payment by the patient's payer? For example, perhaps the claim is missing the patient's social security number or health care plan identification number. Second, does the claim meet logical standards and is it complete? For example, a claim may have a charge for laboratory panel, but there may be no charge for a blood draw to collect the sample. Editing is critical to accurate and timely payment by third-party payers.

REGISTRATION

In most cases, a patient or their representative will provide a basic set of patient information prior to the actual delivery of services. In a physician's office this may be done just prior to medical service performance. For an elective hospital inpatient admission, it may be done a week or more prior to admission. A number of clinical and financial sets of information are collected at this point. From the financial perspective, three activities are especially important in the billing and collection process.

Perhaps the most important activity is insurance verification. If the patient has indicated that they have third-party insurance coverage, it is important to have this coverage verified by the payer. The patient may also have secondary coverage from another health plan. Verification of that coverage is also critical to accurate and timely billing. The critical piece of information to collect from the patient in this regard is their health plan identification number, which may sometimes be their social security number. Queries addressed to the

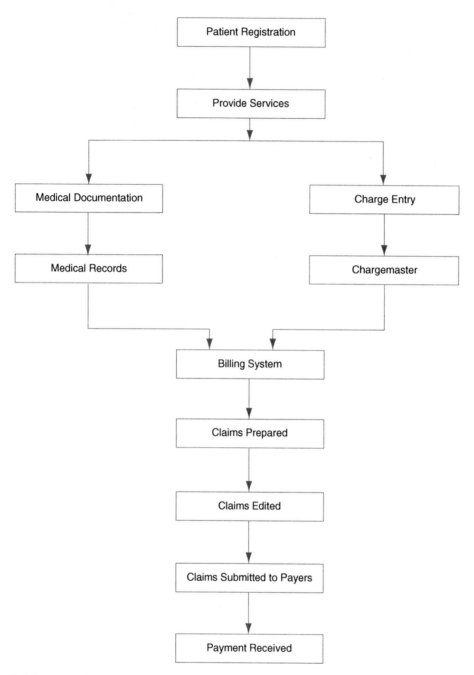

Figure 2–2 Detailed Revenue Cycle

third-party insurance company prior to service can validate the type of coverage provided by the health plan and the eligibility of the patient for the scheduled service. In today's current environment insurance verification is often done online. Sometimes prior approval for elective services is required by the health plan before a claim can be submitted. This prior verification is often referred to as pre-certification. Information regarding

coverage for large governmental programs such as Medicare and Medicaid is not often needed because the benefit structure is standardized. It is important however to verify the existence of current coverage.

The second activity in registration is often related to the computation of co-payment or deductible provisions that may be applicable for the patient. Once insurance coverage has been determined, it is usually possible to calculate the required amount that may still be due from the patient. For example, a Medicare patient without supplemental coverage may report to a hospital for a scheduled CT scan. It is possible for the registration staff to calculate the amount of co-payment that will be due by the patient. The registration staff can then advise the patient regarding the amount of payment due and try to make arrangements for payment at the point of service.

The third activity in this registration process relates to financial counseling. Patients who have no coverage may be eligible for some discount through the health care firm's charity care policy. Any residual that may still be due can be discussed with the patient and financing may be arranged prior to the point of service. It is also possible that an uninsured patient may be eligible for some governmental programs, especially Medicaid. Staff at the health care firm can advise the patient regarding eligibility and help them to complete the necessary documents required for coverage.

LEARNING OBJECTIVE 2

Understand the role of coding information in health care organization claims generation.

MEDICAL RECORD/CODING

Information regarding the services provided to the patient is recorded in the patient's medical record. Critical pieces of information contained in that record are utilized in the billing process and are communicated to the payers to trigger payment. The Health Insurance Portability and Accountability Act (HIPAA) of 1996 designated two specific coding systems to be used in reporting to both public and private payers:

- International Classification of Diseases 9th Revision–Clinical Modification
- Healthcare Common Procedure Coding System

HIPAA requires that two categories of information be reported to payers: diagnosis codes and procedure codes. The International Classification of Diseases 9th Revision–Clinical Modification (ICD–9–CM) has sets of codes that provide information for both diagnosis and procedures. The Healthcare Common Procedure Coding System (HCPCS) provides information in the procedure area, but does not provide information regarding diagnosis. HIPAA therefore requires that ICD–9 codes be used for diagnosis reporting for all health care providers including hospitals and physicians. ICD–9 procedure codes are required for procedure reporting for hospital inpatients, while HCPCS codes are used for procedure reporting by hospitals for outpatient services and also by physicians (See Table 2–1).

ICD–9 diagnosis codes are three digits, which may be followed by a decimal point with two additional digits. For example, all ICD–9 codes that have 428 as their first three digits refer to the primary diagnosis of heart failure. Additional digits following a 428 would further specify the patient's exact condition. For example, 428.1 would refer to left heart failure. Table 2–2 provides a listing of the top ten inpatient diagnoses reported by Medicare in Fiscal Year 2004.

ICD–9 procedure codes are used to report hospital inpatient procedures. These codes may be up to four digits in length, with a decimal point following the first two digits. For example, a code with 37 as the first two digits would refer to procedures on the heart and pericardium. A code of 37.23 would refer to a combined right and left heart cardiac catheterization. Table 2–3 shows a listing of the top ten inpatient ICD–9 procedure codes reported by Medicare in Fiscal Year 2004.

Table 2–1 HIPAA-Designated Coding

| Provider | Inpatient | | Outpatient | |
	Diagnosis	Procedure	Diagnosis	Procedure
Physician	ICD–9–CM	CPT	ICD–9–CM	CPT
Facility	ICD–9–CM	ICD–9–CM	ICD–9–CM	HCPCS (CPT and HCPCS Level II)

Table 2–2 2004 Public Data—Primary Diagnosis Frequency

Dx1	Definition	Frequency	% of Total
4280	Congestive Heart Failure	698,697	5.1
486	Pneumonia, Organism Unspecified	606,396	4.5
41401	Coronary Atherosclerosis of Native Coronary Artery	517,405	3.8
49121	Obstructive Chronic Bronchitis, with Acute Exacerbation	355,457	2.6
V5789	Care Involving Other Specified Rehabilitation Procedure	337,664	2.5
41071	Subendocardial Infarction, Initial Episode of Care	231,249	1.7
5990	Urinary Tract Infection, Site Not Specified	229,076	1.7
42731	Atrial Fibrillation	207,119	1.5
78659	Other Chest Pain	193,757	1.4
2765	Volume Depletion Disorder	190,991	1.4

ICD–9 diagnosis and procedure codes are very important in the assignment of a Diagnosis Related Group (DRG). DRG payment is widely used by many payers, especially Medicare. Coding therefore has a critical link to provider payment.

HCPCS codes are used for reporting procedures by physicians for both inpatient and outpatient procedures. They are also used by facilities for reporting outpatient procedures, but they use ICD–9 procedure codes for reporting inpatient procedures. There are two tiers used in HCPCS coding, Level I and Level II. Level I codes are referred to as CPT (Current Procedure Terminology) codes that have been developed and maintained by the American Medical Association. Level I and CPT are used interchangeably to describe these sets of codes. Six main categories of CPT codes are currently used:

- Evaluation & Management (99201 to 99499)
- Anesthesia (01000 to 01999)
- Surgery (10040 to 69979)
- Radiology (70010 to 79999)

- Pathology and Laboratory (80002 to 89399)
- Medicine (90701 to 99199)

The five digit CPT code may also contain a "modifier," which is a two digit numeric or alphanumeric that may provide additional information essential to process a claim. For example, modifier 91 is used to indicate that a laboratory procedure was repeated. Table 2–4 provides a list of the top ten hospital outpatient CPT codes reported to Medicare in Fiscal Year 2004.

Level II HCPCS codes were developed by CMS to report services, supplies, or procedures that were not present in the Level I (CPT) codes. There are two groups within the Level II HCPCS codes: permanent and temporary. Permanent codes are five digit codes that begin with an alpha character. Table 2–5 provides a list of the top ten Level II permanent HCPCS codes reported to Medicare in Fiscal Year 2004 for hospital outpatients.

Level II temporary HCPCS codes are used to meet a temporary need for a new code. These codes are also five digit codes that begin with an alpha character.

Table 2–3 2004 Public Data—Primary Procedure Frequency

Px1	Definition	Frequency	% of Total
36.01	Ptca-1 Ves/Ath w/o Agent	292,085	3.9
99.04	Packed Cell Transfusion	285,906	3.8
37.22	Left Heart Cardiac Cath	257,270	3.4
81.54	Total Knee Replacement	241,381	3.2
45.16	Egd With Closed Biopsy	230,779	3.1
38.93	Venous Cath Nec	218,295	2.9
39.95	Hemodialysis	207,926	2.8
45.13	Sm Bowel Endoscopy Nec	142,572	1.9
81.51	Total Hip Replacement	116,364	1.5
96.71	Cont Mech Vent < 96 Hrs	113,965	1.5

Table 2–4 2004 Public Data—CPT Frequency

CPT	Definition	Frequency	% of Total
85025	Automated hemogram	8,988,187	4.7
93005	Electrocardiogram, tracing	5,820,832	3.1
71020	Chest x-ray	5,223,746	2.7
80048	Basic metabolic panel	4,855,852	2.5
80053	Comprehen metabolic panel	4,646,886	2.4
99213	Office/outpatient visit, est	4,202,313	2.2
85610	Prothrombin time	4,148,100	2.2
99283	Emergency dept visit	3,623,782	1.9
99211	Office/outpatient visit, est	2,790,103	1.5
88305	Tissue exam by pathologist	2,706,423	1.4

These codes can exist for a long time, but they may be replaced with a permanent code. Table 2–6 provides a list of the top ten Level II temporary HCPCS codes reported to Medicare in Fiscal Year 2004 for hospital outpatients.

HCPCS/CPT codes have a significant effect on provider payment for both facilities and physicians. CPT codes are often linked to fee schedules for many physicians by a large number of payers, which makes coding by medical groups especially critical. CPT and Level II HCPCS codes are also used by Medicare to define payment for many hospital outpatient services in the APC system.

LEARNING OBJECTIVE 3

Define the two major bill types used in health care firms.

CHARGE ENTRY/CHARGEMASTER

Performing actual medical services is the lifeblood of a health care firm's revenue cycle. Without the provision of services there is no revenue, but it is imperative that charges for those services be captured. A service that is performed, but not billed, will not produce revenue. The three greatest concerns in billing are:

- Capture of charges for services performed
- Incorrect billing
- Billing late charges

Charge capture is usually accomplished in one of two ways. For a number of providers actual paper documents or charge slips are used to identify services that are performed. These charge slips are then posted to a patient's account in a batch processing mode by data processing or the business office. Alternatively, an order entry system could be used, which may involve

Table 2–5 2004 Public Data—Level II (Perm) Frequency

Level II (Perm)	Definition	Frequency	% of Total
J3010	Fentanyl citrate injection, .1	1,509,269	8.8
J2250	Inj midazolam hydrochloride	1,321,476	7.7
A4646	Contrast 300-399 MGs iodine	670,868	3.9
J2175	Meperidine hydrochl/100 MG	455,294	2.7
J2405	Ondansetron hcl inj 1 mg	406,727	2.4
A9500	TC 99M sestamibi, per syringe	384,467	2.3
J0690	Cefazolin sodium injection	338,973	2.0
J2550	Promethazine hcl injection	312,201	1.8
J2270	Morphine sulfate injection	302,017	1.8
J1885	Ketorolac tromethamine inj	291,196	1.7

Table 2–6 2004 Public Data—Level II (Temp) Frequency

Level II (Temp)	Definition	Frequency	% of Total
G0001	Drawing blood for specimen	9,823,049	60.8
Q0081	Infusion ther other than che	2,562,493	15.9
Q0136	Non esrd epoetin alpha inj	634,901	3.9
Q0084	Chemotherapy by infusion	467,230	2.9
G0239	Therapeutic procedures	281,637	1.7
G0202	Screening mammography	199,681	1.2
Q0137	Darbepoetin alfa, non esrd	172,803	1.1
Q0083	Chemo by other than infusion	168,884	1.0
G0008	Admin influenza virus vac	143,824	0.9
G0103	Psa, total screening	110,263	0.7

direct entry of charges to the patient's account through a computer terminal. Scanning of bar codes may also be used.

Sometimes health care firms may use a "charge explosion" system to better organize charge entry for selective services. For example, a specific type of surgery may routinely require a standardized set of supplies. Rather than entering all these supplies, one code may be used that then explodes into the list of supply codes used for that surgery.

LEARNING OBJECTIVE 4

Describe the basic characteristics of chargemasters.

The key link between charge capture and the billing process is the "charge code," which is reflected in the order entry system or the charge slips and is also represented on the firm's chargemaster. The chargemaster is the list of services, supplies, and drugs that the firm bills. For hospitals, some chargemasters can have up to 100,000 items. Every chargemaster will usually have the following six common elements:

- Charge code
- Item description
- Department Number
- Charge/Price
- Revenue Code
- CPT/HCPCS code

Table 2–7 provides a sample of selected codes in a hospital's chargemaster. The first column in the chargemaster is the charge code or item code for the specific service or product that is to be billed. The second column provides a short description of the specific item code. For example, item code 3023001 is "Daily Care Fourth North." The third column contains the department number and may reference a specific department within the firm, and which might also relate to their accounting system or general ledger. The fourth column is the current price or standard price for the service or product. In some cases, there may be multiple prices for a given code. For example, a hospital might price a laboratory procedure at one rate for inpatient care, and it may have a different price for outpatient care. These differences may reflect differences in cost or competitive price pressure. Competition for outpatient laboratory procedures may be intense and the hospital may believe that it must discount its price if it wants to maintain its market share for outpatient laboratory services. The fifth column is the revenue code. Revenue codes are a required field in any hospital claim that is submitted on a UB–92. The current categories used have been mandated by CMS and the current list is presented in Table 2–8. The last column that is included in many chargemasters is the field for the HCPCS code. In our sample chargemaster not all entries have a HCPCS code. For example, the first two entries that relate to room and board charges do not have a HCPCS code. Also notice that surgery and anesthesia codes do not have a HCPCS code. Most hospitals bill for a great majority of their surgeries on a time/level basis. Someone from Health Information Management (HIM) will assign a CPT code or an

Table 2–7 Partial Chargemaster File

Item Code	Item Description	Dept Num	Standard Price ($)	Revenue Code	HCPCS
3023001	DAILY CARE FOURTH NORTH	13030	665.50	111	
3120000	DAILY CARE ICU	13120	1,172.50	200	
4156159	MINERAL OIL 30ML	13190	11.50	250	
4400206	SINGLE TOWEL	14430	2.25	270	
4440302	HEP C ANTIBODIES-0288	14440	53.50	300	86803
4470220	HAND XRAY-0183	14470	102.50	320	73130
4472538	C/T PELVIS W & W/O ENHANCEMENT	14302	1,069.75	350	72194
4416000	LASIK SURGERY—PER EYE	13190	2,105.25	360	66999
4416013	O.R. MINOR CHARGE—0.5 HOUR	13190	556.75	360	
4416014	O.R. MINOR CHARGE—1 HOUR	13190	770.75	360	
4416015	O.R. MINOR CHARGE—1.5 HOURS	13190	983.00	360	
4416016	O.R. MINOR CHARGE—2 HOURS	13190	1,197.25	360	
4416017	O.R. MINOR CHARGE—2.5 HOURS	13190	1,409.25	360	
4416018	O.R. MINOR CHARGE—3 HOURS	13190	1,622.25	360	
4520013	ANESTHESIA MINOR—0.5 HOUR	14520	110.25	370	
4520014	ANESTHESIA MINOR—1 HOUR	14520	151.25	370	
4520015	ANESTHESIA MINOR—1.5 HOURS	14520	192.75	370	
4520016	ANESTHESIA MINOR—2 HOURS	14520	233.00	370	
4520017	ANESTHESIA MINOR—2.5 HOURS	14520	274.75	370	
4520018	ANESTHESIA MINOR—3 HOURS	14520	317.00	370	
3167020	BLOOD TRANSFUSION	13160	303.25	391	36430
4532057	MASSAGE <8 MINS	14532	21.00	420	97124
3050717	EVALUATION—OT	13050	130.00	430	97003
3160001	EMERG DEPT OBSERVATION 0–3HRS	13160	241.25	450	99218
3160002	EMERG DEPT OBSERVATION 3–6HRS	13160	406.00	450	99218
3160003	EMERG DEPT OBSERVATION 6–12HRS	13160	492.00	450	99219
3160004	EMERG DEPT OBSERV. OVER 12 HRS	13160	592.75	450	99220
4465350	OUTPAT VISIT LEVEL 1 (NEW)	14465	78.50	510	99201
4465351	OUTPAT VISIT LEVEL 2 (NEW)	14465	92.25	510	99202
4465352	OUTPAT VISIT LEVEL 3 (NEW)	14465	112.50	510	99203
4465353	OUTPAT VISIT LEVEL 4 (NEW)	14465	159.75	510	99204
4465354	OUTPAT VISIT LEVEL 5 (NEW)	14465	$209.00	510	99205

ICD–9 procedure code to the procedure at a later point in time prior to billing. Where a HCPCS code is present in the chargemaster, less time is required in coding claims at the back end, but care needs to be taken that appropriate charge codes are used at charge entry. Direct coding of HCPCS codes into the chargemaster is referred to as static coding. When codes are left off the chargemaster and entered later by HIM personnel, the process is referred to as dynamic coding. Many ancillary procedures such as laboratory or radiology procedures can be coded statically, that is HCPCS codes can be placed in the chargemaster. In contrast, many surgery codes are dynamically coded and HIM staff

will assign the appropriate HCPCS code after the procedure.

BILLING/CLAIMS PREPARATION

For most health care providers medical claims fall into one of two types:

- CMS–1500
- HCFA–1450 (UB–92)

The CMS–1500 form is used by noninstitutional providers and suppliers to submit claims to Medicare and many other payers. The HCFA–1450 or UB–92 is

Table 2–8 Revenue Code Categories

Accommodation Revenue Codes

010X	All-Inclusive Rate
011X	R&B–Private (Medical or General)
012X	R&B–Semiprivate (2 Beds) (Medical or General)
013X	Semiprivate (3 and 4 Beds)
014X	Private (Deluxe)
015X	R&B–Ward (Medical or General)
016X	Other R&B
017X	Nursery
018X	LOA
019X	Subacute Care
020X	Intensive Care
021X	Coronary Care

Ancillary Services Revenue Codes

022X	Special Charges
023X	Incremental Nursing Care Rate
024X	All-Inclusive Ancillary
025X	Pharmacy (See also 063X, an extension of 025X)
026X	IV Therapy
027X	Medical/Surgical Supplies and Devices (See also 062X, an extension of 027X)
028X	Oncology
029X	DME (Other than Renal)
030X	Laboratory
031X	Laboratory Pathological
032X	Radiology–Diagnostic
033X	Radiology–Therapeutic and/or Chemotherapy Administration
034X	Nuclear Medicine
035X	Computed Tomographic TCPScans
036X	Operating Room Services
037X	Anesthesia
038X	Blood
039X	Blood and Blood Component Administration, Processing and Storage
040X	Other Imaging Services
041X	Respiratory Services
042X	Physical Therapy
043X	Occupational Therapy
044X	Speech-Language Pathology
045X	Emergency Room
046X	Pulmonary Function
047X	Audiology
048X	Cardiology
049X	Ambulatory Surgical Care
050X	Outpatient Services
051X	Clinic
052X	Freestanding Clinic
053X	Osteopathic Services
054X	Ambulance
055X	Skilled Nursing
056X	Medical Social Services

Table 2–8 *continued*

Ancillary Services Revenue Codes

057X	Home Health—Home Health Aide
058X	Home Health—Other Visits
059X	Home Health—Units of Service
060X	Oxygen (Home Health)
061X	Magnetic Resonance Technology (MRT)
062X	Medical/Surgical Supplies (Extension of 027X)
063X	Pharmacy—Extension of 025X
064X	Home IV Therapy Services
065X	Hospice Service
066X	Respite Care
067X	Outpatient Special Residence Charges
068X	Trauma Response
069X	Not Assigned
070X	Cast Room
071X	Recovery Room
072X	Labor Room/Delivery
073X	EKG/ECG (Electrocardiogram)
074X	EEG (Electroencephalogram)
075X	Gastrointestinal Services
076X	Treatment or Observation Room
077X	Preventive Care Services
078X	Telemedicine
079X	Extra-Corporeal Shock Wave Therapy
080X	Inpatient Renal Dialysis
081X	Acquisition of Body Components
082X	Hemodialysis—Outpatient or Home
083X	Peritoneal Dialysis—Outpatient or Horne
084X	CAPD—Outpatient or Home
085X	CCPD—Outpatient or Home
086X	Reserved for Dialysis (National Assignment)
087X	Reserved for Dialysis (State Assignment)
088X	Miscellaneous Dialysis
089X	Reserved for National Assignment
090X	Behavioral Health Treatments/Services (See also 091X, an extension of 090X)
091X	Behavioral Health Treatments/Services—extension of 090X
092X	Other Diagnostic Services
093X	Medical Rehabilitation Day Program
094X	Other Therapeutic Services
095X	Other Therapeutic Services—Extension of 094X
096X	Professional Fees (See also 097X and 098X)
097X	Professional Fees (Extension of 096X)
098X	Professional Fees (Extension of 096X and 097X)
099X	Patient Convenience Items
100X	Behavioral Health Accommodations
101X–209X	Reserved for National Assignment
210X	Alternative Therapy Services
211X–300X	Reserved for National Assignment
310X	Adult Care
311X–999X	Reserved for National Assignment

used by institutional providers to submit claims to Medicare and most other payers. Sample copies of both a CMS–1500 and a UB–92 are shown in the Appendix to this chapter.

Most claims in today's environment are submitted in an electronic format. Usually, claims are submitted directly to the payer, or indirectly to a "clearinghouse" where the claims are grouped and then sent to the appropriate payer. The Health Insurance Portability and Accountability Act (HIPAA) administrative simplification provisions direct the Secretary of Health and Human Services to adopt standards for administrative transactions, code sets, and identifiers, as well as standards for protecting the security and privacy of health data. After October 16, 2003, providers who are not small providers (institutional organizations with fewer than 25 full-time employees or physicians with fewer than ten full-time employees) must send all claims electronically in the HIPAA format.

The electronic format required under HIPAA is 837 I for the UB–92 and 837 P for the CMS–1500. These formats specify both the nature of data exchange, as well as the required data fields. There have been a few additional data elements included in the 837 I and 837 P protocols that were not in the current CM–1500 and UB–92 claim forms.

Two of the primary payment grouping algorithms are DRGs and APCs, both of which are used by Medicare for hospital payment and also many commercial payers. Both DRGs and APCs are assigned based on data in the UB–92. A DRG is often assigned depending upon values found in the UB–92 for ICD–9 procedure codes and ICD–9 diagnosis codes. Surgical procedures require an ICD–9 procedure code and may also require a ICD–9 diagnosis code. A medical DRG will require one or more ICD–9 diagnosis codes. Note that in the UB–92 form in the Appendix, there are allowed spaces for a principal diagnosis code and up to eight additional diagnosis codes. There is also a field for the principal procedure and up to five additional procedures may be coded. Many diagnosis and procedure codes may group to more than one DRG. A complete review of the DRG title is necessary to understand the correct DRG assignment. To illustrate this concept, let's examine the following three related DRGs:

- DRG 320 Kidney and Urinary Tract Infections, Age Greater than 17 with Complications or Comorbidities
- DRG 321 Kidney and Urinary Tract Infections, Age Greater than 17 without Complications or Comorbidities
- DRG 322 Kidney and Urinary Tract Infections, Age 0–17

All three of the above DRGs have a common set of diagnosis codes of which one must be present to assign a patient to one of these DRGs. ICD–9 diagnosis code 599.0 (Infection, urinary tract, site not specified) is one of a list of diagnosis codes that would qualify. If the patient was older than 17 they would be assigned to DRG 320 or 321, depending upon the presence of any complications or comorbidities. Examples of common complications or comorbidities would be congestive heart failure, diabetes, and anemia. If the patient was 17 years of age or younger with an ICD–9 diagnosis code that mapped to DRG 320, they would be assigned to DRG 322 with or without the presence of any complications or comorbidities.

Medicare payment for hospital outpatient services shifted to APC payment in 2000. Each APC is related to one or more HCPCS/CPT codes. The assignment of HCPCS/CPT codes is presented in the UB–92 claim form in field locator (FL) #44 HCPCS/Rates. For many inpatient claims, there may be no HCPCS/CPT codes presented. The sample claim in the Appendix is for an inpatient claim and no HCPCS codes are presented. Items are aggregated at the revenue code level. For example, all laboratory procedures are grouped under Revenue Code 300. Outpatient claims will however show detailed procedures and HCPCS/CPT codes will be present. For example, APC 0005 (Level II Needle Biopsy/Aspiration Except Bone Marrow) may be assigned if one of the following CPT codes is present: 19100, 19102, 20206, 32400, 38505, 42400, 47011, 47399, 48511, 48999, 50021, 54500, and 62269. The key point to remember is that for an APC to be assigned, a HCPCS code must be present. Multiple HCPCS codes may map to one APC code, but any given HCPCS code will map to one and only one APC.

LEARNING OBJECTIVE 5

Appreciate the role of claims editing in the bill submission process.

CLAIMS EDITING

Both providers and payers will employ claims editing software to detect possible errors in claim submission. From the provider's perspective, two major objectives are of interest. First, they want to ensure that they receive the maximum payment for the medical services delivered to their patients. Second, providers want to shorten the amount of time from claim submission to actual payment. Payers have a similar set of incentives except they are reversed. Payers do not want to make payment in an amount that is greater than the amount of their obligation. In addition, payers prefer to delay payment as long as possible without violating state payment laws or contract discount terms.

Most large providers use some type of automated software for editing claims that are to be submitted to payers. These software packages check for a large number of possible errors. First, the software will determine if the requisite information for submitting a "clean claim" is present in the claim. Is the patient's name spelled correctly? Is the social security or health care plan identification present? Are diagnosis and procedure codes present? Is the date of service included? And so on. The second set of conditions that are often tested deal with the internal validity of the claim. Is the procedure consistent with the gender of the patient? Was there an injection procedure included in the claim, but no injectable drug listed? Many of these edit checks may be internally developed, but a large number of them may also be related to uniform claim edits developed by Medicare.

The Center for Medicare and Medicaid Services (CMS) developed the National Correct Coding Initiative (NCCI) to promote national correct coding methodologies and to control improper coding that leads to inappropriate payment of Part B health insurance claims. The coding policies developed are based on coding conventions defined in the American Medical Association's CPT codes, national and local policies and edits, coding guidelines developed by national societies, analysis of standard medical and surgical practice, and review of correct coding practice.

The National Correct Coding Initiative edits identify pairs of services that normally should not be billed by the same physician for the same patient on the same day. The NCCI includes two types of edits: comprehensive/component edits and mutually exclusive edits.

- Comprehensive/Component edits identify code pairs that should not be billed together because one service inherently includes the other.
- Mutually Exclusive edits identify code pairs that, for clinical reasons, are unlikely to be performed on the same patient on the same day. For example, a mutually exclusive edit might identify two different types of testing that yield equivalent results.

CMS has designated a series of specific edit checks that are used in determining hospital outpatient claim status. These edit checks are referred to as Outpatient Code Edits (OCE) and at the time of this writing included 73 specific edit checks.

The OCE utilizes claim level and line item level information in the editing process. The claim level information includes such data elements as "from" and "through" dates, ICD–9–CM diagnosis codes, type of bill, age, sex, etc. The line level information includes such data elements as HCPCS codes with up to two modifiers, revenue code, service units, etc.

Each OCE edit results in one of six different dispositions. The dispositions help to ensure that all fiscal intermediaries are following similar procedures. There are four claim level dispositions, which include:

- Rejection—Claim must be corrected and resubmitted
- Denial—Claim cannot be resubmitted, but can be appealed
- Return to provider (RTP)—Problems must be corrected and claim resubmitted
- Suspension—Claim requires further information before it can be processed

There are two line item level dispositions which include:

- Rejection—Claim is processed, but line item is rejected and can be resubmitted later
- Denial—Claim is processed, but line item is rejected and cannot be resubmitted

This area of coding edits is very complex, but extremely important to the provider's ultimate payment. Sometimes the code edits do not appear to be consistent. For example, OCE edit #43 specifies that when a blood transfusion procedure code is present in the claim but there was no related blood product present, the claim will be returned to the provider. There is no related OCE edit to detect the reverse situation, that is when a blood product may be present but no transfusion procedure is included. In this situation, Medicare would pay for the blood product, but the provider would have lost payment for the transfusion procedure. This is an example of an edit that is most likely added to many hospital claims editor programs.

SUMMARY

Accurate billing and coding are essential to a health care firm's financial survival. This is a very complex area that requires the input of billing and coding professionals. In many health care firms, the billing and coding functions may report to the chief financial officer because of their integral relation to revenue generation. Failure to capture all charges associated with a patient encounter can result in significant revenue loss. Some estimates of lost charges run as high as five percent of total charges. Given the relatively low margins for most health care firms, this could be a catastrophic loss. Most claims are submitted electronically to payers and must now be consistent with HIPAA provisions that govern EDI (Electronic Data Interchange) submissions. Health care claims are unique in many respects, but coding is an area of special importance. In most other business settings, a bill would simply list the items purchased or services rendered. In health care firms, the charge codes describing the services or products must be related to standard procedure codes and supplemented with diagnosis codes to document the legitimacy of the services. These codes can and do play a major role in not only the amount of payment received, but also the timeliness of that payment. Claims editing software is widely used by health care providers to ensure the accuracy of their claims prior to submission.

ASSIGNMENTS

1. A hospital submitting an outpatient claim would use a UB–92 claim form. What source of coding information would be used to report diagnosis codes? What source of coding information would be used to report procedures?

2. Elective procedures often require prior approval from the patient's insurance company. What is this approval process often called?

3. From what types of coding information must the following codes be derived?

   • 453.41 Venous embolism and thrombosis of deep vessels of proximal lower extremity
   • 84.55 Insertion of bone void filler
   • 69090 Ear Piercing
   • A4646 Supply of Low Osmolar Contrast Material

4. Including a HCPCS/CPT code directly in the chargemaster is called what?

5. Many DRGs are in pairs that differ by the term with complications or comorbidities (cc), or without cc. The DRG that has the cc is usually paid at a higher rate. What can cause a DRG "without cc" to be changed to a DRG "with cc"?

6. A payer may delay or deny payment because of inaccurate or missing information in a submitted claim. Many contracts require payment within a specified period of time, e.g. 30 days from submission of a "clean claim." How can health care service providers avoid claims rejections?

7. The Medicare intermediary has returned a claim to a hospital because of Outpatient Code Edit (OCE) violation Number 1—invalid diagnosis code. This would imply that the procedure performed is not supported by the diagnosis code. What action can the provider take to ensure payment?

SOLUTIONS AND ANSWERS

1. ICD–9 diagnosis codes would be used to report diagnosis information on a UB–92 for both hospital inpatient and outpatient claims. HCPCS codes would be used to report procedure codes for hospital outpatient claims.

2. Pre-certification.

3. 453.41(ICD–9 Diagnosis Code), 84.55 (ICD–9 Procedure Code), 69090 (Level I HCPCS/ CPT Code), A4646 (Level II HCPCS Code).

4. Static coding.

5. While there are a number of factors that may lead to the designation of "with cc," the presence of additional diagnosis codes, such as anemia or diabetes can often change the coding to a "with cc" designation. This illustrates the importance of good physician documentation in the medical record and accurate transcription from the medical record to the claim form.

6. Insuring a clean claim submission often starts at registration. Accurate collection of patient and related insurance information is critical in the claims submission process. Claims editing software can also check for issues that may result in claims denial prior to submission.

7. Because this is an OCE violation where the claim is returned to the provider, the provider can correct the diagnosis code and resubmit for payment. Ideally, a good claims editing system would have caught this problem prior to submission.

Appendix

Sample UB–92 Form and Sample CMS–1500 Form

SAMPLE UB–92 FORM

ABC Medical Center PO Box 1713 Columbus OH 43210 614-722-9614	2							3 PATIENT CONTROL NO. 13504295			4 TYPE OF BILL 111

5 FED. TAX NO.	6 STATEMENT COVERS PERIOD		7 COV D.	8 N-C D.	9 C-I D.	10 L-R D.	11
	FROM	THROUGH					
311054871	080906	081406	5				

12 PATIENT NAME	13 PATIENT ADDRESS
Brutus Buckeye	00 Buckeye Lane, Columbus OH 43210

14 BIRTHDATE	15 SEX	16 MS	ADMISSION				21 D HR	22 STAT	23 MED. RECORD NO.	CONDITION CODES							31
			17 DATE	18 HR	19 TYPE	20 SRC				24	25	26	27	28	29	30	
01301960	M	S	080906	06	3	1	14	01	404390000003								

32 OCCURRENCE		33 OCCURRENCE		34 OCCURRENCE		35 OCCURRENCE		36 OCCURRENCE SPAN			37
CODE	DATE	CODE	DATE	CODE	DATE	CODE	DATE	CODE	FROM	THROUGH	

38					39 VALUE CODES		40 VALUE CODES		41 VALUE CODES	
					CODE	AMOUNT	CODE	AMOUNT	CODE	AMOUNT
Brutus Buckeye 00 Buckeye Lane Columbus OH 43210					01	444.00				

42 REV. CD.	43 DESCRIPTION	44 HCPCS/RATES	45 SERV. DATE	46 SERV. UNITS	47 TOTAL CHARGES	48 NON-COVERED CHARGES	49
110	Room board, pvt	447.00		5	2,235.00	15.00	
250	Pharmacy			61	674.87		
253	Drugs, take home			65	88.75	88.75	
259	Other pharmacy			27	151.38		
270	Medsur supplies			40	1,603.82		
278	Supply implants			5	2,969.55		
300	Laboratory			3	228.50		
310	Path lab			6	569.00		
360	OR services			29	7,662.00		
370	Anesthesia			3	1,108.05		
410	Respiratory services			1	8.65		
710	Recovery room			2	391.00		
999	Pt convenience			1	7.20	7.20	
001	Total				17,697.77	110.95	

50 PAYER	51 PROVIDER NO.	52 REL. INFO	53 ASG BEN	54 PRIOR PAYMENTS	55 EST. AMOUNT DUE	56
Central Benefits	230147	Y	Y			

57	DUE FROM PATIENT ▶

58 INSURED'S NAME	59 P. REL	60 CERT. - SSN - HIC. - ID NO.	61 GROUP NAME	62 INSURANCE GROUP NO.
Brutus Buckeye	08	000 00 000		

63 TREATMENT AUTHORIZATION CODES	64 ESC	65 EMPLOYER NAME	66 EMPLOYER LOCATION

57 PRIN. DIAG. CD.	68 CODE	69 CODE	OTHER DIAG. CODES 70 CODE	71 CODE	72 CODE	73 CODE	74 CODE	75 CODE	76 ADM. DIAG. CD.	77 E-CODE	78
52469	5180	52461	72210						52469		

79 P.C.	80 PRINCIPAL PROCEDURE		81 OTHER PROCEDURE		OTHER PROCEDURE		82 ATTENDING PHYS. ID
	CODE	DATE	CODE	DATE	CODE	DATE	T Z AC 198x
9	765	081406	247	081406			83 OTHER PHYS. ID
	OTHER PROCEDURE		OTHER PROCEDURE		OTHER PROCEDURE		
	CODE	DATE	CODE	DATE	CODE	DATE	OTHER PHYS. ID

84 REMARKS	
	85 PROVIDER REPRESENTATIVE 86 DATE X

UB-92 HCFA 1450

SAMPLE CMS–1500 FORM

HEALTH INSURANCE CLAIM FORM

1. MEDICARE MEDICAID CHAMPUS CHAMPVA GROUP HLTH PLAN FECA BLK LUNG OTHER	1a. INSURED'S I.D. NUMBER (FOR PROGRAM IN ITEM 1)
☐ (Medicare #) ☐ (Medicaid #) ☐ (Sponsor SSN) ☐ (VA File #) ☐ (SSN or ID) ☐ (SSN) ☐ (ID)	

2. PATIENT'S NAME (Last, First, MI)	3. PATIENT'S DATE OF BIRTH MM DD YY SEX M ☐ F ☐	4. INSURED'S NAME (Last, First, MI)

5. PATIENT'S ADDRESS (No., Street)	6. PATIENT RELATIONSHIP TO INSURED Self ☐ Spouse ☐ Child ☐ Other ☐	7. INSURED'S ADDRESS (No., Street)
CITY STATE	8. PATIENT STATUS Single ☐ Married ☐ Other ☐	CITY STATE
ZIP CODE TELEPHONE (Incl Area Code)	Employed ☐ Full-Time ☐ Part-Time ☐ Student Student	ZIP CODE TELEPHONE (Incl. Area Code)

9. OTHER INSURED'S NAME (Last, First, MI)	10. IS PATIENT'S CONDITION RELATED TO:	11. INSURED'S POLICY GROUP OR FECA NUMBER
a. OTHER INSURED'S POLICY OR GROUP NUMBER	a. EMPLOYMENT? (Current or Previous) YES ☐ NO ☐	a. INSURED'S DATE OF BIRTH MM DD YY SEX M ☐ F ☐
b. OTHER INSURED'S DATE OF BIRTH MM DD YY SEX M ☐ F ☐	b. AUTO ACCIDENT? PLACE (State) YES ☐ NO ☐	b. EMPLOYER'S NAME OR SCHOOL NAME
c. EMPLOYER'S NAME OR SCHOOL NAME	c. OTHER ACCIDENT? YES ☐ NO ☐	c. INSURANCE PLAN NAME OR PROGRAM NAME
d. INSURANCE PLAN NAME OR PROGRAM NAME	10d. RESERVED FOR LOCAL USE	d. IS THERE ANOTHER HEALTH BENEFIT PLAN? YES ☐ NO ☐ If yes, return to and complete item 9a–d

READ BACK OF FORM BEFRE COMPLETING & SIGNING THIS FORM. 12. PATIENT'S OR AUTHORIZED PERSON'S SIGNATURE I authorize the release of any medical or other information necessary to process this claim. I also request payment of government benefits either to myself or to the party who accepts assignment below. SIGNED _____ DATE _____	13. INSURED'S OR AUTHORIZED PERSON'S SIGNATURE I authorize payment of medical benefits to the undersigned physician or Supplier for services described below. SIGNED _____

14. DATE OF CURRENT: ILLNESS (First symptom) OR MM DD YY INJURY (Accident) OR PREGNANCY (LMP)	15. IF PATIENT HAS HAD SAME OR SIMILAR ILLNESS, GIVE FIRST DATE MM DD YY	16. DATES PATIENT UNABLE TO WORK IN CURRENT OCCUPATION MM DD YY MM DD YY FROM TO
17. NAME OF REFERRING PHYSICIAN	17a. ID NUMBER OF REFERRING PHYSICIAN	18. HOSPITALIZATION DATES RELATED TO CURRENT SERVICES MM DD YY MM DD YY FROM TO
19. RESERVED FOR LOCAL USE		20. OUTSIDE LAB? $ CHARGES ☐ YES ☐ NO

21. DIAGNOSIS OR NATURE OF ILLNESS OR INJURY (RELATE ITEMS 1,2,3 OR 4 TO ITEM 24E BY LINE) 1. 3. 2. 4.	22. MEDICAID RESUBMISSION CODE ORIGINAL REF. NO. 23. PRIOR AUTHORIZATION NUMBER

24.	A DATE(S) OF SERVICE From To MM DD YY MM DD YY	B Place of Service	C Type of Service	D PROCEDURES, SERVICES, OR SUPPLIES (Explain Unusual Circumstances) CPT/HCPCS MODIFIER	E DIAGNOSIS CODE	F $ CHARGES	G DAYS OR UNITS	H EPSDT Family Plan	I EMG	J COB	K RESVD FOR LOCAL USE

25. FEDERAL TAX ID NUMBER SSN EIN ☐ ☐	26. PATIENT'S ACCOUNT NO.	27. ACCEPT ASSIGNMENT? (For govt. claims, see back) ☐ YES ☐ NO	28. TOTAL CHARGE $	29. AMOUNT PAID $	30. BALANCE DUE $

31. SIGNATURE OF PHYSICIAN OR SUPPLIER INCLUDING DEGREES OR CREDENTIALS (I certify that the statements on the reverse apply to this bill and are made a part thereof.) SIGNED _____ DATE _____	32. NAME AND ADDRESS OF FACILITY WHERE SERVICES WERE RENDERED (If other than home or office)	33. PHYSICIAN'S, SUPPLIER'S BILLING NAME, ADDRESS, ZIP CODE & PHONE # PIN # GRP #

FORM HCFA-1500

Chapter 3

Financial Environment of Health Care Organizations

After studying this chapter, you should be able to do the following:

1. Describe factors that influence the financial viability of a health care organization.
2. Describe the financial environment of the largest segments of the health care industry.
3. Discuss the major reimbursement methods that are used in health care.
4. Discuss the major aspects of Medicare benefits.
5. Describe how Medicare reimburses the major types of providers, and be able to discuss the implications of these methods for an organization's resource management.

REAL-WORLD SCENARIO

Joshua Douglas, Chief Financial Officer at Marshall Regional Hospital, was exploring an option to convert his hospital to Critical Access Hospital (CAH) status under the Medicare program. The CEO of the hospital, Mikaela Grace, had directed Josh to investigate this possible option at the last hospital board meeting. The hospital has been losing money for the last four years and cash positions have been eroding to the point of possible default on a small debt issue.

Marshall Regional is a 20-bed acute-care hospital with a 120-bed skilled-nursing facility. It is located in a rural area of a western state and is 50 miles from the nearest hospital. The current economic climate in the region is not good and is not expected to improve in the near future. Because of its low volume, Marshall's cost per unit for acute inpatient and outpatient procedures is very high. As a result, the hospital has been losing large sums of money on its sizable Medicare volume. The situation has only worsened since Medicare shifted to prospective payment for outpatient services in August 2000. Josh estimates that his hospital loses 45 cents for every dollar of Medicare payment. Because a high percentage of the local population is elderly, Medicare is the hospital's largest source of business. Medicare represents 50 percent of all outpatient revenue and 65 percent of inpatient revenue. Most inpatient procedures are not complex, and severely ill patients are transferred to a larger hospital 50 miles up the interstate.

Mikaela Grace had been to a recent seminar and learned that her hospital might be eligible for Critical Access Hospital status. If the hospital was successful in its application for CAH status, it would no longer be paid under prospective payment. Instead, Marshall Regional would receive the cost incurred in delivering services to Medicare patients plus one percent. Joshua Douglas estimated that this change in payment could result in a substantial improvement in operating margins and should help the hospital to secure its financial future.

Upon Josh's review of CAH materials, he learned that over 1100 hospitals in the U.S. were designated as CAH in June 2005. While there are a number of criteria that must be met, it seemed that the hospital would be eligible. It was under the 25-bed maximum and it was more than 35 miles from the nearest hospital. It also maintained an acute-care length of stay of less than 96 hours. While there were other criteria, Josh was very optimistic about Marshall's chances of achieving CAH status, and he prepared a memo to Mikaela Grace recommending that they move forward with an application.

Almost any measure of size would indicate that the health care industry is big business. Its proportion of the gross domestic product (GDP) has been steadily increasing for several decades and now represents nearly 16 percent of the GDP and approximately two trillion dollars in expenditures. Paralleling this growth, the pressures for cost control within the system have increased tremendously, especially at the federal and state levels for control of Medicare and Medicaid. Health care organizations (HCOs) that are not able to deal effectively with these pressures face an uncertain future. In short, as the expected demand for health services continues to increase during the next several decades as our population ages, successful HCOs must become increasingly cost efficient.

LEARNING OBJECTIVE 1

Describe factors that influence the financial viability of a health care organization.

FINANCIAL VIABILITY

An HCO is a basic provider of health services, but it is also a business. The environment HCOs viewed from a financial perspective could be schematically represented as depicted in Figure 3–1.

In the long run, the HCO must receive dollar payments from the community in an amount at least equal to the dollar payments it makes to its suppliers. In very simple terms, this is the essence of financial viability.

The community in Figure 3–1 is the provider of funds to the HCO. The flow of funds is either directly or indirectly related to the delivery of services by the HCO. For our purposes, the community may be categorized as follows:

- Patients
  1. Self-payer
  2. Third-party payer
     –Blue Cross and Blue Shield
     –Commercial insurance, including managed care
     –Medicaid
     –Medicare
     –Self-insured employer
     –Other
- Non-patients
  1. Grants
  2. Contributions
  3. Tax support
  4. Miscellaneous

In most HCOs, the greater proportion of funds is derived from patients who receive services directly. The largest percentage of these payments usually comes from third-party sources such as Blue Cross, Medicare, Medicaid, and managed-care organizations. In addition, some non-patient funds are derived from government sources in the form of grants for research purposes or direct payments to subsidized HCOs, such as county facilities. Some HCOs also receive significant sums of money from individuals, foundations, or corporations in the form of contributions. Although these sums may be small relative to the total amounts of money received from patient services, their importance in overall viability should not be understated. In many HCOs, these contributed dollars mean the difference between net income and loss.

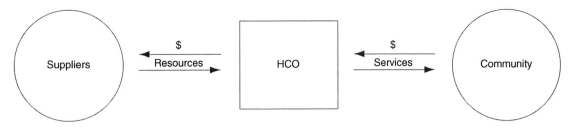

Figure 3–1 Financial Environment of Health Care Organizations

The suppliers in Figure 3–1 provide the HCO with resources that are necessary in the delivery of quality health care. The major categories of suppliers are the following:

- employees
- equipment suppliers
- service contractors
- vendors of consumable supplies
- lenders

Payments for employees usually represent the largest single category of expenditures. For example, in many hospitals, payments for employees represent about 60 percent of total expenditures. Table 3–1 is an example of a statement of operations (similar to an income statement for a for-profit firm) that shows percentages of revenues and expenses for a hospital. Payments for physicians' services also represent important financial requirements. In addition, lenders such as commercial banks or investment bankers supply dollars in the form of loans and receive from the HCO a promise to repay the loans with interest according to a defined repayment schedule. This financial requirement has grown steadily as HCOs have become more dependent on debt financing.

LEARNING OBJECTIVE 2

Describe the financial environment of the largest segments of the health care industry.

SOURCES OF OPERATING REVENUE

Table 3–2 provides a historical breakdown of the relative size of the health care industry and its individual industrial segments. The largest segment is the hospital industry, which absorbs about 33 percent of all health care expenditure dollars (in per capita terms). This per-

centage has been declining over the last few years and is expected to decline further as other industry segments grow more quickly. The physician segment absorbs approximately 20 percent of total health care expenditures; this has been steady in recent years, but still represents a modest increase over the prior decade when expressed as a percentage of total health care expenditures. Prescription drugs represent the third largest health care segment, reflecting the rapid rise in prescription drug use. Whereas in the past nursing homes represented the third largest health care segment, prescription drugs have overtaken nursing homes. Prescription drugs now constitute about 12 percent of all per capita health care expenditures and are projected to have one of the highest expenditure growth rates in the coming years. The once-rapid increases in Medicare spending for skilled nursing facilities (SNFs) have been tempered by the change to prospective payment (explained later in the chapter). Annual growth rates in spending for nursing home care have been cut almost in half in recent years, as providers reacted to the changes in reimbursement method. Demographic factors, however, will still tend to put upward pressure on national nursing home expenditures. Many people believe that the nursing home segment will grow faster as the population ages.

Table 3–3 depicts the sources of operating funds for the four largest health care segments: hospitals, physicians, prescription drugs and nursing homes. It is easy to see dramatic differences in financing among these four segments.

The hospital industry derives more than 50 percent of its total funding from public sources, largely from Medicare and Medicaid. Of the two, Medicare is by far the larger, representing about 30 percent of all hospital revenue. This gives the federal government enormous control over hospitals and their financial positions. Few hospitals can choose to ignore the Medicare program because of its sheer size. Another 34 percent of total hospital funding results from private insurance,

Table 3–1 Statement of Operations for Memorial Hospital, Year Ended 2007 (000s Omitted)

	2007	%
Unrestricted revenues, gains, and other support:		
Net patient service revenue	$85,502	85.84
Premium revenue	11,195	11.24
Other operating revenue	2,913	2.92
Total operating revenue	$99,610	100.0
Expenses		
Salaries and benefits	40,258	40.41
Medical supplies and drugs	27,542	27.65
Professional fees	16,857	16.92
Insurance	5,568	5.59
Depreciation and amortization	3,952	3.97
Interest	1,456	1.46
Provision for bad debts	1,152	1.16
Other	523	0.53
Total expenses	$97,308	97.69
Operating income	2,302	2.31
Investment income	1,846	1.86
Excess of revenues, gains, and other support over expenses	4,148	4.17
Net assets released from restrictions used for purchase of property and equipment	192	0.19
Increase in unrestricted net assets	$ 4,340	4.36

largely from Blue Cross, commercial insurance carriers, managed care organizations, and self-insured employers. Direct payments by patients to hospitals represent approximately three percent of total revenue. The implication of this distribution for hospitals is the creation of an oligopsonistic marketplace. The buying power for hospital services is concentrated in relatively few third-party purchasers, namely the federal government, the state government, Blue Cross, a few commercial insurance carriers, and some large self-insured employers.

The physician marketplace is somewhat different from the marketplace for hospital services. A much larger percentage of physician funding is derived from direct payments by patients (approximately ten percent). And compared with hospital funding, a slightly larger percentage of physician funding results from private insurance sources, largely from Blue Cross and commercial insurance carriers. Physicians derive approximately 51 percent of their total funds from this source; the hospital segment derives 34 percent of total funds from this source. Public programs, although still significant, are the smallest source of physician funding, representing 33 percent of total funds. This situation results because more physician services, such as routine physical examinations and many deductible and copayment services, are excluded from Medicare payment.

Similar to the market for physicians, most of the payments (46 percent) for prescription drugs come from private insurance sources. The impact of Medicare coverage can be clearly seen in Table 3–3. By 2010, projections show that Medicare will be funding 28 percent of all prescription drug costs. Many state Medicaid plans (which are more than 50 percent federally funded) do provide prescription drug benefits. Medicaid represents over 19 percent of the prescription drug payments.

The nursing home segment receives almost no funding from private insurance sources. The major public program for nursing homes is Medicaid, not Medicare. However, the federal government pays more than 50 percent of all Medicaid expenditures. Medicare payments to nursing homes are largely restricted to skilled nursing care, whereas the majority of Medicaid payments to nursing homes are for intermediate-level (custodial) care.

LEARNING OBJECTIVE 3

Discuss the major reimbursement methods that are used in health care.

HEALTH CARE PAYMENT SYSTEMS

One of the most important financial differences between health care firms and other businesses is the way in which their customers or patients make payment for the services they receive. Most businesses have only one basic type of payment: billed charges. Each cus-

Table 3–2 National Health Care Expenditures—2003 and Projected 2010.

	2003	(Projected) 2010	Annual Growth Rate (%)
National health care expenditures (billions)	$ 1,679	$ 2,754	7.3
Population (millions)	296	315	0.9
Per capita expenditures			
Personal health care			
Hospital care	$ 1,742	$ 2,529	5.5
Physician services & clinical services	1,249	1,904	6.2
Dental services	251	370	2.6
Other professional services	164	250	6.2
Home health care	135	234	8.2
Prescription drugs	605	1,172	9.9
Other nondurable medical products	110	144	3.9
Durable medical equipment	69	83	2.7
Nursing home care	374	500	4.2
Other personal health care	167	294	8.4
Total personal health care	$ 4,866	$7,480	6.3
Program administration and insurance cost	586	939	7.0
Government public health activities	99	160	7.1
Research and construction	119	175	5.7
Total national health care expenditures	$ 5,670	$ 8,754	6.2

Source: Centers for Medicare & Medicaid Services, Office of Financial and Actuarial Analysis, Division of National Cost Estimates.

tomer is presented with a bill that represents the product and the quantity of goods or services received and their appropriate prices. Some selective discounting of the price may take place to move slow inventory during slack periods or to encourage large volume orders. The basic payment system, however, remains the same: a fixed price per unit of service that is set by the business, not the customer.

In contrast, the typical health care firm may have several hundred different contractual relationships with payers, which specify different rates of payment for an identical basket of services. While different payers may negotiate different rates of payment, the critical distinction is the unit of payment. For example, some payers will pay physicians a discount from their charges, other payers will pay on fee schedule, Medicare will pay on a relative value scale referred to as RBRVS (Resource-Based Relative Value Scale), and some HMOs may pay on an enrolled or capitated

basis. Similar scenarios would apply in other sectors of the health care industry. Alternative payment units have a different effect on the firm's financial position and might lead to different conclusions with respect to business strategy. Thus, it is extremely important to understand the financial implications of the various payment units used to pay health care firms. Four major payment units are discussed:

1. Historical cost reimbursement
2. Specific services (charge payment)
3. Bundled services
4. Capitated rates

Historical Cost Reimbursement

Until the early 1980s, cost reimbursement was the predominant form of payment by Medicare for most hospitals and other institutional providers. In addition

Table 3–3 Sources of Health Services Funding—2003 and Projected 2010

Source	Hospitals		Physicians		Prescription Drugs		Nursing Homes	
	2003	2010	2003	2010	2003	2010	2003	2010
Private payments (%)								
Out of pocket	3	3	10	10	30	20	28	28
Private insurance	34	34	50	51	46	37	8	7
Other private	4	4	7	6	0	0	4	3
Total private payments	41	41	67	67	76	57	40	38
Government payments (%)								
Medicare	30	32	20	19	2	28	12	12
Medicaid	17	18	7	8	19	11	46	48
Other	12	9	6	6	3	4	2	2
Total government payments	59	59	33	33	24	43	60	62
Total payments (%)	100	100	100	100	100	100	100	100

Source: Centers for Medicare & Medicaid Services, Office of Financial and Actuarial Analysis, Division of National Cost Estimates.

to Medicare, most state Medicaid plans and a large number of Blue Cross plans paid hospitals on the basis of "reasonable" historical costs. Today, the major payers have abandoned historical cost reimbursement and substituted other payment systems. We provide some discussion of cost reimbursement for two reasons. First, it is used in some limited settings for payment. For example, Medicare still pays on a cost basis for services performed in Comprehensive Cancer Centers and critical-access hospitals. Second, some policy analysts have suggested that "regulated cost reimbursement" might be a legitimate way to maintain the quality of patient care.

Two key elements in historical cost reimbursement are reasonable cost and apportionment. Reasonable cost is simply a qualification introduced by the payer to limit its total payment by excluding certain categories of cost or placing limits on costs that the payer deems reasonable. Examples of costs often defined as unreasonable and therefore not reimbursable are costs for charity care, patient telephones, and nursing education. Apportionment refers to the manner in which costs are assigned or allocated to a specific payer, such as Medicaid. For example, assume that a nursing home has total reasonable costs of $10 million, which represent the costs of servicing all patients. If Medicaid is a historical cost reimbursement payer, an allocation or

apportionment of that $10 million is necessary to determine Medicaid's share of the total cost. Quite often, the apportionment is related to billed charges. For example, if charges for services to Medicaid patients were $3 million and total charges to all patients were $15 million, then, 3/15 or 20 percent of the $10 million cost would be apportioned to Medicaid.

Several important financial principles of cost reimbursement should be emphasized. First, cost reimbursement can insulate management somewhat from the financial results of poor financial planning. New clinical programs that do not achieve targeted volume or exceed projected costs may still be viable because of extensive cost reimbursement. This assumes that the payer does not regard the costs as unreasonable. Second, cost reimbursement can often be increased through careful planning, just as taxes can often be reduced through tax planning. The key objective is to maximize the amount of cost apportioned to cost payers subject to any tests for reasonableness.

Specific Services

Most health care firms have some master price list that identifies the appropriate charge for a defined unit of service. These master price lists are often referred to as Charge Description Masters or CDMs (See Chapter 2).

The charges that are applicable for specific services may bear no relationship to amounts actually paid. For example, a hospital may have charges for a patient categorized as Diagnosis Related Group #127 (Heart Failure and Shock) for $15,000, but Medicare could determine that the applicable rate of payment was $4,000. While the charges for specific services of $15,000 are recorded on the patient's bill, the actual charges for specific services are not the basis for payment.

Most institutional providers, such as hospitals and nursing homes, record their charges for specific services on a CMS–1450 or Uniform Bill 1992 (UB–92). Physician bills are often submitted on a CMS–1500. A sample of both the UB–92 and the CMS–1500 are presented in the appendix to Chapter 2. Both of these forms are designed by the Centers for Medicare & Medicaid Services and are standard for claims submission that are required by most payers.

Many medical and surgical procedures often have an assigned code that is either a CPT (Current Procedural Terminology developed and maintained by the American Medical Association) or a HCPCS (HCFA Common Procedure Coding System) developed and maintained by the Centers for Medicare & Medicaid Services. Supply and pharmaceutical items do not usually have CPT codes but may have specific HCPCS codes. However the vast majority of supply and pharmaceutical items do not have a HCPCS or CPT code. The sample UB–92 in the appendix to Chapter 2 consolidates individual charges for specific services by departmental or revenue code. Note that there is no listing of specific services in this bill because the services are consolidated to a revenue code level. If the patient or their insurance plan requested a detailed bill, then the specific services provided would be listed.

Payers who pay on a specific-service basis usually fall into three categories. First, they could be patients who do not have any insurance coverage or lack coverage for the procedures performed. These patients are usually responsible for the total billed charges represented on the claim. Second, the patients could have coverage from an insurance firm that does not have any formal contract with the provider. In the absence of a contract, the patient and/or his carrier would be responsible for the entire amount of billed charges. This often happens when a provider that is out of the carrier's network treats a patient. Third, some insurance firms negotiate contracts with providers on a discounted-charge basis. The carrier agrees to make payment based

upon the total billed charges for the claim, but they will pay something less than 100 percent.

Payment for specific services has several important implications for financial management. First, revenue from specific services may represent the major source of profit for many health care firms. In these situations, pricing or rate setting becomes an important policy (rate setting is addressed in Chapter 5). Second, the firm's rate structure should be based on projected volume and cost. Any unexpected deviation from the projections may require pricing changes. If these changes are not made, there could be a significant effect on the firm's cash flow.

Capitated Rates

Capitated rates represent a new type of payment for many health care providers. In some respects, a capitated rate is a form of bundled service because the unit of payment is based on the individual enrollee. A medical group, hospital, or some association of providers may agree to provide some or all health care services for enrollees during a specified period of time. Most often the provider will agree to pay only for specific services that they perform. For example, a cardiology group might agree to provide all cardiology services to an employer or an HMO for a fixed fee per member per month (PMPM). It is rare that a single health care provider will agree to provide all medical services to an enrolled population. When this does occur, the term global capitation is used to describe the nature of the contractual relationship. Global capitation rates are very uncommon because most health care firms are not in a position to control all health care costs. Capitation arrangements were more common in the mid 1990s and have been declining since then.

In a capitated-payment environment, financial planning and control are critical—even more critical than in a bundled-services payment situation. In a capitated-payment arrangement, the provider is responsible not only for the costs of services provided, but also their utilization. Changes in either costs or utilization can have a dramatic effect on profitability. Unexpected increases in costs will not usually be a basis for contract renegotiation. Therefore, it is imperative that management know what it costs to provide a unit of service required in the contract. For example, if the negotiated rate is to provide all hospital services to subscribers of a health maintenance organization for a fixed fee per subscriber (or capitation), the hospital must know both the utilization and the cost per unit of the required services. Sometimes management may assess the financial desirability of a capitation contract on an incremental basis. This simply means that management is interested in the change in costs and change in revenue that will result if the contract is signed. The firm's cost accounting system should be able to define the incremental costs likely to be incurred in a given contract so that they can be compared to the incremental revenue likely to result from the contract.

Bundled Services

Many of the payment plans used to pay health care providers in today's environment could be classified as bundled-services arrangements. A bundled-services payment plan has two key features. First, payments to the provider are not necessarily related to the list of specific services provided the patient and identified in the UB–92 or the CMS–1500. Instead payment is grouped into a mutually exclusive set of services categories. For example, hospitals are paid by some health care plans on a per-diem or per-case payment rate. Both are examples of bundled services payment. Second, bundled-services arrangements have a fixed fee specified per unit of service. For example, in the per diem arrangement, revenue from treating a patient would be equal to the length of stay times the negotiated per-diem rate.

Medicare has developed bundled-services payment plans for most health care providers. We will discuss some of these plans in detail later in this chapter. Medicare's payment methods have a profound impact on the rest of the industry because they tend to become the standard for payment by many health plans. For example, Medicare pays physicians on an RBRVS basis, which is often used as the payment basis by many

health care plans with one slight wrinkle. Most often these plans will not pay 100 percent of Medicare's rates, but some greater or lesser percentage, such as 110% of RBRVS. The payment units used by Medicare in a variety of health care sectors are presented below in Table 3–4.

Health care providers who are paid under bundled-service arrangements need to understand and monitor their costs of production. A bundled-service unit is simply a set of specific services that may be grouped or classified into a bundled unit of some kind. Total cost of producing the bundled-services unit is therefore a product of two factors:

- Services provided
- Cost per unit of services provided

First, the set of specific services that comprise a bundled unit form the basis for the cost computation. It is important to recognize, however, that the set of services may not always be fixed. For example, home health firms are paid on a 60-day-episode-of-care basis. The number of specific visits per episode is not necessarily fixed. In some cases there may be 30 individual case visits to the patient in the 60-day episode, while in other cases 45 individual visits may be necessary. Second, the cost of producing each of the specific services that comprise the bundled unit is multiplied times the number of units required. Whether 30 or 45 visits of care are required, management must control the unit cost of individual visits by monitoring the productivity of nursing staff. Management's overall objective is to minimize the total cost of production, which means keeping total units of service provided at a minimum and producing each unit of service at an efficient level of cost. Naturally, all this must happen within a quality-of-care constraint.

Table 3–4 Medicare Payment Units for Health Care Sectors

Health Care Sector	Payment Unit
Hospital Inpatient	Diagnosis-Related Groups (DRGs)
Hospital Outpatient	Ambulatory Patient Classifications (APCs)
Physicians	Resource-Based Relative Value Scale (RBRVS)
Skilled Nursing Facilities	Resource Utilization Groups (RUGs)
Home Health Agencies	Home Health Resource Groups (HHRGs)

Discuss the major aspects of Medicare benefits.

MEDICARE BENEFITS

Medicare has three basic benefit programs for its beneficiaries: Part A, Part B, and a prescription-drug benefit, Part D. Part A, or Hospital Insurance, typically is provided free to all beneficiaries if they have 40 or more covered quarters of Medicare employment. Part B, or Medical Insurance, usually requires a monthly payment by the beneficiary. In 2006, this payment was $88.50 per month. Medicare benefits are provided to three categories of individuals. Far and away the largest single group is the aged, beneficiaries over 65 years of age. The second group consists of disabled individuals, and the third group includes people with end-stage renal disease.

There are two primary ways that Medicare beneficiaries receive care through the system. The most popular method is the so-called traditional or original plan. In this plan, Medicare beneficiaries can go to any hospital, doctor, or specialist that accepts Medicare to receive care. The second method is a Medicare Managed Care Plan (Medicare Advantage). Under this method, beneficiaries are enrolled in a private health care plan or HMO, and they are usually limited in terms of the providers that they can visit for care to those included in the plan's network. Usually, Medicare Managed Care Plans provide a wider range of benefits, such as routine physicals and prescription drugs, to offset their restricted networks.

Benefits under Part A include hospital stays, skilled nursing care, home health care, hospice care, and blood received during a hospital stay. Under Part A, there is a deductible, which means that the patient is responsible for this dollar amount prior to any payment by Medicare. In 2006, the hospital deductible was $952. Coinsurance arrangements also exist under Part A coverage. Patients who stay beyond 60 days in a hospital were required to pay $238 per day in 2006. Patients in Skilled Nursing Facilities had no deductible but were required to pay an additional $119 per day for lengths of stay between 21 to 100 days.

Benefits under Part B include a wide range of services, such as doctor's fees, hospital outpatient services, clinical laboratory tests, durable medical equipment, and a number of other preventive medical services. There was a $124 deductible for medical services received under Part B in 2006. Part B benefits also require a coinsurance payment in many cases. This coinsurance is 20 percent of approved amounts. This coinsurance amount can be no less than 20 percent of the total payment due to the provider of services, which includes Medicare's payment and the coinsurance. For example, Medicare may determine that total payment for APC #83 (Coronary Angioplasty) is $3,300. The required coinsurance on this claim may be $1,650 as set by Medicare, which represents 50 percent of the total payment.

Part D, the Medicare drug plan, was initiated on January 1, 2006. The basic plan provides drug coverage that will limit the maximum amount of personal expenditures to $3,600 per year. The minimum coverage plan has an initial $250 deductible, followed by a 25 percent co-pay from $250 to $2,250, followed by a 100% co-pay from $2,250 to $5,100. Expenditures beyond $5,100 are subject to a five percent co-pay.

Many Medicare beneficiaries purchase additional insurance from private insurance firms to pay for deductibles and coinsurance amounts that exist in the Medicare program. This coverage is often referred to as supplemental or Medigap coverage and may also provide limited coverage for other health care services.

For a more complete picture of specific benefits under the Medicare program, visit Medicare's web site, www.medicare.gov.

Describe how Medicare reimburses the major types of providers, and be able to discuss the implications of these methods for an organization's resource management.

MEDICARE PAYMENT: HOSPITAL INPATIENT

Medicare pays hospitals for inpatient care on a bundled-services unit basis referred to as PPS (Prospective Payment System). Medicare officially launched PPS on October 1, 1983. All hospitals participating in the Medicare program are required to participate in PPS, except those excluded by statute. These include:

- children's hospitals.
- distinct psychiatric and rehabilitation units.
- hospitals outside the 50 states.
- hospitals in states with an approved waiver.
- critical-access hospitals.

PPS provides payment for all hospital non-physician services provided to hospital inpatients. This payment also covers services provided by outside suppliers, such as laboratory or radiology units. Medicare makes one comprehensive payment to the hospital, which is then responsible for paying outside suppliers or non-physician services.

The basis of PPS payment is the DRG system developed by Yale University. The DRG system takes all possible diagnoses from the *International Classification of Diseases, 9th Revision, Clinical Modification* (ICD–9–CM) system and classifies them into 25 major diagnostic categories based on organ systems. These 25 categories are further broken down into 559 distinct medically meaningful groupings or DRGs (Appendix 3 in this chapter contains a list of the 559 DRGs). Medicare contends that the resources required to treat a given DRG entity should be similar for all patients within a DRG category.

Total payments to a hospital under Medicare can be split into the following elements (See Figure 3–2):

- Prospective payments
  1. DRG operating payment
  2. DRG capital payment
- Reasonable cost payments

The DRG operating payment results from the multiplication of the hospital dollar rate and the specific case weight of the DRG. Appendix 3 provides the most recent case weight for the 559 DRGs. The case weight for DRG 001, Craniotomy, Age > 17 with cc, is 3.4347. This measure indicates that in terms of expected cost, DRG 001 would cost about 3.4347 times more than the average case. A specific weight is assigned to each of the 559 DRGs.

The dollar rate is broken down into a labor and non-labor component. The labor component is adjusted for cost of living. Table 3–5 provides hypothetical rates which might be defined by Medicare.

Every hospital in the United States has a wage index value assigned to it. That wage index is multiplied by

Table 3–5 Hypothetical Medicare Rates According to Hospital Status

Rate	
Labor	Non-labor
$3,500	$1,600

the labor component of the Medicare standardized payment to yield the DRG operating payment. If we assume that a hospital has a wage index of 1.2509, its DRG operating payment for DRG 001 would be calculated as follows:

$$\text{Payment} = \text{DRG weight} \times [(\text{labor amount} \times \text{wage index}) + \text{non-labor amount}]$$

$$\text{Payment} = 3.4347 [(\$3,500 \times 1.2509) + \$1,600]$$
$$= \$20,533.15$$

This dollar payment may be further increased by additional payments to cover the following areas:

- Indirect medical education
- Disproportionate share
- Outlier payments

The add-on to a teaching hospital is referred to as an indirect medical education adjustment. This allowance is related to the numbers of interns and residents at the hospital and the number of beds. The allowance is over and above salaries paid to interns and residents, which are already covered as a reasonable cost. The additional payment is meant to cover the additional costs that the teaching hospital incurs in the treatment of patients.

A separate payment is also provided to a hospital that treats a large percentage of Medicaid and Medicaid-eligible patients. This payment is referred to as a disproportionate share payment.

Outlier payments are additional payments for patients who use an unusually large amount of resources. We will discuss their computation shortly.

There is still a portion of the total Medicare payment that is related to reasonable cost, as shown in Figure 3–2. Costs that are still paid on this basis include:

- direct medical education costs.
- kidney acquisition costs.
- bad debts for copayments and deductibles (reimbursed at 60%).

There is a national standardized federal payment rate for capital costs that is similar to the national rates

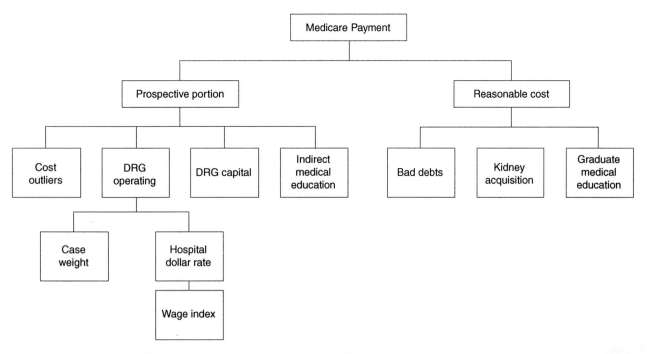

Figure 3–2 Breakdown of Medicare Inpatient Payments to a Hospital

for labor and non-labor costs discussed earlier. In 2006, the federal rate for capital costs was $421.00. This rate would be adjusted for the following factors:

- case mix, using the DRG relative weight
- indirect medical education
- outlier adjustments (the adjustment is much lower than before, to recognize the presumed fixed-cost nature of capital costs)
- disproportionate share adjustment
- geographic adjustment, using the wage index to impute higher costs to higher wage areas
- large urban adjustment of three percent, to reflect higher costs

As an illustration, assume that we wish to calculate capital payment for DRG 001 when the federal payment rate for capital was approximately $421.00. We will also assume that our hospital is in a large urban area with a geographical adjustment factor of 1.194. Please note that a hospital's geographical adjustment factor and its wage index are not usually the same. We will assume that no other adjustments are applicable. The amount of payment would be:

Capital payment = DRG wt. × [standard amount × large urban adjustment × geographical adjustment factor]

Capital payment = 3.4347 × [$421 × 1.03 × 1.194]
          = $1,778.33

We will now conclude our discussion of Medicare DRG payment with the incorporation of the outlier adjustment. An additional payment for a cost outlier is made when the actual cost of the case exceeds DRG payment by $23,600, the required amount. To determine if this threshold is met, one must define actual costs for the specific case under consideration. Costs are defined using the hospital's overall ratio of cost to charges. For example, a claim with $100,000 of charges in a hospital with a ratio of cost to charges of 0.75 would have a designated cost of $75,000. If this cost were above the threshold, Medicare would make payment at 80 percent of the difference. The reason that Medicare does not pay 100 percent of the difference relates to the concept of marginal cost. Medicare believes that additional costs incurred to treat outlier patients are not 100 percent of average cost.

To give the reader some idea of payment composition for an average U.S. hospital, Table 3–6 presents the median payment by category in 2004 for all U.S. hospitals for a DRG with a case weight of 1.00.

There are a number of ways that a hospital can try to increase its total payment under Medicare inpatient PPS payment rules. For example, it can try to get the

Table 3–6 Median Medicare Payment for U.S. Hospitals, DRG Case Weight of 1.00—2004

DRG Operating Payment	$ 4,488
DRG Capital Payment	471
Indirect Medical Education	275
Disproportionate Share	416
Coinsurance and Deductible	472
Outlier Payments	160
Other	115
Total	$ 6,397

hospital reclassified to a higher wage index, document bad debts better on Medicare patients, change its ratio of residents to beds to increase its indirect medical education payment, and change the DRG assignment. Far and away the most likely source of increased payment is DRG reclassification. DRGs are assigned by a software package referred to as a grouper. That grouper assigns a DRG based upon the patient's age, the principal diagnosis, procedures performed, and secondary diagnosis. In many cases, missed secondary diagnoses can cost the hospital significant amounts of reimbursement.

DRG 079 (Respiratory Infections) carries a DRG weight of 1.6238 while DRG 089 (Simple Pneumonia and Pleurisy) carries a weight of 1.0320. For a hospital with an average payment of $5,000 per case weight of 1.000, a patient erroneously assigned to DRG 089 instead of DRG 079 would cost the hospital $2,959 [$5,000 × (1.6238 − 1.0320)]. What would cause a patient with an assignment of DRG 089 to be moved to DRG 079? Very simply, is there a specified cause for the pneumonia? For example, if the physician identified salmonella as the bacterial cause, the patient could be legitimately coded as DRG 079. Medical record coders must be on the alert for this information in the physician's notes and other documents, and physicians must be educated about the importance of accurate documentation.

There are literally hundreds of situations like this within a hospital. The importance of accurate coding cannot be overstated in today's payment environment. On the other hand, hospitals should seek to accurately code and not to over code to maximize reimbursement. Hospital executives who intentionally upcode may fall under the government's fraud and abuse regulations, which can impose some severe civil and criminal penalties.

At the time of this writing, Medicare has proposed to modify its DRG system in Fiscal Years 2007 and 2008. In FY 2007, the DRG weights will be established based upon costs, not charges as has been previously done. This change will increase the relative weights for medical DRGs and reduce the weights for many surgical DRGs. In FY 2008, the DRGs will be adjusted to reflect severity levels. This change will increase the number of DRGs significantly and will provide a boost in payment to those hospitals who treat more severely ill patients.

MEDICARE PAYMENT: PHYSICIANS

Beginning in January 1992, Medicare began paying for physician services using a new resource-based relative value scale (RBRVS). This new payment system replaced the old reasonable-charge method that had been the basis for physician payment since the inception of the Medicare program in the 1960s. Medicare pays the lesser of the actual billed charge or the fee-schedule amount.

From Medicare's perspective, physicians are categorized as participating or non-participating physicians. A participating physician is a physician who agrees to accept Medicare's payment for a service as payment in full and will bill the patient for the copayment portion only. The copayment portion is usually 20 percent of the charge. For example, assume that a patient received a service from a physician that had an approved fee schedule of $100.00. The participating physician would receive $80.00 directly from Medicare and would bill the patient for $20.00, which would represent the copayment portion of the bill. If the physician's bill for the service was only $80.00, Medicare would pay 80 percent, or $64.00, and the patient would be billed 20 percent, or $16.00. A participating physician agrees to accept assignment on each and every Medicare patient that he or she treats.

A non-participating physician can choose to accept assignment on a case-by-case basis. While this arrangement initially might seem advantageous, there are several major drawbacks. First, a non-participating physician has a lower fee schedule. The limiting charge is equal to 95 percent of the approved fee schedule. If the physician in the illustration just discussed were non-participating, the amount of the Medicare payment would be $95.00, not $100.00. This difference may not seem all that important if the physician can recover any of the difference from the patient. However, Medicare has placed some limits on the amount that a non-participating physician can recover from the patient. Medicare sets a maximum fee for a non-participating physician equal to 115 percent of the approved fee for non-participating physician, which is already only 95 percent of the approved fee schedule for a participating physician.

A simple illustration may better explain this narrative. Assume that a non-participating physician provides services to a patient resulting in charges of $200.00, but Medicare's approved schedule for a participating physician is only $100.00. How much can the physician collect? The answer depends on whether the physician accepts or rejects Medicare assignment. First, assume that the physician rejects assignment. The maximum amount that can be collected from this service is:

$$\$109.25 = [.95 \times \$100] \times 1.15$$

The entire amount will come from the patient directly. No check will be sent to the physician from Medicare. The final total payment could be allocated as follows:

Medicare payment to patient (.8 × $95.00)	$76.00
Patient's copayment (.2 × $95.00)	19.00
Additional patient payment	14.25
Total payment to physician	$109.25

The non-participating physician can also choose to accept assignment on a case-by-case basis. The advantage realized with assignment is that Medicare will now pay the physician directly for his or her portion of the bill. The disadvantage is that the physician must accept the fee schedule for non-participating physicians, which will only be 95 percent of the fee approved for participating physicians. In the example above, the non-participating physician who agreed to accept assignment on this patient would receive the following payments:

Medicare payment to physician (.8 × $95.00)	$76.00
Patient's copayment (.2 × $95.00)	19.00
Total payment to physician	$ 95.00

The participating physician would be able to receive $100.00 for this service because of the higher approved-fee schedule. Of the total $100.00 in payment, $80.00 would come directly from Medicare and $20.00 from the patient as the copayment portion.

At the present time, there are Medicare payment rates for more than 10,000 physician services, which are usually broken out by CPT or HCPCS code. There are specific values for those codes that vary by region; presently there are distinct values for each of the Medicare carrier localities. These payment rates result from the multiplication of three relative values and regional cost indexes. For every procedure there are three components that together reflect the cost of a particular procedure:

1. Work (RVUw)—This factor represents not only physician time involved, but also skill levels, stress, and other factors.
2. Practice expense (RVUpe)—This factor represents non-physician costs, excluding malpractice costs.
3. Malpractice (RVUm)—This factor represents the cost of malpractice insurance.

Each of the individual relative values is then multiplied by a region-specific set of price indexes. To illustrate this adjustment, the weighted value for excision of neck cyst (CPT # 42810) for Los Angeles is presented in Table 3–7. To determine the payment rate for this procedure in Los Angeles, the index-adjusted relative value would be multiplied by a conversion factor. If we assume that the conversion factor is $40.00, the approved charge for excision of neck cyst in Los Angeles would be $309.20 (7.73 x $40.00).

Medicare also differentiates the payment by the setting in which the procedure was performed. If the procedure was performed in a facility setting (generally a hospital, SNF, or Ambulatory Surgery Center), the amount allowed for Practice expense is reduced compared to what it would be if the procedure were performed in a non-facility setting. For example, the allowed practice-expense weight for excision of neck cyst in a facility setting is 3.55, but if the procedure were performed in a non-facility setting, the allowed weight would be 5.73. The rationale for these differences is related to the additional payment that Medicare would make to the facility. A procedure performed in a hospital would involve a payment to the hospital, as well as to the physician.

Table 3–7 Components of Price Adjustment for Excision of Neck Cyst in Los Angeles

	RVU	Geographical Cost Index for Los Angeles	Product
Work	3.25	1.043	3.39
Practice expense	3.55	1.144	4.06
Malpractice	0.29	0.954	.28
Total			7.73

MEDICARE PAYMENT: HOSPITAL OUTPATIENT

The Balanced Budget Act of 1997 (BBA) directed CMS to implement a prospective payment system (PPS) under Medicare for hospital outpatient services. All services paid under the new PPS are classified into groups called Ambulatory Payment Classifications, or APCs. Services in each APC are similar clinically and in terms of the resources they require. A payment rate is established for each APC. Depending on the services provided, hospitals may be paid for more than one APC for an encounter. Not all hospital outpatient procedures have an assigned APC code; some procedures are paid on a fee-schedule basis, such as lab tests. Others may not be paid at all because they are considered incidental services, such as some drugs and medical supply items.

The BBA also changed the way beneficiary coinsurance is determined for the services included under the PPS. A coinsurance amount will initially be calculated for each APC based on 20 percent of the national median charge for services in the APC. The coinsurance amount for an APC will not change until the amount becomes 20 percent of the total APC payment. In addition, no coinsurance amount can be greater than the hospital inpatient deductible in a given year. This is a major change for Medicare and will mean that the total burden of payment will shift more to Medicare in the future. A similar change for physician payment was made in 1992.

Both the total APC payment and the portion paid as coinsurance will be adjusted to reflect geographic wage variations using the hospital wage index. It is assumed that 60 percent of the total payment is labor related and thus subject to the wage-index adjustment. Each APC is assigned a relative weight and then that weight is multiplied by the current conversion factor to determine total payment. This same methodology

framework is used throughout most of Medicare's payment plans.

To illustrate the details discussed, assume that APC # 80 (Left Heart Catheterization) has a relative weight of 37.00 when the national conversion rate is $60.00. The total amount paid for this APC would be $2,220 (37 × $60.00). We will further assume that Medicare has set the national coinsurance for APC#80 at $840.00. To adjust actual payment for a hospital with a wage index of 1.200, the following computations would be made to adjust both the total and the coinsurance payments:

Total Payment = [.60 × $2,220 × 1.200] + [.40 × $2,220] = $2,486.40

Coinsurance = [.60 × $840.00 × 1.200] + [.40 × $840] = $940.80

Medicare payment for a specific outpatient claim is illustrated in the following example taken from a hospital-submitted UB–92. The claim relates to a patient who had a left heart cardiac catheterization (See Table 3–8).

The example claim shows that total payment for this claim would be $2,289.75 with $845.00 coming from the patient as coinsurance. A large number of the items have a status code of "N" or incidental services that are packaged into the APC rate. Many of these procedures are either imaging procedures or injections that are considered to be a part of CPT 93510 (Left Heart Catheterization). This procedure has a "T" status indicator code, which indicates that it would be discounted at 50 percent if another "T"-coded procedure were performed. In our example, there is no other "T"-coded procedure present in the claim, so the procedure would not be discounted. When multiple "T"-coded procedures are performed, the highest-value procedure is paid at 100 percent, but all other "T"-coded procedures would be paid at 50 percent. The lab procedures are all coded as "A," which in this case means they are clini-

Table 3–8 Example of Medicare Payment for Outpatient Left Heart Cardiac Catheterization

APC Reimbursement
APC # 80

Revenue Code	Description	HCPCS	Units	Total Charges	Status Code	APC Total Payment	Copayment
300	Lab	80051	1	$27.42	A	$10.00	$0
301	Lab	82565	1	7.42	A	7.25	0
301	Lab	84520	1	6.46	A	10.00	0
305	Lab	85027	1	20.77	A	9.00	0
305	Lab	85730	1	14.21	A	8.50	0
460	Pulmonary	94760	1	16.46	N	0	0
481	Cath Lab	93510	1	1711.17	T	2,220.00	840.00
481	Cath Lab	93539	1	607.79	N	0	0
481	Cath Lab	93540	1	607.79	N	0	0
481	Cath Lab	93543	1	1288.48	N	0	0
481	Cath Lab	93545	1	607.79	N	0	0
481	Cath Lab	93555	1	718.29	N	0	0
481	Cath Lab	93556	1	718.29	N	0	0
636	Drugs	J7040	1	7.13	N	0	0
710	Recovery		6	373.13	N	0	0
730	EKG	93005	1	60.74	X	25.00	5.00
				$6,793.34		$2,289.75	$845.00

cally diagnostic laboratory services that are paid from a fee schedule with no coinsurance payments. There are other examples of "A"-coded procedures, which are described in Table 3–9. The EKG is coded as an "X" procedure, which implies that it is an ancillary service.

It is also important to note that Medicare provides additional payments to hospitals for outliers. Outlier payments are made on an APC basis and are equal to 50 percent of the cost of the APC that is above 175 percent of the actual APC payment. For example, if an APC had a total payment, including the coinsurance, of $1,000 and the estimated cost of the APC was $4,000, then Medicare would pay an additional $1,125 [.50 × ($4,000 − $1,750)]. Please recognize that the cost of the APC does include incidental services or "N"-status items, which makes it important to include these items and to charge for them, even if Medicare does not recognize them as APC or fee-schedule items.

Resource management under APC reimbursement is more difficult than it is under DRGs because payment is not fixed. In a DRG-payment environment, once the patient is classified, cost minimization is the optimal

financial strategy because payment will not increase if additional services are provided. In an APC payment situation, payments may increase when more services are provided. Management must determine from a financial perspective if the marginal revenue of additional services is greater than the marginal cost of providing those services.

MEDICARE PAYMENT: SKILLED NURSING FACILITIES (SNFS)

As you can tell from our discussion of Medicare payments for hospital-inpatient, hospital-outpatient, and physician services, Medicare payment involves a complex set of rules. Medicare has paid Skilled Nursing Facilities (SNFs) on a prospective basis since July 1, 1998. The rate that is paid is a per-diem rate that is calculated to include the costs of all services, including routine, ancillary, and capital. Per-diem payments for each admission are case-mix adjusted using a resident classification system known as Resource Utilization Groups III (or RUG III). As with most CMS payments, the actual payment amounts are adjusted for differences

Table 3–9 Status Codes

Indicator	Service	Status
A	Clinical laboratory, ambulance, physical & occupational therapy	Fee schedule
B	Non-recognized codes	Not paid
C	Inpatient procedure	Not paid
D	Discontinued codes	Not paid
E	Non-allowed item or service	Not paid
F	Acquisition of corneal tissue	Reasonable cost
G	Current drug / biological pass-through	Additional payment
H	Device pass-through	Additional payment
K	Non-pass-through drug / biological	APC rate
L	Vaccine	Reasonable cost
N	Incidental service	Packaged
P	Partial hospitalization	Paid per diem
S	Significant procedure	APC rate
T	Significant procedure, reduced when multiple	APC rate
V	Clinic or ED visit	APC rate
X	Ancillary service	APC rate
Y	Non-implant DME	Not paid under OPPS

in cost of living by the hospital wage index on the labor portion of the payment.

There are seven major categories of patients under RUG III with 54 distinct payment categories, as follows (See Table 3–10):

Patients are assigned to one of the payment categories by a "RUGs III Grouper" based upon six key determinants:

*   Number of minutes per week needed for rehabilitation services
*   Number of different rehabilitation disciplines needed
*   Specific treatments received
*   Resident's ability to perform activities of daily living (ADL)

Table 3–10 Number of Payment Categories for Major Resource Utilization Groups III

Major RUG III Group	Number of Payment Categories
Rehabilitation	23
Extensive Services	3
Special Care	3
Clinically Complex	6
Impaired Cognition	4
Behavioral Problems	4
Reduced Physical Function	11

*   ICD-9 diagnoses
*   Resident's cognitive performance

To properly classify residents, SNFs must complete resident assessments on the 5th, 14th, 30th, 60th, and 90th days after admission. These forms are extensive and require another layer of administrative support to properly record information and report it to CMS.

To see how the payment system would operate, let us assume that a rehabilitation patient has been categorized as "Ultra high with treatment minimum of 720 minutes per week." Payment per day for this patient would be computed as shown in Table 3–11.

The rates used in the example will be updated over time as most Medicare rates are adjusted to reflect inflation.

MEDICARE PAYMENT: HOME HEALTH AGENCIES (HHAS)

The Balanced Budget Act of 1997 called for the development and implementation of a prospective payment system (PPS) for Medicare home health services to be implemented starting October 1, 2000. Under prospective payment, Medicare will pay HHAs a predetermined base payment. The payment will be adjusted for the health condition and care needs of the beneficiary. The payment will also be adjusted for the geographic differences in wages for HHAs across

Table 3–11 Components of Payment Under RUG III Categorization of "Ultra High plus Extensive Services, High (RUX)"

Category	Dollar Amount
Nursing Care	$261.42
Occupational, Physical, and Speech Therapies	233.19
Capital and General and Administrative	70.22
Total Allowed per Diem	$564.83
x Labor %	.75922
Labor per Diem	$428.83
x Wage Index	.9907
Labor Adjusted per Diem	$424.84
Non-labor per Diem	136.00
Case-Mix Adjusted per Diem	$560.84

the country. The adjustment for the health condition, or clinical characteristics, and service needs of the beneficiary is referred to as the case-mix adjustment. The home health PPS will provide HHAs with payments for each 60-day episode of care for each beneficiary. If a beneficiary is still eligible for care after the end of the first episode, a second episode can begin; there are no limits to the number of episodes a beneficiary who remains eligible for the home health benefit can receive. While payment for each episode is adjusted to reflect the beneficiary's health condition and needs, a special outlier provision exists to ensure appropriate payment for those beneficiaries who need the most expensive care. Adjusting payment to reflect the HHA's cost in caring for each beneficiary, including the sickest, should ensure that all beneficiaries have access to home health services for which they are eligible.

The home health PPS is composed of six main features:

1) 60-Day episode

The unit of payment under HHA PPS will be for a 60-day episode of care. An agency will receive half of the estimated base payment for the full 60 days, as soon as the fiscal intermediary receives the initial claim. This estimate is based upon the patient's condition and care needs (case-mix assignment). The agency will receive the residual half of the payment at the close of the 60-day episode unless there is an applicable adjustment to that amount. The full payment is the sum of the initial and residual percentage pay-

ments, unless there is an applicable adjustment. This split-percentage-payment approach provides reasonable and balanced cash flow for HHAs. Another 60-day episode can be initiated for longer-stay patients.

2) Case-mix adjustment

After a physician prescribes a home health plan of care, the HHA assesses the patient's condition and likely needs for skilled nursing care, therapy, medical, social services, and home health aide service needs. The assessment must be done for each subsequent episode of care a patient receives. A nurse or therapist from the HHA uses the Outcome and Assessment Information Set (OASIS) instrument to assess the patient's condition. (All HHAs have been using OASIS since July 19, 1999.) OASIS items describing the patient's condition, as well as the expected therapy needs (physical, speech-language pathology, or occupational) are used to determine the case-mix adjustment to the standard payment rate. Eighty case-mix groups, or Home Health Resource Groups (HHRGs), are available for patient classification using three classification criteria.

Classification Categories	Severity Levels
Clinical Severity	4 Levels (0–3)
Functional Severity	5 Levels (0–4)
Service Utilization Severity	4 Levels (0–3)

The HHRG system in the proposed rule uses data from a large-scale case-mix research project conducted between 1997 and 1999.

3) Outlier payments

Additional payments will be made to the 60-day case-mix-adjusted episode payments for beneficiaries who incur unusually large costs. These outlier payments will be made for episodes whose imputed cost exceeds a threshold amount for each case-mix group. The amount of the outlier payment will be a proportion of the amount of imputed costs beyond the threshold. Outlier costs will be imputed for each episode by applying standard per-visit amounts to the number of visits by discipline (skilled nursing visits, or physical, speech-language pathology, occupational therapy, or home health aide services) reported on the claims. Total national outlier payments for home health services annually will be no more than five percent of estimated total payments under home health PPS.

4) Adjustments for beneficiaries who require only a few visits during the 60-day episode

The proposed home health PPS has a low-utilization payment adjustment for beneficiaries whose episodes consist of four or fewer visits. These episodes will be paid the standardized, service-specific per-visit amount multiplied by the number of visits actually provided during the episode. For 2006, the national payments unadjusted for wage index were as follows:

Discipline	Per-Visit Rate
Home Health Aide	$45.88
Medical Social Service	162.41
Occupational Therapy	111.53
Physical Therapy	110.78
Skilled Nursing	101.32
Speech Pathology	120.38

5) Adjustments for beneficiaries who experience a significant change in their condition

When a beneficiary experiences a significant change in condition during the 60-day episode not envisioned in the original physician's plan of care and original case-mix assignment, a Significant Change in Condition (SCIC) adjustment can occur. This requires that a new payment amount be determined. The SCIC payment adjustment occurs within a given 60-day episode.

6) Adjustments for beneficiaries who change HHAs

The home health PPS will include a partial episode payment adjustment. A new episode clock will be triggered when a beneficiary elects to transfer to another HHA or when a beneficiary is discharged and readmitted to the same HHA during the 60-day episode. The partial episode payment will provide a simplified approach to the episode definition that takes into account key intervening health events in a patient's care. The partial episode payment allows the 60-day episode clock to end and a new clock to begin if a beneficiary transfers to another HHA or is discharged, but returns

to the same HHA because of a decline in his condition within the 60-day episode. When a new 60-day episode begins, a new plan of care and a new assessment are necessary. The original 60-day episode payment is proportionally adjusted to reflect the length of time the beneficiary remained under the agency's care before the intervening event. An initial episode payment of one half of the new case mix group is paid at the start of the new episode, and the 60-day clock is restarted.

To illustrate the actual payment determination for an episode of care under the HHA PPS program, assume that a patient has been classified as 0 severity for clinical, 1 severity for functional, and 2 severity for services utilization (C0F1S2). Payment for this patient under the PPS program would be calculated as follows:

National Standardized Payment Rate	$2,320.89
Case Weight	× 1.5769
Case-Mix Adjusted Payment	$3,659.81

This amount would then be adjusted for the actual wage index of the provider. Under the HHA PPS program, 77.7 percent of the payment is assumed to be labor-related, while the remaining 22.3 percent is assumed to be non-labor-related. Actual payment for a provider with a wage index of 1.2000 would be $4,228.54:

$$[\$3,659.81 \times .777 \times 1.2000] + [\$3,659.81 \times .223] = \$4,228.54$$

SUMMARY

Compared with most businesses, health care organizations are financially complex. Not only do they provide a large number of specific services, but also their individual services often have different effective price structures. Services may be bundled in different ways to determine prices, according to the agreements in place with each specific payer. One customer may choose to pay on the basis of cost while another may pay full charges. Prices may be determined prospectively or may be capitated for broad scopes of care. This variation in payment patterns creates problems in the establishment of prices for products and services. Indeed, the revenue function of a typical health care entity is usually much more complex than that of a comparably sized non-health care business. Further, organizations within different segments of the health care industry are affected by changes in payment arrangements in different ways.

Health care entities also depend quite heavily on a very limited number of key clients for most of their operating funding. Their largest client is often the federal government or the state government. Doing business with the government involves a significant amount of reporting to ensure compliance and adherence to governmental regulations. Moreover, since the federal government is such a large purchaser of services, a thorough understanding of the nature and implications of the Medicare payment system's rules and regulations is a must for effective management of a health care organization. Important differences exist in setting rates and bundling services between hospital inpatient and outpatient care, physician services, skilled nursing facilities, and home health care. Each system has differing implications for the management of resources by the HCO.

The revenue function of a typical health care entity is usually much more complex than that of a comparably sized non-health care business. Organizations can have vastly different revenue structures, depending on the segments of the health care industry in which they are active. Government commands enormous influence as a purchaser of health care services and maintains complex payment systems. Because payment arrangements are determined primarily by the payer, an effective health care administrator must have a firm understanding of the various systems that exist, both public and private. Although health care organizations may be complex from a financial perspective, they are still businesses. Their financial viability requires the receipt of funds in amounts sufficient to meet their financial requirements.

ASSIGNMENTS

1. From the following data, determine the amount of revenue that needs to be generated to meet hospital financial requirements.

Volume

Medicare cases	1,000
Cost-paying cases	400
Charity care and bad-debt cases	100
Charge-paying cases	500
Total cases	2,000

Financial data

Budgeted expenses	$6,000,000
Debt principal payment	200,000
Working capital increase	250,000
Capital expenditures	400,000

Present payment structure

☐ Medicare pays only $2,800 per case, or a total of $2,800,000.

☐ All other cost payers pay their share of existing expenses.

2. Why is the accumulation of funded reserves for capital replacement more critical for non-profit health care entities than for investor-owned health care facilities?

3. Teaching hospitals receive an additional payment to recognize the indirect costs of medical education. What rationale might be used to justify this extra payment?

4. Depreciation expense is recognized as a reimbursable cost by a number of payers who pay prospective rates for operating costs. Would you prefer accelerated depreciation (sum of the year's digits) or price-level depreciation for a five-year life asset with a $150,000 cost? Assume that inflation is projected to be six percent per year.

5. Evaluate the statement that non-profit organizations should not make a profit. Is this true?

6. Using the data from Assignment 1 above, calculate the impact of a ten percent reduction in operating expenses, that is, down to $5,400,000, on the required revenue and rate structure. Discuss the implications of your findings.

7. Calculate the RBRVS rate for CPT 33426, repair of mitral valve for a physician in Chicago, Illinois. Assume the conversion factor is 40.7986. The following table provides relevant values to complete this calculation:

Repair of Mitral Valve
(33426)

RVU	Chicago Index	Product	
Work	26.07	1.028	26.80
Practice expense	31.96	1.080	34.52
Malpractice	5.80	1.382	8.02
			69.34

8. Medicare currently reimburses hospitals for 70 percent of bad debts written-off on Medicare patients, copayments, and deductibles. If a hospital had $1,000,000 in Medicare deductibles and copayments, what amount might Medicare pay for its bad debts?

9. Discussions with a group of physicians regarding employment status of your hospital are taking place. If the physicians were employed by your hospital, they would be performing all surgical procedures at your hospital instead of their current offices. This could mean a sizable change in total revenue, especially from Medicare patients. To see the effect of this change, assume the example in Table 3-7 for CPT # 42810, excision of a neck cyst. If Medicare would pay the hospital $1,600 for the facility fee and the physicians would receive $309.10, calculate the amount the physicians would lose if the procedure were paid in a non-facility setting. Assume the non-facility practice expense weight is 5.73.

10. Your hospital is reviewing its DRG coding patterns for Medicare. It has focused on two DRGS: 296 (Nutritional and Misc Metabolic Disorders w/ cc) and 297 (Nutritional and Metabolic Disorders w/o cc). There were 100 patients assigned to these two DRGs: 50 to 296 and 50 to 297. National averages suggest that 85 should have been assigned to DRG 296 and 15 to DRG 297. Assuming an average payment of $6,000 per DRG with a case weight of 1.0, how much lost payment from Medicare may be resulting from poor coding and documentation? Use case weight values from the Appendix in this chapter.

SOLUTIONS AND ANSWERS

1. The relevant calculation is as follows:

   Revenue =

   $$\frac{\text{Budgeted expense} + \text{Desired net income} - \text{Noncharge-paying payments}}{\text{Proportion of charge-paying patients}}$$

   Revenue =

   $$\frac{\$6,000,000 + \$850,000 - \$4,000,000}{.25} = \$11,4000,000 \text{ or } \$5,700 \text{ per case}$$

   Desired net income = $850,000 = $200,000 + $250,000 + $400,000

   Non-charge-paying patient payments = Medicare payments + Cost-paying patient payments

   $$\$2,800,000 + \left(\frac{400}{2,000} \times \$6,000.00\right) = \$4,000,000$$

   $$\text{Proportion of charge-paying patients} = \frac{500}{2,000} = .25$$

2. A non-profit entity does not have the same opportunities for capital formation that an investor-owned organization does. Specifically, the non-profit entity cannot sell new shares or ownership interests. Its sources of capital are limited to its accumulated funded reserves and to new debt. In some special situations, non-profit organizations may receive contributions, but these amounts are usually not significant.

3. Part of the rationale used is related to severity of patients. It is widely believed that teaching hospitals treat more severely ill patients. The currently used DRG classification system does not incorporate severity adjustments. The proposed changes to the DRG classification system by Medicare in Fiscal Year 2008 incorporate severity in the DRG assignments and could result in lower payments for indirect medical education.

4. The relevant comparative data would be as follows:

	Price Level Depreciation*	Sum-of-the-Years Digits Depreciation**
Year 1	$ 31,800	$ 50,000
Year 2	33,708	40,000
Year 3	35,730	30,000
Year 4	37,874	20,000
Year 5	40,147	10,000
	$179,259	$150,000

*Depreciation in year t = 150,000/5 $(1.06)^t$. This term reflects compounding of straight-line depreciation at 6 percent per year.

**Depreciation in year t of an N-year life asset is equal to the historical cost times $2(N + 1 - t)/N(N + 1)$.

In year 1, the depreciation would be: $150,000 × 10 ÷ 30, or $50,000.

In most cases, price-level-adjusted depreciation would be better. However, for short-lived assets, accelerated depreciation may provide greater levels of reimbursement in earlier years to offset lower returns in later years. The lower the rate of asset inflation, the more desirable accelerated depreciation becomes.

5. Profit is essential to most business organizations because accounting expenses do not equal cash requirements. Additional funds or profits must be available to meet the financial requirements of debt principal payments, increases in working capital, and capital expenditures.

6. The relevant calculation would be as follows:

$$\text{Revenue} = \frac{\$5,400,000 + \$850,000 - \$3,880,000}{.25} = \$9,480,000, \text{ or } \$4,740 \text{ per case}$$

A ten percent reduction in operating expenses permitted a 17 percent reduction in rates ($5,700 to $4,740 per case). Cost control is critical in health care entities, especially in those with relatively low levels of cost payers. A reduction in rates is especially important when competing for major contracts in which price is a predominant determinant.

7. The RBRVS rate for this procedure would be:

$$\$2,829 = \$40.7986 \times 69.34$$

8. While the total Medicare deductible and copayment amount is $1,000,000, a small percentage will most likely remain unpaid. Many Medicare beneficiaries have supplemental insurance that pays for deductibles and copayments. In addition, many Medicare patients do pay for their deductibles and copayments. In 2004, the average reported Medicare bad debt was approximately 15 percent of deductibles and copayments. In our example, this would mean $150,000 of reported bad debts. Medicare would then pay 70 percent ($105,000).

9. The current practice expense weight in a facility setting is 3.55 per Table 3–7. The weight in a non-facility setting is 5.73 per discussion in the text. The lost payment that the doctors would experience would be:

$$(5.73 - 3.55) \times 1.144 \times \$40 = \$99.76$$

The net difference in payment would be $1,500.24 ($1,600.00 − $99.76). The dilemma is the distribution of payments. The hospital would gain $1,600, but the physicians would lose $99.76.

10. If the hospital had the same coding percentages as the national average, it would have had 35 more cases coded as 296 and 35 fewer cases coded as 297. Using the case weights in Appendix 3 and the $6,000 payment per case weight of 1.0, the additional payment would be:

$$35 \text{ cases} \times (0.8187 - 0.4879) \times \$6,000 = \$69,468$$

Appendix 3

List of Diagnosis-Related Groups (DRGs) and Relative Weights for Fiscal Year 2006

Drg	Mdc	Type	Drg Title	Weights	Mean LOS	Arithmetic Mean LOS
001	01	Surg	Craniotomy Age >17 W CC	3.4347	7.6	10.1
002	01	Surg	Craniotomy Age >17 W/O CC	1.9587	3.5	4.6
003	01	Surg *	Craniotomy Age 0–17	1.9860	12.7	12.7
004	01	Surg	No Longer Valid	0.0000	0.0	0.0
005	01	Surg	No Longer Valid	0.0000	0.0	0.0
006	01	Surg	Carpal Tunnel Release	0.7878	2.2	3.0
007	01	Surg	Periph & Cranial Nerve & Other Nerv Syst Proc W CC	2.6978	6.7	9.7
008	01	Surg	Periph & Cranial Nerve & Other Nerv Syst Proc W/O CC	1.5635	2.0	3.0
009	01	Med	Spinal Disorders & Injuries	1.4045	4.5	6.4
010	01	Med	Nervous System Neoplasms W CC	1.2222	4.6	6.2
011	01	Med	Nervous System Neoplasms W/O CC	0.8736	2.9	3.8
012	01	Med	Degenerative Nervous System Disorders	0.8998	4.3	5.5
013	01	Med	Multiple Sclerosis & Cerebellar Ataxia	0.8575	4.0	5.0
014	01	Med	Intracranial Hemorrhage Or Cerebral Infarction	1.2456	4.5	5.8
015	01	Med	Nonspecific Cva & Precerebral Occlusion W/O Infarct	0.9421	3.7	4.6
016	01	Med	Nonspecific Cerebrovascular Disorders W CC	1.3351	5.0	6.5
017	01	Med	Nonspecific Cerebrovascular Disorders W/O CC	0.7229	2.5	3.2
018	01	Med	Cranial & Peripheral Nerve Disorders W CC	0.9903	4.1	5.3
019	01	Med	Cranial & Peripheral Nerve Disorders W/O CC	0.7077	2.7	3.5
020	01	Med	Nervous System Infection Except Viral Meningitis	2.7865	8.0	10.4
021	01	Med	Viral Meningitis	1.4451	4.9	6.3
022	01	Med	Hypertensive Encephalopathy	1.1304	4.0	5.2
023	01	Med	Nontraumatic Stupor & Coma	0.7712	3.0	3.9
024	01	Med	Seizure & Headache Age >17 W CC	0.9970	3.6	4.8
025	01	Med	Seizure & Headache Age >17 W/O CC	0.6180	2.5	3.1
026	01	Med	Seizure & Headache Age 0–17	1.8191	3.4	6.3
027	01	Med	Traumatic Stupor & Coma, Coma >1 Hr	1.3531	3.2	5.2
028	01	Med	Traumatic Stupor & Coma, Coma <1 Hr Age >17 W CC	1.3353	4.4	5.9

Source: Reprinted from Centers for Medicare & Medicaid Services.

Drg	Mdc	Type	Drg Title	Weights	Mean LOS	Arithmetic Mean LOS
029	01	Med	Traumatic Stupor & Coma, Coma <1 Hr Age >17 W/O CC	0.7212	2.6	3.4
030	01	Med *	Traumatic Stupor & Coma, Coma <1 Hr Age 0–17	0.3359	2.0	2.0
031	01	Med	Concussion Age >17 W CC	0.9567	3.0	4.0
032	01	Med	Concussion Age >17 W/O CC	0.6194	1.9	2.4
033	01	Med *	Concussion Age 0–17	0.2109	1.6	1.6
034	01	Med	Other Disorders Of Nervous System W CC	1.0062	3.7	4.8
035	01	Med	Other Disorders Of Nervous System W/O CC	0.6241	2.4	3.0
036	02	Surg	Retinal Procedures	0.7288	1.3	1.6
037	02	Surg	Orbital Procedures	1.1858	2.7	4.2
038	02	Surg	Primary Iris Procedures	0.6975	2.5	3.5
039	02	Surg	Lens Procedures With Or Without Vitrectomy	0.7108	1.7	2.4
040	02	Surg	Extraocular Procedures Except Orbit Age >17	0.9627	3.0	4.1
041	02	Surg *	Extraocular Procedures Except Orbit Age 0–17	0.3419	1.6	1.6
042	02	Surg	Intraocular Procedures Except Retina, Iris & Lens	0.7852	2.0	2.8
043	02	Med	Hyphema	0.6141	2.4	3.1
044	02	Med	Acute Major Eye Infections	0.6874	3.9	4.8
045	02	Med	Neurological Eye Disorders	0.7474	2.5	3.1
046	02	Med	Other Disorders Of The Eye Age >17 W CC	0.7524	3.2	4.2
047	02	Med	Other Disorders Of The Eye Age >17 W/O CC	0.5203	2.3	2.9
048	02	Med *	Other Disorders Of The Eye Age 0–17	0.3012	2.9	2.9
049	03	Surg	Major Head & Neck Procedures	1.6361	3.1	4.4
050	03	Surg	Sialoadenectomy	0.8690	1.5	1.8
051	03	Surg	Salivary Gland Procedures Except Sialoadenectomy	0.8809	1.9	2.8
052	03	Surg	Cleft Lip & Palate Repair	0.8348	1.5	1.9
053	03	Surg	Sinus & Mastoid Procedures Age >17	1.3269	2.4	3.9
054	03	Surg *	Sinus & Mastoid Procedures Age 0–17	0.4882	3.2	3.2
055	03	Surg	Miscellaneous Ear, Nose, Mouth & Throat Procedures	0.9597	2.0	3.1
056	03	Surg	Rhinoplasty	0.8711	1.8	2.6
057	03	Surg	T&A Proc, Except Tonsillectomy &/Or Adenoidectomy Only, Age >17	1.0428	2.3	3.6
058	03	Surg *	T&A Proc, Except Tonsillectomy &/Or Adenoidectomy Only, Age 0–17	0.2772	1.5	1.5
059	03	Surg	Tonsillectomy &/Or Adenoidectomy Only, Age >17	0.8082	1.8	2.6
060	03	Surg *	Tonsillectomy &/Or Adenoidectomy Only, Age 0–17	0.2110	1.5	1.5
061	03	Surg	Myringotomy W Tube Insertion Age >17	1.2867	3.3	5.4
062	03	Surg *	Myringotomy W Tube Insertion Age 0–17	0.2989	1.3	1.3
063	03	Surg	Other Ear, Nose, Mouth, & Throat O.R. Procedures	1.3983	3.0	4.5
064	03	Med	Ear, Nose, Mouth, & Throat Malignancy	1.1663	4.1	6.1
065	03	Med	Dysequilibrium	0.5991	2.3	2.8
066	03	Med	Epistaxis	0.5958	2.4	3.1
067	03	Med	Epiglottitis	0.7725	2.9	3.7
068	03	Med	Otitis Media & Uri Age >17 W CC	0.6611	3.2	4.0
069	03	Med	Otitis Media & Uri Age >17 W/O CC	0.4850	2.5	3.0
070	03	Med	Otitis Media & Uri Age 0–17	0.4210	2.1	2.3
071	03	Med	Laryngotracheitis	0.7524	3.2	4.0
072	03	Med	Nasal Trauma & Deformity	0.7449	2.6	3.4
073	03	Med	Other Ear, Nose, Mouth, & Throat Diagnoses Age >17	0.8527	3.3	4.4

Drg	Mdc	Type	Drg Title	Weights	Mean LOS	Arithmetic Mean LOS
074	03	Med *	Other Ear, Nose, Mouth, & Throat Diagnoses Age 0–17	0.3398	2.1	2.1
075	04	Surg	Major Chest Procedures	3.0732	7.6	9.9
076	04	Surg	Other Resp System O.R. Procedures W CC	2.8830	8.4	11.1
077	04	Surg	Other Resp System O.R. Procedures W/O CC	1.1857	3.3	4.7
078	04	Med	Pulmonary Embolism	1.2427	5.4	6.4
079	04	Med	Respiratory Infections & Inflammations Age >17 W CC	1.6238	6.7	8.5
080	04	Med	Respiratory Infections & Inflammations Age >17 W/O CC	0.8947	4.4	5.5
081	04	Med *	Respiratory Infections & Inflammations Age 0–17	1.5383	6.1	6.1
082	04	Med	Respiratory Neoplasms	1.3936	5.1	6.8
083	04	Med	Major Chest Trauma W CC	0.9828	4.2	5.3
084	04	Med	Major Chest Trauma W/O CC	0.5799	2.6	3.2
085	04	Med	Pleural Effusion W CC	1.2405	4.8	6.3
086	04	Med	Pleural Effusion W/O CC	0.6974	2.8	3.6
087	04	Med	Pulmonary Edema & Respiratory Failure	1.3654	4.9	6.4
088	04	Med	Chronic Obstructive Pulmonary Disease	0.8778	4.0	4.9
089	04	Med	Simple Pneumonia & Pleurisy Age >17 W CC	1.0320	4.7	5.7
090	04	Med	Simple Pneumonia & Pleurisy Age >17 W/O CC	0.6104	3.2	3.8
091	04	Med	Simple Pneumonia & Pleurisy Age 0–17	0.8124	3.4	4.4
092	04	Med	Interstitial Lung Disease W CC	1.1853	4.8	6.1
093	04	Med	Interstitial Lung Disease W/O CC	0.7150	3.1	3.9
094	04	Med	Pneumothorax W CC	1.1354	4.6	6.2
095	04	Med	Pneumothorax W/O CC	0.6035	2.9	3.6
096	04	Med	Bronchitis & Asthma Age >17 W CC	0.7303	3.6	4.4
097	04	Med	Bronchitis & Asthma Age >17 W/O CC	0.5364	2.8	3.4
098	04	Med *	Bronchitis & Asthma Age 0–17	0.5560	3.7	3.7
099	04	Med	Respiratory Signs & Symptoms W CC	0.7094	2.4	3.1
100	04	Med	Respiratory Signs & Symptoms W/O CC	0.5382	1.7	2.1
101	04	Med	Other Respiratory System Diagnoses W CC	0.8733	3.3	4.3
102	04	Med	Other Respiratory System Diagnoses W/O CC	0.5402	2.0	2.5
103	Pre	Surg	Heart Transplant Or Implant Of Heart Assist System	18.5617	23.7	37.7
104	05	Surg	Cardiac Valve & Oth Major Cardiothoracic Proc W Card Cath	8.2201	12.7	14.9
105	05	Surg	Cardiac Valve & Oth Major Cardiothoracic Proc W/O Card Cath	6.0192	8.4	10.2
106	05	Surg	Coronary Bypass W Ptca	7.0346	9.5	11.2
107	05	Surg	No Longer Valid	0.0000	13.5	13.5
108	05	Surg	Other Cardiothoracic Procedures	5.8789	8.6	11.0
109	05	Surg	No Longer Valid	0.0000	12.1	12.1
110	05	Surg	Major Cardiovascular Procedures W CC	3.8417	5.7	8.4
111	05	Surg	Major Cardiovascular Procedures W/O CC	2.4840	2.6	3.4
112	05	Surg	No Longer Valid	0.0000	0.0	0.0
113	05	Surg	Amputation For Circ System Disorders Except Upper Limb & Toe	3.1682	10.8	13.7
114	05	Surg	Upper Limb & Toe Amputation For Circ System Disorders	1.7354	6.7	8.9
115	05	Surg	No Longer Valid	0.0000	15.8	15.8

Drg	Mdc	Type	Drg Title	Weights	Mean LOS	Arithmetic Mean LOS
116	05	Surg	No Longer Valid	0.0000	9.3	9.3
117	05	Surg	Cardiac Pacemaker Revision Except Device Replacement	1.3223	2.6	4.2
118	05	Surg	Cardiac Pacemaker Device Replacement	1.6380	2.1	3.0
119	05	Surg	Vein Ligation & Stripping	1.3456	3.3	5.5
120	05	Surg	Other Circulatory System O.R. Procedures	2.3853	5.9	9.2
121	05	Med	Circulatory Disorders W Ami & Major Comp, Discharged Alive	1.6136	5.3	6.6
122	05	Med	Circulatory Disorders W Ami W/O Major Comp, Discharged Alive	0.9847	2.8	3.5
123	05	Med	Circulatory Disorders W Ami, Expired	1.5407	2.9	4.8
124	05	Med	Circulatory Disorders Except Ami, W Card Cath & Complex Diag	1.4425	3.3	4.4
125	05	Med	Circulatory Disorders Except Ami, W Card Cath W/O Complex Diag	1.0948	2.1	2.7
126	05	Med	Acute & Subacute Endocarditis	2.7440	9.4	12.0
127	05	Med	Heart Failure & Shock	1.0345	4.1	5.2
128	05	Med	Deep Vein Thrombophlebitis	0.6949	4.4	5.2
129	05	Med	Cardiac Arrest, Unexplained	1.0404	1.7	2.6
130	05	Med	Peripheral Vascular Disorders W CC	0.9425	4.4	5.5
131	05	Med	Peripheral Vascular Disorders W/O CC	0.5566	3.2	3.9
132	05	Med	Atherosclerosis W CC	0.6273	2.2	2.8
133	05	Med	Atherosclerosis W/O CC	0.5337	1.8	2.2
134	05	Med	Hypertension	0.6068	2.4	3.1
135	05	Med	Cardiac Congenital & Valvular Disorders Age >17 W CC	0.8917	3.2	4.3
136	05	Med	Cardiac Congenital & Valvular Disorders Age >17 W/O CC	0.6214	2.2	2.8
137	05	Med *	Cardiac Congenital & Valvular Disorders Age 0–17	0.8288	3.3	3.3
138	05	Med	Cardiac Arrhythmia & Conduction Disorders W CC	0.8287	3.0	3.9
139	05	Med	Cardiac Arrhythmia & Conduction Disorders W/O CC	0.5227	2.0	2.4
140	05	Med	Angina Pectoris	0.5116	2.0	2.4
141	05	Med	Syncope & Collapse W CC	0.7521	2.7	3.5
142	05	Med	Syncope & Collapse W/O CC	0.5852	2.0	2.5
143	05	Med	Chest Pain	0.5659	1.7	2.1
144	05	Med	Other Circulatory System Diagnoses W CC	1.2761	4.1	5.8
145	05	Med	Other Circulatory System Diagnoses W/O CC	0.5835	2.1	2.6
146	06	Surg	Rectal Resection W CC	2.6621	8.6	10.0
147	06	Surg	Rectal Resection W/O CC	1.4781	5.2	5.8
148	06	Surg	Major Small & Large Bowel Procedures W CC	3.4479	10.0	12.3
149	06	Surg	Major Small & Large Bowel Procedures W/O CC	1.4324	5.4	6.0
150	06	Surg	Peritoneal Adhesiolysis W CC	2.8061	8.9	11.0
151	06	Surg	Peritoneal Adhesiolysis W/O CC	1.2641	4.0	5.1
152	06	Surg	Minor Small & Large Bowel Procedures W CC	1.8783	6.7	8.0
153	06	Surg	Minor Small & Large Bowel Procedures W/O CC	1.0821	4.5	5.0
154	06	Surg	Stomach, Esophageal & Duodenal Procedures Age >17 W CC	4.0399	9.9	13.3
155	06	Surg	Stomach, Esophageal & Duodenal Procedures Age >17 W/O CC	1.2889	3.1	4.1

Drg	Mdc	Type	Drg Title	Weights	Mean LOS	Arithmetic Mean LOS
156	06	Surg *	Stomach, Esophageal, & Duodenal Procedures Age 0–17	0.8535	6.0	6.0
157	06	Surg	Anal & Stomal Procedures W CC	1.3356	4.1	5.8
158	06	Surg	Anal & Stomal Procedures W/O CC	0.6657	2.1	2.6
159	06	Surg	Hernia Procedures Except Inguinal & Femoral Age >17 W CC	1.4081	3.8	5.1
160	06	Surg	Hernia Procedures Except Inguinal & Femoral Age >17 W/O CC	0.8431	2.2	2.7
161	06	Surg	Inguinal & Femoral Hernia Procedures Age >17 W CC	1.1931	3.1	4.4
162	06	Surg	Inguinal & Femoral Hernia Procedures Age >17 W/O CC	0.6785	1.7	2.1
163	06	Surg	Hernia Procedures Age 0–17	0.6723	2.2	2.9
164	06	Surg	Appendectomy W Complicated Principal Diag W CC	2.2476	6.6	8.0
165	06	Surg	Appendectomy W Complicated Principal Diag W/O CC	1.1868	3.6	4.2
166	06	Surg	Appendectomy W/O Complicated Principal Diag W CC	1.4521	3.3	4.5
167	06	Surg	Appendectomy W/O Complicated Principal Diag W/O CC	0.8929	1.9	2.2
168	03	Surg	Mouth Procedures W CC	1.2662	3.3	4.9
169	03	Surg	Mouth Procedures W/O CC	0.7297	1.8	2.3
170	06	Surg	Other Digestive System O.R. Procedures W CC	2.9612	7.8	11.0
171	06	Surg	Other Digestive System O.R. Procedures W/O CC	1.1905	3.1	4.1
172	06	Med	Digestive Malignancy W CC	1.4125	5.1	7.0
173	06	Med	Digestive Malignancy W/O CC	0.7443	2.7	3.6
174	06	Med	G.I. Hemorrhage W CC	1.0060	3.8	4.7
175	06	Med	G.I. Hemorrhage W/O CC	0.5646	2.4	2.9
176	06	Med	Complicated Peptic Ulcer	1.1246	4.1	5.2
177	06	Med	Uncomplicated Peptic Ulcer W CC	0.9166	3.6	4.4
178	06	Med	Uncomplicated Peptic Ulcer W/O CC	0.7013	2.6	3.1
179	06	Med	Inflammatory Bowel Disease	1.0911	4.5	5.9
180	06	Med	G.I. Obstruction W CC	0.9784	4.2	5.4
181	06	Med	G.I. Obstruction W/O CC	0.5614	2.8	3.3
182	06	Med	Esophagitis, Gastroent, & Misc Digest Disorders Age >17 W CC	0.8413	3.4	4.4
183	06	Med	Esophagitis, Gastroent, & Misc Digest Disorders Age >17 W/O CC	0.5848	2.3	2.9
184	06	Med	Esophagitis, Gastroent, & Misc Digest Disorders Age 0–17	0.5663	2.5	3.3
185	03	Med	Dental & Oral Dis Except Extractions & Restorations, Age >17	0.8702	3.2	4.5
186	03	Med *	Dental & Oral Dis Except Extractions & Restorations, Age 0–17	0.3253	2.9	2.9
187	03	Med	Dental Extractions & Restorations	0.8363	3.1	4.2
188	06	Med	Other Digestive System Diagnoses Age >17 W CC	1.1290	4.2	5.6
189	06	Med	Other Digestive System Diagnoses Age >17 W/O CC	0.6064	2.4	3.1
190	06	Med	Other Digestive System Diagnoses Age 0–17	0.6179	3.1	4.4

Drg	Mdc	Type	Drg Title	Weights	Mean LOS	Arithmetic Mean LOS
191	07	Surg	Pancreas, Liver, & Shunt Procedures W CC	3.9680	9.0	12.9
192	07	Surg	Pancreas, Liver, & Shunt Procedures W/O CC	1.6793	4.3	5.7
193	07	Surg	Biliary Tract Proc Except Only Cholecyst W Or W/O C.D.E. W CC	3.2818	9.9	12.1
194	07	Surg	Biliary Tract Proc Except Only Cholecyst W Or W/O C.D.E. W/O CC	1.5748	5.6	6.7
195	07	Surg	Cholecystectomy W C.D.E. W CC	3.0530	8.8	10.6
196	07	Surg	Cholecystectomy W C.D.E. W/O CC	1.6031	4.9	5.7
197	07	Surg	Cholecystectomy Except By Laparoscope W/O C.D.E. W CC	2.5425	7.5	9.2
198	07	Surg	Cholecystectomy Except By Laparoscope W/O C.D.E. W/O CC	1.1604	3.7	4.3
199	07	Surg	Hepatobiliary Diagnostic Procedure For Malignancy	2.4073	6.8	9.5
200	07	Surg	Hepatobiliary Diagnostic Procedure For Non-Malignancy	2.7868	6.5	9.8
201	07	Surg	Other Hepatobiliary Or Pancreas O.R. Procedures	3.7339	9.9	13.7
202	07	Med	Cirrhosis & Alcoholic Hepatitis	1.3318	4.7	6.2
203	07	Med	Malignancy Of Hepatobiliary System Or Pancreas	1.3552	4.9	6.5
204	07	Med	Disorders Of Pancreas Except Malignancy	1.1249	4.2	5.6
205	07	Med	Disorders Of Liver Except Malig, Cirr, Alc Hepa W CC	1.2059	4.4	6.0
206	07	Med	Disorders Of Liver Except Malig, Cirr, Alc Hepa W/O CC	0.7292	3.0	3.9
207	07	Med	Disorders Of The Biliary Tract W CC	1.1746	4.1	5.3
208	07	Med	Disorders Of The Biliary Tract W/O CC	0.6895	2.3	2.9
209	08	Surg	No Longer Valid	0.0000	17.1	17.1
210	08	Surg	Hip & Femur Procedures Except Major Joint Age >17 W CC	1.9059	6.1	6.9
211	08	Surg	Hip & Femur Procedures Except Major Joint Age >17 W/O CC	1.2690	4.4	4.7
212	08	Surg	Hip & Femur Procedures Except Major Joint Age 0–17	1.2877	2.4	2.9
213	08	Surg	Amputation For Musculoskeletal System & Conn Tissue Disorders	2.0428	7.2	9.7
214	08	Surg	No Longer Valid	0.0000	0.0	0.0
215	08	Surg	No Longer Valid	0.0000	0.0	0.0
216	08	Surg	Biopsies Of Musculoskeletal System & Connective Tissue	1.9131	3.3	5.8
217	08	Surg	Wnd Debrid & Skn Grft Except Hand, For Muscskelet & Conn Tiss Dis	3.0596	9.3	13.2
218	08	Surg	Lower Extrem & Humer Proc Except Hip, Foot, Femur Age >17 W CC	1.6648	4.4	5.6
219	08	Surg	Lower Extrem & Humer Proc Except Hip, Foot, Femur Age >17 W/O CC	1.0443	2.6	3.1
220	08	Surg *	Lower Extrem & Humer Proc Except Hip, Foot, Femur Age 0–17	0.5913	5.3	5.3
221	08	Surg	No Longer Valid	0.0000	0.0	0.0
222	08	Surg	No Longer Valid	0.0000	0.0	0.0
223	08	Surg	Major Shoulder/Elbow Proc, Or Other Upper Extremity Proc W CC	1.1164	2.3	3.2

Drg	Mdc	Type	Drg Title	Weights	Mean LOS	Arithmetic Mean LOS
224	08	Surg	Shoulder, Elbow, Or Forearm Proc, Exc Major Joint Proc, W/O CC	0.8185	1.6	1.9
225	08	Surg	Foot Procedures	1.2251	3.7	5.2
226	08	Surg	Soft Tissue Procedures W CC	1.5884	4.5	6.5
227	08	Surg	Soft Tissue Procedures W/O CC	0.8311	2.1	2.6
228	08	Surg	Major Thumb Or Joint Proc, Or Oth Hand Or Wrist Proc W CC	1.1459	2.8	4.1
229	08	Surg	Hand Or Wrist Proc, Except Major Joint Proc, W/O CC	0.6976	1.9	2.5
230	08	Surg	Local Excision & Removal Of Int Fix Devices Of Hip & Femur	1.3174	3.7	5.6
231	08	Surg	No Longer Valid	0.0000	0.0	0.0
232	08	Surg	Arthroscopy	0.9702	1.8	2.8
233	08	Surg	Other Musculoskelet Sys & Conn Tiss O.R. Proc W CC	1.9184	4.6	6.8
234	08	Surg	Other Musculoskelet Sys & Conn Tiss O.R. Proc W/O CC	1.2219	2.0	2.8
235	08	Med	Fractures Of Femur	0.7768	3.8	4.8
236	08	Med	Fractures Of Hip & Pelvis	0.7407	3.8	4.6
237	08	Med	Sprains, Strains, & Dislocations Of Hip, Pelvis, & Thigh	0.6090	3.0	3.7
238	08	Med	Osteomyelitis	1.4401	6.7	8.7
239	08	Med	Pathological Fractures & Musculoskeletal & Conn Tiss Malignancy	1.0767	5.0	6.2
240	08	Med	Connective Tissue Disorders W CC	1.4051	5.0	6.7
241	08	Med	Connective Tissue Disorders W/O CC	0.6629	3.0	3.7
242	08	Med	Septic Arthritis	1.1504	5.1	6.7
243	08	Med	Medical Back Problems	0.7658	3.6	4.5
244	08	Med	Bone Diseases & Specific Arthropathies W CC	0.7200	3.6	4.5
245	08	Med	Bone Diseases & Specific Arthropathies W/O CC	0.4583	2.5	3.1
246	08	Med	Non-Specific Arthropathies	0.5932	2.8	3.6
247	08	Med	Signs & Symptoms Of Musculoskeletal System & Conn Tissue	0.5795	2.6	3.3
248	08	Med	Tendonitis, Myositis, & Bursitis	0.8554	3.8	4.8
249	08	Med	Aftercare, Musculoskeletal System, & Connective Tissue	0.7095	2.7	3.9
250	08	Med	Fx, Sprn, Strn, & Disl Of Forearm, Hand, Foot Age >17 W CC	0.6974	3.2	3.9
251	08	Med	Fx, Sprn, Strn, & Disl Of Forearm, Hand, Foot Age >17 W/O CC	0.4749	2.3	2.8
252	08	Med *	Fx, Sprn, Strn, & Disl Of Forearm, Hand, Foot Age 0–17	0.2567	1.8	1.8
253	08	Med	Fx, Sprn, Strn, & Disl Of Uparm, Lowleg Ex Foot Age >17 W CC	0.7747	3.8	4.6
254	08	Med	Fx, Sprn, Strn, & Disl Of Uparm, Lowleg Ex Foot Age >17 W/O CC	0.4588	2.6	3.1
255	08	Med *	Fx, Sprn, Strn, & Disl Of Uparm, Lowleg Ex Foot Age 0–17	0.2990	2.9	2.9
256	08	Med	Other Musculoskeletal System & Connective Tissue Diagnoses	0.8509	3.9	5.1

Drg	Mdc	Type	Drg Title	Weights	Mean LOS	Arithmetic Mean LOS
257	09	Surg	Total Mastectomy For Malignancy W CC	0.8967	2.0	2.6
258	09	Surg	Total Mastectomy For Malignancy W/O CC	0.7138	1.5	1.7
259	09	Surg	Subtotal Mastectomy For Malignancy W CC	0.9671	1.8	2.8
260	09	Surg	Subtotal Mastectomy For Malignancy W/O CC	0.7032	1.2	1.4
261	09	Surg	Breast Proc For Non-Malignancy Except Biopsy & Local Excision	0.9732	1.6	2.2
262	09	Surg	Breast Biopsy & Local Excision For Non-Malignancy	0.9766	3.3	4.8
263	09	Surg	Skin Graft &/Or Debrid For Skn Ulcer Or Cellulitis W CC	2.1130	8.6	11.4
264	09	Surg	Skin Graft &/Or Debrid For Skn Ulcer Or Cellulitis W/O CC	1.0635	5.0	6.5
265	09	Surg	Skin Graft &/Or Debrid Except For Skin Ulcer Or Cellulitis W CC	1.6593	4.4	6.8
266	09	Surg	Skin Graft &/Or Debrid Except For Skin Ulcer Or Cellulitis W/O CC	0.8637	2.3	3.2
267	09	Surg	Perianal & Pilonidal Procedures	0.8962	2.8	4.2
268	09	Surg	Skin, Subcutaneous Tissue, & Breast Plastic Procedures	1.1326	2.4	3.5
269	09	Surg	Other Skin, Subcut Tiss, & Breast Proc W CC	1.8352	6.2	8.6
270	09	Surg	Other Skin, Subcut Tiss, & Breast Proc W/O CC	0.8313	2.7	3.9
271	09	Med	Skin Ulcers	1.0195	5.6	7.1
272	09	Med	Major Skin Disorders W CC	0.9860	4.5	5.9
273	09	Med	Major Skin Disorders W/O CC	0.5539	2.9	3.7
274	09	Med	Malignant Breast Disorders W CC	1.1294	4.7	6.3
275	09	Med	Malignant Breast Disorders W/O CC	0.5340	2.4	3.3
276	09	Med	Non-Malignant Breast Disorders	0.6892	3.5	4.5
277	09	Med	Cellulitis Age >17 W CC	0.8676	4.6	5.6
278	09	Med	Cellulitis Age >17 W/O CC	0.5391	3.4	4.1
279	09	Med *	Cellulitis Age 0–17	0.7822	4.2	4.2
280	09	Med	Trauma To The Skin, Subcut Tiss, & Breast Age >17 W CC	0.7313	3.2	4.1
281	09	Med	Trauma To The Skin, Subcut Tiss, & Breast Age >17 W/O CC	0.4913	2.3	2.9
282	09	Med *	Trauma To The Skin, Subcut Tiss, & Breast Age 0–17	0.2600	2.2	2.2
283	09	Med	Minor Skin Disorders W CC	0.7423	3.5	4.6
284	09	Med	Minor Skin Disorders W/O CC	0.4563	2.4	3.0
285	10	Surg	Amputat Of Lower Limb For Endocrine, Nutrit, & Metabol Disorders	2.1831	8.2	10.5
286	10	Surg	Adrenal & Pituitary Procedures	1.9390	4.0	5.5
287	10	Surg	Skin Grafts & Wound Debrid For Endoc, Nutrit, & Metab Disorders	1.9470	7.8	10.4
288	10	Surg	O.R. Procedures For Obesity	2.0384	3.2	4.1
289	10	Surg	Parathyroid Procedures	0.9315	1.7	2.6
290	10	Surg	Thyroid Procedures	0.8891	1.6	2.1
291	10	Surg	Thyroglossal Procedures	1.0877	1.6	2.8
292	10	Surg	Other Endocrine, Nutrit, & Metab O.R. Proc W CC	2.6395	7.3	10.3
293	10	Surg	Other Endocrine, Nutrit, & Metab O.R. Proc W/O CC	1.3472	3.2	4.5
294	10	Med	Diabetes Age >35	0.7652	3.3	4.3

Drg	Mdc	Type	Drg Title	Weights	Mean LOS	Arithmetic Mean LOS
295	10	Med	Diabetes Age 0–35	0.7267	2.8	3.7
296	10	Med	Nutritional & Misc Metabolic Disorders Age >17 W CC	0.8187	3.7	4.8
297	10	Med	Nutritional & Misc Metabolic Disorders Age >17 W/O CC	0.4879	2.5	3.1
298	10	Med	Nutritional & Misc Metabolic Disorders Age 0–17	0.5486	2.5	3.9
299	10	Med	Inborn Errors Of Metabolism	1.0329	3.7	5.2
300	10	Med	Endocrine Disorders W CC	1.0922	4.6	6.0
301	10	Med	Endocrine Disorders W/O CC	0.6118	2.7	3.4
302	11	Surg	Kidney Transplant	3.1679	7.0	8.2
303	11	Surg	Kidney, Ureter, & Major Bladder Procedures For Neoplasm	2.2183	5.8	7.4
304	11	Surg	Kidney, Ureter, & Major Bladder Proc For Non-Neopl W CC	2.3761	6.1	8.6
305	11	Surg	Kidney, Ureter, & Major Bladder Proc For Non-Neopl W/O CC	1.1595	2.6	3.2
306	11	Surg	Prostatectomy W CC	1.2700	3.6	5.5
307	11	Surg	Prostatectomy W/O CC	0.6202	1.7	2.1
308	11	Surg	Minor Bladder Procedures W CC	1.6349	3.9	6.1
309	11	Surg	Minor Bladder Procedures W/O CC	0.9085	1.6	2.0
310	11	Surg	Transurethral Procedures W CC	1.1898	3.0	4.5
311	11	Surg	Transurethral Procedures W/O CC	0.6432	1.5	1.9
312	11	Surg	Urethral Procedures, Age >17 W CC	1.1159	3.2	4.8
313	11	Surg	Urethral Procedures, Age >17 W/O CC	0.6783	1.7	2.2
314	11	Surg *	Urethral Procedures, Age 0–17	0.5012	2.3	2.3
315	11	Surg	Other Kidney & Urinary Tract O.R. Procedures	2.0823	3.6	6.8
316	11	Med	Renal Failure	1.2692	4.9	6.4
317	11	Med	Admit For Renal Dialysis	0.7942	2.4	3.5
318	11	Med	Kidney & Urinary Tract Neoplasms W CC	1.1539	4.2	5.8
319	11	Med	Kidney & Urinary Tract Neoplasms W/O CC	0.6385	2.1	2.8
320	11	Med	Kidney & Urinary Tract Infections Age >17 W CC	0.8658	4.2	5.2
321	11	Med	Kidney & Urinary Tract Infections Age >17 W/O CC	0.5652	3.0	3.6
322	11	Med	Kidney & Urinary Tract Infections Age 0–17	0.5498	2.9	3.4
323	11	Med	Urinary Stones W CC, &/Or Esw Lithotripsy	0.8214	2.3	3.1
324	11	Med	Urinary Stones W/O CC	0.5050	1.6	1.9
325	11	Med	Kidney & Urinary Tract Signs & Symptoms Age >17 W CC	0.6436	2.9	3.7
326	11	Med	Kidney & Urinary Tract Signs & Symptoms Age >17 W/O CC	0.4391	2.1	2.6
327	11	Med *	Kidney & Urinary Tract Signs & Symptoms Age 0–17	0.3748	3.1	3.1
328	11	Med	Urethral Stricture Age >17 W CC	0.7079	2.6	3.5
329	11	Med	Urethral Stricture Age >17 W/O CC	0.4701	1.5	1.8
330	11	Med *	Urethral Stricture Age 0–17	0.3227	1.6	1.6
331	11	Med	Other Kidney & Urinary Tract Diagnoses Age >17 W CC	1.0619	4.1	5.5
332	11	Med	Other Kidney & Urinary Tract Diagnoses Age >17 W/O CC	0.6160	2.4	3.1
333	11	Med	Other Kidney & Urinary Tract Diagnoses Age 0–17	0.9669	3.5	5.3
334	12	Surg	Major Male Pelvic Procedures W CC	1.4368	3.5	4.3

Drg	Mdc	Type	Drg Title	Weights	Mean LOS	Arithmetic Mean LOS
335	12	Surg	Major Male Pelvic Procedures W/O CC	1.1004	2.4	2.7
336	12	Surg	Transurethral Prostatectomy W CC	0.8425	2.5	3.3
337	12	Surg	Transurethral Prostatectomy W/O CC	0.5747	1.7	1.9
338	12	Surg	Testes Procedures, For Malignancy	1.3772	3.9	6.2
339	12	Surg	Testes Procedures, Non-Malignancy Age >17	1.1866	3.2	5.1
340	12	Surg *	Testes Procedures, Non-Malignancy Age 0–17	0.2868	2.4	2.4
341	12	Surg	Penis Procedures	1.2622	1.9	3.2
342	12	Surg	Circumcision Age >17	0.8737	2.5	3.4
343	12	Surg *	Circumcision Age 0–17	0.1559	1.7	1.7
344	12	Surg	Other Male Reproductive System O.R. Procedures For Malignancy	1.2475	1.7	2.7
345	12	Surg	Other Male Reproductive System O.R. Proc Except For Malignancy	1.1472	3.1	4.8
346	12	Med	Malignancy, Male Reproductive System, W CC	1.0441	4.2	5.7
347	12	Med	Malignancy, Male Reproductive System, W/O CC	0.6104	2.2	3.1
348	12	Med	Benign Prostatic Hypertrophy W CC	0.7188	3.2	4.1
349	12	Med	Benign Prostatic Hypertrophy W/O CC	0.4210	1.9	2.4
350	12	Med	Inflammation Of The Male Reproductive System	0.7289	3.5	4.5
351	12	Med *	Sterilization, Male	0.2392	1.3	1.3
352	12	Med	Other Male Reproductive System Diagnoses	0.7360	2.9	4.0
353	13	Surg	Pelvic Evisceration, Radical Hysterectomy, & Radical Vulvectomy	1.8504	4.7	6.3
354	13	Surg	Uterine, Adnexa Proc For Non-Ovarian/Adnexal Malig W CC	1.5135	4.6	5.7
355	13	Surg	Uterine, Adnexa Proc For Non-Ovarian/Adnexal Malig W/O CC	0.8824	2.8	3.1
356	13	Surg	Female Reproductive System Reconstructive Procedures	0.7428	1.7	1.9
357	13	Surg	Uterine & Adnexa Proc For Ovarian Or Adnexal Malignancy	2.2237	6.5	8.1
358	13	Surg	Uterine & Adnexa Proc For Non-Malignancy W CC	1.1448	3.2	4.0
359	13	Surg	Uterine & Adnexa Proc For Non-Malignancy W/O CC	0.7948	2.2	2.4
360	13	Surg	Vagina, Cervix, & Vulva Procedures	0.8582	2.0	2.6
361	13	Surg	Laparoscopy & Incisional Tubal Interruption	1.0847	2.2	3.0
362	13	Surg *	Endoscopic Tubal Interruption	0.3057	1.4	1.4
363	13	Surg	D&C, Conization & Radio-Implant, For Malignancy	0.9728	2.7	3.8
364	13	Surg	D&C, Conization Except For Malignancy	0.8709	3.0	4.2
365	13	Surg	Other Female Reproductive System O.R. Procedures	2.0408	5.3	7.7
366	13	Med	Malignancy, Female Reproductive System W CC	1.2348	4.8	6.6
367	13	Med	Malignancy, Female Reproductive System W/O CC	0.5728	2.3	3.0
368	13	Med	Infections, Female Reproductive System	1.1684	5.2	6.7
369	13	Med	Menstrual & Other Female Reproductive System Disorders	0.6310	2.4	3.3
370	14	Surg	Cesarean Section W CC	0.8974	4.1	5.2
371	14	Surg	Cesarean Section W/O CC	0.6066	3.1	3.4
372	14	Med	Vaginal Delivery W Complicating Diagnoses	0.5027	2.5	3.2
373	14	Med	Vaginal Delivery W/O Complicating Diagnoses	0.3556	2.0	2.2
374	14	Surg	Vaginal Delivery W Sterilization &/Or D&C	0.6712	2.5	2.8

Drg	Mdc	Type	Drg Title	Weights	Mean LOS	Arithmetic Mean LOS
375	14	Surg *	Vaginal Delivery W O.R. Proc Except Steril &/Or D&C	0.5837	4.4	4.4
376	14	Med	Postpartum & Post Abortion Diagnoses W/O O.R. Procedure	0.5242	2.6	3.4
377	14	Surg	Postpartum & Post Abortion Diagnoses W O.R. Procedure	1.6996	2.9	4.5
378	14	Med	Ectopic Pregnancy	0.7472	1.9	2.3
379	14	Med	Threatened Abortion	0.3578	2.0	2.8
380	14	Med	Abortion W/O D&C	0.3925	1.6	2.1
381	14	Surg	Abortion W D&C, Aspiration Curettage Or Hysterotomy	0.6034	1.6	2.2
382	14	Med	False Labor	0.2070	1.3	1.4
383	14	Med	Other Antepartum Diagnoses W Medical Complications	0.5053	2.6	3.7
384	14	Med	Other Antepartum Diagnoses W/O Medical Complications	0.3225	1.8	2.6
385	15	Med *	Neonates, Died Or Transferred To Another Acute Care	1.3930	1.8	1.8
386	15	Med *	Extreme Immaturity Or Respiratory Distress Syndrome, Facility Neonate	4.5935	17.9	17.9
387	15	Med *	Prematurity W Major Problems	3.1372	13.3	13.3
388	15	Med *	Prematurity W/O Major Problems	1.8929	8.6	8.6
389	15	Med *	Full Term Neonate W Major Problems	3.2226	4.7	4.7
390	15	Med *	Neonate W Other Significant Problems	1.1406	3.4	3.4
391	15	Med *	Normal Newborn	0.1544	3.1	3.1
392	16	Surg	Splenectomy Age >17	3.0459	6.5	9.2
393	16	Surg *	Splenectomy Age 0–17	1.3645	9.1	9.1
394	16	Surg	Other O.R. Procedures Of The Blood And Blood Forming Organs	1.9109	4.5	7.4
395	16	Med	Red Blood Cell Disorders Age >17	0.8328	3.2	4.3
396	16	Med *	Red Blood Cell Disorders Age 0–17	0.8323	2.6	4.3
397	16	Med	Coagulation Disorders	1.2986	3.7	5.1
398	16	Med	Reticuloendothelial & Immunity Disorders W CC	1.2082	4.4	5.7
399	16	Med	Reticuloendothelial & Immunity Disorders W/O CC	0.6674	2.7	3.3
400	17	Surg	No Longer Valid	0.0000	0.0	0.0
401	17	Surg	Lymphoma & Non-Acute Leukemia W Other O.R. Proc W CC	2.9678	8.0	11.3
402	17	Surg	Lymphoma & Non-Acute Leukemia W Other O.R. Proc W/O CC	1.1810	2.8	4.1
403	17	Med	Lymphoma & Non-Acute Leukemia W CC	1.8432	5.8	8.1
404	17	Med	Lymphoma & Non-Acute Leukemia W/O CC	0.9265	3.0	4.2
405	17	Med *	Acute Leukemia W/O Major O.R. Procedure Age 0–17	1.9346	4.9	4.9
406	17	Surg	Myeloprolif Disord Or Poorly Diff Neopl W Maj O.R.Proc W CC	2.7897	7.0	9.9
407	17	Surg	Myeloprolif Disord Or Poorly Diff Neopl W Maj O.R.Proc W/O CC	1.2289	3.0	3.8
408	17	Surg	Myeloprolif Disord Or Poorly Diff Neopl W Other O.R.Proc	2.2460	4.8	8.2
409	17	Med	Radiotherapy	1.2074	4.3	5.8

Drg	Mdc	Type	Drg Title	Weights	Mean LOS	Arithmetic Mean LOS
410	17	Med	Chemotherapy W/O Acute Leukemia As Secondary Diagnosis	1.1069	3.0	3.8
411	17	Med	History Of Malignancy W/O Endoscopy	0.3635	2.5	3.3
412	17	Med	History Of Malignancy W Endoscopy	0.8451	1.8	2.8
413	17	Med	Other Myeloprolif Dis Or Poorly Diff Neopl Diag W CC	1.3048	5.0	6.8
414	17	Med	Other Myeloprolif Dis Or Poorly Diff Neopl Diag W/O CC	0.7788	3.0	4.0
415	18	Surg	O.R. Procedure For Infectious & Parasitic Diseases	3.9890	11.0	14.8
416	18	Med	Septicemia Age >17	1.6774	5.6	7.5
417	18	Med	Septicemia Age 0–17	1.1689	3.2	4.1
418	18	Med	Postoperative & Post-Traumatic Infections	1.0716	4.8	6.2
419	18	Med	Fever Of Unknown Origin Age >17 W CC	0.8453	3.4	4.4
420	18	Med	Fever Of Unknown Origin Age >17 W/O CC	0.6077	2.7	3.4
421	18	Med	Viral Illness Age >17	0.7664	3.1	4.1
422	18	Med	Viral Illness & Fever Of Unknown Origin Age 0–17	0.6171	2.6	3.7
423	18	Med	Other Infectious & Parasitic Diseases Diagnoses	1.9196	6.0	8.4
424	19	Surg	O.R. Procedure W Principal Diagnoses Of Mental Illness	2.2773	7.3	12.4
425	19	Med	Acute Adjustment Reaction & Psychosocial Dysfunction	0.6191	2.6	3.5
426	19	Med	Depressive Neuroses	0.4656	3.0	4.1
427	19	Med	Neuroses Except Depressive	0.5135	3.2	4.7
428	19	Med	Disorders Of Personality & Impulse Control	0.6981	4.6	7.3
429	19	Med	Organic Disturbances & Mental Retardation	0.7919	4.3	5.6
430	19	Med	Psychoses	0.6483	5.8	7.9
431	19	Med	Childhood Mental Disorders	0.5178	4.0	5.9
432	19	Med	Other Mental Disorder Diagnoses	0.6282	2.9	4.3
433	20	Med	Alcohol/Drug Abuse Or Dependence, Left Ama	0.2776	2.2	3.0
434	20	Med	No Longer Valid	0.0000	0.0	0.0
435	20	Med	No Longer Valid	0.0000	0.0	0.0
436	20	Med	No Longer Valid	0.0000	0.0	0.0
437	20	Med	No Longer Valid	0.0000	0.0	0.0
438	20		No Longer Valid	0.0000	0.0	0.0
439	21	Surg	Skin Grafts For Injuries	1.9398	5.4	8.9
440	21	Surg	Wound Debridements For Injuries	1.9457	5.9	9.2
441	21	Surg	Hand Procedures For Injuries	0.9382	2.3	3.4
442	21	Surg	Other O.R. Procedures For Injuries W CC	2.5660	6.0	8.9
443	21	Surg	Other O.R. Procedures For Injuries W/O CC	0.9943	2.6	3.4
444	21	Med	Traumatic Injury Age >17 W CC	0.7556	3.2	4.1
445	21	Med	Traumatic Injury Age >17 W/O CC	0.5033	2.2	2.8
446	21	Med *	Traumatic Injury Age 0–17	0.2999	2.4	2.4
447	21	Med	Allergic Reactions Age >17	0.5569	1.9	2.6
448	21	Med *	Allergic Reactions Age 0–17	0.0987	2.9	2.9
449	21	Med	Poisoning & Toxic Effects Of Drugs Age >17 W CC	0.8529	2.6	3.7
450	21	Med	Poisoning & Toxic Effects Of Drugs Age >17 W/O CC	0.4282	1.6	2.0
451	21	Med *	Poisoning & Toxic Effects Of Drugs Age 0–17	0.2663	2.1	2.1

Drg	Mdc	Type	Drg Title	Weights	Mean LOS	Arithmetic Mean LOS
452	21	Med	Complications Of Treatment W CC	1.0462	3.5	4.9
453	21	Med	Complications Of Treatment W/O CC	0.5285	2.2	2.8
454	21	Med	Other Injury, Poisoning, & Toxic Effect Diag W CC	0.8141	2.9	4.1
455	21	Med	Other Injury, Poisoning, & Toxic Effect Diag W/O CC	0.4725	1.7	2.2
456	22		No Longer Valid	0.0000	0.0	0.0
457	22	Med	No Longer Valid	0.0000	0.0	0.0
458	22	Surg	No Longer Valid	0.0000	0.0	0.0
459	22	Surg	No Longer Valid	0.0000	0.0	0.0
460	22	Med	No Longer Valid	0.0000	0.0	0.0
461	23	Surg	O.R. Proc W Diagnoses Of Other Contact W Health Services	1.3974	3.0	5.1
462	23	Med	Rehabilitation	0.8700	8.9	10.8
463	23	Med	Signs & Symptoms W CC	0.6960	3.1	3.9
464	23	Med	Signs & Symptoms W/O CC	0.5055	2.4	2.9
465	23	Med	Aftercare W History Of Malignancy As Secondary Diagnosis	0.6224	2.4	3.8
466	23	Med	Aftercare W/O History Of Malignancy As Secondary Diagnosis	0.7806	2.8	5.3
467	23	Med	Other Factors Influencing Health Status	0.4803	2.0	2.7
468			Extensive O.R. Procedure Unrelated To Principal Diagnosis	4.0031	9.7	13.2
469		**	Principal Diagnosis Invalid As Discharge Diagnosis	0.0000	0.0	0.0
470		**	Ungroupable	0.0000	0.0	0.0
471	08	Surg	Bilateral Or Multiple Major Joint Procs Of Lower Extremity	3.1391	4.5	5.1
472	22	Surg	No Longer Valid	0.0000	0.0	0.0
473	17	Med	Acute Leukemia W/O Major O.R. Procedure Age >17	3.4231	7.4	12.7
474	04	Surg	No Longer Valid	0.0000	0.0	0.0
475	04	Med	Respiratory System Diagnosis With Ventilator Support	3.6091	8.1	11.3
476		Surg	Prostatic O.R. Procedure Unrelated To Principal Diagnosis	2.1822	7.4	10.5
477		Surg	Non-Extensive O.R. Procedure Unrelated To Principal Diagnosis	2.0607	5.8	8.7
478	05	Surg	No Longer Valid	0.0000	0.0	0.0
479	05	Surg	Other Vascular Procedures W/O CC	1.4434	2.1	2.8
480	Pre	Surg	Liver Transplant And/Or Intestinal Transplant	8.9693	13.7	18.0
481	Pre	Surg	Bone Marrow Transplant	6.2321	18.2	21.7
482	Pre	Surg	Tracheostomy For Face, Mouth, & Neck Diagnoses	3.3387	9.6	12.1
483	Pre	Surg	No Longer Valid	0.0000	0.0	0.0
484	24	Surg	Craniotomy For Multiple Significant Trauma	5.1438	9.3	12.8
485	24	Surg	Limb Reattachment, Hip And Femur Proc For Multiple Significant Trauma	3.4952	8.4	10.2
486	24	Surg	Other O.R. Procedures For Multiple Significant Trauma	4.7323	8.5	12.5
487	24	Med	Other Multiple Significant Trauma	1.9459	5.3	7.3
488	25	Surg	HIV W Extensive O.R. Procedure	4.4353	11.8	16.4
489	25	Med	HIV W Major Related Condition	1.8058	5.9	8.4
490	25	Med	HIV W Or W/O Other Related Condition	1.0639	3.8	5.4

Drg	Mdc	Type	Drg Title	Weights	Mean LOS	Arithmetic Mean LOS
491	08	Surg	Major Joint & Limb Reattachment Procedures Of Upper Extremity	1.6780	2.6	3.1
492	17	Med	Chemotherapy W Acute Leukemia Or W Use Of Hi Dose Chemoagent	3.5926	8.8	13.7
493	07	Surg	Laparoscopic Cholecystectomy W/O C.D.E. W CC	1.8333	4.5	6.1
494	07	Surg	Laparoscopic Cholecystectomy W/O C.D.E. W/O CC	1.0285	2.1	2.7
495	Pre	Surg	Lung Transplant	8.5736	14.0	17.3
496	08	Surg	Combined Anterior/Posterior Spinal Fusion	6.0932	6.4	8.8
497	08	Surg	Spinal Fusion Except Cervical W CC	3.6224	5.0	5.9
498	08	Surg	Spinal Fusion Except Cervical W/O CC	2.7791	3.4	3.8
499	08	Surg	Back & Neck Procedures Except Spinal Fusion W CC	1.3831	3.1	4.3
500	08	Surg	Back & Neck Procedures Except Spinal Fusion W/O CC	0.9046	1.8	2.2
501	08	Surg	Knee Procedures W Pdx Of Infection W CC	2.6462	8.5	10.4
502	08	Surg	Knee Procedures W Pdx Of Infection W/O CC	1.4462	4.9	5.9
503	08	Surg	Knee Procedures W/O Pdx Of Infection	1.2038	2.9	3.8
504	22	Surg	Exten. Burns Or Full Thickness Burn W/Mv 96+ Hrs W/Skin Gft	11.8018	21.7	27.3
505	22	Med	Exten. Burns Or Full Thickness Burn W/Mv 96+ Hrs W/O Skin Gft	2.2953	2.4	4.6
506	22	Surg	Full Thickness Burn W Skin Graft Or Inhal Inj W CC Or Sig Trauma	4.0939	11.2	15.9
507	22	Surg	Full Thickness Burn W Skin Grft Or Inhal Inj W/O CC Or Sig Trauma	1.7369	5.8	8.5
508	22	Med	Full Thickness Burn W/O Skin Grft Or Inhal Inj W CC Or Sig Trauma	1.2767	5.1	7.4
509	22	Med	Full Thickness Burn W/O Skin Grft Or Inh Inj W/O CC Or Sig Trauma	0.8217	3.6	5.2
510	22	Med	Non-Extensive Burns W CC Or Significant Trauma	1.1817	4.4	6.4
511	22	Med	Non-Extensive Burns W/O CC Or Significant Trauma	0.7424	2.6	4.1
512	Pre	Surg	Simultaneous Pancreas/Kidney Transplant	5.3660	10.7	12.8
513	Pre	Surg	Pancreas Transplant	5.9669	8.9	9.9
514	05	Surg	No Longer Valid	0.0000	0.0	0.0
515	05	Surg	Cardiac Defibrillator Implant W/O Cardiac Cath	5.5205	2.6	4.3
516	05	Surg	No Longer Valid	0.0000	0.0	0.0
517	05	Surg	No Longer Valid	0.0000	0.0	0.0
518	05	Surg	Perc Cardio Proc W/O Coronary Artery Stent Or Ami	1.6544	1.8	2.5
519	08	Surg	Cervical Spinal Fusion W CC	2.4695	3.0	4.8
520	08	Surg	Cervical Spinal Fusion W/O CC	1.6788	1.6	2.0
521	20	Med	Alcohol/Drug Abuse Or Dependence W CC	0.6939	4.2	5.6
522	20	Med	Alc/Drug Abuse Or Depend W Rehabilitation Therapy W/O CC	0.4794	7.7	9.6
523	20	Med	Alc/Drug Abuse Or Depend W/O Rehabilitation Therapy W/O CC	0.3793	3.2	3.9
524	01	Med	Transient Ischemia	0.7288	2.6	3.2
525	05	Surg	Other Heart Assist System Implant	11.4282	7.2	13.6

Drg	Mdc	Type	Drg Title	Weights	Mean LOS	Arithmetic Mean LOS
526	05	Surg	No Longer Valid	0.0000	0.0	0.0
527	05	Surg	No Longer Valid	0.0000	0.0	0.0
528	01	Surg	Intracranial Vascular Proc W Pdx Hemorrhage	7.0505	13.8	17.2
529	01	Surg	Ventricular Shunt Procedures W CC	2.3160	5.3	8.3
530	01	Surg	Ventricular Shunt Procedures W/O CC	1.2041	2.4	3.1
531	01	Surg	Spinal Procedures W CC	3.1279	6.5	9.6
532	01	Surg	Spinal Procedures W/O CC	1.4195	2.8	3.7
533	01	Surg	Extracranial Procedures W CC	1.5767	2.4	3.8
534	01	Surg	Extracranial Procedures W/O CC	1.0201	1.5	1.8
535	05	Surg	Cardiac Defib Implant W Cardiac Cath W Ami/Hf/Shock	7.9738	7.9	10.3
536	05	Surg	Cardiac Defib Implant W Cardiac Cath W/O Ami/Hf/Shock	6.9144	5.9	7.6
537	08	Surg	Local Excis & Remov Of Int Fix Dev Except Hip & Femur W CC	1.8360	4.8	6.9
538	08	Surg	Local Excis & Remov Of Int Fix Dev Except Hip & Femur W/O CC	0.9833	2.1	2.8
539	17	Surg	Lymphoma & Leukemia W Major Or Procedure W CC	3.2782	7.0	10.8
540	17	Surg	Lymphoma & Leukemia W Major Or Procedure W/O CC	1.1940	2.6	3.6
541	Pre	Surg	Ecmo Or Trach W Mv 96+Hrs Or Pdx Exc Face, Mouth, & Neck W Maj O.R.	19.8038	38.1	45.7
542	Pre	Surg	Trach W Mv 96+Hrs Or Pdx Exc Face, Mouth, & Neck W/O Maj O.R.	12.8719	29.1	35.1
543	01	Surg	Craniotomy W/Implant Of Chemo Agent Or Acute Complx Cns Pdx	4.4184	8.5	12.3
544	08	Surg	Major Joint Replacement Or Reattachment Of Lower Extremity	1.9643	4.1	4.5
545	08	Surg	Revision Of Hip Or Knee Replacement	2.4827	4.5	5.2
546	08	Surg	Spinal Fusion Exc Cerv With Curvature Of The Spine Or Malig	5.0739	7.1	8.8
547	05	Surg	Coronary Bypass W Cardiac Cath W Major Cv Dx	6.1948	10.8	12.3
548	05	Surg	Coronary Bypass W Cardiac Cath W/O Major Cv Dx	4.7198	8.2	9.0
549	05	Surg	Coronary Bypass W/O Cardiac Cath W Major Cv Dx	5.0980	8.7	10.3
550	05	Surg	Coronary Bypass W/O Cardiac Cath W/O Major Cv Dx	3.6151	6.2	6.9
551	05	Surg	Permanent Cardiac Pacemaker Impl W Maj Cv Dx Or Aicd Lead Or Gnrtr	3.1007	4.4	6.4
552	05	Surg	Other Permanent Cardiac Pacemaker Implant W/O Major Cv Dx	2.0996	2.5	3.5
553	05	Surg	Other Vascular Procedures W CC W Major Cv Dx	3.0957	6.6	9.7
554	05	Surg	Other Vascular Procedures W CC W/O Major Cv Dx	2.0721	4.0	5.9
555	05	Surg	Percutaneous Cardiovascular Proc W Major Cv Dx	2.4315	3.4	4.7
556	05	Surg	Percutaneous Cardiovasc Proc W Non-Drug-Eluting Stent W/O Maj Cv Dx	1.9132	1.6	2.1
557	05	Surg	Percutaneous Cardiovascular Proc W Drug-Eluting Stent W Major Cv Dx	2.8717	3.0	4.1

Drg	Mdc	Type	Drg Title	Weights	Mean LOS	Arithmetic Mean LOS
558	05	Surg	Percutaneous Cardiovascular Proc W Drug-Eluting Stent W/O Maj Cv Dx	2.2108	1.5	1.9
559	01	Med	Acute Ischemic Stroke With Use Of Thrombolytic Agent	2.2473	5.8	7.2

Medicare Data Have Been Supplemented By Data From 19 States For Low Volume Drgs.

Drgs 469 And 470 Contain Cases Which Could Not Be Assigned To Valid Drgs.

Note: Geometric Mean Is Used Only To Determine Payment For Transfer Cases.

Note: Arithmetic Mean Is Presented For Informational Purposes Only.

Note: Relative Weights Are Based On Medicare Patient Data And May Not Be Appropriate For Other Patients.

Chapter 4

Legal and Regulatory Environment

After studying this chapter, you should be able to do the following:

1. Explain the financial risks to an organization that could result from a failure to plan for the health care legal and regulatory environment.
2. Explain the difference between fraud and abuse.
3. Describe how the False Claims Act has been applied in health care.
4. Describe the managerial and organizational implications of the Emergency Medical Transfer and Active Labor Act (EMTALA).
5. Explain the major objectives of U.S. antitrust law, as applied to the health care industry.
6. Describe the managerial and organizational implications of the Health Insurance Portability and Accountability Act (HIPAA).
7. List some of the penalties for non-compliance with HIPAA.
8. Describe the major provisions of the Stark II laws and of the safe harbor regulations.
9. List the major components of compliance and internal control programs.

REAL-WORLD SCENARIO

Anne Stewart, CEO of Hufford Community Hospital, is reviewing a letter that she received from the Office of Inspector General (OIG) of the Department of Health and Human Services (DHHS). In that letter, the OIG has requested access to medical record data for a large number of Medicare patients treated during the last three years at Hufford. The OIG is specifically concerned about the relative frequency of Medicare patients grouped to DRG 79 (respiratory infections and inflammations for age > 17 with complications and comorbidities) compared to the number of Medicare patients grouped to DRG 89 (simple pneumonia and pleurisy, age > 17 with complications and comorbidities). Hufford receives approximately $8,500 from Medicare for each DRG 79 case compared with $5,400 for DRG 89. Hufford had a total of 168 Medicare DRG 79 patients in the last year and 40 Medicare DRG 89 patients. State comparative data suggest that Hufford should have had 55 DRG 79 patients and 153 DRG 79 patients. The OIG is investigating Hufford because of a *qui tam* complaint filed by a Hufford employee alleging that medical record coders were instructed to upcode patients to DRG 79.

Ms. Stewart is not aware of any illegal or fraudulent activity on the part of any member of her staff, but is very concerned about the potential legal and administrative costs involved in defending both her and the hospital. Ron Olsen, Director of Medical Records, explains to Stewart that the primary criterion used to classify patients into DRG 79 or DRG 89 is whether the bacteria causing the pneumonia is specified or unspecified, but not represented by an ICD–9 (*International Classification of Diseases, Ninth Revision*) code. If the bacteria is specified, but not represented by a code, then 482.89 should be used and the patient will be classified as a DRG 79. If the physician does not specify the bacteria, then 482.9 should be used and the patient will be classified as DRG 89. The critical question for Ms. Stewart and Mr. Olsen is whether the physicians specified the bacteria in the medical record.

Hospital attorneys have explained that the hospital may be liable for repayment of prior reimbursement if the OIG finds insufficient documentation to justify current coding. Criminal penalties may also be involved if it can be shown that hospital management or staff encouraged miscoding. Both scenarios are unpleasant and Ms. Stewart hopes that adequate physician documentation exists. Among other worries, Ms. Stewart is concerned that the hospital could be liable under the False Claims Act, which provides for treble damages, unless the hospital has an effective compliance plan. The OIG lays out a model compliance plan in its guidelines.

While the federal government has long been concerned with Medicare and Medicaid fraud and abuse, the May 1995 launch of Operation Restore Trust (ORT) ushered in a new era of investigation and enforcement of these crimes. In recent years, fiscal responsibility and accountability have been hallmarks of the government's stance toward health providers, primarily because of Medicare's uncertain financial future. The Department of Health and Human Services' Office of Inspector General reported overpayments of $20 billion (or 11 percent of Medicare payments) to hospitals, physicians, and other health care providers in fiscal year 1997 (DOJ, 1998). In that same year, estimates suggest that more than $500 in improper payments were made for each Medicare beneficiary. Whatever the reason for the government's zealous pursuit of fraud and abuse, the playing field for health care providers has been irrevocably altered.

As a result of their decentralized delivery system and relatively lax controls, home health care agencies were an early target of the government's fraud investigations. Hospitals and health systems, where large payments and deep pockets would make fraud investigations particularly lucrative, were also targeted. Financial executives in health care can no longer consider the legal and regulatory environment to be solely the purview of corporate counsel. The financial risks to health care organizations resulting from noncompliance or poor compliance with health laws are so great that they must be proactively planned for by all financial management personnel.

LEARNING OBJECTIVE 1

Explain the financial risks to an organization that could result from a failure to plan for the health care legal and regulatory environment.

From the government's perspective, the initiatives associated with Operation Restore Trust have been an unqualified success. In one year alone, $1.2 billion was awarded or negotiated as a result of civil settlements, fines, or judgments surrounding health care fraud. Some 363 defendants were convicted of fraud, and over 1000 businesses and individuals were excluded from federal health programs for fraud convictions (DOJ, 1998).

The health care industry has responded with deliberation and dispatch. A whole new classification of health care professional has emerged in the compliance officer, an individual responsible for ensuring that the organization complies with governmental regulations surrounding Medicare and Medicaid. Organization-wide compliance programs have quickly become operational, and health care professionals' awareness of the financial risks and ethical issues surrounding fraud and abuse has increased dramatically.

LEARNING OBJECTIVE 2

Explain the difference between fraud and abuse.

Fraud consists of intentional acts of deception, whereas abuse involves improper acts that are unintentional, but which are inconsistent with standard practice. Fraud and abuse can take many forms. Providers can bill for services not delivered or not medically necessary (false claims). Double-billing for a single procedure can occur, as can improper upcoding to receive a higher reimbursement rate. Kickbacks for referrals or medical procedures are another frequently cited form of fraud.

The Medicare program involves claims for services submitted by thousands of providers on behalf of more than 40 million beneficiaries. The cumulative effect of even small overpayments can translate into significant program losses because of the number of claims and providers involved. The Justice Department's recent multistate initiatives address this particular vulnerability of the Medicare program.

LEARNING OBJECTIVE 3

Describe how the False Claims Act has been applied in health care.

The False Claims Act (FCA) is the federal government's primary civil remedy for improper or fraudulent claims[1]. Under the FCA, health care providers who knowingly make false or fraudulent claims to the government are fined $5,500 to $11,000 per claim, plus up to three times the amount of the damages caused to the federal program. This can result in significant fines because some health care providers routinely submit thou-

[1] In 2000, the U.S. Supreme Court ruled that state-owned providers could not be subject to damages under the False Claims Act, effectively shielding state-owned health care providers from the FCA.

sands of claims to the government each year. For example, on March 10, 2000, the Department of Justice filed claims under FCA seeking recovery of over $1 billion from Vencor Inc., a long-term health care provider, for its alleged knowing submission of false claims. The FCA has been applied to cases of improper billing practices; claims for services not rendered; provision of medically unnecessary services; misrepresenting eligibility or credentials; and substandard quality of care.

Although the FCA applies to all federal programs, not just to health care benefits, it increasingly has been applied in health care, due mainly to the large dollar amounts involved. Originally enacted in 1863, the FCA was amended significantly in 1986. With these changes, specific intent to defraud the government is not required; the government needs only establish that the claim submitted is false and that it was submitted knowingly. Thus, the FCA covers activity that would not be included under the traditional definition of fraud, which requires actual knowledge and the intent to defraud. As with most other civil actions, the government must establish its case by presenting a preponderance of the evidence, rather than by meeting the higher burden of proof that applies in criminal cases.

To prove that a provider knowingly submitted a false claim, the government must establish that the person submitted the claim with actual knowledge, in deliberate ignorance, or with reckless disregard for the claim's truth or falsity. The 1986 amendments clarify that the statute is not intended to apply to honest mistakes and negligence. Yet, one of the goals of the amendments was to obligate those doing business with the government to make at least limited inquiries as to the accuracy of the claims they submit.

The number of civil health care fraud matters pending at the Justice Department rose from 270 at the end of fiscal year 1992 to more than 4000 in fiscal year 1997, yet the quantity has moderated in recent years. In 1999, 2278 civil matters were pending, and 91 civil cases were filed; and a total of 396 defendants were convicted of health care fraud-related crimes.

Each U.S. Attorney's Office now has a health care fraud coordinator, and there is increasingly closer coordination among the Departments of Justice and Health and Human Services, the Office of the Inspector General, the Federal Bureau of Investigation, State Medicaid fraud units, and a number of other federal agencies.

Operation Restore Trust

The perception of widespread abuse in health care billing led the Clinton Administration to initiate the pilot program Operation Restore Trust (ORT) on May 3, 1995. This anti-fraud and anti-abuse initiative started in five states: California, Florida, New York, Texas, and Illinois. At the time, these states accounted for 40 percent of the nation's Medicare and Medicaid beneficiaries. Within two years, ORT had recovered nearly $190 million from fraudulent health care schemes. On May 20, 1997, the Secretary of the Department of Health and Human Services announced the next phase of ORT, which expanded investigations into 12 additional states. The program has since been expanded nationwide and is targeting additional provider groups.

In ORT, the DHHS assembled an interdisciplinary project team with representatives from the federal and state governments, as well as the private sector. The team focused on home health care, nursing home care, hospice, and durable medical equipment, which are four of the fastest growing areas in Medicare. Three agencies within the DHHS—the Office of the Inspector General (OIG), the Centers for Medicare & Medicaid Services[2] (CMS), and the Administration on Aging—are involved, along with the Department of Justice (DOJ).

In addition to identifying and penalizing those who willingly defraud the government, the project has alerted the public and the health care industry to the existence and prevention of fraud schemes.[3] Operation Restore Trust has also helped to identify and to correct the vulnerabilities in the Medicare and Medicaid programs. The program uses sophisticated statistical methods to identify providers for investigations and audits. The activities in ORT include:

- financial audits by the OIG and CMS.
- criminal investigations and referrals by OIG to appropriate law enforcement officials.
- civil and administrative sanctions and recovery actions by the OIG and other appropriate law enforcement officials.

- surveys and inspections of long-term care facilities by CMS and state officials in search of fraudulent activities.
- studies and recommendations by the OIG and CMS for program adjustments to prevent fraud and reduce waste and abuse.
- issuance of special fraud alerts to notify the public and the health care community about schemes by fraudulent providers of home health services, nursing care, and medical equipment and supplies.

Criminal-Disclosure Provision of the Social Security Act (SSA)

Providers also must consider their liabilities under the criminal-disclosure provision of the Social Security Act (SSA). This provision makes it a felony, punishable by up to five years in prison and/or a fine of up to $25,000, for a health care provider (or a beneficiary) who possesses

> knowledge of the occurrence of any event affecting (A) his initial or continued right to any such benefit or payment, or (B) the initial or continued right to any such benefit or payment of any other individual in whose behalf he has applied for or is receiving such benefit or payment; . . . [to] conceal . . . or fail . . . to disclose such event with an intent fraudulently to secure such benefit or payment either in a greater amount or quantity than is due or when no such benefit or payment is authorized. 42 U.S.C. 1320a-7b(a)(3)

The criminal-disclosure provision of the Social Security Act imposes an obligation to disclose overpayments to the government regardless of the provider's good faith at the time the claim was submitted. This provision is meant to compel disclosure of overpayments so that the government may initiate collection efforts. A provider's good-faith submission of its payment claim may provide a partial or complete defense if the government attempts recovery under the False Claims Act, but it does not negate criminal liability under the criminal-disclosure provision of the Social Security Act.

Providers should be especially aware of the potentially harsh penalties related to the interaction of the Social Security Act's criminal-disclosure provision with the Stark II law, which prohibits physicians from referring patients to providers with which the physician has a

---

[2]The name of the Health Care Financing Administration (HCFA) was changed on June 14, 2001, to the Centers for Medicare & Medicaid Services.

[3]Institutions have been fined for instances of overbilling, even where there was counterbalancing underbilling. Some have criticized this aspect of the federal government's efforts.

financial relationship. The law clearly states that a provider is not entitled to Medicare payments for services or items rendered in violation of the Stark II restrictions on self-referrals, regardless of the provider's state of mind. Thus, a provider that belatedly discovers it had a prohibited relationship with a referring physician and knows it received payment on Medicare claims for treating patients that were referred to it by that physician, is in violation of Stark II and faces potential criminal liability if it does not disclose such circumstances. This scenario highlights the importance of identifying restricted financial relationships with physicians as early as possible.

Definitions of a prohibited relationship could include the more obvious, such as payments for referrals, or the less obvious, such as a hospital renting office space to physicians at below-market levels. It has even been construed that free parking for physicians at a hospital where others are charged is an impermissible benefit for referring physicians.

Until recently, no prosecutions had been based on the criminal-disclosure statute, suggesting, perhaps, that the Department of Justice viewed it as difficult to prove the illicit intent to secure fraudulent overpayments. At least two indictments based (at least in part) on this provision have been handed down. In California, three individuals were charged with conspiracy to defraud the United States in connection with a scheme to submit fraudulent certificates of medical necessity for certain medical equipment. Elsewhere, another indictment alleged a conspiracy among defendants to knowingly misstate certain interest expenses on provider cost reports filed with the government. Included in the description of the conspiracy is the defendants' deliberate failure to notify the government of the fiscal intermediary's audit error concerning interest expense. The government obtained convictions on the conspiracy count, but the jury was not required to make a separate finding on the failure-to-disclose allegations.

These indictments indicate that the government does not view the monies at issue in these cases to have been obtained innocently or in good faith. Thus, whether the government will use this statute to prosecute those who fail to disclose monies obtained by mistake remains an open question. These indictments should be of interest to all officers and directors of corporate health care providers because they underscore the government's willingness to prosecute individuals under this previously unused statute for alleged nondisclosures made by a corporation.

Most false claim statutes impose liability on persons who "submit or cause to be submitted" false statements to obtain payment from the government. This precise language is not found in the criminal-disclosure provision of the Social Security Act, but the circumstances of the indictments noted above make it abundantly clear that government prosecutors will seek to impose personal criminal responsibility on officers (and possibly directors) of corporate providers who know, but fail to disclose, that the provider is not entitled to some Medicare payments it received.

LEARNING OBJECTIVE 4

Describe the managerial and organizational implications of the Emergency Medical Transfer and Active Labor Act (EMTALA).

The Emergency Medical Treatment and Active Labor Act (EMTALA) requires all Medicare- or Medicaid-participating hospitals with an emergency department to provide appropriate medical screening to each patient requesting emergency care to determine if the patient requires such care. Originally passed by Congress in 1985 as part of the Consolidated Omnibus Budget Reconciliation Act of 1985 (COBRA), EMTALA often is referred to as the "antidumping law" because it prohibits hospitals from transferring an emergency patient to another hospital simply because of the patient's inability to pay.

If emergency care is needed, the statute requires the hospital to medically stabilize the patient (assuming the hospital has the medical capabilities to do so), irrespective of the patient's ability to pay. Hospitals are prohibited from posting payment information in their emergency rooms. Patients who have medical conditions that the hospital is incapable of stabilizing (as certified by a physician) or who ask to be transferred to another facility before the hospital can stabilize their condition, must be transferred to another facility in accordance with specific requirements of the EMTALA law. If, after evaluation, the patient is found not to have a medical emergency, the hospital's obligation to the patient under EMTALA ends.

EMTALA also requires that a Medicare- or Medicaid-participating hospital ensure that emergency department staff does not engage the patient in discussion regarding his or her financial or insurance information before conducting the medical screening examination and stabilization of the emergency condition. Hospitals may, however, commence normal registration procedures, which may include asking whether the patient carries insurance, as long as such procedures do not delay screening and stabilization.

Hospital Compliance with EMTALA

To avoid EMTALA violations, hospitals should:

* require all clinical, administrative, and contract staff to review and understand the EMTALA requirements.
* ensure that all patients who decide to leave the hospital without receiving treatment or withdraw their request for emergency treatment, are offered a medical examination and treatment within the hospital facilities before they leave, and that staff who can identify and stabilize a patient's medical condition always are available in the hospital to provide these services (that is, within the limits of the hospital staff's medical capabilities).
* ensure that all reasonable steps are taken to obtain the patient's written informed consent to refuse any examination or treatment services, and that the patient's medical record contains a description of the examination, treatment, or both, as well as documentation of the patient's refusal to receive emergency care.
* ensure that emergency department staff has reviewed and understand all statutory requirements regarding transfer of patients to another facility.
* instruct hospital staff to refrain from asking patients to complete financial forms or inquiring about patients' financial or insurance status (even if the patient engages the staff in conversation) until the medical screening examination has been conducted and the patient's emergency medical condition has been stabilized.

LEARNING OBJECTIVE 5

Explain the major objectives of U.S. antitrust law, as applied to the health care industry.

The purpose of antitrust laws is to promote a competitive, free marketplace; they are intended to protect the public from the adverse effects of monopoly power. The federal government and virtually all state governments have antitrust laws, which reflect a public policy principle that a competitive marketplace will protect consumers, restrain private economic power, and generally produce the best allocation of quality goods and services at the lowest prices.

There are three main sources of U.S. antitrust law: the Sherman Act, the Clayton Act, and the Federal Trade Commission Act. Section 1 of the Sherman Act prohibits all conspiracies or agreements that restrain trade. Section 7 of the Clayton Act prohibits all mergers and acquisitions of stock or assets that may substantially lessen competition or that tend to create a monopoly. Section 5 of the Federal Trade Commission Act prohibits unfair methods of competition.

Sherman Act

As interpreted by the courts, Section 1 of the Sherman Act applies to agreements that unreasonably restrain trade, which may include agreements or conspiracies to fix prices, divide market territories or groups of customers, boycott other firms, or to use coercive tactics with the intent and effect of injuring competition. Ironically, many hospital administrators argue that what has caused merger-mania among hospitals has been the onset of managed care, and the inability of hospitals to evenhandedly negotiate with those companies, which, like insurance companies, are exempt from antitrust laws.

The Sherman Act applies to virtually all businesses in the country, including health care providers. It condemns any conduct that causes inefficiencies resulting in higher prices or lower quality of services to the ultimate consumer. Most business practices that are condemned under the Sherman Act are justified from a business standpoint, but deemed illegal because they "unreasonably" restrain trade (i.e., the anticompetitive effect of the business practices outweigh their pro-business justifications). An example of such a practice would be a noncompete clause prohibiting the seller of a business from ever engaging in a similar business activity. Although such a noncompete clause would be justified on business grounds for the buyer, the clause's provision could unreasonably restrain trade. Some practices, however, are condemned because there are no acceptable justifications for the conduct. An example of such a practice is an agreement among competitors to fix prices.

A traditional Integrated Delivery System (IDS) does not violate the Sherman Act. Integrated delivery systems, which link hospitals with physicians and other medical service providers, are also exempt from the anti-referral provisions of Stark. As an IDS acquires physician practices and other providers, the group becomes a single legal entity with almost complete discretion to coordinate the activities of the providers whose businesses or practices it owns. It therefore cannot conspire with itself to restrain trade.

Similarly, a virtual IDS runs few antitrust risks. Because each provider participating in such an organization has its own separate payer contracts established in arm's-length transactions, the IDS constituents do not collectively set prices for health care services.

Nonetheless, under exceptional circumstances, the federal government may bring antitrust challenges against such virtual arrangements. On April 10, 2000, a federal court ruled that two virtually integrated hospitals in Poughkeepsie, New York, committed per se (or by rule of reason) illegal price-fixing and market allocation. Notwithstanding such exceptions, however, as long as a virtual IDS refrains from collective price setting and market allocation, the risks of condemnation under Section 1 of the Sherman Act are limited.

By contrast, a partially-integrated IDS faces significant risk of being challenged under the Sherman Act. In forming a partially-integrated IDS, the hospital, physicians, and other providers pay a price in the form of increased antitrust risk by collectively contracting with a payer, and yet maintaining their independence as separate legal entities. From an antitrust perspective, these providers may be viewed as competitors that are jointly setting the price they will charge for their services, which is a classic violation of Section 1 of the Sherman Act. Therefore, to minimize their antitrust exposure, providers considering this model should be careful to structure the IDS in accordance with Section 1 of the Sherman Act, taking into account the federal antitrust agencies' various guidelines and enforcement policies.

Enforcement of antitrust laws is jointly shared by the Department of Justice (DOJ) and the Federal Trade Commission (FTC). The DOJ has responsibility of enforcing the Sherman Act, while the FTC enforces the

Federal Trade Commission Act. Both agencies have jurisdiction under the Clayton Act. Some actions by providers, such as agreements among firms to fix prices or divide markets, are on their face antitrust violations, and are called "*per se*" violations. Actions not considered *per se* violations are evaluated under the "rule of reason."

A merger or joint venture between two or more hospitals may be investigated by either the DOJ or the FTC under the Clayton Act. The procedure established for deciding which agency will investigate a particular merger or joint venture is based on staff expertise, prior dealings with the parties involved, and caseload. While either agency may investigate a merger or joint venture for civil violations, once criminal conduct is suspected, the case is referred to the DOJ. Private parties and State Attorney Generals may also sue to block mergers or joint ventures under either the Sherman or Clayton Act.

Depending on the degree of state supervision and control of hospital activities, hospitals may be immune from federal antitrust enforcement under the state action immunity doctrine. For private anticompetitive conduct to be immune from federal antitrust liability under this doctrine, the state must (1) clearly articulate and affirmatively express a policy to displace competition with regulation, and (2) actively supervise and control the private anticompetitive conduct.

FEDERAL ENFORCEMENT ACTIONS

The Hart-Scott-Rodino Antitrust Improvements Act of 1976 requires that parties notify both the FTC and the DOJ of certain mergers, acquisitions, joint ventures, or tender offers before consummation of the agreements. This filing requirement applies to all parties engaged in such activities, including hospitals, and covers agreements in which the acquiring hospital has net sales or total assets of at least $100 million, and the hospital being acquired has assets of at least $10 million. Based on information provided in these filings, the DOJ and the FTC decide whether to allow the proposed merger to proceed or to open a preliminary investigation. If the preliminary investigation indicates that a potential violation exists, the FTC or DOJ may issue a second request for additional information to review before deciding whether to challenge the proposed merger or collaboration.

Reviews of mergers might include interviews of competitors and analysis of the marketplace. When weak competitors are interviewed by the DOJ, however, they are often cowed by the specter of the larger competitor that could be either their future partner, or a monolith ready to put them out of business. Other providers might be inclined to give unwarranted opposition because they do not want the increased competition.

For the 13-year period covering fiscal years 1981 through 1993, the DOJ and FTC received 397 Hart-Scott-Rodino filings involving acute care hospital mergers and acquisitions. After initial review of the filings, the two agencies conducted preliminary investigations in 68 cases, or about 17 percent, of the total filings. Less than half of these resulted in second requests for information. In five cases, the parties voluntarily agreed to withdraw the Hart-Scott-Rodino Act filing. Seven cases resulted in a court or administrative challenge. In three cases, the parties agreed to a consent decree.

In August 1996, the Antitrust Division of the U.S. Department of Justice and the Federal Trade Commission issued their current guidelines, "Statements of Antitrust Enforcement Policy in Health Care," consisting of nine statements that outline general enforcement policies regarding certain types of practices of health care providers. The 1996 Statements, which revised earlier guidelines, specify how agencies will apply the antitrust laws to nine types of conduct of hospitals, physicians, nursing homes, and other providers, such as joint purchasing, information exchange, and formation of physician-hospital organizations.

The ninth policy statement applies to any organization composed of various types of providers that combine to jointly offer health care services. The agencies recognize that the most common form of this type of organization is the physician–hospital organization (PHO), but the statement also provides considerable insight into how the agencies would assess the competitive effects of a partially-integrated IDS.

According to the statement, if members of the network offer only complementary or unrelated services, they do not compete and there will be no antitrust concerns. If the network is formed by a group composed of competing providers, however, the antitrust agencies are concerned that the network may interfere with competition and with the market efficiencies that competition protects.

The antitrust agencies therefore may challenge a partially-integrated IDS if it is composed of providers that otherwise would compete for the services that the IDS provides. The agencies also may be concerned that the IDS's operational integration in delivering services to patients under the IDS contracts increases the likelihood that the participating providers will compete less aggressively in delivering services to patients outside the network. To address these concerns, the antitrust agencies identified ways in which a partially-integrated IDS may be structured to create incentives for providers to operate efficiently even in the absence of competition.

Creation of a Risk-Sharing Integrated Delivery System

From an antitrust perspective, providers in a partially-integrated IDS must share "substantial" financial risk. The antitrust agencies will regard these providers as risk-sharing if the compensation each receives through the IDS depends on the overall performance of the IDS as a whole.

Although many different types of compensation structures could be established to ensure an appropriate level of risk-sharing, the 1996 Statements identify at least four different financial structures that might satisfy this requirement. In one way or another, all of these financial structures are designed so that the ultimate profitability of the IDS and its members will depend on their efficient delivery of care.

- The IDS could agree to accept a capitation payment for each enrollee, agreeing to furnish all services that each enrollee requires under that payment, regardless of the amount of services required.
- The IDS could agree to furnish specified services to members of a health plan for a predetermined percentage of the revenues of the plan.
- The IDS could use a modified fee-for-service compensation system that includes significant financial incentives (e.g., fee withholds or financial penalties) to induce its members, as a group, to meet certain cost-containment goals defined, for example, in terms of utilization or costs.
- The IDS could receive a fixed amount for a "package" of complex or extended services delivered by its participating providers, even though

services may require numerous providers and the aggregate cost of furnishing services might vary significantly from patient to patient.

Perhaps the best example of the fourth of these arrangements is the formation of a system consisting of a hospital, OB/GYNs, pediatricians, and anesthesiologists that collectively agree to furnish all necessary prenatal, delivery, and postdelivery services to enrollees for a fixed fee.

As an alternative, the antitrust agencies suggest that an IDS may be able to adopt and strictly enforce clinical standards that would guarantee the efficient delivery of care, even in the absence of risk-sharing or competition. Multispecialty providers have been wary of clinical integration, however, because self-policing of compliance with clinical standards is financially and professionally burdensome. The problem is that it is difficult, if not impossible, to apply a single set of standards to the practice patterns of many different types of providers. Therefore, to date, no IDS (partially- or fully-integrated) has been formed using clinical integration as a surrogate for competition or for risk-sharing.

Antitrust Evaluation of a Risk-Sharing IDS

In the ninth policy statement the agencies also set forth the standards they will use to determine whether a risk-sharing IDS unreasonably restrains competition. The agencies identified three groups—individual providers, traditional insurance and managed care plans, and multiprovider organizations—on whose operations a risk-sharing IDS could have anticompetitive effects, and they have outlined how the agencies will evaluate the markets for these groups.

Individual providers. The agencies will examine if an IDS will limit competition in the markets for services furnished by its member hospitals and physicians. For example, the participating hospitals and physicians could surreptitiously use the IDS to fix prices for services they furnish not only to IDS enrollees, but also to nonenrollees. Similarly, if the IDS enrolls a large percentage of the area's population, it could effectively limit the competitive strength of providers that do not participate in the IDS by excluding them from participation in the IDS.

A partially-integrated IDS can reduce these antitrust risks in three ways:

- Ensure that participation in the IDS does not involve an unnecessarily large number of the hospitals, general practitioners, specialists, or other providers in the area
- Have participating providers agree to give the IDS's central administration exclusive access to all pricing data that they must submit for use in the bidding process and in setting payment levels to individual members
- Ensure that limiting participation in the IDS does not prevent nonparticipating providers from effectively competing in the delivery of health care services to non-IDS enrollees. For example, if an IDS enters into exclusive contracts with too many payers, a non-IDS provider may be precluded from marketing its services to enough patients to become or remain a viable business.

Insurance and managed care plans. The antitrust agencies are concerned that certain conditions that an IDS might impose for participation in its network, such as exclusive contracts, could have an anticompetitive effect on traditional insurance and managed care plans in the IDS's market. Depending on the number of specialists in an area, the use of exclusive contracts may make it more difficult for other insurance plans to compete with the IDS.

The agencies have stated explicitly that they will examine numerous factors to determine if an IDS is truly nonexclusive. Thus, for example, even if the IDS's organizational documents do not contain exclusivity provisions, the antitrust agencies will evaluate if the participating providers actually contract with other payers or whether they earn a significant portion of their income from other payers.

Multiprovider organizations. The antitrust agencies may assess whether an IDS will limit the formation and competition of other IDSs. In urban areas, this situation can arise if the IDS is formed by more providers than are truly necessary to furnish covered services to its enrollees. The excessive participation of any type of provider in an individual IDS—more than one hospital, an unusually large percentage of general practitioners in the area, or all of a particular specialty—will make the formation of other IDSs more difficult, thus impairing competition.

The partially-integrated IDS model appeals to providers because it allows them the flexibility to pursue risk contracts as a single entity that can provide the continuum of service, while maintaining the operational independence to pursue other contracts as individual organizations. However, providers considering formation of this type of IDS should be aware of the attendant antitrust issues and carefully structure both their negotiations and the organization, and seek advice of legal counsel, to minimize their antitrust risks. Although the 1996 Statements appear to give providers a degree of flexibility in creating such an organization, providers should be extremely cautious in taking advantage of this apparent flexibility and be prepared for close scrutiny of the arrangement by antitrust agencies.

Clayton Act

Section 7 of the Clayton Act prohibits mergers and acquisitions that may substantially lessen competition "in any line of commerce . . . in any section of the country (The Clayton Antitrust Act of 1914)." Enacted in 1914, the Clayton Act made price discrimination, tying and exclusive dealing contracts, mergers of competing companies, and interlocking directorates illegal, but not criminal.

In 1950, Congress modified Section 7 of the Clayton Act with the Celler-Kefauver Act, proscribing one company from acquiring part or all of assets of a competitor where such an action could result in substantially lessening competition or creating a monopoly. In 1980, Congress further modified Section 7 of the Clayton Act, extending its reach to any person subject to Federal Trade Commission (FTC) jurisdiction, thus adding partnerships and sole proprietorships.

Unlike the Sherman Act, enforcement of the Clayton Act involves only civil remedies. Whereas the Department of Justice directly enforces actions of the Sherman Act, both the Department of Justice and the Federal Trade Commission enforce the Clayton Act. The Department of Justice can bring equitable actions in federal district courts to prevent and hinder acts limiting competition, and the FTC may enforce its actions through both its own agency, administrative hearings, and the federal district courts. Also, private parties may bring their own treble damages actions for injuries resulting from Section 7 violations.

As an example, consider Glaxo's 1995 acquisition of Wellcome. The FTC was concerned that the companies were competitors in a highly-concentrated market for a specific type of advancement in migraine treatment. The Commission alleged that the acquisition would eliminate actual competition between the two companies in researching and developing migraine remedies. The Commission also alleged that the acquisition would reduce the number of research and development tracks for these migraine remedies and increase Glaxo's unilateral ability to reduce research and development of these drugs.

Glaxo and Wellcome reached an agreement with the Commission that allowed them to proceed with their merger. The agreement required the combined firm to divest Wellcome's assets related to the research and development of the migraine remedy. Among those assets were patents, technology, manufacturing information, testing data, research materials, and customer lists. The assets also included inventory needed to complete all trials and studies required to obtain FDA approval. The acquirer, Zeneca Pharmaceuticals, had to be approved by the Commission. The Commission's purpose in requiring this divestiture was to ensure continued research and development of Wellcome's potential product in the same manner in which the product would be developed without the merger. The Commission believed the remedy would lessen the anticompetitive effects of the merger.

The Glaxo merger remedy has been successful. Zeneca received FDA approval for its migraine drug, marketed under the name Zomig, within fifteen months after the Commission approved Glaxo's application to divest its migraine drug assets to Zeneca.

ANTITRUST POLICY STATEMENTS

1992 DOJ/FTC Horizontal Merger Guidelines

Because the Department of Justice and Federal Trade Commission have joint antitrust enforcement duties, the two agencies issued joint guidelines in 1992 to demonstrate their uniformity in approach in the application of standards of review. The agencies' intention was to provide guidance to merger participants on the agencies' analytical approach to protecting free-market competition by preventing anticompetitive activities, while simultaneously reducing barriers to efficiency-enhancing activities designed to promote competition. The agencies stated their joint view: merger enforcement must prevent anticompetitive mergers without interfering with pro-competitive or neutral mergers.

In the guidelines, the agencies described their enforcement policy relative to the Sherman, Clayton, and Federal Trade Commission Acts, and emphasized the need to apply the guidelines to the specific facts of each case. Unlike the courts, the agencies did not assign burdens of production or proof to the parties, but instead applied a five-step methodology outlined in the guidelines for analyzing the specific facts of each merger.

The guidelines provide a general analytical methodology used by the agencies in deciding if the agencies will challenge a merger. First, the agencies determine whether the merger will increase concentration in a market already concentrated. If not, then the analysis generally will not proceed any further. However, if so, then the agencies will assess if increased concentration raises anticompetitive concerns. Next, the agencies will consider whether another competitor can make a timely market entry, to deter or counteract the competitive concern. Then, the agencies will assess any efficiencies that would be gained solely as a result of the proposed merger. Finally, the agencies will ask if either merging party would fail absent the merger, resulting in the failing party's assets exiting the market.

The guidelines describe a positive relationship between market concentration and power: the greater the market concentration, then generally the greater the market power a firm can exert. The agencies must define the product market (the same products or services produced or sold by competitive firms, close substitutes, or other firms which could produce the products or services with little effort), and the relevant product market (the smallest group of products for which a seller can impose a "small but significant and non-transitory" increase in price). Then the agencies will determine for each product market, the geographic market in which the firms operate (this geographic market being a region where a hypothetical monopolist could cause a small, but significant nontransitory increase in price).

After determining the product and geographic markets, the agencies will determine the market shares held by the participants in those markets, and then examine those shares using the Herfindahl-Hirshman Index (HHI). The agencies will consider both the pre-merger HHI, and the post merger increase in HHI. In a highly concentrated market (HHI over 1800), an increase of over 50 points raises concern; an increase over 100 points creates a presumption of market power

—that the ability to influence market prices. The agencies have noted market share and market concentration represent only a starting point for analysis.

The guidelines identify market ease-of-entry as one factor mitigating anticompetitive concerns created by high HHIs or increases in HHIs. The agencies note that if participants can enter the market easily, in a timely fashion, and with sufficient force, then they could deter the anticompetitive effect of high concentrations, and the market power of the merged firms.

The guidelines suggest that if a merger the agencies might otherwise challenge can demonstrate significant efficiencies, then the agencies will not challenge that merger. Examples of suggested acceptable efficiencies include economies of scale, reduction in expenses, or integration of facilities. However, the guidelines note if the merging firms could achieve those efficiencies by other means than a merger, then the agencies will reject those efficiencies.

As a final element in merger analysis, the agencies will consider if one of the merging firms will fail if the merger does not take place, and whether that firm's assets will exit the relevant market. If so, then the merger likely will not create or enhance market power, and the agencies would not challenge the merger. However, the agencies will closely assess whether the failing firm has thoroughly explored all other alternatives to merger or acquisition.

1993 National Association of Attorneys General (NAAG) Horizontal Merger Guidelines

The Horizontal Guidelines of the National Association of Attorneys General (NAAG) generally parallel the DOJ/FTC Horizontal Merger Guidelines with respect to market definition and market entry analyses. However, NAAG guidelines differ significantly by giving efficiencies much less weight, reflecting NAAG's belief that Congress intended the Clayton Act to lessen market concentration. The NAAG guidelines expressly reject efficiencies as a defense, and question whether merging firms could demonstrate efficiencies with any accuracy.

1996 Statements of Antitrust Enforcement Policy in Health Care

In 1996, the Department of Justice and the Federal Trade Commission revised the Statements of Antitrust

Enforcement Policy in Health Care, updating and expanding the previous 1993 and 1994 versions. The agencies recognized the need for specific guidelines in the health care area to prevent antitrust concerns from deterring activities that could potentially result in lower health care costs, increased competition, and increased consumer choice.

The agencies have suggested that many potential hospital mergers pose little competitive concerns and require less analysis. In fact, some providers argue that the increase in enforcement has been concurrent with the federal government's desire to lower costs in the health care environment. The providers' desire to obtain higher payments banded them together. Thus, increased enforcement leads to the balance of power being shifted to the payors.

To further facilitate competitive analysis, the agencies created so-called "antitrust safety zones" in which the agencies will not challenge mergers if the hospitals meet certain requirements.

The agencies have stressed that if the merging hospitals fall outside the safety zone, they may still not challenge the proposed merger and they will apply the five-step analytical process described earlier in the 1992 Horizontal Merger Guidelines. After applying this rule of reason analysis, the agencies have not challenged mergers in the following situations: where the merger did not increase market power because of the post-merger presence of strong competitors; where the merged hospitals could achieve cost savings not otherwise possible; and, where the merger would include a failing hospital likely to exit the market otherwise. Hospitals falling outside the safety zone can seek agency review by the DOJ or the FTC prior to the merger, for a preliminary determination of the agencies' probability of challenging the mergers.

LEARNING OBJECTIVE 6

Describe the managerial and organizational implications of the Health Insurance Portability and Accountability Act (HIPAA).

Concerns about possible misuse of individuals' health data have long plagued the health care industry. As a result, network security, privacy, and confidentiality have attracted increasing attention in recent years. This is due in equal parts to public perceptions about use of information technology in health care, and to a growing sense of dissatisfaction with managed care delivery models. Federal and state laws guarding confidentiality of medical information on paper also apply to electronic modes. As more health care organizations move their transactions online, confidentiality, security and privacy become much more critical.

The implementation of the Health Insurance Portability and Accountability Act (HIPAA), passed by Congress in 1996, requires that health care organizations take common-sense rules of privacy a step further. The new rules address every aspect of electronic medical communications—from confidentiality tenets to privacy assurances for electronic data interchange. HIPAA forces health care providers and the government to pay attention to these concerns by enacting a range of regulations against unauthorized access to electronically-stored or electronically-transmitted patient records and misuse of personal health care data.

In general, the HIPAA privacy standards were designed to accomplish three broad objectives:

- To define and limit the circumstances under which entities subject to the standards (covered entities) may use and disclose protected health information
- To establish certain individual rights regarding protected health information
- To require covered entities to adopt administrative safeguards to protect the confidentiality and privacy of protected health information

Although the law does not require the collection or electronic transmission of any health information, it does require that the standards be followed any time the transactions are conducted electronically. Becoming compliant with HIPAA rules was one of the most time-consuming tasks that health care organizations faced through 2002, when most HIPAA provisions were in place. The final rule for the HIPAA standards for privacy of individually identifiable health information was published in the *Federal Register* on December 28, 2000.

Another aspect of the HIPAA requirements, Administrative Simplification, intends to reduce the costs and administrative burdens of health care by making possible the standardized, electronic transmission of certain administrative and financial transactions that previously were carried out manually on paper. To accomplish this, the law requires the Secretary of Health and Human Services to adopt national uniform standards for these transactions. Many health care executives are concerned, however, that health care organizations will incur significant costs to meet the new requirements for safeguarding electronically-transmitted personal health information. Some providers argue that some of the same bodies that are concerned about cost containment and quality of care are forcing both providers and payers to incur additional expenses, the bulk of which are non-patient care-related expenses.

The effective date of the final rule for the HIPAA standards for electronic transactions, which is part of the requirements of the Administrative Simplification section, was October 16, 2002, for most health care organizations. This rule adopts standards for eight electronic transactions and for code sets to be used in those transactions. It also contains requirements concerning the use of these standards by health plans, health care clearinghouses, and certain health care providers. Proponents believe that the use of these standard transactions and code sets will improve the effectiveness and efficiency of the health care industry in general, by simplifying the administration of the system and enabling efficient electronic transmission of certain health information.

Some theorize that these new rules eventually will lead to the development of the computerized universal patient record. This is probably the direction in which the federal government is headed, because there is a belief that it would cut down on unnecessary, duplicative treatment. Although many facilities are contributing to the development of an electronic medical record, few institutions have fully implemented one. Meanwhile, there is no reimbursement mechanism to pay for its development.

According to the Department of Health and Human Services, about 75 percent of consumers surveyed are concerned that the use of electronic medical records will negatively affect their privacy. Even industry trade groups, such as the Medical Records Institute, agree that legislation must be passed that includes at least three critical elements:

1. The patient's right to access and correct his/her own health records
2. A requirement that health care providers maintain audit trails of who has accessed the patient record
3. The patient's right to view the audit trail of his/her records

The Joint Commission on Accreditation of Healthcare Organizations (JCAHO) also has concerned itself with the privacy of the medical record, electronic and otherwise. The JCAHO could cite an institution for not taking adequate precautions with patient data.

The HIPAA regulations are based on standard security policies found in most other industries. Adapting those rules for health care, however, poses special problems. In particular, there is a the challenge of ensuring the policies' applicability to a range of venues, from a one-physician office to a multinational corporation with 400 hospitals, all exchanging information.

In brief, the rules require that hospitals, physicians, clinics—basically any entity that uses electronic means for patient transactions—address the following areas:

* *Administration*: Develop and document policies for restricted data access, staff security training, auditing procedures, contingency plans for recovering data during disasters, and certification that third-party partners are managing patient data with the same diligence. Penalties for deliberate violations of these policies include $250,000 fines and up to ten years in prison; accidental violations incur a $100 fine per incident.
* *Confidentiality*: The issue is complicated and political, involving not just physician management of patient information, but also the myriad channels medical data traverse in the course of a typical patient encounter. For example, in addition to actual patient treatment, health care information is used for health care funding, reimbursement, quality reporting, accreditation, physician peer review, disease management, and monitoring for Medicare and Medicaid fraud and abuse.
* *Electronic signature*: Develop and implement secure, public-key/private-key encryption for security of electronic signature programs. Few commercial products, however, use this scheme due to its technical complexity. Violation penalties are the same as those for administrative infractions.
* *National identifiers*: Health care organizations must use unique identification numbers for providers, health plans, and employers. (The national unique patient identifier was placed on hold by the U.S. Congress.) The penalty for violating the rule is denial of claims.

- *Electronic data interchange*: Physicians and health care providers must adopt nine new standards for secure transmission of data between hospitals and payers. The compliance deadline was October 16, 2002 for most health care organizations.

The HIPAA privacy standards (45 CFR Part 160 Subparts A and E of Part 164) prohibit all "covered entities" from using or disclosing "individually identifiable health information" that is or has been transmitted or maintained electronically, except in certain circumstances. Unlike many medical records statutes, this requirement is not limited to the record in which the information appears, but applies to the information itself. Thus, any information transmitted by fax, telephone, computer, electronic handheld device, or any other electronic means is protected by the HIPAA standards thereafter in whatever form it might appear, including oral communications.

"Individually identifiable health information" refers to information created by or received from a health care provider, health plan, employer, or health care clearinghouse that relates to the past, present, or future physical or mental health or condition of an individual who is either identified directly or could reasonably be identified using the information.

"Covered entities" include "health care providers," "health plans," and "health care clearinghouses." "Health care provider" refers to any provider of health care services as defined in relevant Medicare provisions and to any other person or organization that furnishes, bills, or is paid for health care services or supplies in the normal course of business. "Health plan" is defined broadly to include any individual or group plan that provides or pays the cost of medical care. "Health care clearinghouse" is defined as a public or private entity that processes or facilitates the processing of nonstandard data elements of health information into standard data elements. Billing companies are considered to be health care clearinghouses.

The regulations also affect business partners of covered entities. A "business partner" is a person (or other entity) to whom the covered entity discloses protected health information to enable that person to carry out or assist with the performance of a function for the covered entity, or to perform the function on behalf of the covered entity. Examples of business partners include independent contractors or other persons or entities receiving information for the purposes noted above, including lawyers, accountants, auditors, consultants, billing firms, and other covered entities.

The rule specifies that covered entities may not disclose protected health information to business partners without "satisfactory assurances" that the business partner complies with relevant standards. Satisfactory assurances include certain contractual language that must be included in all contracts between the covered entities and the business partners. Accordingly, covered entities need to consider HIPAA provisions when drafting contracts with independent contractors.

Covered entities are required to take "reasonable steps" to ensure business partners are in compliance with the proposed regulations. Such steps are important, as a covered entity would be liable for the misdeeds of a business partner if it knew, or should have known, of those misdeeds.

LEARNING OBJECTIVE 7

List some of the penalties for non-compliance with HIPAA.

The deadline for compliance with the HIPAA Security Rule was April 2005, and the deadline for HIPAA Privacy Rule compliance was April 2003. Non-compliance with HIPAA privacy standards are punishable by civil fines of up to $25,000 per calendar year for each violation, and criminal penalties that would increase in severity based on intent (e.g., whether the entity intended to sell the information or reap personal gain from the disclosure). The latter includes a fine of up to $250,000, a 10-year prison term, or both.

Among 324 health care executives responding to a semi-annual survey by Phoenix Health Systems and the Healthcare Information and Management Systems Society (HIMSS), only 55 percent of providers and 72 percent of payers were compliant with the Security Rule as of January 2006. In the same survey, 80 percent of providers and 86 percent of payers reported that they are compliant with HIPAA Privacy Rule requirements (HIMSS, 2006).

Exceptions to HIPAA Data Disclosure Provisions

The proposed HIPAA standards set forth three general exceptions to the general prohibition of disclosure:

- Permissive disclosures
- Mandatory disclosures
- Disclosure of de-identified information

Permissive disclosures. A covered entity is permitted to disclose protected information without authorization if it is necessary to do so to carry out treatment, payment, or health care operations. This exception, however, does not apply to disclosure of psychotherapy notes or to information for purposes of research unrelated to treatment. Disclosure of protected information is also permitted without authorization for certain public-policy purposes (e.g., law enforcement, health fraud, national security, research, public health, and oversight).

The HIPAA standards were designed to make disclosure of information relatively easy for patient care purposes and more difficult for purposes other than direct health care. For example, the standards do not require authorization of disclosures that are necessary to maintain a provider's medical record, for consultation with other providers about diagnosis or treatment, or to make a referral to another provider. In addition, consent is not required for disclosure of information for payment purposes, such as description of a service that is required upon submission of a claim to ensure that payment reflects the appropriate service. Disclosure is also permitted as necessary to conduct health care operations, such as internal quality assurance.

In addition, the proposed standards include a number of policy exceptions, each having specific conditions for disclosure. These exceptions are too numerous to describe here, but an example is an allowance without individual authorization for research, provided that an institutional review board (or equivalent) has approved the research protocol and has determined that the protocol meets specified criteria regarding protected health information.

Mandatory disclosures. Covered entities are required to respond to requests by individuals to inspect or obtain a copy of their own protected information and to requests connected with a DHHS enforcement action or compliance review.

The aforementioned right of an individual applies to information held by the covered entity and any information in a business partner's record that is not duplicative of the covered entity's record. The rule states that health care providers and health plans are required to have procedures in place to enable such access, in accordance with general guidelines set forth in the HIPAA standards. A covered entity is permitted to deny an individual access to his or her own health information only in certain limited circumstances, such as where disclosure might endanger the life of the individual or another person.

De-identified information. Covered entities are allowed to strip identifiers from protected information and use and disclose such information if:

- the mechanism that would enable re-identification is not disclosed.
- the disclosing entity had no reason to think the use or disclosure of the pared-down information would lead to use or disclosure of protected information.

Minimum necessary information. Even where the DHHS proposes that disclosure be permitted, however, covered entities are required to make all reasonable efforts not to use or disclose more than the minimum amount of protected health information needed to achieve the purpose for making the disclosure. Thus, disclosure is not an all-or-nothing proposition. Rather, each disclosure is tailored on a case-by-case basis to achieve the desired purpose with the minimum amount of disclosure necessary.

This requirement has been the subject of criticism: some argue that it is excessively burdensome and costly to implement, while others suggest that it is deleterious to patient care.

Individual Rights

The rule accounts for the following rights of individuals:

A right to notice of the covered entity's information practices. This notice must include a description of:

- the uses and types of disclosures and the covered entity's policies and procedures regarding such uses and disclosures.
- certain required statements.
- the name and phone number of the covered entity's "information disclosure" contact person or office.
- the date the version of the notice was produced.

Notably, although an individual may request that certain uses and disclosures be restricted, the covered entity is not required to agree with the request. If the covered entity agrees to honor the request, however, it is legally bound to do so.

A right of access to inspect and copy protected information for as long as the information is maintained. This right correlates with the aforementioned mandatory disclosure requirement for covered entities and their business partners.

A right to receive an accounting of all disclosures made by the covered entity. This right does not apply to disclosures made for treatment, payment, or health care operations or to health oversight or law enforcement agencies. A required accounting must include:

* the date of each disclosure.
* the name and address of the recipient of the information.
* a brief description of the information disclosed.
* the purpose of the disclosure (if it was made for a purpose requested by the individual).

More importantly, the DHHS proposes that a covered entity must track all disclosures of protected information and be able to provide a list of all such disclosures to the affected individual. Although this task would be comparatively manageable as it pertains to maintenance of paper medical records, it is extremely difficult when it comes to tracking disclosures of protected information made orally in person or via telephone, computer, fax, or other electronic devices. In addition, covered entities are required to ensure that business partners meet their requirement to provide such an accounting of all disclosures upon request.

A right to request amendment and correction of inaccurate or incomplete information. An individual may request that a health plan or health care provider amend or correct protected health information for as long as the entity maintains the information.

A covered entity may deny the request if the information:

* was not created by the covered entity.
* would not be available for inspection and copying under the HIPAA standards.
* is accurate and complete.

Administrative Safeguards

Regarding the HIPAA objective that covers entities adopting administrative safeguards for protected health information, the rule established compliance guidelines that include requirements to:

* designate a privacy officer with primary responsibility for ensuring compliance with the regulations.
* establish training programs for all employees of the covered entity who may have access to protected information.
* implement appropriate policies and procedures to prevent intentional and accidental disclosures of protected information.
* establish a system for receiving and responding to complaints regarding the covered entity's privacy practices.
* implement appropriate sanctions for violations of the privacy guidelines.

The current HIPAA standards also attempt to account for differences between health care enterprises by allowing covered entities, which vary in size and type, to decide for themselves the details of the policies and procedures to use to comply with the HIPAA administrative requirements. For example, although HIPAA standards require each covered entity to appoint a privacy officer, the DHHS has left it to the covered entity to decide whether the designated person might have other responsibilities as well. A small physicians' group might have its office manager also serve as privacy officer, while a large entity may create a position with sole responsibility for privacy. Similarly, although HIPAA standards require all covered entities to implement a method of receiving complaints, a smaller entity might use a less formal process.

Implications of HIPAA for the Health Care Industry

Although the Health Insurance Portability and Accountability Act (HIPAA) was enacted in part to simplify administrative processes and reduce costs associated with claims transactions, implementation of the act initially resulted in increased operating costs for most institutions and for individuals. A large portion of these increased costs are due to consulting and legal fees, additional operations personnel, and information systems development and integration. Once the requisite processes and integrated information systems are in place, however, health care organizations should begin to enjoy the intended administrative simplification benefits.

By contrast, the continuing efforts required to ensure compliance with HIPAA privacy standards, unlike the efforts to meet the HIPAA's administrative simplification requirements, represent significant costs to health care organizations for implementation and ongoing maintenance of compliance systems and processes that may not necessarily be offset by future savings.

The HIPAA standards also impede the flow of information because of the limits they impose on access to information. Moreover, the need to comply with the new standards adds complexities to ensuring the free flow of information among certain health care professionals and institutions trying to coordinate patient care.

Another difficult challenge involves ensuring HIPAA compliance of the individuals, business partners, and associates with which health care organizations often must share patient information (e.g., vendors, attorneys, and consultants). It is difficult for health care organizations to monitor or to influence the compliance of these outside entities even though they will have the potential to create compliance problems for health care organizations. To address this concern, health care organizations need to craft written contracts governing privacy issues where none may exist today. Moreover, numerous amendments to existing contracts have been effected to ensure compliance. New terms and conditions have to be negotiated, and legal counsel needs to be consulted.

Among the most difficult issues are the requirements that covered entities provide individuals with effective notice and an accounting of all disclosures, and that they submit to requests by individuals to amend or correct information. Meeting these requirements is a herculean administrative task, especially if compliance must extend to e-communications.

Finally, the implications of the standards for e-health companies are particularly significant. Telemedicine, videostreaming, e-connectivity, and other e-health activities are affected in that e-health companies that provide such services to covered entities are required to enter into written agreements obligating them to abide by HIPAA requirements.

The privacy standards seek to provide necessary protections for individuals with respect to personal information about their health status and other health-related concerns. The hope is that such protections will facilitate the free flow of information without being unreasonably obtrusive. One of the biggest challenges is to ensure that these much-needed protections do not interfere with the standardization, consistency, and information sharing that health care providers require to ensure the provision of effective care.

LEARNING OBJECTIVE 8

Describe the major provisions of the Stark II laws and the safe harbor regulations.

Stark II Laws

Two distinct, but overlapping federal statutes are designed to prevent conflicts of interest in Medicare patient referrals. The Stark II law prohibits physicians from referring patients to providers with which the physician has a financial relationship and the anti-kickback statute is designed to prevent the offer or payment of bribes or other remuneration as an inducement to refer Medicare patients for treatment or services.

Both statutes are very technical and employ broad definitions that tend to ensnare providers who may be engaging in conduct that is not inherently illegal. Indeed, Congress was so concerned about the potential reach of the anti-kickback statute that it adopted legislation requiring the Centers for Medicare & Medicaid Services to promulgate safe harbor regulations.

Briefly, Stark II provides that if a physician (or an immediate family member of a physician) has a specified financial relationship with an entity (such as a health care organization), the physician may not refer Medicare or Medicaid patients to the entity to receive designated health services (e.g., clinical laboratory services, radiology services, durable medical equipment, and inpatient or outpatient hospital services), and the recipient of the referral may not present a claim for any designated health services furnished pursuant to a prohibited referral. Penalties for providers that receive prohibited referrals include denial of Medicare and Medicaid claims resulting from the referral and mandatory refunds of any amounts collected in violation of the statute. Any person who presents or causes to be presented a bill or claim for services "that such person knows or should know" is covered by the prohibition is subject to a civil monetary penalty of up to $15,000 per service, treble damages, and exclusion from Medicare and Medicaid programs.

Anti-kickback Statute

A referral that violates Stark II does not necessarily involve the payment of an illegal kickback; however, the financial relationship between the referral source and the provider that triggers the Stark II prohibition also may yield impermissible "remuneration" under the anti-kickback statute. The federal anti-kickback statute makes it a crime to knowingly and willfully offer, pay, solicit, or receive any remuneration to induce a person (1) to refer an individual to a person for the furnishing of any item or service covered under a federal health care program; or (2) to purchase, lease, order, arrange for, or recommend any good, facility, service, or item covered under a federal health care program. The term "any remuneration" encompasses any kickback, bribe, or rebate, direct or indirect, overt or covert, in cash or in kind, and any ownership interest or compensation interest.

Knowing and willful conduct is a necessary element of this criminal offense. The burden of proving intent beyond a reasonable doubt makes criminal prosecution difficult but not impossible, and the government has demonstrated some willingness to bear the criminal burden of proof. Pursuant to a 1987 congressional mandate, safe harbor regulations have been promulgated in 14 general areas to protect health care providers from an extremely vague statute.

On November 19, 1999, the Department of Health and Human Services' Office of the Inspector General ("OIG") published an array of long-awaited and widely-anticipated safe harbors to the federal anti-kickback statute. They contain (1) eight new, final safe harbors based on proposed safe harbors issued in 1993 and 1994, (2) clarification of six of the original eleven safe harbors published in 1991, and (3) two new, interim final safe harbors implementing the statutory exception to the anti-kickback statute for shared risk arrangements. As of late 2005, there were twenty-four safe harbors, in addition to three proposed safe harbors.

It is thought that the new safe harbors will provide their greatest benefit to managed care relationships, physician investments in ambulatory surgery centers, and a variety of arrangements in medically underserved areas (e.g., physician recruitment, joint ventures and hospital acquisitions of physician practices).

The clarification of certain existing safe harbors will be useful for (1) discount arrangements, because the clarifications have also expanded that safe harbor and (2) leases and personal services contracts, because the OIG is now explicitly permitting "for cause" termination provisions, even though the safe harbors otherwise require terms of at least one year.

Arrangements that come within a safe harbor are immune from prosecution under the anti-kickback statute, which is a criminal statute prohibiting the knowing and willful offer, payment, receipt, or solicitation of any remuneration to induce referrals of federal health care program-related business. Arrangements outside of any safe harbor do not necessarily violate the anti-kickback statute, but may be subject to scrutiny and potential prosecution. Historically, the OIG's safe harbors have been narrowly drawn to protect only a limited range of conduct. Although the new safe harbors continue this tradition of conservative rulemaking, they do offer significant relief in selected areas. Furthermore, in the preamble to the safe harbors, the OIG repeatedly invites parties who cannot meet a safe harbor to seek an advisory opinion on whether their arrangement is nonetheless permissible under the anti-kickback statute. The following discussion presents highlights and clarifications of the new safe harbors, but does not attempt to address every requirement in each safe harbor.

New Safe Harbors

These eight new safe harbors became effective immediately upon publication in 1999.

Investments in Ambulatory Surgical Centers

The proposed safe harbor, as originally issued, would have protected investment interests in Medicare-certified ambulatory surgical centers ("ASCs") only if they were held entirely by surgeons. The new, final safe harbor has substantially broadened this exception. Four categories of ASCs are now protected: (1) surgeon-owned ASCs, (2) single-specialty ASCs (e.g., those owned by gastroenterologists), (3) multi-specialty ASCs, and (4) hospital/physician ASCs. In each case, physician investors must disclose their investments to their patients.

The safe harbor is generally designed to protect ASCs that function as extensions of physician office practices, and will not protect investments by physicians who might refer to the ASC, but who do not personally perform ASC-covered procedures. Accordingly, physician investors are generally protected only if they are in a position to refer to the ASC, and, in fact, perform procedures there. In contrast, to meet the safe harbor for hospital/physician ASCs, *hospital* investors must *not* be in a position to make or influence referrals to the ASC. The meaning of this requirement is not clear, because according to discussion in the preamble to the safe harbor, ASCs may be located near or even on the hospital's campus (if rent is fair market value and other conditions are met). Unfortunately, the OIG offers little guidance on this issue, other than suggesting that hospitals may be able to influence the referrals of physicians employed by the hospital or by a medical practice owned by the hospital

Joint Ventures in Underserved Areas

In recognition of the fact that "medically underserved" areas (MUAs, as defined by separate regulation) often have difficulty attracting the capital necessary to build and operate health care facilities, the OIG has relaxed the conditions for the existing small entity investment safe harbor. Joint ventures in MUAs are permitted to have a higher percentage of physician ownership (up to 50 percent instead of the 40 percent limitation applicable to other geographic areas) and to allow the ventures unlimited revenues from referring investors (instead of the 40 percent limitation applicable in other geographic areas). The new, final safe harbor also expands on the earlier, proposed safe harbor by including underserved urban, as well as rural, areas.

Practitioner Recruitment in Underserved Areas

This safe harbor protects payments to recruit new and relocating physicians who establish their practice in rural or urban health professional shortage areas (HPSAs), which are designated by the Health Resources and Services Administration (the earlier, proposed safe harbor was limited to rural areas). On a helpful note, the OIG has eliminated a requirement from the proposed safe harbor that the physician must be relocating from at least 100 miles away. In addition, although the safe harbor limits the time period for recruitment payments to three years, it does not regulate the nature of the payments, such as whether they may include income guaranties, moving expenses, etc. However, the OIG specifically declined to protect (1) payments by hospitals to existing group practices to re-

cruit new physicians to the group, and (2) payments to retain physicians.

Unfortunately, the interplay between the anti-kickback statute and the federal anti-referral statute (commonly known as "Stark") will continue to complicate compliance efforts. For example, the exception for physician recruitment, as set forth in the proposed regulations to Stark, issued January 9, 1998, permits payments by a hospital to an existing medical group to recruit physicians, even though these payments are specifically excluded from the new anti-kickback statue safe harbor.

Sales of Physician Practices to Hospitals in Underserved Areas

This safe harbor allows a hospital in a HPSA to buy and "hold" the practice of a retiring physician pending recruitment of a physician to replace the one retiring. The safe harbor requires that the purchase be completed within three years and that the hospital undertake good faith efforts to recruit a replacement physician. Also, the recruitment of the replacement physician must satisfy the conditions of the safe harbor for physician recruitment.

Subsidies for Obstetrical Malpractice Insurance in Underserved Areas

This safe harbor allows hospitals (and other entities) in primary care HPSAs to pay some or all of the obstetrical malpractice insurance premiums for practitioners engaging in obstetrical practice; this includes certified nurse midwives, as well as physicians. If a practitioner engages in obstetrics part time, the safe harbor protects only payments attributable to the obstetrical portion of the practitioner's practice.

Investments in Group Practices

This safe harbor protects physician investments in their own medical group, that is if it meets the Stark definition of a "group practice." (Unfortunately, the Stark definition of a group practice is intricate, complex, and not yet established in final regulations.) This new safe harbor does not protect investments made by the group in other entities (e.g., laboratories, imaging centers). Unfortunately, this new safe harbor potentially creates as many problems as it resolves. This is because, particularly before the promulgation of the Stark legislation, it was widely believed that for purposes of the anti-kickback statute there was no such thing as a referral among physicians within an integrated medical group. This was because the patients were patients of the group, a single legal entity. Even the OIG states elsewhere in the preamble to the new safe harbors that "the anti-kickback statute is not implicated when payments are transferred within a single corporate entity . . ." (CFR, November 19, 1999, p. 63520). In fact, the OIG notes in the preamble that most public commenters questioned the need for a safe harbor to protect physician investments in their own medical groups. The OIG, however, states that the anti-kickback statute "is implicated" (CFR, November 19, 1999, p. 63524) by physician ownership interests in medical groups, and even ownership interests in single shareholder professional corporations, although the OIG does not consider either of these investment interests to be "suspect per se" (CFR, November 19, 1999, p. 63540). Physicians, no doubt, will take little comfort from the OIG's statement that owning a medical practice is not, in and of itself, suspect under the anti-kickback statute. Unfortunately, physicians that do not meet the definition of a group practice under Stark (even if they comply with Stark because they meet other Stark exceptions) must now consider whether they may be violating the anti-kickback statute because they are outside of the applicable safe harbor.

Specialty Referral Arrangements Between Providers

This safe harbor protects certain arrangements whereby one provider (which may be any individual or entity) refers a specific patient to another provider for specialty services, with the understanding that the specialty services provider will refer the patient back to the original provider when the course of treatment by the specialist is completed (assuming it is clinically appropriate to do so). Among other things, the safe harbor requires that (1) the services be within the expertise of the referred party and not the referring party, (2) the parties receive no payments from each other for the referral, and (3) the only payments either party receives are from the patient or third-party payors for services that party performs.

Cooperative Hospital Services Organizations

This safe harbor protects cooperative hospital service organizations (CHSOs) that qualify for tax exemption under Section 501(e) of the Internal Revenue Code. CHSOs are formed by two or more tax-exempt hospitals to provide certain shared services (e.g., purchasing, billing or clinical services) to the hospitals that form them. The safe harbor will protect certain payments between the CHSO and the hospitals that form the CHSO from scrutiny under the anti-kickback statute.

Clarification of Existing Safe Harbors

In 1994, the OIG issued a proposed clarification of six of the original eleven safe harbors, which had been issued in 1991. In addition, the proposed clarification would have added a rule providing that sham transactions "entered into or employed for the purpose of appearing to fit within a safe harbor when the substance of the transaction or device is not accurately reflected by the form" (42 CFR Part 1001, Sec. 1001.954) would not qualify for immunity from prosecution under the anti-kickback statute. The OIG has withdrawn this proposed rule, which engendered a firestorm of criticism from the health care industry when it was issued, and was widely derided as the "unsafe" harbor. However, the OIG continues to caution that it will look at both the form and the substance of an arrangement to determine whether it meets a safe harbor. For example, a services contract that otherwise appears to meet the safe harbor will not protect the parties if they do not intend the services described in the contract to actually be provided, and they are not, in fact, provided.

Large and Small Entity Investments

The existing safe harbor for investments in large and small entities has been refined in five ways: (1) only assets or revenues relating to health care will count toward the $50,000,000 asset requirement for "large" entities or the 60-40 revenue test for small entities (i.e., the requirement that no more than 40 percent of revenue may come from referrals or business generated by investors); (2) the prohibition of small entities loaning funds to investors to acquire their interests is extended to prohibit loans to an investor from other investors or persons acting "on behalf of" the entity or an investor; (3) the current prohibition of more than 40 percent of "each class" of a small entity's investors being in a position to refer to the entity has been modified to permit equivalent classes of investment to be aggregated; (4) the 60-40 revenue test for small entities has been modified so that it counts only referred business toward the 40 percent limitation, i.e., it no longer counts revenue from items or services furnished by an investor to the venture; and (5) interests acquired in "large" entities must be on terms available to the general public with regard to (a) restrictions on transferability, and (b) price. These changes to the existing safe harbor closely follow the proposed clarification issued in 1994. These changes tighten requirements in some areas and loosen them in others, but by and large they constitute "fine tuning" that is unlikely to have a major impact on the manner in which investment interests are structured, except for businesses for whom health care is only a small sideline. In these cases, the business may be somewhat handicapped by the exclusion of non-health assets and revenues in satisfying applicable requirements.

Space and Equipment Rentals and Personal Services and Management Contracts

The OIG is making the same two changes to each of (1) the space rental safe harbor, (2) the equipment rental safe harbor, and (3) the safe harbor for personal services and management contracts. These two changes are already reflected in the comparable Stark exceptions for these types of arrangements. The first change expands the existing requirement that the lease or contract specify the premises, equipment, or services covered, with a requirement that the lease or contract cover all of the premises, equipment, or services leased or provided between the parties during the term of the lease or contract. The OIG explains that this new requirement is to prevent "schemes involving the use of multiple overlapping contracts." The second change is the addition of a new requirement that the aggregate space, equipment, or services provided must be reasonably necessary to accomplish "commercially reasonable business" practices. The latter requirement is meant to prevent parties from renting space or equipment or purchasing services that have no intrinsic value to the lessee or purchaser other than as a way of paying for referrals.

Referral Services

This safe harbor receives one minor change, which was proposed in 1994. The preamble indicates that the one public comment received regarding the proposed change was favorable. The change is from a prohibition of referral service charges based on "referrals to or business otherwise generated by the participants for the referral service" to a prohibition of charges based on referrals of business generated by either party for the other party. The world will continue much as it did

before this clarification became law (CFR, November 19, 1999, p. 63526).

Discount Arrangements

The discount safe harbor, which is probably the most complex and confusing of the 23 safe harbors, has been significantly modified in a number of respects to make it easier to use and to broaden its application. This is welcome relief for those who struggle to apply this exception to the myriad of commercially common discounting arrangements. In recognition that some parties that offer discounts are intermediaries, and not, strictly speaking, buyers or sellers, the safe harbor has been expanded to include "offerors." All parties to discount transactions (i.e., buyers, sellers and offerors) can now come within the safe harbor by meeting the separate requirements applicable to them. One of the greatest concerns raised by the original safe harbor was that a seller's ability to come within the safe harbor was contingent on the buyer's compliance, which, of course, is not within the seller's control. Now, a seller can satisfy the safe harbor, even if its buyers do not, so long as the seller informs the buyer "in a manner reasonably calculated to give the buyers notice of their reporting obligations" (CFR, November 19, 1999, p. 63527) of the buyer's reporting obligations under the safe harbor.

Another change from the original rule permits discounts to be offered to a beneficiary, if other requirements of the safe harbor are met. (Previously, discounts to beneficiaries were ineligible under the safe harbor.) Routine waivers of deductibles or coinsurance, however, are not protected. Another significant, beneficial change modifies the old rule's prohibition of discounts offered on one good or service to induce the purchase of a different good or service. As modified, the rule permits mixing discounts on different goods and services so long as "the goods and services are reimbursed by the same Federal health care program using the same methodology and the reduced charge is fully disclosed to the Federal health care program and accurately reflected where appropriate, and as appropriate, to the reimbursement methodology. . ." (CFR, November 19, 1999, p. 63554).

A number of other changes are of a more editorial variety, such as correcting a "technical error" from the original rule (these are generally referred to by those outside of the government as "typos"). Over all, the changes made to the discount safe harbor are among the more significant of the clarifications to the original safe harbors.

Shared Risk Safe Harbors

In 1996, Congress added a statutory exception to the anti-kickback statute for certain shared risk arrangements, and directed the OIG to develop regulations to implement the exception through a negotiated rulemaking process. Comprised of industry and government representatives, a negotiated rulemaking committee developed a joint committee statement, issued in January 1998, to reflect the committee's agreement and serve as guidance for the OIG's rulemaking. The OIG has now issued two interim, final rules based on the committee statement.

The first interim final rule protects virtually any financial arrangement between an eligible managed care organization (EMCO) (i.e., one that is compensated on a capitated basis by a federal health care program), and any of its direct contracting providers. In addition, the rule protects any of their next tier "downstream" direct contracting sub-providers, so long as certain requirements are met. These requirements are that the agreement between the EMCO or "upstream" provider and the "downstream" sub-provider must: (1) be set out in writing and signed by the parties, (2) specify the items and services covered by the agreement, (3) be for a period of at least one year, and (4) specify that the "downstream" provider cannot claim payment in any form from a federal health care program. In addition, remuneration under (or outside of) the agreement may not be used in return for or to induce referral of federal health care program-covered business (other than that covered under the arrangement) for which payment is made on a fee-for-service basis. This rule will protect a substantial portion of managed care arrangements involving federal health care program business.

The second final interim rule protects contracting arrangements between certain qualified managed care plans (QMCPs) and their contractors and subcontractors when the latter mentioned parties are at "substantial financial risk" for the cost or utilization of items or services they provide or order for federal health care program beneficiaries. The term "substantial financial risk" is defined in two basic ways under the new rule: by payment methodology (e.g., capitation, percentage of premium and DRG payments) and by a numeric standard (i.e., if a certain percentage of the provider's compensation is subject to a withhold). The numeric

threshold is met for hospitals and nursing homes if their total potential compensation is at least 10% greater than their minimum compensation. For all other providers, maximum potential compensation must be at least 20% greater than minimum compensation.

Ultimately, this second "shared risk" safe harbor may have very limited use. In fact, the OIG candidly admits this. The reason is that in most managed care arrangements (except for arrangements that are downstream from federal health care program managed care plans and thus already covered by the first interim final rule), virtually all providers are reimbursed on a fee-for-service basis by federal health care programs.

Criminal penalties for violations of the Stark II and anti-kickback statute include up to five years imprisonment, plus fines up to $25,000 for each violation. In addition, all claims for reimbursement made while an illegal kickback arrangement exists may constitute false claims under the False Claims Act. This is because the provider would have falsely certified that it is in compliance with all Medicare billing requirements by submitting claims and filing cost reports, whether or not the related services were induced by the legal remuneration. Thus, providers are exposed to *qui tam* actions for anti-kickback and Stark violations because private plaintiffs can use the Medicare certification of compliance procedures to bootstrap claims that are actionable under the False Claims Act.

New Civil Monetary Penalty

In addition to the criminal penalties and the sanction of exclusion from the Medicare program, the Balanced Budget Act of 1997 (BBA) created a civil monetary penalty for anti-kickback violations. The civil penalty is treble damages (three times the illegal remuneration), plus $50,000 per violation, plus possible exclusion from Medicare. The government can now impose exorbitant fines for anti-kickback violations that it proves with a simple preponderance of the evidence, a standard much easier to satisfy than the criminal standard of "beyond a reasonable doubt." The government is more likely to pursue anti-kickback prosecutions now that a lower civil burden of proof applies.

Stacked Penalties

The government has successfully contended that violating either Stark II or the anti-kickback statute also may constitute making a false statement or the submission of false claim under the False Claims Act. The primary theory in these cases is that a provider that submits a claim to the government (e.g., in a cost report) is certifying, either implicitly or explicitly, that all services or items were provided in accordance with applicable laws, such as Stark II or the anti-kickback statute.

Under this characterization, the violation of the statute or regulation is a material fact that, if disclosed, would have affected the government's payment of the claim, thus making it actionable under the False Claims Act. Although the merits of this "stacking" concept are not yet fully developed, a provider must consider False Claims Act implications whenever a possible Stark II or anti-kickback statute violation is discovered. It is important to understand that linking Stark II and the anti-kickback statute with the False Claims Act greatly increases the likelihood that the provider will be sued. Under the *qui tam* provisions of the False Claims Act, an employee or other person (i.e., a relator), who is aware that false claims have been made, may bring an action in the name of the government and, if successful, retain a portion of the recovery.

By the time news of a Stark II problem reaches a provider's executives or counsel, it is highly likely that many other people within the organization know of the problem. The longer a provider waits to resolve the problem, the greater the likelihood that a whistleblower will file an action under the False Claims Act. In these situations, management must act quickly to determine if violations have occurred.

Counsel should be contacted as early as possible to assist in evaluating the issues and minimizing the dissemination of potentially damaging information among nonprivileged persons. Management and counsel need to determine whether to publicly disclose the violations and/or repay any overpayments or, if warranted, explain to the investigators why violations have not occurred.

Although most providers are aware of the False Claims Act's *qui tam* provisions, senior management rarely considers the threat of a *qui tam* lawsuit when the underlying compliance issues do not involve fraud in the traditional sense, such as upcoding or fraudulent invoices. A provider now must consider if its failure to comply with technical, prophylactic regulations, such as those under the Stark II law, has created an incentive for an employee, competitor, patient, or other person to bring a false claims action based solely on such regulatory violations.

In addition, stacking greatly increases the extent of the defendant's exposure and, conversely, the government's leverage. Violators of the False Claims Act face civil monetary penalties of $5,000 to $10,000 per violation, plus treble damages. The criminal penalties include up to five years in prison and/or a fine. A corporate official who uncovers potential violations of Stark II or the anti-kickback statute must consider the potential for these additional penalties when evaluating a provider's exposure and planning a corrective course of action.

LEARNING OBJECTIVE 9

List the major components of compliance and internal control programs.

MANAGEMENT RESPONSIBILITY FOR COMPLIANCE

Internal Control

As described by the American Institute of Certified Public Accountants (AICPA), "internal control is a process effected by an entity's board of directors, management, and other personnel designed to provide reasonable assurance regarding the achievement of objectives in the following categories: reliability of financial reporting, effectiveness and efficiency of operations, and compliance with applicable laws and regulations" (AICPA, p. 68). This definition emphasizes the fact that internal control is a function of the board, management, and other personnel within the organization. The responsibility for internal control rests squarely on management's shoulders.

The AICPA identifies the five interrelated components of internal control as:

- Control environment sets the tone of an organization, influencing the control consciousness of its people. It is the foundation for all other components of internal control, providing discipline and structure.
- Risk assessment is the entity's identification and analysis of relevant risks to achievement of its

objectives, forming a basis for determining how the risks should be managed.

- Control activities are the policies and procedures that help ensure that management directives are carried out.
- Information and communication are the identification, capture, and exchange of information in a form and time frame that enable people to carry out their responsibilities.
- Monitoring is a process that assesses the quality of internal control performance over time.

Corporate Compliance Programs

The Office of the Inspector General (OIG) of the Department of Health and Human Services strongly recommends adopting a corporate compliance plan because it helps reduce the risk of compliance errors and can limit the liability of directors and management. An effective plan can also reduce liability under the Federal Sentencing Guidelines. Best of all, a corporate compliance plan helps employees follow the laws and enables management to know that the laws are being followed.

The OIG has suggested that an effective corporate compliance plan contain the following elements:

1. Adoption of reasonable compliance standards of conduct and procedures. The provider must organize its compliance materials, learn what laws and regulations govern its practices, and put in writing the steps necessary for a high-level compliance officer to ensure the provider obeys the law.
2. Appointment of a high-level compliance officer. For the plan to be effective, this officer must be someone who can insist upon compliance from anyone in the organization, therefore, this role should be by someone at the highest level of management.
3. Education and systematic compliance training of employees.
4. Development of effective lines of communication. There must be easy access to the compliance officer so that problems can be reported and corrected. There must also be the guarantee that employees can report compliance issues without fear of retaliation. In larger organizations, experts

suggest a 24-hour hotline so employees can report problems anonymously.

5. Consistent and continuous enforcement of compliance standards through well-publicized disciplinary standards. The OIG suggests that every plan contain disciplinary standards so there are consequences for serious deviations from the organization's standards of conduct. Disciplinary standards should apply not just for the employee who erred, but also for the supervisor who failed to detect the problem. The OIG also suggests that employers use background checks for new employees to ensure that they have not previously been involved in health care fraud. The OIG is setting up a national data bank that lists people who have been sanctioned for health care fraud.
6. Development of auditing and monitoring programs. A monitoring program should include regular reports to the compliance officer and to senior management. For larger organizations, this program will probably include compliance audits by internal or by outside auditors who are expert in federal billing regulations.
7. Development of a mechanism for reporting detected violations to the appropriate agency and for correcting the problem prospectively. Information about the guidelines for compliance can be found at the OIG website, http://oig.hhs.gov/fraud/complianceguidance.html.

To have an effective compliance plan, all employees must be aware of it. The OIG will survey employees when auditing an institution.

To develop an effective plan, the first step should be to assess areas of risk facing the organization. For example, while almost any health care provider could legitimately worry about tax, antitrust, environmental, employment, intellectual property, confidentiality, licensing and controlled substance issues, designing an all-encompassing compliance plan is likely to be too difficult to achieve at one time.

The greatest risk for most organizations is erroneous or fraudulent billing. In these cases, the first phase of plan development should be to get a snapshot of the organization's billing practices. The risk analysis should usually be made under the supervision of the organization's lawyers.

Problems will develop at an institution when their employee-agents perpetuate frauds that are relatively commonplace, such as billing for services of physicians who inadequately supervise medical residents, or spend inadequate time with patients. The facility will be culpable unless it has an adequate compliance plan and it did not know or should have known about their employees' behavior.

After the risk areas are identified, a written compliance plan should be developed. The plans are most effective when everyone who is part of the billing process gives his input and the values of the individual organization are included in the code of standards. The written plan should then be distributed to all personnel and training should commence.

Once the plan is operative, it will be effective only if it includes management support, effective communication, continuous monitoring, and individual accountability. Federal prosecutors have made it clear that simply having an elegant, but unused plan on the shelf of the practice manager will be regarded as worse than having no plan at all. Developing a plan can take anywhere from several months for a small medical practice to about a year for a large hospital. The protection afforded by such a plan makes the investment of time and resources well worth the effort.

SUMMARY

This chapter provides an overview of the major rules and regulations related to health care. This material should give the financial manager an appreciation for the increasing complexity of the legal and regulatory environment in health care. A prudent manager must plan for and adapt to this environment. As shown in the examples cited in the chapter, failure to comply can put an organization at significant financial risk. Proper planning, implementation, execution, and evaluation of corporate compliance programs is vital for the financial security of today's health care organizations.

REFERENCES

United States Department of Justice, Office of the Deputy Attorney General (1998) *Health Care Fraud Report: Fiscal Year 1997*, http://www.justice.gov/dag/pubdoc/health97.htm

Social Security Act, Title XI, §1128B [42 U.S.C. 1320a-7b(a)(3). "Criminal Penalties for Acts Involving Federal Health Care Programs." http://www.ssa.gov/OP_Home/ssact/title11/1128B.htm

The Clayton Act of 1914, 15 U.S.C. § 12-27, 29 U.S.C. § 52-53

Health Insurance Portability and Accountability Act of 1996 (HIPAA), Public Law 104–191.

U.S. Department of Health and Human Services, Office for Civil Rights, 45 CFR Parts 160 and 164. "Standards for Privacy of Individually Identifiable Health Information Regulation Text; Security Standards for the Protection of Electronic Protected Health Information; General Administrative Requirements Including, Civil Money Penalties: Procedures for Investigations, Imposition of Penalties, and Hearings." December 28, 2000 as amended: May 31, 2002, August 14, 2002, February 20, 2003, and April 17, 2003. Available on the Internet: http://www.hhs.gov/ocr/combinedregtext.pdf

HIMSS and Phoenix Health Systems. (Winter 2006). "US Healthcare Industry HIPAA Compliance Survey Results: Winter 2006." Available on the Internet: http://www.hipaadvisory.com/action/surveynew/results/Winter2006.htm

U.S. Department of Health and Human Services, Office of Inspector General. (November 19, 1999). 42 CFR Part 1001, "Medicare and State Health Care Programs: Fraud and Abuse; Clarification of the Initial OIG Safe Harbor Provisions and Establishment of Additional Safe Harbor Provisions Under the Anti-Kickback Statute; Final Rule. Vol. 64, No. 223. Available on the Internet: http://oig.hhs.gov/fraud/docs/safeharborregulations/getdoc1.pdf

U.S. Department of Health and Human Services, Office of Inspector General. (July 21, 1994). 42 CFR Part 1001, Sec. 1001.954, "Medicare and State Health Care Programs: Fraud and Abuse; Clarification of the OIG Safe Harbor Anti-Kickback Provisions." Available on the Internet: http://oig.hhs.gov/fraud/docs/safeharborregulations/072194.htm

The American Institute of Certified Public Accountants. (2005). Healthcare Organizations Audit and Accounting Guide. New York. http://oig.hhs.gov/fraud/complianceguidance.html.

ASSIGNMENTS

1. What is the distinction between fraud and abuse? Give four examples of fraud or abuse.

2. What is the required behavior of hospitals under EMTALA law? How can the obligation to the patient be ended?

3. What is the purpose of antitrust laws? Identify and describe the main sources of antitrust law in the U.S.

4. What is HIPAA? What are the objectives of the HIPAA privacy standards?

5. What is the purpose of the Stark II law?

1. Fraud consists of intentional acts of deception, whereas abuse involves improper acts that are unintentional, but which are inconsistent with standard practice.

    Four examples of fraud and/or abuse:
    - Billing for services not delivered or not medically necessary (false claims)
    - Double-billing for a single procedure
    - Improper upcoding to receive a higher reimbursement rate
    - Kickbacks for referrals or medical procedures

2. If emergency care is needed, the statute requires the hospital to medically stabilize the patient (assuming the hospital has the medical capabilities to do so), irrespective of the patient's ability to pay. Hospitals are prohibited from posting payment information in their emergency rooms. Patients who have medical conditions that the hospital is incapable of stabilizing (as certified by a physician), or who ask to be transferred to another facility before the hospital can stabilize their condition, must be transferred to another facility in accordance with specific requirements of the EMTALA law. If, after evaluation, the patient is found not to have a medical emergency, the hospital's obligation to the patient under EMTALA ends.

3. The purpose of antitrust laws is to promote a competitive, free marketplace; they are intended to protect the public from the adverse effects of monopoly power. The federal government and virtually all state governments have antitrust laws, which reflect a public policy principle that a competitive marketplace will protect consumers, restrain private economic power, and generally produce the best allocation of quality goods and services at the lowest prices.

    There are three main sources of U.S. antitrust law: the Sherman Act, the Clayton Act, and the Federal Trade Commission Act. Section 1 of the Sherman Act prohibits all conspiracies or agreements that restrain trade. Section 7 of the Clayton Act prohibits all mergers and acquisitions of stock or assets that may substantially lessen competition or that tend to create a monopoly. Section 5 of the Federal Trade Commission Act prohibits unfair methods of competition.

4. In general, the Health Insurance Portability and Accountability Act (HIPAA) privacy standards were designed to accomplish three broad objectives:

    - To define and limit the circumstances under which entities subject to the standards (covered entities) may use and disclose protected health information
    - To establish certain individual rights regarding protected health information
    - To require covered entities to adopt administrative safeguards to protect the confidentiality and privacy of protected health information

5. Stark II provides that if a physician (or an immediate family member of a physician) has a specified financial relationship with an entity (such as a health care organization), the physician may not refer Medicare or Medicaid patients to the entity to receive designated health services (e.g., clinical laboratory services, radiology services, durable medical equipment, and inpatient or outpatient hospital services), and the recipient of the referral may not present a claim for any designated health services furnished pursuant to a prohibited referral.

Chapter 5

Revenue Determination

LEARNING OBJECTIVES

After studying this chapter, you should be able to do the following:

1. Define basic methods of payment for health care firms.
2. Understand the general factors that influence pricing.
3. Define the basic health care pricing formula.
4. Determine if prices are defensible.
5. List some of the important considerations when negotiating a managed-care contract.

REAL-WORLD SCENARIO

Gary Bentham, CFO of Bartlett Community Hospital, is preparing for contract negotiation with his largest nongovernmental payer, Antrim Healthcare. Antrim currently accounts for approximately 30 percent of all patient-care revenue at Bartlett and this percentage is growing. The current contract has been in force for three years and expires on June 30th of this year. Gary has given Antrim the required 180-day notification of his intent to terminate, but is alarmed by the position taken by Antrim's chief negotiator, Alice Mullins. Alice told Gary that Antrim is unwilling to increase its present payment schedule beyond five percent. Currently, Antrim pays for inpatient care on a DRG basis, using the relative weights employed by CMS. The base payment for a case with weight of 1.0 is $2,600. Gary knows that Medicare currently pays the hospital $4,800 for a case with a weight of 1.0. While the outpatient payment from Antrim is more reasonable, Gary is concerned about the hospital's long-term financial position if the Antrim inpatient rate cannot be increased substantially.

Alice told Gary that she believes the current inpatient rate is reasonable because Medicare patients are much more resource intensive than Antrim's younger health management organization (HMO) patient population. To test this hypothesis, Gary compared the average charge by DRG for Medicare traditional patients and Antrim's HMO patients. Gary was amazed at the similarity when the data analysis was completed. He discovered that on average an Antrim patient consumed 94.5 percent of the resources of a traditional Medicare patient. Gary further concluded that since the average cost of a traditional Medicare patient with a case weight of 1.0 was $4,600, he would need a payment of $4,347 (.945 × $4,600) from Antrim to break even. If Alice is serious about her company's maximum rate increase of five percent, then the best rate that Gary could expect would be $2,730 (1.05 × $2,600, which is well below his estimated cost).

Even after Gary shared his cost analysis with Alice, Alice remained firm in her position. The best inpatient rate that Antrim will offer is $2,730. Alice told Gary that any rate higher will compromise Antrim's market position and either destroy its margins or lead to a loss of market share.

Gary must now determine what position his hospital system should take with Antrim. He knows that his system controls about 40 percent of the capacity in their market, with the remaining 60 percent controlled by a competitive system. Both systems have some excess capacity, but that excess capacity has narrowed in the last few years as both hospitals have purchased smaller hospitals and consolidated them into their operations. There are also two major health plans that compete with Antrim. Both of these plans, as well as Antrim have contracts with both systems. Gary knows that his present rates of payment from the other health plans are higher than Antrim's. He is also fairly certain that Antrim's rate of payment to his competitor is higher.

Gary is attempting to answer the following questions before his next scheduled meeting with Alice: What is his marginal or incremental cost for the Antrim book of business? Could his competitor handle his present Antrim volume, and at what cost? If Gary's system were not in Antrim's network, what percentage of his present Antrim volume would he retain? These issues and others are central to his negotiation posture with Alice and have profound implications for his hospital system.

LEARNING OBJECTIVE 1

Define basic methods of payment for health care firms.

PAYMENT METHODS AND THEIR RELATIONSHIP TO PRICE SETTING

In Chapter 3 we discussed four generic methods of payment for health care firms: historical cost, bundled services, billed charges, and capitated rates. Table 5–1 presents a scheme for categorizing payment plans by their payment basis and the unit of payment used for reimbursement. There are three payment-determination bases: cost, fee schedule, and price related. A cost-payment basis simply means that the underlying method for payment will be the provider's cost. A fee-schedule basis means that the actual payment will be pre-determined and will be unrelated to either the provider's cost or the provider's actual prices. Usually these fee schedules are negotiated in advance with the payment party or are accepted as a condition of participation in programs such as Medicare and Medicaid. A

price-related payment basis means that the provider will be paid for services based upon some relationship to its total charges or price for the services delivered to the patient. These three payment bases may have two different units of payment, either bundled services or specific services. For example, many managed-care contracts often pay for inpatient services on a per diem or DRG basis. Payment is fixed in advance, based upon an agreed fee schedule—for example, $1,000 per day to cover all services provided—and is a bundled unit of payment because the provider does not receive additional payment for provided ancillary services. This same contract may also make payment for outpatient services based upon a discount from billed charges, for example, 75 percent of billed charges. This outpatient provision is related to the provider's prices and it is based upon the prices of specific services that constitute the total claim for the patient, including radiology procedures, lab tests, and other procedures provided to the patient.

In many cases, managed-care contracts will have elements that may appear in more than one of the six cells displayed in Table 5–1. Many contracts that pay hospitals on a DRG basis will have a separate provision for outliers. Payment for outliers is often related

Table 5–1 Health Care Payment Methods

Payment-Determination Basis

Unit of Payment	Cost	Fee Schedule	Price Related
Specific services	• high-cost drugs • devices	• RBRVS • APCs	• no contract • self pay
Bundled services	• critical-access hospitals	• DRGs	• outpatient
		• per diem • OP surgery groups	• outliers

to charges. For example, a contract may stipulate that for all claims in excess of $75,000 in billed charges, the payer will pay the claim not on a DRG basis, but at 80 percent of billed charges. Assume that a claim had a DRG payment of $15,000, but the patient incurred total charges of $90,000. The payer in this case would not pay $15,000, but 80 percent of $90,000, or $72,000. An interesting case is a health plan that has not negotiated a contract with a provider. In that situation, the payment method would be billed charges and it would be related to the specific services provided. The apportionment of payment responsibility between the patient and its plan would need to be worked out because the patient may have gone out of network, but the hospital in this case would expect payment based upon billed charges.

Health care providers have three major ways that they can control their revenue function in today's economic climate. First, they can set their prices in a manner to generate the required level of revenue that they need to sustain their operations. Pricing by health care firms is still a very important element of the revenue function even though the majority of revenue may not be related to prices. For example, a nursing home may have 80 percent of its revenue derived from Medicare and Medicaid that make payments on a fixed-fee-schedule basis that is unrelated to specific prices. The remaining 20 percent of the nursing home's business is affected by its set prices, and these prices may well mean the difference between a profit and a loss. Second, contract negotiation is a critical activity for all health care firms that derive substantial portions of their revenue from commercial insurers. Any provider that negotiates rates that are lower than its costs is digging itself a deep hole from which it may not be able to recover. Finally, billing and coding issues are very

important in the current world of health care payment. Providers that fail to include delivered services on a claim will not be paid for those services. For example, if an injectable drug is administered to a patient, but the drug administration for that drug is not coded, lost payment will result. In a similar fashion, if secondary diagnosis codes are not included on a hospital claim, then the claim may be assigned to a lower-weighted DRG, resulting in lost payment.

While coding and billing issues were addressed in Chapter 2, our focus now is on the first two areas of revenue determination: pricing and managed-care contract negotiation. Improving performance in these areas will have a very positive impact on the firm's total revenue function.

LEARNING OBJECTIVE 2

Understand the general factors that influence pricing.

GENERIC FACTORS OF PRICING

Figure 5–1 provides a schematic depicting the generic factors that influence pricing in any business. The three identified factors are: desired net income, competitive position, and market structure. All of these factors influence how a firm can change its prices and to what extent they are likely to control their pricing function. The first factor, desired net income, is the starting block for most short- and long-term pricing decisions. Every business must be able to generate enough revenue through its sales of products and services to sustain its operations and provide for the

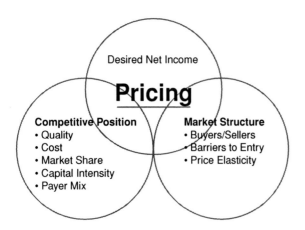

Figure 5–1 Factors Influencing Pricing

replacement of its physical assets, as well as provide a return to its investors. Failure to realize adequate levels of pricing will result in eventual business failure. Deficiencies in levels of net income can be tolerated for short time frames, but long-term continuation of inadequate pricing will eventually result in business termination.

The position of a business relative to its competitors has a significant influence upon pricing policy. One of the most important factors in any business, but especially health care, is the perceived quality of the firm's products and services. Firms with higher perceived levels of quality can often price their products and services at a slightly higher level. Specific health care providers that are perceived as quality leaders in a market place often can realize higher prices in several ways. First, these firms may be able to negotiate more favorable payment terms with major health plans in the area. Second, if the general community perceives one provider to be higher quality, employers may desire to have that provider in the plan's network of providers. It is also likely that the provider can establish prices that are above its local competitors because it knows that it has a premium quality advantage.

Lower-cost providers can afford to sell their products at lower prices and still generate adequate levels of profit, or they can sell their products at a competitive price and realize even higher profits. In either case, it usually means market expansion for the lower-cost provider. If they establish lower prices, then they should be able to increase their market share. If they maintain competitive prices, the realization of greater profit may lead to expansion in the marketplace be-

cause of better access to capital, and as a result they may even be in a position to acquire local competitors.

Market share is a critical determinant of price for any business. Most health care markets are regional in nature, and there are travel limits beyond which most consumers will not venture. Greater market share leads to greater leverage when negotiating managed-care contracts. For example, if a hospital controlled 85 percent of the acute-care capacity in the region, virtually every health plan would be required to include that hospital in its network. This gives the hospital tremendous leverage when negotiating payment terms.

Capital intensity can also have an influence on pricing. Firms that are heavily capital intensive often have higher levels of fixed costs. It is also likely that their variable cost of production as a percentage of total cost may be lower, which may lead to marginal cost pricing in markets that have excess capacity. This behavior was seen in many urban hospital markets in the early days of managed-care growth. Many hospitals would sign agreements with health plans at payment levels below their average total cost, but above their variable or marginal cost. These hospitals were afraid that they might be excluded from a plan's network and lose critical volume so they agreed to payment levels that just barely covered their variable costs.

Of all the factors discussed to this point, none has a more pervasive influence on prices than does payer mix, at least in the health care market place. Providers with heavy percentages of Medicaid and uninsured patients will usually experience large losses on these patients no matter how efficiently they produce health care services. These providers must then be in a situation where they can increase prices paid by other patients to offset losses from Medicaid and uninsured patients. This point will be emphasized later in this chapter.

The market structure in which a firm exists also influences pricing in a variety of ways. The number of buyers and sellers is a key dynamic that impacts pricing. Increasing the ratio of providers to health plans reduces the pricing flexibility of the provider. A worst-case scenario for a provider would be to be located in a market with many providers and only one buyer. In most health care markets, the government is the major buyer through its Medicare and Medicaid programs. Providers have virtually no control over payment terms. Their only choice is either to participate in the program and accept the payment rates, or to exit and seek business with non-government patients. Given the sheer size of the Medicare and Medicaid programs, this is not a choice for many providers. It is the private market that represents the major area for pricing discretion. Ideally, providers would like to operate in a market where there were no or few other providers and many small health plans. Most health care markets are not like this, and there are usually a limited number of both providers and health plans. As health plans merge and consolidate, most providers feel a similar need to merge with other provider to maintain a level negotiation playing field.

Most businesses would ideally like to operate in an environment in which significant barriers to entry exist, thus protecting them from new competitors. Large capital investment often serves as a barrier to entry. The actual level of investment required to either buy or build a hospital in an existing market can be more than $100 million. This level of capital will cause many potential competitors to think twice before entering a market in which present excess capacity exists. Certificate-of-Need regulations can also prevent new health care providers from entering a market, as well as restrict growth for existing providers. Certificate-of-Need (CON) programs are utilized by approximately 37 states to help maintain quality of care, to control a portion of the health care costs of communities, and to promote rational distribution of certain health care services. CON regulations require that individuals or health care facilities seeking to initiate or expand services submit applications to the State. Approval must be obtained before initiating projects that require capital expenditures above certain dollar thresholds, introduce new services, or expand beds or services.

The final factor affecting pricing under the market-structure umbrella is price elasticity. The concept of price elasticity describes the relationship between a change in price and demand for the service or product. Products or services for which ultimate demand is strongly influenced by price are said to be price elastic. Most products or services have some degree of price elasticity. Consumers will usually purchase fewer goods or services as prices increase. For example, if the price of coffee rises, consumption would be expected to fall. Health care services, while not immune from the pressures of price elasticity, are usually less affected than other products. When someone needs to have his appendix removed, he is concerned less about price than he would be about the cost of a cup of coffee. The

presence of health insurance has further insulated many from the effects of price in health care markets. The cost of many procedures is either completely paid or is subject to relatively small deductibles and co-payments. The rise of consumer-directed health plans has begun to affect price elasticity in health care markets. Many of these plans call for large initial deductibles of $1,000 or more. Patients in these types of plans are no longer insulated from the cost of health services, and price can become a more important factor in the decision to seek medical services.

LEARNING OBJECTIVE 3

Define the basic health care pricing formula.

PRICE SETTING FOR HEALTH CARE SERVICES

Health care firms must set rates at levels sufficient to maintain their financial viability. Prices must be set to cover the individual areas identified in Figure 5–2. Failure to develop pricing to cover all of these areas will result in eventual failure.

It hardly seems necessary to state that any price must be set to cover the average cost of producing the product or service. If it costs $500 to perform a specific-imaging procedure, pricing that service at $400 would be a sure-fire formula for insolvency. We discussed earlier that on some occasions, firms may price a product at less than cost, but more than average marginal cost. In our imaging-procedure example, the marginal cost of producing the image might be $250. In this case, the firm might price the procedure at $250 or slightly more. This price would cover the marginal cost of production, but would not cover the fixed costs of operation, such

- Average costs
- Losses on third-party fee-schedule payments
  - Medicaid
  - Medicare
  - Other
- Write-offs on billed-charge patients
  - Self-pay
  - Commercial
- Reasonable return on investment
  - Sustainable growth

Figure 5–2 Four Elements of Pricing

as depreciation, interest expense on debt, and administrative costs. So-called marginal-cost pricing would, however, cover the incremental cost of production, assuming excess capacity would contribute something to the coverage of fixed costs. In the long run, however, prices must be established to cover full costs of production.

In setting health care prices, one must also recognize that some payers may pay values less than full or average cost. For example, Medicaid may pay a nursing home $80 per day when the cost of one day of care is $100. Any price that is set not only must cover the cost of providing the service, but also must cover losses incurred on other patients such as Medicare and Medicaid. It is not just governmental programs that may have payment rates below cost. A number of major health plans may have contracts that call for payment at levels below full cost. All of the collective losses incurred on these patients must be included in the price which is finally set. Losses incurred on patients create an additional layer of cost, which ultimately raises the overall set price.

Prices must also reflect discounts from billed charges that may be granted to health plans or uninsured patients. For example, a health plan may agree to pay a provider 85 percent of billed charges. A patient's claim with $100 of charges would therefore be paid 85 percent or $85. If $100 was needed to cover costs and losses from other third-party payers, the provider would need to set a price at $117.65, which when paid at 85 percent of billed charges, would equal $100. Uninsured patients are a growing problem for many health care providers, especially hospitals. Most hospitals in the United States collect only a small percentage of the billed charges for these patients, usually five percent or less. The vast majority of the charges are written off as either charity care or bad debt. These patients create the same type of pricing issue that was just discussed. Uninsured patients are really patients who pay on a discount from billed charges, except their discount is usually very large.

The last requirement that needs to be included in price setting is some factor for profit. Health care providers with either tax-exempt or taxable status need some return to insure their financial survival. A nursing home that only recovered the historical cost of its plant and equipment through depreciation expense would be unable to replace its plant and equipment if the replacement prices of those assets increased. In ad-

dition, all businesses need to cover so-called working capital costs, which are not recognized as expenses in a financial statement. Collections for many health care providers average 60 days or more, but payroll expenses and supply payments to vendors are paid on a more frequent basis. This difference, though not an accounting cost, must be financed, adding another element for required profit. Ultimately, any firm needs to generate a return on investment (ROI) that will meet its requirement for sustainable growth. We will talk more about this topic in Chapter 10.

With this background on how prices should be set, let's examine a simple example to incorporate the four requirements for pricing just listed. We will use the data in Table 5–2 to illustrate the methodology of pricing. Note at the outset that we must set a price that will generate $105,000 of revenue, $100,000 of cost and $5,000 of profit. We also know, given the current estimates of volume by payer and present payer rates, that we will receive $38,000 from Medicare (400 × $95), $7,500 from Medicaid (100 × $75), and $33,000 from Managed Care Plan # 1 (300 × $110). The total of these three fixed-fee schedule payers is $78,500. This means that we need to recover $26,500 from the two remaining payers that pay on a price or billed-charge basis. Managed Care Plan # 2 has 100 patients that will pay 80 percent of billed charges and the 100 uninsured patients will pay 10 percent of billed charges. Another way to look at the billed-charge payers would be to state that we will have 80 patients from Managed Care Plan # 2 that will pay 100 percent of their charges and 20 patients who will pay nothing. We also have 10 uninsured patients who will pay 100 percent of the charges and 90 who will pay nothing. Viewed from

---

Table 5–2 Price-Setting Example

Total cost	$100,000
Total volume	1,000
Average cost	$100
Payer volumes	
Medicare (payment rate = $95)	400
Medicaid (payment rate = $75)	100
Managed Care # 1 (payment rate = $110)	300
Managed Care # 2 (pay 80% of charges)	100
Uninsured (pay 10% of charges)	100
Total all payers	1,000
Desired net income	$5,000

this perspective, we will have 90 (80 +10) patients who must cover the $26,500 of remaining financial requirement. Dividing the $26,500 by 90 yields a required price of $294.44. Table 5–3 shows an income statement that proves the accuracy of our calculations.

The actual method for pricing can be reduced to a formula that is presented in Figure 5–3. The formula states that the average required price is derived from a series of computations. First, the price must be set to include the average cost of production. Figure 5–4 inserts the value of $100 into the average cost field using the example of Table 5–2. Second, the required level of net income must be defined, which was $5,000 in our example. Third, the total loss incurred on fixed-fee-schedule patients must be calculated. The loss on fee schedule patients is $1,500 and is derived as follows:

- Loss on Medicare = 400 patients × $5.00 per patient is $2,000
- Loss on Medicaid = 100 patients × $25.00 per patient is $2,500
- Gain on Managed Care Plan # 1 = 300 patients × $10.00 is $3,000

It is important to note that the $3,000 gain from the managed-care plan offsets the $4,500 loss incurred on Medicare and Medicaid patients. The total loss on the three fixed-payer groups is thus $1,500 and is inserted in Figure 5–4. In some situations, this term can be negative, which means that there is no overall loss, but a gain on fixed-fee-schedule patients. When this situation occurs, the actual required price that must be set can be decreased because the fixed-fee payers make a contribution toward the required profit level. The next step is to determine the number of total patients who pay on a charge basis. In our example, this value is 200, 100 managed-care plan #2 patients and 100 unin-

sured patients. The final step is to derive the actual discount that is experienced on charge-paying patients. This figure is defined by weighting the proportion of charge patients in a specific payer category to total charge patients by the appropriate discount rate of that charge payer. The value for our example is .55 and its computation is shown below:

$$[(100/200) \times .20] + [(100/200) \times .90] = .55$$

The formula yields a required price of $294.44, as we have previously determined. In this example, note that our markup from cost is 294 percent, which simply means that our charges ($294.44) are 2.94 times our average cost ($100). This seems like a very high markup and would cause many people to think that the health care firm is making an excessive amount of profit, when in fact their margin is fairly small: $5,000 on a total cost of $100,000 (5%).

The formula of Figure 5–3 helps us to understand the effects of critical drivers on a health care firm's prices. In general, prices will increase when:

1. costs increase.
2. governmental programs pay less than cost.
3. managed-care plans adopt fee schedules that do not pay at levels above cost.
4. the firm's required profit increases because of financial needs, such as debt-service obligations or capital replacement.
5. the proportion of charge-paying patients drops.
6. levels of uninsured patients increase.

It might be useful to see the effects of a system where every payer except the uninsured patients paid 100 percent of billed charges. If this were the situation, the required price in our example would fall to

Table 5–3 Income Statement for Case Example

Revenue	Computation	Amount
Medicare	400 × $95	$38,000
Medicaid	100 × $75	7,500
Managed Care # 1	300 × $110	33,000
Managed Care # 2	100 × 80% × $294.44	23,555
Uninsured	100 × 10% × $294.44	2,944
Total		$105,000
less Costs		100,000
Profit		$5,000

Figure 5–3 Pricing Formula

$$\text{Price} = \frac{\text{Average cost} + \dfrac{\text{Required net income} + \text{Loss on fee-schedule payers}}{\text{Volume of charge payers}}}{1 - \text{Average discount experienced on charge payers}}$$

$115.38. This of course means that Medicare, Medicaid, and all managed-care plans would pay 100 percent of billed charges, and we would still experience a 90 percent write-off on the uninsured patients. Figure 5–5 shows the computation of price in this revised-payment scheme.

The results in our example are painfully obvious to every health care executive. Health care firms that lose money on Medicare, Medicaid, and managed-care contracts must raise rates sharply to a limited charge-related payer base. Large write-offs or discounts to the charge-related payer base can and often do escalate prices to levels that are well above costs. This is the nature of the economic environment facing health care firms today. Wishing it were not so will not change the facts. Unless major payment system changes take place, prices will always be a large multiple of costs. Health care providers must educate the public that these high prices are the result of payer methodology and are not related to provider profiteering.

LEARNING OBJECTIVE 4

Determine if prices are defensible.

JUSTIFYING HEALTH CARE FIRM PRICES

The rising visibility of health care firm prices in general, and hospital prices in particular have focused attention on how best to both communicate and justify prices to the general public. There has been a dramatic increase in hospital prices over the last 20 years. Figure 5–6 demonstrates that the relationship between hospital cost and hospital price has changed markedly during the period 1996–2004. From our earlier discussion of pricing we learned that actual cost is but one factor that impacts price. Payer-mix variables such as percentage of billed-charge patients, level of uninsured patients, losses on Medicare and Medicaid, and payment patterns of managed-care plans have a much more pervasive influence on prices than costs. This of course explains why the level of markups (price divided by cost) in the hospital industry has increased from 1.6 in 1996 to 2.20 in 2004.

The term "reasonable charges" is used by many people when they review health care firm pricing. Oftentimes, there is disagreement about the issue of reasonableness when the underlying data is the same. It is critical to bring a structured framework that may be used to assess the issue of reasonableness as it pertains to health care pricing. There are two generic ways that reasonableness of charges or prices has been used in the health care industry:

1. **Return-on-investment adequacy.** Most public utility regulatory models permit the earning of a reasonable rate of return on investment to ensure that capital can be replaced. Without adequate rates of return, capital will not be available to replace and renovate plant and equipment. Health care firms have a heavy investment in plant and equipment and must maintain and/or replace it periodically to keep pace with advances in medical technology.

   In addition, health care firms have sizable working capital needs that are not recognized as expenses, but require cash outlays. For example, most health care firms pay employees on a bi-weekly basis, but collect patient receivables on a 60-plus-day basis. Health care firms must set prices to generate a reasonable level of profit that will permit them to replace their capital-asset

$$\text{Price} = \frac{\$100 + \dfrac{\$5,000 + \$1,500}{200}}{1 - .55} = \$294.44$$

Figure 5–4 Pricing Formula

$$\text{Price} = \frac{100 + \dfrac{5,000}{1,000}}{1 - .09} = \$115.38$$

Figure 5–5 Pricing Formula for Revised Payment Scheme

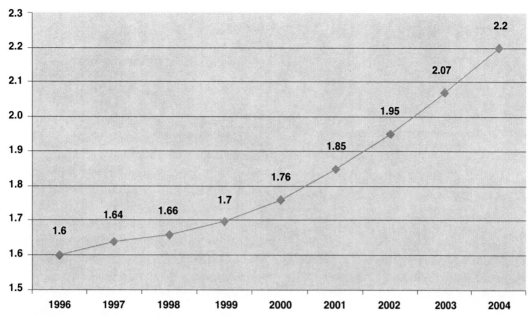

Figure 5–6 Median Hospital Mark-Ups 1996–2004
Source: Cleverley & Associates

bases in a timely manner and to provide for working capital needs.

2. **Comparison with other health care firms.** Oftentimes both payers and health care firms will assess the reasonableness of health care charges based upon comparisons with similar and/or other health care firms in the same geographic region. A number of states and local communities have reporting mechanisms for health care firms to report charges for either specific procedures or some aggregate measure of hospital output, such as discharges. One of the difficulties with comparing hospital charges is that they may vary significantly across hospitals, not necessarily because of operating cost differences, but because of payer differences. Hospitals with heavy percentages of Medicare, Medicaid, and indigent patients will need to have higher prices in order to realize minimal levels of profitability. Size, complexity, and teaching status will also impact charges.

Using the two methods described above, the following section will include a specific hospital example with which to develop a framework for assessing the reasonableness of charges.

REASONABLENESS OF CHARGES FOR CASE HOSPITAL – ROI METHOD

Historically, many public utility rates were based upon the fair- return-on-fair-value concept, manifested in an 1898 Supreme Court decision (Smyth vs. Ames et al.). Implicitly, this permits a reasonable profit on the firm's underlying investment.

$$\text{Return on Investment} = \frac{\text{Revenue} - \text{Cost}}{\text{Investment}}$$

Using the above model to assess the reasonableness of Case Hospital's charges, we will address three issues:

- Is the return on investment (ROI) at Case Hospital reasonable?
- Are costs at Case Hospital reasonable?
- Is investment at Case Hospital reasonable?

The first question to be raised is whether returns at Case Hospital are high in relation to hospital industry averages. Case Hospital is a major academic medical center, and it will be compared with two peer groups of academic medical centers, one being a state group and the other a regional group. Figures 5–7 and 5–8 display values derived from Medicare Cost Reports for

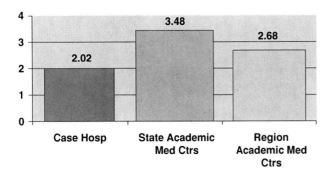

Figure 5–7 Return on Assets (Net Income/Assets) 5-Year Average − 2000–2004

two comparative groups and Case Hospital for the period 2000–2004. The data suggest that Case Hospital has not realized excessive levels of profit based upon values reported here.

The second question to be answered is the reasonableness of costs at Case Hospital. In general, there are two methods of assessing hospital cost at the facility level. One method uses an adjusted-patient day or adjusted-discharge method. A second method relies on individual assessment of cost for inpatient and outpatient services. In our opinion, the second method provides superior accuracy for reasons that we will discuss later in Chapter 10. The methodology for defining a facility-wide measure of hospital cost involves weighting two measures:

1. Medicare cost per discharge (MCPD) – Case-mix- and wage-index adjusted
2. Medicare cost per outpatient claim (MCPC) – relative-weight and wage-index adjusted

The hospital cost index (HCI) is then constructed as follows:

$$HCI = \% \text{ Inpatient revenue} \times \frac{MCPD}{U.S. \text{ avg}} +$$
$$\% \text{ Outpatient revenue} \times \frac{MCPC}{U.S. \text{ avg}}$$

Values for these cost measures are presented in Figures 5–9, 5–10, and 5–11. The data in Figure 5–9 show that Case Hospital has an overall cost structure that is very similar to that of the state academic medical centers and the median value for regional academic medical centers. Case Hospital appears to have slightly higher inpatient costs, as seen in Figure 5–10, but its outpatient costs are considerably lower than those of the comparison groups. We can conclude that Case Hospital is providing health services at levels of cost consistent with expected values. Therefore, based on this analysis, we can conclude that Case Hospital's costs are reasonable.

The third and final question relates to investment levels at Case Hospital. Review of investment levels shows Case Hospital to have above-average efficiency with respect to investment in plant, property, and equipment (see Figure 5–12).

All of these data indicate the following:

1. Case Hospital is not realizing excessive profits.
2. Costs at Case Hospital are consistent with expected values and are reasonable.
3. Investment at Case Hospital is reasonable and not excessive.

These three points show clearly that revenue and prices at Case Hospital are reasonable. This does not

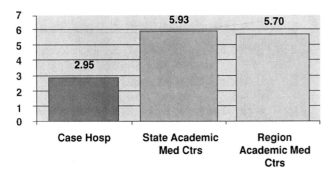

Figure 5–8 Return on Equity (Net Income/Equity) 5-Year Average − 2002–2004

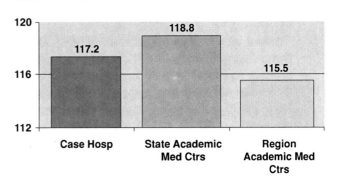

Figure 5–9 Hospital Cost Index – 2004

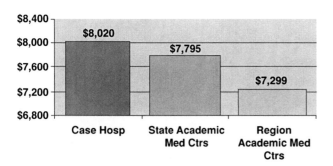

Figure 5–10 Medicare Cost per Discharge (CMI & WI Adj) – 2004

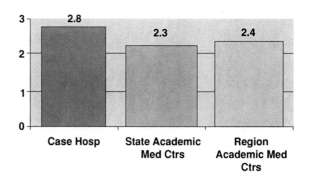

Figure 5–12 Fixed Asset Turnover (Revenue/Net Fixed Assets) – 2004

mean that its individual prices for some services will not be higher than those at local, comparative hospitals. Hospitals can have different levels of Medicaid and indigent-care, or managed-care contracts with differences in payment. Whatever the underlying cause or causes, however, it is clear that Case Hospital's charges are reasonable.

REASONABLENESS OF CHARGES FOR CASE HOSPITAL – COMPARISON-OF-CHARGES METHOD

Frequently, both payers and hospitals will assess the reasonableness of their prices based upon comparisons with similar hospitals and/or other hospitals in the same geographic region. A number of state and local communities have mechanisms for hospitals to report charges for either specific procedures or some aggregate measure of facility output, such as discharges. Most recently, some states, including California, have made portions of hospital Charge Description Masters publicly available. One of the difficulties with compar-

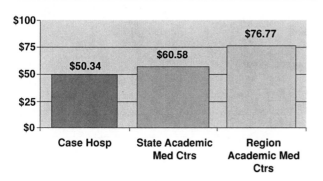

Figure 5–11 Cost per Medicare Visit (RW & WI Adj) – 2004

ing hospital charges is that they may vary significantly across hospitals, not necessarily because of operating cost differences but because of payer differences. Hospitals with heavy percentages of Medicare, Medicaid, and indigent patients will have higher prices in order to realize minimal levels of profitability, as we previously discussed.

To provide some basis for comparison of charges at Case Hospital, we selected all academic medical centers in Case Hospital's state. We also included the regional average for academic medical centers, adjusting for cost-of-living differences. Academic medical centers often have both higher costs and charges because their patients are often more severely ill. Medicare has recognized this reality and provides greater levels of payment to compensate them for their greater costs.

We examined the relative level of charges at Case Hospital from a global facility-level basis, using the same construction discussed earlier for costs. These comparisons are presented in Figures 5–13, 5–14, and 5–15. The data reflected in these three graphs show charges at Case Hospital to be above those of the comparative groups. We believe that Case Hospital's charges are above the comparative groups because of its higher level of care provided to Medicaid and indigent patients. To see the effects of this patient mix on charges, refer to Figure 5–16, which shows the Medicare inpatient disproportionate (DSH) percentage for Case Hospital and the two comparative groups. High values for the ratio indicate the relationship of Medicaid and Medicaid-eligible days to total days. The DSH percentage at Case Hospital is 26 percent above the state academic medical center average and 80 percent above the regional academic medical center average.

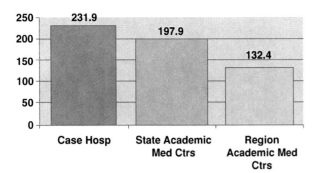

Figure 5–13 Hospital Charge Index – 2004

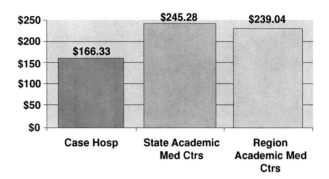

Figure 5–15 Average Charge per APC (RW & WI Adj) – 2004

In summary, we believe Case Hospital's charges are reasonable when compared to similar hospitals after payer-mix differences are considered.

LEARNING OBJECTIVE 5

List some of the important considerations when negotiating a managed-care contract.

MANAGED-CARE CONTRACT NEGOTIATION

Having discussed pricing, we will now focus our attention on the last area of revenue management, the negotiation of managed-care contracts. This particular type of negotiation has become much more intense in recent years. When managed-care plans were in their infancy in the early and mid-1980s, many providers would sign contracts that covered less than their full costs, but greater than their marginal cost to gain market share and foster competition among health care plans. Blue Cross/Blue Shield plans were the dominant

health insurers at that point and were perceived by many providers as the enemy. As managed-care plans grew and gained market share, they began to consolidate as a result of a number of acquisitions and mergers. Table 5–4 shows the consolidation of the health care insurance market in recent years.

After the surge in payer merger activity, providers began to feel significant financial pressures that resulted from managed-care contracts that were perceived as one sided. To counter these pressures, many provider groups, including hospitals and medical groups, began to consolidate themselves through mergers, affiliation arrangements, and outright acquisitions. Without provider consolidation, many managed-care plans would threaten to exclude them from their provider networks if they did not accept the terms established by the managed-care plans. In economic terminology, the existence of health care plan oligopsonies produced health care provider oligopolies. This balance of market power has made it more difficult for both providers and insurers to walk away from contract negotiations. Providers must contract with the smaller

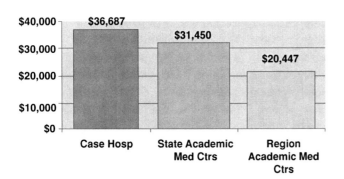

Figure 5–14 Medicare Charge per Discharge (CMI & WI Adj) – 2004

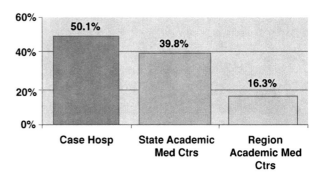

Figure 5–16 Medicare Inpatient Disproportionate (DSH) % Average Value – 2001–2004

Table 5–4 Health Maintenance Organizations (HMOs) and Enrollment, 1976–2003

	Number of HMOs	*HMO Enrollment (millions)*
1976	174	6.0
1980	235	9.1
1990	572	33.0
1995	562	50.9
1998	651	76.6
1999	643	81.3
2000	568	80.9
2001	541	79.5
2002	500	76.1
2003	454	71.8

Source: Center for Medicare and Medicaid Services (CMS)

number of payers, and payers must contract with the smaller number of providers if they are to maintain market presence.

In any managed-care contract, there are two critical elements. First, there is the payment schedule, which describes the basis of payment and actual payment/fee schedules. Second, there is the actual contract language, which describes the administration of the contractual arrangement that determines how services are provided and paid. Most attention is focused on the actual payment schedules, but the actual administrative language is becoming more important. In the remainder of this section, we will describe ten important areas of managed-care contract language.

1. **Remove contract ambiguity.** It seems that a hallmark of many business relationships is to establish written agreements that no one except attorneys can understand. If contract language is unclear, it should be clarified.

2. **Eliminate retroactive denials.** It has become increasingly common for health plans to deny claims for services that were either directly or indirectly approved by the plan. Contract clauses which permit retroactive denials should be removed from contract documents. An example of a retroactive denial clause follows:

   The Company, on its behalf and on behalf of other payers, reserves the right to perform utilization review (including retrospective review) and to adjust or

deny payment for medically inappropriate services.

3. **Establish a reasonable appeal process.** Medical necessity of services is a key element in payment approval. When services have been approved by the plan or the plan has been notified and did not protest the provision of services, claims should be paid. This is the basis of "retroactive denials," which we just discussed. In some cases, services may be provided because the member's physician believed they were necessary, but the plan protested. In these cases, a reasonable appeal process should be established that is not one-sided. The following contract language came from an actual managed-care contract and does not provide for any provider representation. These types of appeal arrangements should be modified to include both provider and plan representation on any appeal board.

Level 1 Appeal

Part 1: The matter will be reviewed by a physician selected by ABC. If the physician determines that the decision to deny payment is in error, payment of the Claim will be authorized. If the decision to deny payment is affirmed by the physician, the Case will then automatically proceed to Part 2 of the Level 1 Appeal procedure.

Part 2: The matter will be reviewed by a physician selected by ABC, who is currently practicing in a specialty relevant to the Case in question. If the physician determines that the decision to deny payment is in error, the payment of the Claim will be authorized. If the decision to deny payment is affirmed by the physician, no payment will be made.

Level 2 Appeal

If HOSPITAL continues to dispute the payment decision, a Level 2 Appeal shall be available within the same time frames as set forth above. The matter will be reviewed by a physician selected by ABC, who is practicing in a specialty relevant to the Case in question and who was not involved in the Level 1 Appeal. If this reviewing physician determines that the decision to deny payment is in error, the payment of the Claim will be authorized. If the decision to deny payment is affirmed by the physician, no payment will be made. This level of appeal shall become final and binding upon both parties.

4. **Define clean claims.** In most managed-care contracts, providers are required to submit claims on a standard form, usually an HCFA 1450 or UB-92 for institutional providers, or an HCFA 1500 for medical professionals. Some health plans often reject claims and return them to the provider for reasons that are not material to claim payment. For example, the claim may be missing the provider's address or it might have an incorrect patient zip code. While the claims may be paid eventually, it can cause cash flow hardships for providers. Many states have legislation requiring health plans to make payment for "clean claims" within specified time periods, for example 30 days. Claim denial for missing data is sometimes used as a stalling tactic.

   The following is language from a typical contract. Notice that it is the plan that determines if the claim is complete, and no specific standards are identified.

   Any amount owing under this agreement shall be paid within thirty (30) days after receipt of a complete claim, unless additional information is requested within the thirty (30) day period.

5. **Remove most favored nation (MFN) clauses.** Some managed-care contracts contain provisions that preclude a provider from contracting with any other health plan at rates lower than those defined in the current contract. This is commonly referred to as a "most favored nation" clause. These provisions are very hard to enforce and impair the provider's ability to conduct its business affairs in a reasonable manner.

A simple response to the inclusion of a MFN clause in a contract is to make it reciprocal and require the health plan not to pay more for services to any other provider. While the health plan may argue this would be a violation of antitrust, it does point out the inequity of a one-sided MFN clause. The MFN clause can make it very difficult to negotiate new contracts. To illustrate this, assume a provider has just negotiated a new three-year contract with a sizable price increase. If the new prices are above existing contract provisions in other older managed-care contracts, the inclusion of a MFN could roll back payment terms to an existing old contract. MFN clauses are also very difficult to test. Payment terms are usually not identical across plans. One plan may pay on a per-diem basis and another on a case basis. The following actual contract language illustrates the difficulty of administration of MFN clauses.

Except as provided herein, during the term of this Agreement and any renewal thereafter, HOSPITAL agrees that it will not accept a Modified Rate from an Other Payer. Hospital will conduct annual audits of its agreements to determine whether a Modified Rate has inadvertently been accepted with an Other Payer. Except as provided herein, if a Modified Rate is accepted, HOSPITAL agrees to concurrently give written notice to ABC of the acceptance of the Modified Rate and offer the same Modified Rate to ABC and the Modified Rate shall become the new ABC Rate and shall be weighted across all networks.

6. **Prohibit silent PPO arrangements.** A common practice in the health care insurance marketplace is the leasing of networks. One health insurance plan may lease or rent its network to another plan for a sum of money. Members in that plan may then present themselves for medical services at the provider and claim the negotiated payment rate of the leased network. This will often extend payment discounts to a much larger group than originally intended. There should be specific contract language prohibiting this ar-

rangement. Without specific language, it is inferred that the lease arrangement is valid. The contract language below extends the definition of the "Plan" to a potentially broad group, thereby allowing a large number of individuals access to favorable rates.

Plan. Any health benefit product or plan issued, administered, or serviced by the company or one of its affiliates, including but not limited to HMO, preferred provider organizations, indemnity, Medicaid, Medicare, and Workers' Compensation.

7. **Include terms for outliers or technology-driven cost increases.** Ideally, the contract will contain provisions allowing for increases in payments as time passes and costs increase. Sometimes market forces or technology-driven changes in medical practice can cause major increases in costs. The use of stents in angioplasty is an example of a technology-driven change. Stents are used in most angioplasty cases today, but were seldom used in the past. One possible way to objectively link payment increases to costs is to relate actual payment to Medicare fee schedules. Payments for outliers should also be included to avoid the losses that result from treating catastrophic cases.

8. **Establish ability to recover payment after termination.** Most managed-care contracts will establish a term for the contract, usually three to five years. After that term, the contract will automatically renew for a year unless terminated. Termination in the initial term is often difficult unless there is a default or breach of the contract. After the initial term, either party can usually terminate the contract without cause, provided proper notification is given. A critical question to address is: How will payment be made to the providers after the contract period? Providers must be careful to ensure that payment terms in the contract are not carried forward for a prolonged period of time after termination. The following contract language permits the plan to utilize existing payment terms for up to a full year in certain circumstances. This is not an ideal situation for the provider because it permits the plan an opportu-

nity to seek other providers for their network without creating additional cost and it keeps members content because existing patient/provider relationships can be maintained.

Upon Termination. Upon termination of this Agreement for any reason, other than termination by Company, Hospital shall remain obligated at Company's sole discretion to provide Hospital Services to: (a) any Member who is an inpatient at Hospital as of the effective date of termination until such Member's discharge or Company's orderly transition of such Member's care to another provider; and (b) any Member, upon request of such Member or the applicable Payer, until the anniversary date of such Member's respective Plan or for one (1) calendar year, whichever is less. The terms of this Agreement shall apply to all services.

9. **Preserve the ability to be paid for services.** Health plans are naturally interested in shielding their members from additional medical costs that are associated with services that were not medically necessary. The critical question is: How will services that were deemed not medically necessary or not covered by the plan's benefits be paid? We have already discussed the importance of removing the plan's ability to retroactively deny claims. In some situations, pre-certification by the plan for a member's treatment has been clearly denied. The provider in these situations should be free to provide services if requested by the patient and bill the patient directly. The following contract language appears to limit the provider's ability to do this without unnecessary bureaucracy. These kinds of clauses should be modified to maintain patient protection, but not destroy the legitimate right of the provider to be paid for services provided to the patient when consent is granted.

HOSPITAL may seek payment from the Covered Individual for Health Services which are not provided in the Covered Individual's Health Benefit Plan when the non-coverage is due to reasons other than lack of Medical Necessity. HOSPITAL may seek payment from the Covered Individual for Health Services which are non-Covered Services because the services have been deemed not Medically Necessary, only if the Covered Individual has requested the Health Services to be provided notwithstanding Plan's determination, and only if HOSPITAL has provided Covered Individual notice in writing prior to the rendition of services of the approximate cost said Covered Individual will incur, and Covered Individual has agreed to the rendition of the service having had the benefit of said information. In such event, HOSPITAL may bill the Covered Individual at its customary rate for such services.

10. **Minimize health plan rate differentials.** It is an interesting economic twist that providers seem to reward the worst-paying customers and punish their best-paying customers. The health plan that has negotiated the best rate or largest discount has a cost advantage over other health plans in the market. This should enable them to gain market share and drive out competitive plans. In turn, this gives the plan more negotiating leverage in establishing even steeper discounts, which further enhances the plan's market position. The plans with smaller discounts—which means higher payments to providers—are forced out. Rather than continue this cycle, it may make sense for providers to establish a rate structure for all plans and grant discounts for administrative efficiencies only. This, of course, is much easier said than done, especially where a provider is facing financial ruin if 20 percent of its business is lost. Payment equity across plans is a goal, however, and should be pursued where economically feasible.

MANAGED-CARE PAYMENT SCHEDULES

From most providers' perspectives, the key element in a managed-care contract is the payment or compensation schedule. Table 5–5 presents a 2005 summary of over 200 managed-care contract payment provisions for U.S. hospitals. The numbers presented are an average for all plans that make payments based upon the unit identified. For example, the average percentage of billed charges paid for hospital inpatient services was 78 percent. Hospitals that were paid on a billed-charge basis would most likely not have any separate payments on a per-diem or case basis. The data in Table 5–5 state that the average payment per case or DRG was $5,457 for a case weight of 1.0. For hospitals, the predominant unit of payment for inpatient care is usually a per-day basis. Sometimes a mix of the two may be present. For example, the plan may pay a per-diem rate for all inpatients except a case rate for selected DRGs; most often these are high-cost surgical cases, such as DRG 107 (coronary artery by-pass). Outpatient care is often paid on either a fee-schedule or discount-from-charges basis. Again, a mix of the two may be present, and selected surgical and radiology procedures may be fee schedule, with all others being discounted charges.

Many hospital contracts have outlier or stop-loss provisions. This provision specifies that the hospital may pay on a basis other than per diem or case if charges exceed a specific limit. For example, Table 5–5 states that the average stop-loss threshold is $77,856, and any inpatient claim that has more than $77,856 would be paid at a discount from billed-charge basis. In some cases, the entire claim would be paid as a discount from billed charges, for example, 66 percent. In other cases, only the charges that exceed the threshold would be paid at a billed-charge basis. For example, assume a claim with $100,000 of charges and a stop loss at $70,000 with payment at 70 percent of excess charges. Payment for this claim would consist of the original DRG fee and then an additional stop-loss payment of $21,000 [70% × ($100,000 – $70,000)].

Many managed-care contracts that provide for payment of claims on a discount from billed charges include rate-increase-limit clauses. The overall objective of a price-increase-limit provision is fairly straightforward. The price-increase-limit provision is intended to prevent a hospital from raising its prices beyond reasonable levels. Significant increases in prices could cause a payer to lose large sums of money on existing negotiated contracts with employers and weaken the health plan's financial viability. In most cases, the presence of a price-increase limit can modify the historical discount from billed charges contained in the contract. The key contract provision is the allowed rate

Table 5–5 HMO/PPO Contract Comparison (All U.S.)

*213 Comparison Plans

	Average Value*
Inpatient Rates	
All Services % of Billed Charges	78%
DRG Base Rate	$5,457
Per Diem Rates	
Medical	$1,562
Surgical	$1,189
Med/Surg 1 Day Stay	$2,893
TCU/Telemtry	$1,799
ICU/CCU	$2,447
PTCA	$4,057
Cardiac Surgery 1st Day	$3,671
Cardiac Surgery Add'l Days	$3,798
Psych	$667
Alcohol/Chemical Dependency	$598
SNF	$579
Rehab	$1,032
Case Rates	
PTCA	$6,366
Pacemaker Implant	$12,517
Cardiac Cath	$4,272
Cardiac Surgery	$18,243
Cardiac Surg - CARVE OUT (% BC)	74%
Lithotripsy	$4,378
DRG 104	$29,164
DRG 105	$24,445
DRG 106	$27,076
DRG 107	$24,708
DRG 108	$23,698
DRG 109	$21,577
DRG 110	$20,536
DRG 111	$17,609
DRG 116	$11,829
DRG 124	$5,788
DRG 125	$4,475
DRG 209	$11,819
DRG 210	$16,837
DRG 471	$13,903
DRG 496	$25,672
DRG 497	$18,976
DRG 498	$16,882
DRG 499	$9,247
DRG 500	$7,264
DRG 493	$6,397
DRG 494	$5,940
DRG 514	$27,758
DRG 515	$25,625
DRG 516	$11,034
DRG 517	$9,343
DRG 518	$17,420
DRG 526	$12,856
DRG 527	$1,992

*213 Comparison Plans	Average Value*
OB/Nursery	
Normal Vag. Del. Case Rate (or 2 Day Stay)	$3,185
1 Day Stay or PD	$1,905
3 Day Stay	$5,255
Add'l Days	$1,264
C-Section Case Rate (or 3 Day Stay)	$4,576
1 Day Stay or PD	$2,502
2 Day Stay	$3,800
4 Day Stay	$6,223
Addt'l Days	$1,242
Nursery Level 1 - Boarder	$510
Nursery Level 2	$1,536
Nursery Level 3	$1,858
Nursery Level 4 - NICU	$2,113
Outpatient Rates	
All Services % of Billed Charges	73%
Emergency Department (% BC)	76%
Flat Fee	$492
Level 1	$155
Level 2	$274
Level 3	$626
Level 4	$788
Level 5	$944
Observation (% BC)	67%
Obs Flat Fee Case Rate	$612
Physical Therapy (% BC)	69%
PT Flat Fee Per Hour	$112
Occupational Therapy (% BC)	77%
OT Flat Fee Per Hour	$118
Speech Therapy (% BC)	70%
ST Flat Fee Per Hour	$120
MRI (% BC)	67%
MRI Case Rate	$778
CT Scan (% BC)	74%
CT Scan Case Rate	$518
Outpatient Surgery % of Billed Charges	73%
Surgery Group - Case Rate	$2,145
Group 1- Case Rate	$1,032
Group 2- Case Rate	$1,269
Group 3- Case Rate	$1,687
Group 4- Case Rate	$2,023
Group 5- Case Rate	$2,833
Group 6- Case Rate	$2,388
Group 7- Case Rate	$3,275
Group 8- Case Rate	$3,324

continues

Table 5–5 continued

*213 Comparison Plans

	Average Value*
Group 9- Case Rate	$5,285
Ungrouped Case Rate	$1,799
Ungrouped (% BC)	73%
PTCA Case Rate	$5,064
Cardiac Cath Case Rate	$4,550
Cardiac Cath (% BC)	74%
Lithotripsy Case Rate	$3,420
Other (% BC)	71%
Stop Loss: Threshold	$77,856
Total Charges Paid At:	66%
Excess Charges Paid At:	66%
Rate Increase Limit %	6%

Source: Cleverley & Associates

of increase. The allowed rate of increase is used in conjunction with the actual rate of increase to determine whether an adjustment in the discount is necessary, and if so, to what extent. The usual payment adjustment can be stated as follows:

$$\text{New payment \%} = \frac{1 + \text{Allowed rate increase}}{1 + \text{Actual rate increase}} \times \text{Present payment \%}$$

To illustrate this methodology, assume a present contract provides for payment at 70 percent of billed charges. The contract has a price-increase limit of 5 percent, and the hospital has put a 10 percent rate increase into effect. The revised payment percent would be 66.82% (1.05/1.10 × 70%). To see the actual effect of the adjustment, assume a present procedure is priced at $1,000 and its price is increased to $1,100 (a ten percent increase). The hospital would have been paid $700 under the old arrangement (70 percent of $1,000). It will now be paid $735 ($1,100 × 66.82%). The actual payment increase is $35 or a 5 percent increase from the original $700 base payment, which is the maximum price increase allowed under the contract.

Medical groups are often paid on a fee-schedule basis, with capitation arrangements sometimes being used. The fee schedules are usually by CPT and, in come cases, are directly related to Medicare's Resource-Based Relative Value Scale (RBRVS) payment system. The health plan often contracts to pay some percentage, for example, 110 percent of Medicare RBRVS rates. A sample schedule of fees for an OB/GYN medical group is presented in Table 5–6.

Table 5–6 Sample Fee Schedule for OB/GYN Medical Group

Procedure Code	Description	Amount
99201	Off Vst/New	$ 34.50
99202	Off Vst/New	54.20
99203	Off Vst/New	75.60
99204	Off Vst/New	110.40
99205	Off Vst/New	138.00
99212	Off Vst/Est	30.00
99213	Off Vst/Est	41.40
99214	Off Vst/Est	63.10
99215	Off Vst/Est	97.30
99384	New Prevent Vst	112.00
99385	New Prevent Vst	106.40
99386	New Prevent Vst	129.50
99387	New Prevent Vst	141.40
99394	Est. Prevent Vst	98.00
99395	Est. Prevent Vst	93.50
99396	Est. Prevent Vst	104.70
99397	Est. Prevent Vst	116.60
59425	Prenatal Exam	324.50
59426	Prenatal Exam	556.90
19000	Aspiration of Breast	54.70
57500	Cervical biopsy	65.70
57452	Colposcopy	71.40
57454	Colposcopy	101.20
57460	Colposcopy	188.20
57522	LEEP w/Tray	269.80
57505	ECC	77.70
59000	Amniocentesis	92.70
59812	D&C–Incompl	277.60
59820	D&C–Missed	311.30
90780	IV Therapy 1	42.40
90781	IV Therapy *--	21.40
59025	Non-Stress Te	43.70
76818	Biophysical P	110.60
76805	Echo	142.50
76810	Echo–Multi Ge	284.20
76815	Echo–Limited	95.80
76700	Abdominal Sc	126.90
76857	Echo (Limited)	64.60
76856	Pelvic Scan	102.20
76830	Vaginal Scan	102.20
76831	Hysterosonography	103.40
51772	Pressure Profile	96.60

SUMMARY

The critical driver of any firm's financial solvency is usually its ability to generate reasonable levels of profit, which can provide for the replacement and growth of capital in the firm. Because profit is simply the difference between revenue and cost, careful attention must be directed at both revenue management and cost control. This chapter has focused on revenue management, leaving the area of cost control to later chapters. Revenue management is directly affected by three key areas: pricing, managed-care contract negotiation, and billing and coding. Our focus in this chapter has been on pricing and managed-care contract negotiation. Prices are currently receiving a lot of exposure in the health care industry, and the public is concerned about the relationship of prices to cost. We have seen

that health care firm prices are a function of four basic factors: costs, payment provisions of large third-party payers, levels of care provided to the uninsured, and required levels of profit. Because of inadequate payments from large governmental programs and the rising levels of uninsured patients, many health care firms have prices that are multiples of cost, but profit levels are only marginal. Managed-care contract negotiation can be a primary means to profit enhancement if reasonable rates of payment can be negotiated. It is also important, however, to examine specific contract language because reasonable payment rates mean very little if significant numbers of claims are denied.

ASSIGNMENTS

1. You have been asked to comment on the reasonableness of a health care firm's prices using the return on investment (ROI) methodology described in this chapter. Your review has determined that the firm's costs are in line with industry averages and its overall investment is similar to other comparable health care firms, but its level of return on investment is 20 percent higher than industry averages. Are there any factors which the firm might use to justify its higher-than-average rate of profitability?

2. You are trying to determine the average discount rate for charge payers to be used in the formula described in Figure 5–3. You have the following three payers with different discount rates: 200 uninsured patients who pay on average 5 percent of charges, 300 managed-care patients who pay 85 percent of billed charges, and another block of 500 managed-care patients who pay 75 percent of billed charges. What is the average discount rate that should be used in Figure 5–3?

3. Quality is usually described as a key factor in pricing. How can a health care firm with perceived higher levels of quality of care benefit from higher quality if 75 percent of its business is derived from Medicare and Medicaid patients who pay on a fixed-fee basis that does not adjust for quality differences?

4. Consumer-driven health plans rely on large deductibles that are often funded via a health savings account framework. How might the presence of a large deductible affect price elasticity for health services?

5. In negotiating a managed-care contract, why is it important to spell out precisely what constitutes a clean claim?

6. Your hospital has a contract with a large national health insurer that provides very favorable payment terms to the insurer. Under the terms of this contract, the insurer may extend its contract terms to other plans when it leases its network to them. Why might it be desirable to remove this provision from your contract?

7. Using the example of Table 5–2, assume that the average cost has jumped from $100 to $105. All other factors in the example will remain the same. What will be the new required price?

8. Modifying the example in #7, assume that all fixed payers will raise their payment levels 5 percent. Medicare will pay $99.75, Medicaid will pay $78.75, and Managed Care Plan # 1 will pay $115.50. If costs have still increased 5 percent to $105, what rate would now be required?

9. Using the data of Table 5–2, assume that a new managed-care plan has approached you with an opportunity to sign a contract with them that would pay on a fixed-fee schedule. The rate of payment would be $95 per unit and 200 new patient units would result. It is also assumed that the additional 200 new units would increase total cost from $100,000 to $112,000. This means that the marginal or variable cost per unit is $60. If the present price cannot be changed and will remain at $294.44 as determined in Table 5–3, what will be the effect on the firm's total profit? Should this contract be signed?

SOLUTIONS AND ANSWERS

1. The best way to review the adequacy of current profit is to examine current and projected uses for the firm's profit. For example, a not-for-profit firm located in a growing market may need to earn above-average levels of profit to provide for larger capital expenditures to meet replacement and growth needs. A firm might also have a very high level of current debt financing, which calls for large payments of debt principal in the short term. Other possible areas might include a need to build current cash reserves because of present inadequacies. Major delays in claim payment might also cause a firm to increase profit levels to finance the larger balances of accounts receivable.

2. $[(200/1000 \times .95] + [(300/1000) \times .15] + [(500/1000) \times .25] = .36$. The average discount rate to be used for the three payers is 36 percent or, alternatively, the average rate of payment would be 64 percent.

3. Two possible benefits of higher quality still exist. First, higher quality may drive more patients to the firm. If the payment from Medicare and Medicaid patients exceeds the marginal cost of service delivery, the incremental profit will go up. Second, higher quality may permit the firm to negotiate more favorable payment rates from the remaining payers in either better managed-care contract terms or higher prices.

4. Large deductibles place the initial cost of many health services upon the patient as opposed to traditional health insurance coverage, which provides payment for many health services. Because payment for health services is now coming directly from the patient and is not being paid by an insurance plan, many patients may delay or avoid seeking health care services or actively seek out the lowest-cost provider.

5. Without a definition of the requirements for a clean claim, payers can delay or avoid completely paying what is otherwise a legitimate claim.

6. This provision is often referred to as a silent PPO arrangement and extends the potential network far beyond the original expected patient population. The original payment terms may have included very low inpatient rates but provided for percentage-of-billed-charge payment for outpatient services. If the insurer's network were leased to a patient population with a much higher inpatient utilization experience, the relative profitability of the contract could be eroded.

7. Note that the increase in average cost will have two effects upon the resulting price. First, it will raise average cost to $105, and second it will increase the loss on fee-schedule payers. The original loss on fee-schedule payers was $1,500, but with the $5.00 increase in average cost, the new loss on fee-schedule payers becomes $5,500 (the original loss of $1,500 + $5.00 × 800 units of Medicare, Medicaid, and Managed Care Plan # 1). The new required price is $350, 18.9 percent above the original price of $294.44.

$$\text{Price} = \frac{\$105 + \dfrac{\$5,000 + \$5,500}{200}}{1 - .55} = \$350.00$$

8. The increase in fixed-fee schedules will impact the loss on fee-schedule payers as follows:

$$\text{Medicare Loss} = 400 \times (\$105.00 - \$99.75) = \$2,100$$

$$\text{Medicaid Loss} = 100 \times (\$105.00 - \$78.75) = \$2,625$$

$$\text{Managed Care Loss} = 300 \times (\$105.00 - \$115.50) = -\$3,150$$

The total loss is now $1,575, which is added to the required net income of $5,000. The new required price is $306.39, 4.1 percent above the original $294.44.

$$\text{Price} = \frac{\$105 + \dfrac{\$5,000 + \$1,575}{200}}{1 - .55} = \$306.39$$

9. Because the contract calls for payment at a rate of $95, which is greater than the marginal cost ($60), we know that the contract will produce more profit, as Table 5–7 shows below. The firm will generate $7,000 in new profit ($12,000 less the original level of profit $5,000). Alternatively, the new profit is simply marginal revenue ($95 per unit) less marginal cost ($60 per unit) times the 200 new units. On the surface this seems like a favorable contract, but it might have negative long-term effects. Most specifically, perhaps the present managed-care plan that pays $110 and provides 300 patient units may discover this payment arrangement and demand a similar rate.

Table 5–7 Income Statement for Case Example

Revenue	Computation	Amount
Medicare	400 × $95	$38,000
Medicaid	100 × $75	$7,500
Managed Care # 1	300 × $110	$33,000
Managed Care # 3	200 × $95.00	$19,000
Managed Care # 2	100 × 80% × $294.44	$23,555
Uninsured	100 × 10% × $294.44	$2,944
Total		$124,000
less Costs		$112,000
Profit		$12,000

Chapter 6

Managed Care

LEARNING OBJECTIVES

After studying this chapter, you should be able to do the following:

1. Define a health maintenance organization (HMO).
2. Describe the four main activities of health plans.
3. List the four types of HMOs and their characteristics.
4. Describe the forces that influenced the development of integrated delivery systems.
5. Describe some of the methods by which providers are paid in a managed-care environment.
6. Describe how managed-care organizations (MCOs) establish their prices.
7. Discuss legal and regulatory issues that affect MCOs.

REAL-WORLD SCENARIO

Archie Griffin, CEO of Cardiology Associates, has been approached by A.J. Hawk, a Vice President of Alpha Health Plans, to accept a capitation arrangement for all professional services associated with enrollees in Alpha's local market area. Currently, Cardiology Associates is being paid on an RBRVS fee schedule that gives them 110 percent of current Medicare rates. Mr. Hawk wants Archie to accept a capitation payment of $10.50 per month for every enrollee in Cardiology Associates' market area. Mr. Hawk has explained the many benefits of this payment methodology, but Archie is not certain whether all of Mr. Hawk's claims are true.

Archie discussed this proposal with the principal partners in the practice and most of them are unclear as to whether this is a wise business move. Currently, Cardiology Associates captures about 40 percent of Alpha Health Plans' local enrollees and this figure would certainly increase to close to 100 percent of their enrollees if they accepted Alpha's proposed capitation plan. The firm believes that they have capacity to service this contract because last year they hired six new physicians who are not 100 percent productive at the present time.

The basic arrangement of the capitation plan is to have Cardiology Associates provide all professional services to the plan's enrollees for the fixed sum of $10.50 per member per month (PMPM). Archie explained to the physicians that this method of payment will essentially shift utilization risk to the physicians and offers them the possibility of greater returns if usage rates are controlled. Archie asked Alpha Health Plans for historical data that will show him historical utilization patterns by procedure code. Archie is especially concerned about the future demographics of Alpha Health Plans' enrollees. Alpha is growing rapidly in the marketplace and has established a qualified managed-care program for Medicare beneficiaries. Mr. Hawk's current proposal does not provide for different levels of payment for enrollees in its Medicare plan from its non-Medicare plans. Cardiology services increase rapidly with age, and a shift in the demographics of Alpha's enrollee population to an older mix could accelerate usage patterns, quickly creating a financial disaster for Cardiology Associates.

Most of the physicians in Cardiology Associates are willing to accept a capitation plan from Alpha because they see a potential for capturing market share; however, they do want some age adjustment included in the capitation rate to protect them from adverse risk selection. Archie has scheduled a future meeting with Mr. Hawk to see if this is a possibility.

Managed-care, health maintenance organizations (HMOs), preferred provider organizations (PPOs), physician organizations (POs), physician hospital organizations (PHOs), capitation, medical service organizations (MSOs), consumer-directed health plans (CDHP), and integrated delivery systems (IDSs) are all terms and acronyms used freely in today's health care arena. These terms often represent different things to different people and often change in meaning over time. There is one common thread running through all of these terms and sweeping the health care industry: the issue of change and market reform. The focus in this chapter will be primarily on the development of managed-care plans and the development of required premium payments for health care coverage.

LEARNING OBJECTIVE 1

Define a health maintenance organization (HMO).

HEALTH MAINTENANCE ORGANIZATIONS (HMOS) AND MANAGED-CARE DEVELOPMENT

Before describing the development of HMOs in the health care market, it is important to define what we mean by an HMO. HMOs are organizations that receive premium dollars from subscribers in exchange for a promise to provide all health care required by that subscriber for a defined period. They assume the risk of delivering both physician and hospital services to their enrolled populations for a fixed sum of money provided on a prepaid basis. HMOs are a type of health plan or health insurance company. In this regard, they are no different than any other type of health insurer.

Figure 6–1 presents a view of the cash flows from health plan subscribers to health care service providers.

Health plans receive premium dollars from buyers who may be employers, groups, or individuals on a prepaid basis in return for a promise to provide payment for covered health care services when needed. Payments for those services can be paid to the subscriber or to the health care provider. Indemnity plans would make payments to the subscriber or indemnify the subscriber for covered health care services; but, in most cases, payments are made directly to the provider.

Health plans must make a profit to remain in business, and it is easy to understand the principles of profitability in the health insurance marketplace. To earn positive profits, health plans must receive payments from subscribers greater than payments to health care providers. They must also cover their own internal administrative costs. In addition, health plans generate some additional revenue from the investment of prepaid health premiums. The amounts of investment income earned by health insurers are relatively small compared to life insurance companies where the premium dollars are received far in advance of payment.

What functions do health plans perform to justify their position in the health care marketplace? There are four primary activities described in the following text.

LEARNING OBJECTIVE 2

Describe the four main activities of health plans.

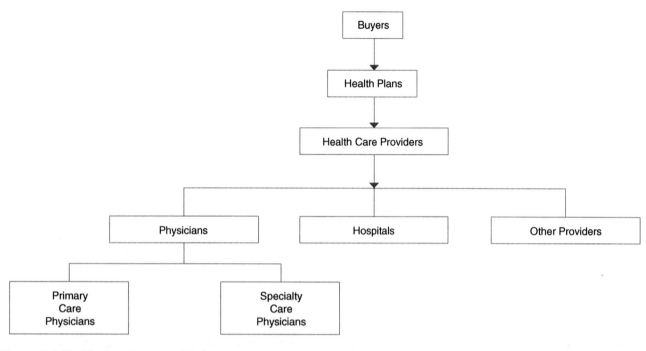

Figure 6–1 Health Care Insurance Market

UNDERWRITING

Health plans accept risk in the same way that any insurance company accepts risk. They agree to provide payment for services that at the time of contract are not certain. Greater-than-expected utilization can easily destroy profits and cause payments to exceed receipts. Underwriting of risk is an important business function. Few of us would be willing to live in homes without homeowner's insurance because the occurrence of a fire could destroy us financially. Even though we may pay the insurance company much more in premiums over our lifetimes than we receive in payments, we are not willing to assume the risk of a fire. Health insurance serves the same purpose. Payment for open heart procedures, kidney transplants, and other sophisticated medical procedures are very expensive, and we all hope that we never need them, but if we do, it is comforting to know that we have a source of payment for these procedures. Our country is different than most other industrialized nations regarding the percentage of private versus public financing. The United States relies on private financing of medical care to a much greater extent than do most other countries. This places a much greater emphasis on health insurance in our country and less on public financing programs, such as Medicare and Medicaid.

MARKETING

Insurance companies, in general, and health insurers, in particular, must communicate the availability of their products to prospective buyers and convince said buyers of the value of the product. Various media are used to accomplish this task: individual salespersons, television promotions, and other media advertising. There are substantial costs associated with these marketing efforts.

UTILIZATION REVIEW

Increasingly, health plans have sought to control escalating costs through a variety of utilization-review techniques. Health plans employ doctors and nurses to review and approve the delivery of non-emergent medical care for necessity and appropriateness. Medical personnel at health plans also work with health care providers to plan discharges from hospitals to less intense, subacute settings as soon as possible. Case management of chronic conditions, such as mental illness is also used by health plans to control costs. Much of the "managed" in managed-care deals with health-plan review and approval of treatment protocols.

CLAIMS ADMINISTRATION

Payments to health care providers for the provision of services to subscribers are a necessary administrative process. The health plan must verify that coverage for the services exists and that the services were in fact performed. In most cases, the health plan also must determine the amount of payment for the services, which is often different than the charges listed on a patient's bill or claim form. Verification of primary coverage also must be determined in cases when the individual has more than one insurer. The process of assigning payment responsibility when multiple insurers exist is called coordination of benefits.

HMOs are a subset of health plans and share all of the functions identified previously; however they are different in several areas, most notably regarding the pattern of relationships with their health care providers. First, most HMOs do not permit their subscribers to select providers who are out of the network. For example, an HMO subscriber who wished to use an orthopedic surgeon not in the HMO's network may not be covered for charges incurred by that surgeon. A hybrid form of an HMO package called point of service (POS) has a provision that permits subscribers to go out of network for services, but in these cases subscribers must pay a greater percentage of the cost. We will review POS options later in the text. Second, most HMOs rely on a primary-care gatekeeper concept. The HMO uses the primary care physician as a central triage point for the referral and approval of services. Before a subscriber can see a specialist, the referral must first be approved by the primary care physician. The use of the primary care physician as a gatekeeper is a central concept underlying HMO success, and has been adopted by other health plans that might not be characterized as HMOs.

HMOs are often categorized by the pattern of provider relationships they maintain, especially physician-provider relationships. HMOs are usually categorized into four types discussed in the next section.

LEARNING OBJECTIVE 3

List the four types of HMOs and their characteristics.

STAFF MODEL HMO

In a staff model HMO, the physicians are either employees of the HMO or they provide most of their services to HMO members through a contractual relationship. The latter alternative is used in states where HMOs cannot employ physicians because of restrictions on employment of physicians by non-physician-owned companies. Not all physicians may be employees, nor may they be under direct contract; but the critical segment is that of the primary care physicians. The HMO must control the primary care physician network to be a true staff model HMO. A staff model also may own other related health care providers such as hospitals, but ownership is not necessary.

GROUP MODEL HMO

In a group model HMO, the HMO contracts with one or more medical groups to provide all necessary services to HMO members. Usually, the groups are not exclusively bound to any one HMO and may provide services to several HMOs. The groups also may be primary care, specialty based, or multiple specialty based. The physicians in the groups, however, must come together and transfer all or most of their medical practice assets and liabilities to the group entity.

INDIVIDUAL PRACTICE ASSOCIATION (IPA) MODEL HMO

An IPA model HMO is a much looser affiliation of independent physicians who have not come together and integrated their practices in any substantive way. The IPA contracts with the HMO for needed medical services, but the individual physicians maintain their own independent practices and use the IPA only to sign contracts with HMOs and other health plans. County medical societies often create an IPA for their physician members.

NETWORK MODEL HMO

Network model HMOs are really a hybrid of the previous three forms. A network model HMO may contract with both medical groups and IPAs, as well as employ individual physicians. The key to their success is the ability to access a pool of cost-effective physicians who can manage care.

ALTERNATIVE HEALTH INSURANCE PLANS

Table 6–1 provides some data on the types and distribution of health care coverage for employees in companies where health care benefits are provided. The most dramatic change between 1993 and 2005 was the reduction in conventional coverage, which is largely indemnity-type plans. The reduction in conventional coverage can be traced to the large increases in PPO and POS plans. Both of these plan types provide greater access to physicians and hospitals. Access to both physicians and hospitals who may be out of network has become critical to many health plan beneficiaries. Table 6–2 summarizes the key characteristics of alternative health plans.

Indemnity plans, which are often referred to as traditional or conventional plans, provide their members with the greatest access to health care. Members are not restricted in terms of whom they can see for treatment of any medical disorders. In short, freedom of choice is the highest in indemnity plans. HMOs are usually the most restrictive in terms of choice and often limit access to hospitals and physicians that are part of the network. PPOs may be as restrictive as HMOs, but usually have larger panels of both doctors and hospitals. They attempt to select providers who have a good track record on both quality and cost effectiveness.

HMOs usually provide the broadest range of medical benefits, whereas indemnity or traditional plans are often the most restrictive. HMO members often have access to liberal outpatient and drug benefits that other health plans do not offer. The cost for increased

---

Table 6–1 Distribution and Premium Cost for Alternative Health Plans among Covered Employees

	Percentage		Average Annual Premium–Single
	1993	2005	2005
Conventional	46	3	$3,782
HMO	21	21	3,767
PPO	26	61	4,150
POS	7	15	3,914
Total	100	100	$4,024

Source: Kaiser/HRET Survey of Employer-Sponsored Health Benefits, 2005.

benefits is most often limited access. HMO members cannot go to any doctor or hospital they wish to visit, but are limited to the panel listed in the benefits directory. Without a POS provision, HMO members are precluded from going out of the network for services. PPOs often will provide provisions for out-of-network services, but require members to pay a portion of the cost for these benefits in the form of higher copayments and deductibles. A copayment is a provision that specifies a percentage of the approved charge that must be paid by the member. For example, a 20-percent copay would require a PPO member to pay 20 percent of the approved charge. The approved charge may be different from the charge made to the member for the service. A doctor may charge $2,000 for a procedure that the PPO says is approved at $1,200. The member would be required to pay the doctor 20 percent of the approved charge of $1,200, or $240, plus the difference between the approved charge and the actual charge, or $800, for a total payment of $1,040.

There is current interest in the recent rise of consumer-directed health plans (CDHP). These plans are relatively new in origin and became viable alternatives with the passage of the 2003 Medicare Prescription Drug, Improvement, and Modernization Act. This act provided for the creation of health-savings accounts (HSA). HSAs can be created by individuals using pre-tax dollars to fund a variety of health care expenses, including large deductibles and copayments. Most of the CDHPs are combined with HSAs and usually have annual deductibles of more than $1,000 per individual or $2,000 per family. The primary objective of these plans is to increase the involvement of patients in selecting cost-effective health care services. Most of the large health plans provide CDHP options, but current enrollment in CDHPs still remains small.

Indemnity or traditional plans usually pay providers, both hospitals and doctors, on the basis of charges. In some cases, there may be a fee schedule in effect that limits payment liability. PPOs usually negotiate some discount with the providers as a condition for participation in the network of providers. HMOs work in much the same way as PPOs and require a discount for participation in the network of providers. There is also a possibility of capitated payment to providers in an HMO arrangement. Capitation simply means the provider is not paid on the basis of services performed, but rather on the basis of the number of HMO members assigned to its organization. This means the provider may

Table 6–2 Health Care Insurance Alternatives

| Parties | Alternative Plans | | |
	HMOs	PPOs	Indemnity (Traditional)
Subscribers	Restricted choice Generous benefits	Choice from panel Copays Out-of-network with reduced benefits and higher cost Broader benefits	Free choice Deductible and 80/20 copays Major medical benefits Limited outpatient coverage
Physicians	Limited access Discounted reimbursement or capitation Utilization review (UR) requirements	Access by contracting Discounted charges or fee schedule UR-mostly hospital-based	All participate Paid charges
Hospitals	Limited access Discounted charges, per diems, case rates, or capitation UR	Limited access Discounted charges, per diem, or case rates UR	All participate Paid charges
Employers	Reduced cost	Reduced cost	Expensive, but most freedom for employees

be paid on a per-member-per-month (PMPM) basis. Finally, HMOs use stringent utilization review (UR) procedures at both the hospital and physician levels to eliminate unnecessary services and to provide cost-effective treatment plans. PPOs use UR procedures, but at the present time most of their efforts are directed at hospitals. Indemnity plans are also beginning to use UR procedures to curtail unnecessary utilization.

Costs of health care coverage to the employer are usually lowest in an HMO plan. The reason for this is simple. HMOs try to reduce unnecessary utilization for both doctors and hospitals and they also try to curtail the amount paid for services to health care providers by restricting the network of providers. PPOs have tried to reduce costs primarily through reduced prices to selected contracted providers, but utilization reductions have not been substantial relative to those achieved in an HMO setting. The big advantage that PPOs have regarding their remarkable growth rate can be attributed to the ease of organization. It takes much less planning and effort, as well as capital, to create a PPO than it does to create an HMO. Some policy experts believe, however, that the evolutionary cycle eventually will

change many of these PPOs to HMOs, as continued cost pressure from major purchasers of health care—employers and the government—force health plans to further decrease costs. Most of the future reductions in health care costs will not likely flow from lower prices per unit of service, but rather from reduced utilization of expensive procedures, especially hospital inpatient procedures.

HMOs are not a new development and have been in existence for many years. Two of the earliest HMOs were Kaiser Permanente and Group Health of Puget Sound. Both of these HMOs could be described as staff model HMOs. Physicians and hospitals that participated in these HMOs derived most, if not all, of their business from the HMO. In the early 1970s, Dr. Paul Elwood of Interstudy, a consulting firm in Minneapolis, coined the term "health maintenance organization" to describe the kind of health plan represented by Kaiser and Group Health. The development of HMOs, although rapid, was not very impressive until the mid-1980s, when HMOs started to develop and grow. Most of the growth occurred in non-staff model HMOs. Newly formed HMOs simply could not put together the ownership structures necessary to employ physicians directly and relied on contractual relationships with groups and IPAs. Physicians also were reluctant to give up their independent status for employee positions. Staff-model enrollment today represents approximately ten percent of all HMO enrollment.

LEARNING OBJECTIVE 4

Describe the forces that influenced the development of integrated delivery systems.

INTEGRATED DELIVERY SYSTEMS

With the growth of HMOs and PPOs, buying power was concentrated in fewer purchasing groups, and hospitals and physicians sought some way to reduce the trend of greater and greater discounts granted for participation in managed-care contracts. To offset this concentration of purchasing power, hospitals and physicians began to develop integrated delivery system (IDS) structures to better position themselves and place themselves closer to the premium dollar. In some cases, these IDS organizations even approached employers directly to sell health insurance coverage. This eliminated the health plan, which they regarded as a middleman in the marketplace.

IDSs, which consisted of at least a hospital and physician component, began to develop in the early 1990s. An IDS was thought of as a strategic alliance among doctors, hospitals, and other ancillary providers to deliver care to a defined population. There are few fully integrated delivery systems presently, and most consist of only hospital and doctor elements. IDS organizations initially sought to develop managed-care contracts on behalf of both the hospitals and the physicians, and served primarily as a contracting vehicle. There were a number of economic factors, however, that created the stimulus for the formation of IDSs. These factors are discussed in the following text.

Negotiation for Health Plan Contracts

One of the key driving forces behind hospital-physician integration has been the present need, or perceived future need, to provide health insurers with a single contract for health services. This will be easier to negotiate if the doctors and hospitals are within the same organizational system. Much of the consolidation now occurring in the health care delivery system is related to this factor.

Growing Importance of Payer Referrals

Physicians receive about 27 percent of each health care dollar in the United States, yet they control most of the expenditures. Hospitals and other institutional providers depend upon physician referrals to keep utilization in their facilities at reasonable levels. Although physician referrals are still the primary source of business for most health care providers, there has been a subtle but growing increase in payer referrals. Physicians and hospitals suddenly have found that they are no longer acceptable providers for some health plans and that they have been dropped. Most of the reasons for their exclusion relate to the high cost of their practice patterns with only minimal, if any, attention presently paid to quality of care. Fear of being excluded has caused many hospitals and doctors to create larger corporate structures. It is believed the sheer size of these hospital-physician combinations will strengthen their negotiating position with health plans.

Increasing Importance of Capitation

Under a capitated payment system, providers are paid a fixed amount for each person living in their covered service area. This is very different from the current practice of most payers, including most HMOs, who pay on the basis of services provided. The speed and extent to which the current system (which is largely dominated by retrospective payment for services) will be replaced with prospective capitation is debatable. It is not clear at the present time whether capitation payments to providers will increase. One thing, however, is very clear. Capitation payments will reverse present incentives that exist in fee-for-service-payment methods. Supporters believe that this will encourage preventive care and reduce unnecessary utilization of services; others worry that it will create incentives for skimping on service or reducing quality.

Shift of Hospital Services to Outpatient

In 1988, about 88 percent of all hospital revenue was derived from traditional inpatient services. By 2004, that figure had fallen to 64 percent. From 2001 to 2004, gross outpatient revenue growth was 43 percent, while gross inpatient revenue growth was only 38 percent. This shift from inpatient to outpatient, though possibly mitigated somewhat by the advent of outpatient prospective payment system (PPS), is related to three factors: (1) tremendous cost pressures to perform procedures on an outpatient basis when possible, (2) technology that has made outpatient procedures more feasible, and (3) a strong desire by patients to be treated on an outpatient basis. The cost pressures have forced hospitals to become more active in outpatient services that were traditionally the domain of the physician office, while new technology has enabled doctors to provide services in their offices that were historically performed in hospitals. The outpatient market can either be an area where hospitals and physicians can productively collaborate, or it can degenerate into a fierce competitive battleground between the two groups. For an integrated delivery system to succeed, it is imperative that collaboration, not competition, occurs. Only then can an appropriate continuum of care be assured for every patient.

Integrated Data Systems

Technology has made it possible to share vast quantities of information among various potential users. Shared clinical data among physicians, hospitals, and other providers can enhance both the quality and effectiveness of medical care. Data that are shared also permit some economics in business functions such as billing. Although shared data is an objective sought by many parties, it is much easier to accomplish in organizations that are formally related either through common ownership or business-related affiliations. Unfortunately, the health care industry is notoriously behind in using the power of modern computer systems to solve business and clinical problems. This is partly because the hospital environment is complex and partly because the system is fragmented. For instance, a person who can get cash instantly from an ATM machine while traveling in the Philippines still cannot access his or her medical records if admitted to a hospital one county away from his or her home. A person can call a travel agent to schedule a complex trip itinerary involving multiple airlines, yet one cannot schedule a day's worth of diagnostic and treatment steps in a hospital without serious risk of delays or cancellations. The most impor-

tant factor in the future success of the integrated delivery system likely will be its ability to use information as a competitive resource.

Vertical and Horizontal Integration Trends

There has been a concerted effort during the last few years to develop new entities that can dominate health care markets in selected areas. Major hospital chains have announced new mergers on a weekly basis that are designed to enhance their market position. HCA—The Healthcare Company (formerly Columbia/HCA)—through its mergers, quickly became the nation's largest hospital provider, with special strengths in certain regions across the country. This is an example of horizontal integration and it can be a successful market strategy. Many other regional systems have chosen vertical integration as a means to market dominance. For example, Sentara Health System in Norfolk, Virginia, includes 6 hospitals, 43 primary-care sites, 7 nursing homes, 3 assisted living centers, and its own HMO. Sentara has concentrated its efforts in one region, but it has also combined many of the individual elements of the delivery system and created its own financing entity. The important lesson that most health care providers have realized is that it is dangerous to be small and unaffiliated in today's competitive markets. There is a major "shake-out" coming in the health care industry, and it will involve hospitals, physicians, and payers. Those who are incorporated into larger systems are the most likely to have greater access to consumer and capital markets, and thus be better positioned for long-term survival.

Productivity

Many economists believe that improvements in productivity are the primary means for realizing increases in the standard of living within a nation. The same is true in an economic enterprise. Over the long term, a hospital, medical group, or insurance company cannot increase its financial performance without continually enhancing productivity. One of the key potential benefits of creating integrated delivery systems is the opportunity to reengineer processes across what were formerly impregnable barriers to communication, thereby reducing redundancy and cost.

Figure 6–2 presents a diagram of an IDS and shows its insertion among the health plan, the providers of

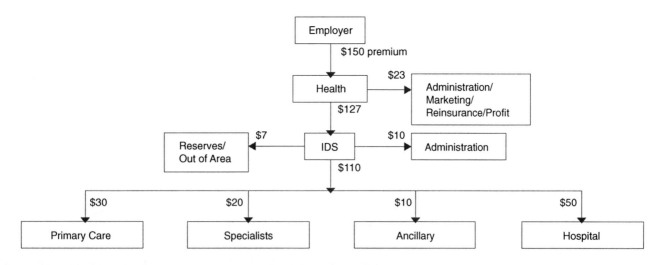

Figure 6–2 Integrated Delivery System Structure Funds Flow in an IDS

medical services, and products that were shown in Figure 6–1. One of the developments discussed earlier that has led to the development of IDS organizations is the increasing importance of capitation as a form of payment to health care providers. As of 2002, it was estimated that 58 percent of the HMOs used capitation for paying primary care physicians, 42 percent used capitation for paying specialty care physicians, and 19 percent used capitation for hospital payment. These percentages have decreased in the last five years as physicians and hospitals gained market leverage and abandoned capitation contracts. It should be noted that these percentages do not reflect the actual percentages of payment made on a capitated basis, only the percentage of HMOs using capitation as a method of payment. For example, the average amount of capitated revenue in a typical hospital is very small, approximately five percent or less. An HMO may use a capitated contract for several of its providers, but the majority of its provider contracts still may be on a fee-for-service basis of some kind.

HMOs have a strong financial incentive to capitate providers whenever possible because this guarantees their profit and locks in a fixed return. For example, the illustration in Figure 6–2 depicts a situation where the HMO could guarantee itself a $23 return PMPM if it could negotiate a fixed PMPM payment of $127 to an IDS for all health care services. Although HMOs have begun to push capitation on health care providers, the providers have asked themselves whether it is to their advantage or not to accept capitation and directly market an insurance product to major employers, thus elim-

inating the middleman health plan from the revenue stream. The health care providers assume that they can perform appropriate utilization review, administer claims, and market their product to employers. The only piece that they may be uncomfortable with is the assumption of risk or underwriting. If HMOs push capitation downward to them, this is no longer an issue. They are already capitated and must assume the medical underwriting risk anyway. This may partially explain why capitation is losing favor with many providers.

It is difficult to answer the question of who controls the IDS. In general, there are three alternatives. Hospitals can seek to control the IDS and protect their position in the health care marketplace as inpatient acute-care utilization falls. Physicians may think that they are in a better position to control the IDS because the emphasis is increasingly on managing care, and this is a role that physicians are uniquely qualified to assume. Finally, organizers of health plans may believe that they are in the best position to control the IDS because of their closeness to the premium dollar and their historical interest in cost control. Health plans also presently have the cash reserves to finance much of the organizational development necessary to make this happen.

The primary vehicle for hospital control has been a physician-hospital organization, or PHO. The PHO may serve as the IDS in Figure 6–2 and contract on behalf of physicians and hospitals. The development of PHOs is relatively new and most were not started until 1993 or later. PHOs are, in theory, a partnership between hospitals and physicians; however, many have been tightly controlled by the hospital and do not always represent a true partnership. Figure 6–3 presents two possible PHO organizational structures. PHOs formed between a hospital and a formal physician organization often are better suited to tackle the issues of managed care because they have a structure in place to encourage hospital-physician dialogues about cost-effective care. PHOs formed without a physician organization simply may represent shareholder interests of individual physicians or groups. This greatly diminishes physician control in the PHO. Significant physician involvement is needed to create an effective integrated delivery system. A loosely organized physician body may give effective control to the hospital, but not really accomplish the physician–hospital integration, which is essential to the success of a PHO.

A PHO may be formed on either a taxable or tax-exempt basis. There are pros and cons for either alternative, but if the objective is the eventual acquisition or employment of physicians, a taxable basis appears to have fewer problems. The creation of a tax exempt nonprofit PHO may raise the issue of inurement, which will be discussed later.

A PHO is not usually a fully integrated delivery system. The major difficulty with many PHOs is determining how to divide the payments from the health plan or HMO among the hospital and its contracting physicians. Each party wants to protect its level of income, and without common ownership or control, this challenge of revenue allocation may doom many PHOs in the long term. Hospital-dominated PHOs are often considered by physicians as an attempt to protect the hospital's declining market share and to perpetuate hospital domination of the health care market.

Medical service organizations (MSOs) are an alternative organizational structure to a PHO that also may serve as an IDS and contract for medical services with a health plan. MSOs are often formed to provide management services to medical groups and may or may not have any hospital ownership or control. If an MSO is formed without hospital interest, the MSO may have to contract with a hospital if the MSO wishes to contract for both hospital and physician services.

Physician organizations (POs) are a relatively recent development. Most POs were developed in large part because of dissatisfaction with hospital-sponsored

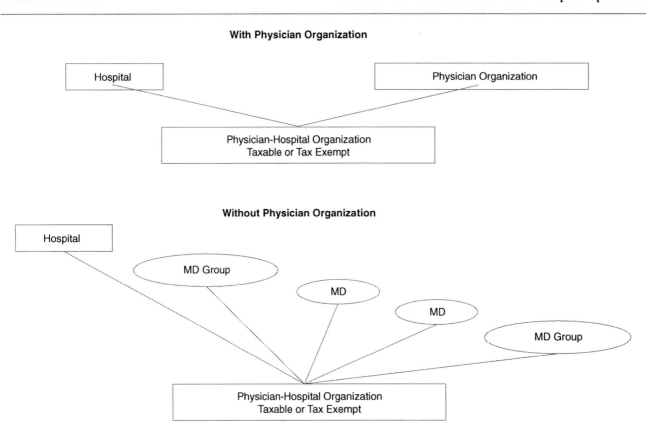

Figure 6–3 Physician-Hospital Organizational Structure

PHOs. They represented an attempt by physicians to take back control in the new managed-care world. The primary problem many physicians encountered when creating a PO was a lack of capital and organizational management skills. Investors have begun to pour capital dollars into the development of POs because they recognize the gigantic opportunities for cost savings in health care, and the pivotal role that physicians play in the realization of those cost savings. National corporations, as well as the American Medical Association, have been aggressively organizing and funding POs to put them in a position where they can begin forming their own managed-care organizations and directly contract for health care services on a capitated basis.

Health insurers and HMOs are also actively entering the IDS arena and beginning to directly provide medical services, especially outpatient services. Acquisition of clinics and the employment of physicians have been undertaken by a number of insurers, and more are considering these types of ventures. Even large employers are beginning to ask the question, "Why should we buy health insurance when we believe that we can make our own delivery system and produce care cheaper than we buy it?" This is most often seen in the development of clinics for employees of a firm.

LEARNING OBJECTIVE 5

Describe some of the methods by which providers are paid in a managed-care environment.

PAYING PROVIDERS IN A MANAGED-CARE ENVIRONMENT

One of the most difficult problems in a less-than-fully-integrated delivery system is splitting the revenue among individual health care providers. Let's assume that the IDS represented in Figure 6–2 does not own the individual health care providers to which it is distributing premium dollars. How does it determine that primary care physicians get $30 PMPM and specialty care physicians get $20 PMPM? Or on an even more basic level, how does the IDS decide if it will pay physicians on a capitated PMPM basis or use a fee schedule?

The decisions referenced previously are related to pricing and are ultimately related to costs. No business

wishes to price its products at levels lower than its costs. If a business continued to do this, it would ultimately be forced to close its doors. Health care providers and insurers are not an exception. The health plan or HMO in Figure 6–2 knows that in its marketplace it can sell health care insurance for $150 on a PMPM basis. Of that $150, $23 is needed to cover internal administrative costs and marketing costs. Additional costs are allocated for reinsurance and profit for the health plan's investors. Reinsurance represents the additional costs paid to other insurers for assumption of unusual risks. For example, the health plan may have to pay the IDS additional payments for treating high-risk patients, such as patients with AIDS.

The health plan then pays the IDS $127 PMPM to provide all health care benefits or some subset of benefits. The IDS needs $10 PMPM to cover its costs of administration and another $7 to create a reserve position to meet out-of-service-area costs. Reserves are needed because the IDS is obligating itself to pay for all health care costs that will be provided during the benefit period. The actual level of utilization is not certain. A reserve position will help them cover costs in situations when actual utilization exceeds estimates. Reserve requirements might also reflect a state requirement that the IDS entity be treated as an insurance company; therefore, statutory reserve levels may be required. Out-of-area costs simply represent those payments that will be made to health care providers out of the service area. A subscriber may be traveling in another state and require emergency medical attention that could not be provided by a network provider.

The IDS now has $110 to pay the providers of health care services that are part of its regional network. Each of those providers will develop a budget of expected costs likely to be incurred for the insured population. For example, assume that the primary care physicians have developed the following schedule to estimate their costs:

Unit of service: Office visits

Annual frequency per 1000 members: 4000

Unit Cost: $75

Net PMPM Cost: $25

The primary care physicians have estimated that approximately 4000 visits per 1000 members will be required per year. At this rate of utilization, approximately four office visits per year will be required per member with an estimated cost of $75 per office visit. Therefore, the average cost per member per year is 4 × $75, or $300 per year. Dividing by twelve, the number of months in a year, yields a PMPM basis of $25. The primary care physicians would be willing to accept any amount greater than $25 PMPM to provide office visits for this insured, especially if they have confidence in their estimated rate of utilization of four visits per year.

Estimating costs under a capitated contract basis is easy to understand from a conceptual basis. Cost can be expressed simply as follows:

$$\text{PMPM cost} = \frac{\text{Expected encounters per year} \times \text{Cost per encounter}}{12}$$

With this framework, the IDS (or the health plan if there is no intermediate IDS entity) has three primary forms of payment. These forms are discussed in the following text.

SALARY OR BUDGET

If the providers are owned by the IDS or health plan or are employees of the organization, there is no real revenue-sharing arrangement in effect. The IDS is merely trying to determine what costs it will incur when it treats the insured population for the budget period. A Kaiser-owned hospital receives a budget based upon expected utilization during the coming year. Salaried physicians are not paid on a volume basis, but are paid a salary with perhaps some incentives for above-average performance. The key relationship in this arrangement is determining the required physician and hospital staffing necessary to meet expected utilization.

FEE FOR SERVICE

Doctors and hospitals in this payment mode are paid on a volume-related basis. For doctors, there are two primary alternatives: charges or fee schedule. In a charge-based payment system, the doctor usually would be paid on the basis of total charges, most often some negotiated percentage of total charges such as 80 percent. In a fee-schedule arrangement, the doctor would be paid based upon some contractually specified fee structure. The Resource-Based Relative Value Scale (RBRVS) described in Chapter 3 would be an example. Hospitals usually are paid on one of three bases: charges, per diems, or per case. As with physicians, a

hospital being paid on a charge basis most likely would not receive 100 percent of charges, but rather some lower percentage. Per-diem payment is common among many HMOs and simply guarantees the hospital so much per patient day, for example $900 for every medical-surgical patient day. Different rates may apply to maternity and intensive-care days. Case payment may be similar to Medicare's diagnosis-related groups (DRGs) and could relate payment to specific DRGs. Case payment could be some aggregation of case categories, such as medical cases, obstetrical cases, and surgical cases. Hospital outpatient services most often are based upon discounted charges, but ambulatory patient classification (APC) groups and other classification methods are becoming more popular and could be used to devise a fee schedule.

CAPITATION

Presently, capitation arrangements are much more common for physicians, especially primary care physicians, than they are for hospitals. Physicians are in a much better position to control and manage costs than are hospitals, which largely provide services ordered and administered by physicians. In a flat-rate capitation arrangement, the provider would receive a flat amount, such as $30 PMPM, to provide all contracted services. A percentage arrangement pays the provider some fixed percentage, for example 25 percent of the PMPM premium payment. Floors or adjustments are sometimes included in capitated arrangements to protect the provider. For example, utilization is usually a function of age, gender, prior health status, and other variables. If an HMO contracted with a primary care group for $30 PMPM, that rate might be sufficient for insured individuals between twenty-five and fifty-five years old, but grossly inadequate for the population older than sixty-five years. The primary care group may therefore adjust its PMPM payment based upon age.

WITHHOLDS AND RISK POOLS

The last element of provider payment that needs to be addressed is the presence of withholds and risk pools. Withholds are most common in fee-for-service arrangements and provide a mechanism for reducing the risk to the IDS or health plan. Table 6–3 presents an example that we will use to illustrate the concept of withholds and risk pools. There are three categories of providers: primary care physicians who are paid $30 PMPM, specialty care physicians who are paid on a fee-schedule basis, and the hospital that is paid $850 per patient day. There are 10,000 people who are insured by the HMO, and budgets are projected for each category.

The hospital budget is projected to be $3,400,000 and is derived as follows, assuming 400 patient days per 1000 members with 10,000 members:

= 4,000 Patient Days × $850

= $3,400,000

The hospital also is subject to a ten percent withhold, which means they will be paid $765 per diem (90 percent of $850). Now assume that actual days were 450 days per 1000 members. Payments would be calculated as follows:

Initial Hospital Payment (4500 Days × $765)	= $3,442,500
Risk Pool (Budget − Paid) ($3,400,000 − $3,442,500)	= −$42,500
Additional Payments to Hospital	= 0

If actual days were 350 instead of 450, the following payments would result:

Initial Hospital Payment (3500 × $765)	= $2,677,500
Risk Pool (Budget − Paid) ($3,400,000 − $2,677,500)	= $722,500
Additional Payments to Hospital (One-third of Risk Pool)	= $180,625

In the first example of excessive utilization, the risk pool is a negative value at the end of the year and the hospital would receive no additional moneys. An inter-

esting question is how the negative risk pool balance would be divided among the primary-care physician, the hospital, and the HMO. We will assume in this example that only the HMO is assuming the negative variance. In the second example, there is a surplus in the risk pool. The balance in the risk pool would be split equally among the four parties: the HMO, the hospital, specialty care physicians, and the primary care physicians. The critical factor in each situation is utilization. Some may wonder why the primary care physicians would be eligible to participate in the hospital risk pool, but these physicians constitute the group that makes the referral and admission decisions that ultimately impact hospital utilization. Sharing in the risk pool gives them an incentive to keep utilization in check. The primary care physicians also share in the specialty care risk pool for the same reason. It is their referral decisions that will determine actual utilization; therefore, they determine the total payments, given a fixed-fee schedule for payment to specialty care physicians.

The use of withholds and risk pools can be confusing to even the most experienced financial analyst. It is important to work out several examples to make certain that all parties understand the contract language. The examples also may be part of the contract to help clarify actual interpretation.

LEARNING OBJECTIVE 6

Describe how managed-care organizations (MCOs) establish their prices.

SETTING PRICES IN CAPITATED CONTRACTS

Pricing in any market is a function of a variety of factors, but it ultimately rests on the relationship between

Table 6–3 HMO Payment Example

	Primary Care Physicians (PCP)	Specialty Care Physicians (SCP)	Hospital
Payment	$30 PMPM	Fee schedule	$850 per diem
Annual budget for 10,000 covered items	$3,600,000	$2,400,000	$3,400,000
Risk pool	0	$240,000	$340,000
Parties splitting risk pool	none	PCP, SCP, HMO	PCP, Hospital, HMO
Withhold	none	none	10%

costs and expected prices. In most markets, prices already are established within some narrow band. An HMO cannot decide to price a policy at $400 PMPM when its closest competitor is pricing a similar product at $300 PMPM. It would have few buyers, if any, and would be forced out of that market. The HMO must therefore decide if it can provide coverage for approximately $300 PMPM to remain competitive in the marketplace.

Table 6–4 presents some hypothetical data and shows average PMPM expenses. The table is useful in identifying the major categories of expense and their relative importance in the cost structures of HMOs.

Revenues for HMOs consist of three categories: premiums, copayments, and coordination of benefits. The largest element is premiums received from HMO subscribers. In addition to those premiums, HMOs also may receive additional revenues from copayments for selected services. For example, the HMO may have a $10 copayment for physician office visits, which is usually collected at the time of the visit. This copayment generates some additional revenue, and it also provides an incentive for subscribers not to overuse physician services. Coordination of benefits relates to the recovery of payments from other insurers when two or more insurance policies are involved. For example, an HMO may have made payments to health care providers on behalf of a member for services rendered, but discovers later that the member also had coverage under a spouse's policy. The two insurance companies would work together to determine the amount that each insurance company is liable to pay and the HMO might receive some payment from the other insurance company for services that it has already paid.

Table 6–4 PMPM Revenue and Expense Averages

Revenue (including copayments and coordination of benefits)	$300.00
Expenses	
Inpatient	$ 80.00
Physician	90.00
Other professional	18.00
Outside referral	15.00
Emergency room and out-of-area	8.00
Other expenses	42.00
Administration	26.00
Total expenses	$ 279.00

The two largest categories of expense for HMOs are inpatient expenses and physician payments. Inpatient expenses are mostly payments to hospitals for covered admissions, whereas physician payments reference amounts paid to both primary care and specialty care physicians. As discussed earlier, these payment types could be fee-for-service or capitation. Other professional services relate to payments for diagnostic lab and radiology, home-health, and other professional services. Outside referral payments are payments to physicians and others for services not contracted with existing providers. Emergency room payments are payments to hospitals for emergency room visits, and out-of-area payments relate to payments for services to members who become ill and need medical attention while traveling outside the plan's service area. Other expenses represent a "catch-all" category designed to include expenses not previously included in the other categories. Lastly, administrative expenses refer to the marketing and administrative costs of plan management. Also included here are premium taxes charged against health insurance sales.

An HMO or an intermediate IDS that is attempting to either set a price or assess the profitability of an existing price will have to determine its expected costs of servicing the defined population. To do this, the following cost relationship would be used:

$$PMPM = \frac{Expected\ encounters\ per\ year \times Cost\ per\ encounter}{12}$$

Cost is a simple function of expected utilization and cost per type of encounter. We will now discuss each of these factors in detail and use the pricing example of Table 6–5. Table 6–5 presents four categories of provider expenses: hospital inpatient, hospital outpatient, physician, and other. Each cost category in the table converts to a budgeted cost on a PMPM basis. To understand this more clearly, let's go through the first item, medical-surgical benefits. It is currently expected that 350 days per 1000 lives will be used and that the HMO will pay the hospital(s) an average rate of $900 per day. To convert this to a PMPM basis, the following calculation would be performed:

$$\$26.25 = \frac{.350 \times \$900}{12}$$

There is also a copayment provision in this insurance package that requires a $100 copayment, but it is not expected that all 350 days will be subject to the copayment provision. Most likely, the copayment is in the form of a deductible payment that is paid upon admission. The expected copayment to be received for medical-surgical patients is .300 times $100, or $30, which is then converted to a PMPM basis of $2.50. The net PMPM cost of medical-surgical benefits is then $23.75 ($26.25–$2.50). The copayment is subtracted from the expected payments to providers because this payment from the subscriber offsets provider payments. The health plan will pay $26.25 per member per month to providers, but it will recover $2.50 in direct payments from the subscriber to the health plan. Similar methodology would be applied to the other cost categories.

The total cost of health care benefits expected to be paid using Table 6–5 is $99.54. This amount is net of copayments, but does not reflect any coordination of benefit (COB) recoveries. COB recoveries are expected to be two percent of the total and reduce the health care cost of this insurance package to $97.55. The HMO needs to mark up this amount by 15 percent to cover administrative costs and reserves, and to build in a profit requirement. The required PMPM price is then $112.18.

The process of pricing is relatively easy as the example shows. The most difficult part is forecasting, especially predicting expected utilization. For example, how certain are we that 350 days of medical-surgical care will be delivered as the forecast states? If 400 days of medical-surgical care were required rather than the budgeted 350, the additional cost would be $3.75 PMPM. This may seem like a small variance, but it should be remembered that margins in most HMOs are not large. Small variations in utilization can have disastrous effects on the financial performance of an HMO.

Table 6–6 provides some utilization averages from the National Center for Health Statistics. The data clearly show the effects of age, gender, and income upon hospital utilization. It is important to carefully assess and estimate utilization, incorporating all of the factors that are likely to drive usage rates.

A policy with liberal benefits for mental health probably would have much greater mental health utilization than one with more stringent benefits. Perhaps the best source of information on expected utilization is prior utilization for the covered population. What were inpatient usage rates last year? How many office visits were made? What kinds of chronic conditions exist in the population? Have physician practice patterns changed or are they likely to change as a result of different financial incentives? The HMO should have data that answer these questions, as well as others, and should be willing to release those data in the contracting phase.

One of the first major effects of managed-care programs is often a reduction in inpatient usage. The biggest area of cost is in inpatient usage, and plans that provide financial incentives for reducing inpatient days almost always experience significant declines in inpatient days per 1000. The use of withholds and risk pools described earlier provides strong financial incentives for physicians to decrease usage rates. Some analysts are predicting that inpatient days per 1000 could drop as low as 100 for the population younger than 65 years in mature managed-care markets.

The cost per unit is not a terribly difficult item to forecast and usually is established in the contract. The HMO knows, for example, they will pay $900 per medical-surgical inpatient day, subject only to a withhold and/or risk pool. The only real issue to confront here is one of negotiation. The HMO wants to get the lowest possible price from the provider, and the provider wants to get the highest possible price from the HMO. If the provider is reasonably certain that dramatic reductions in utilization can occur, it might make sense to negotiate a capitation arrangement. For example, the hospital in Table 6–5 may decide that instead of receiving $900 per day for medical-surgical care, it would rather have $23.75 PMPM, subject to its collection of the copayment. If it can keep usage rates down, the hospital stands to make much more money. However, if usage rates increase above 350 days per 1000, it will lose money. This is a fundamental principle behind risk-return tradeoffs. The entity assuming the risk gets the return or loss.

A provider or the provider's appointed IDS agent, however, needs to make an important decision during negotiation. Namely, the provider must decide whether to provide the services internally or buy contractually required services. For example, the hospital is scheduled to receive $300 per day for inpatient mental health services. Should it provide this service internally, assuming it has the delivery capability, or should it contract this out to a specialized mental health provider? The hospital may decide that it is better off to contract out inpatient mental health benefits for $300 per day and divert its resources to areas where it

Table 6–5 Development of PMPM Rate

Category	Annual Frequency per 1000	Unit Cost	PMPM	Copay Frequency per 1000	Copay Amount	Copay PMPM	Net PMPM
Hospital inpatient							
Medical-surgical	350	$900	$ 26.25	300	$100	$2.50	$ 23.75
Maternity	20	900	1.50	20	100	.17	1.33
Mental Health	30	300	.75	-	-	-	.75
Subtotal			$ 28.50			$2.67	$ 25.83
Hospital outpatient							
Surgery	70	$1,200	$ 7.00	-	-	-	$ 7.00
X-ray & lab	400	250	8.33	-	-	-	8.33
Emergency room	120	250	2.50	80	50	.33	2.17
Subtotal			$ 17.83			$ .33	$ 17.50
Physician							
Inpatient visits	200	$ 100	$ 1.67	-	-	-	$ 1.67
Inpatient surgery	70	1,500	8.75	-	-	-	8.75
Outpatient surgery	400	200	6.67	-	-	-	6.67
Maternity	15	2,000	2.50	15	100	.13	2.37
Office visits	4,000	75	25.00	3,000	10	2.50	22.50
Emergency room	120	100	1.00	-	-	-	1.00
Mental health	350	125	3.65	350	10	.29	3.36
Subtotal			$ 49.24			$2.92	$ 46.32
Other							
Home health	50	$ 200	$ .83	-	-	-	$ .83
Diagnostic X-ray & lab 700	125	7.29	-	-	-		7.29
Durable med. equip.	30	300	.75	-	-	-	.75
Ambulance	35	400	1.17	35	50	.15	1.02
Subtotal			$ 10.04			$ .15	$ 9.89
Total			$105.61			$6.07	$99.54
Coordination of benefits (2%)							(1.99)
							97.55
Net health care cost retention (15%)							14.63
PMPM requirement							$112.18

has a significant competitive advantage, such as cardiology or orthopedics. In some cases, there is no choice because the provider may not have the capability. For example, a primary care medical group that did not have any specialists would be required to negotiate contracts with specialty physicians to provide services if the primary care group contracted for all physician services.

Before we conclude this section on capitation pricing, there are five issues that are of paramount importance to providers or their IDS agents who are negotiating capitated rates with an HMO or directly with an employer.

Delineation of the Set of Covered Services

A provider and health plan should carefully define the set of services covered under their agreement. For example, are transplants and AIDS patients included under the plan? A useful way to summarize this discussion is through the use of a responsibility matrix. The responsibility matrix would list services in the

Table 6–6 Inpatient Utilization Data – 2002

	Days per 1000	Discharges per 1000
Total	541.0	122.9
< 18 years	267.0	80.4
18–44 years	313.4	95.1
45–64 years	573.0	124.1
≥ 65 years	1,738.7	293.1
Male	313.2	72.8
Female	416.2	122.7
Poor	747.9	158.3
Near poor	492.8	124.4
Non-poor	283.3	83.0
Medicare HMO	1,075.4	239.3
Medicare fee for service	1,836.3	258.3
Medicaid	3,286.7	488.5

Source: National Center for Heath Statistics.

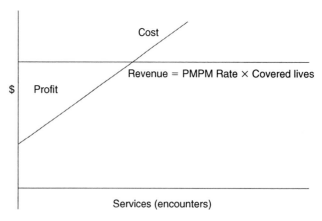

Figure 6–4 Break-Even Analysis in a Capitated Environment

rows and parties responsible in the columns. This matrix could be a part of the formal contract. Included in this category is the specific listing of carve-outs or services that are not included as part of the provider's responsibility, such as mental health.

Determination of Break-Even Service Volumes

Providers that accept a capitation rate have a different break-even structure, as Figure 6–4 shows. In a capitation environment, revenue is fixed, and costs vary with volume. The provider wishes to minimize services or encounters for a fixed number of plan subscribers. The provider accepting a capitation rate must carefully determine the maximum amount of service that could be provided before costs exceeded revenues.

Cost and Use of Stop-Loss Coverage

Providers may have the option of buying stop-loss coverage from the HMO or another insurer to cover costs of patients with catastrophic illnesses. For example, a hospital may negotiate a $75,000 stop loss on inpatient care. Whenever a patient incurred charges greater than $75,000, the stop-loss insurer would pay the hospital for all costs above the threshold. In a like manner, physicians may negotiate lower stop-loss limits of $7,500 per patient for physician charges.

Adverse Selection Provisions

Some reference should be made to adverse selection of HMO members. If a significant number of chronically ill patients, such as patients with AIDS, are attracted to the HMO, both the HMO and the providers may lose. However, if the HMO has subcapitated all its providers with no adverse selection provisions, it might be encouraged to market its policies to anyone at lower-than-required rates because the HMO has a guaranteed cost because it has capitated its providers.

Reporting Requirements

In capitated contracts, providers must closely and frequently monitor utilization rates. Small changes in usage rates can quickly destroy profitability. Data systems must be in place to collect and report this information on a regular basis. Providers also must be aware of the potential for an unrecorded liability referred to as incurred, but not reported (IBNR). This covers situations when services have been delivered, but no claim has been received to date. Providers under capitation may be obligated to pay for services not performed in their network and should be aware of this potential liability. For example, a hospital that contracted out mental health services may not know at any point in time the total outstanding liability. These amounts, although small in relationship to total cost, can produce severe distortions of estimated profitability on contracts unless information about these changes is reported promptly and reasonable estimates of expected costs are made.

MEDICARE AND MEDICAID RISK CONTRACTS

Perhaps the last frontier for major managed-care expansion is the arena of the Medicare and Medicaid markets. Figure 6–5 presents a graph showing the recent growth in managed-care programs. Both Medicare and Medicaid have experienced dramatic growth in managed care, but growth in the Medicare program has begun to decline. Medicare has increased payment for its managed-care program to entice greater participation. The reason for the growth of managed care in Medicare and Medicaid is the potential for cost reduction, especially in inpatient areas. Medicare inpatient days per 1000 average approximately 2000 in the traditional fee-for-service plans, but decrease to 1100 in Medicare risk contracts. Medicaid inpatient days are especially high and might also benefit from a managed-care approach. The potential for cost reduction is enormous, and government fiscal pressure is forcing the movement to managed care.

Because Medicaid is a state-run health care program, there is no nationwide uniform program. Each state has its own defined program and will be different from programs in other states. Most states have received Section 1115 waivers that permit states to engage in Medicaid demonstration projects. These waivers are largely used to expand Medicaid enrollment in HMOs. In many of these contracts, long term care is eliminated or carved out because nursing home expenditures are such a large percentage of the total Medicaid budget, and prediction of utilization can be difficult.

Medicare is encouraging beneficiaries to drop fee-for-service arrangements and switch to its Medicare Advantage plan. The Medicare Advantage plan is at risk for all services provided by Medicare. Medicare reimburses health plans 95 percent of the estimated fee-for-service payment. The base rate is known as the adjusted average per capita cost (AAPCC) and is computed for each county in the United States. The AAPCC is the government's estimate of what fee-for-service costs would have been in the next fiscal year. Individual county rates are published in the Centers for Medicare and Medicaid Services (CMS) AAPCC rate book. Categories include demographic cost factors for Medicare Part A and Part B. These county rates are further adjusted for gender, age, Medicaid eligibility, work status, and institutionalized status. Rates can vary enormously by region of the country. In one recent year, the range was $1,281 PMPM in New Orleans to $620 PMPM in Wyoming. Potential contractors must review their projected costs using a format similar to the one presented in Table 6–5 and compare those with the allowed Medicare AAPCC.

A new risk adjustment payment methodology for Medicare Advantage was required for calendar year (CY) 2000. The approach CMS used to meet the year 2000 mandate for risk-adjusted payments was as follows:

1. It was based on inpatient data.
2. It used individual enrollee risk scores in determining fully capitated payments.
3. It utilized a prospective Principal Inpatient Diagnostic Cost Group (PIP–DCG) risk adjuster to estimate relative beneficiary risk scores.
4. It applied separate demographic-only factors to new Medicare enrollees for whom no diagnostic history was available.
5. It applied a rescaling factor to address inconsistencies between demographic factors in the rate book and the new risk adjusters.

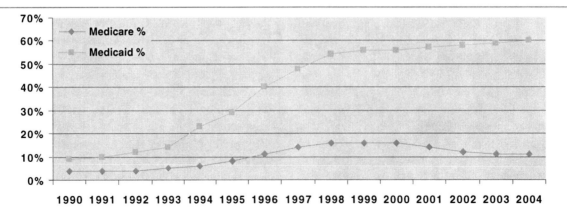

Figure 6–5 Medicare and Medicaid Managed-Care Enrollment Percentage (1990–2004)
Source: Centers for Medicare and Medicaid Services

6. It used 6-month old diagnostic data to assign PIP-DCG categories.
7. It allowed for a reconciliation after the payment year to account for late submissions of encounter data.
8. It phased in the effects of risk adjustment, beginning with a blend of 90 percent of the demographically-adjusted payment rate, and ten percent of the risk-adjusted payment rate in the first year (CY 2000).
9. It implemented processes to collect encounter data on additional services, and moved to a full-risk adjustment model as soon as is feasible.

The previous AAPCC model made no adjustments for level of illness. The goal of the PIP-DCG model is to offer a significant improvement over the previous system by identifying a relatively small group of high-cost, serious illnesses, and provide a marginal additional payment appropriate for those beneficiaries.

Under the previous AAPCC payment system, all enrollees were placed in a base group, which was paid according to demographic characteristics. In the PIP-DCG risk-adjustment system, hospitalizations are used as markers for a particularly ill and high-cost subset of beneficiaries for whom higher payments will be made in the next year. However, the costs associated with beneficiaries who have been hospitalized for conditions used in the PIP-DCG system are no longer in the base payment category. Payments for people in the base payment category decrease as payments are increased for beneficiaries identified as high cost.

Because the initial risk-adjustment methodology is based on data from just one site of service (inpatient hospital encounters), CMS has established a subset of conditions that will be recognized for increased payments. The system will recognize only those admissions for which inpatient care is most frequently appropriate and which are predictive of higher future costs. Admissions for diseases/illnesses most commonly treated on an outpatient basis will remain in the base group and will not be used for upward adjustment. CMS believes that inclusion of these admissions could provide an inappropriate incentive for hospitalization.

LEARNING OBJECTIVE 7

Discuss legal and regulatory issues that affect MCOs.

LEGAL AND REGULATORY ISSUES

There are a number of legal and regulatory issues that affect the formation and operation of provider-based managed-care organizations, especially integrated delivery systems. Among them are the following:

Antitrust

One concern with loose affiliations of physicians, such as an IPA, is the potential for price fixing. If the physicians do not share risk and have not co-mingled their assets and liabilities, the government may view an IPA arrangement that forms to negotiate prices with insurers as an attempt to fix prices. Similar arguments would apply to loose affiliations of hospitals or other providers who are not financially integrated, but who merely created an association to negotiate prices.

Inurement

If a nonprofit entity is involved in the creation of an IDS with physicians, it must be careful to ensure that it is not giving away more than it is receiving in value. This covers situations of physician-practice acquisition, rental of space, or the provision of other services to physicians or other groups. The nonprofit entity must not have its resources used to the benefit of any individual. A "commercially reasonable" test is often used to assess the potential of inurement. Did the nonprofit entity pay more for something that was commercially reasonable or provide services at a price less than commercially reasonable? In the areas of physician-practice acquisition, did the nonprofit entity pay more than fair market value for the practice?

Licensure As an Insurer

It is not clear at this stage whether a provider or provider group, such as an IDS, is required to be licensed as an HMO if it accepts payment on a capitated basis for services that it does not provide. For example, if a primary care group contracted with an HMO for all physician services, not just primary care, would it be required to be licensed by the state as an HMO? Increasingly, many IDS organizations are being required to become licensed as HMOs if they contract out some of the medical services to organizations that are not part of its corporate system.

Incentive Payments to Physicians to Reduce Services

Payments to physicians that provide incentives for fewer services may not be legal if they, in turn offer incentives to provide services less than medically necessary. Practically all current HMO arrangements have financial rewards for reduced services and the pivotal point may be the term "medically necessary."

Intentional Torts

If physicians or other health care providers commit an act of malpractice because they wish to make more money, this may be construed as an intentional tort and their malpractice insurance may not be obligated to pay if wrongdoing was found to have occurred. Physicians may be potentially liable under existing payment arrangements if their malpractice insurer could argue medical services were denied to make more money. For example, a doctor who failed to authorize a mammogram for a woman with a history of family breast cancer may be liable for an intentional tort if the physician were capitated and routinely scheduled mammograms for non-HMO patients with similar histories.

Corporate Practice of Medicine

In some states, physicians are precluded from being employed in corporations that are not physician-owned. This may limit the kind of organizational structure that can be used to acquire physician practices.

There are many other legal and regulatory issues that may affect business practices in managed-care relationships. Outside legal advice should be sought to investigate possible problems and solutions for those areas cited previously, as well as others.

SUMMARY

This chapter has covered the topic of managed care and the evolving issues that affect financial management in managed-care situations. Managed care is not a new development in many respects. Health plans always have been in the business of accepting prepaid dollars in return for the promise to pay for any contractual medical benefits provided to the plan member. The new twist in managed care is really on the payment side. Health plans have historically paid providers, doctors, and hospitals on a fee-for-service basis. The health plan then assumed all the risk for utilization variances, whereas the provider assumed the risk of production, in other words, being able to provide services at costs less than negotiated prices. HMOs and other managed-care organizations are also trying to shift utilization risk to providers by capitating payments to them.

Capitation payment systems require providers to know much more about the populations to which they are obligated to provide health care services and to do a much better job of forecasting utilization. Pricing under a capitation-payment system is easy to conceptualize but difficult to implement, because most providers have little experience with utilization variation in a covered population. Historical-use rates may be available, but managed care has created sizable shifts in utilization rates, and forecasting the magnitude of those changes is difficult.

IDSs have formed to try to place providers closer to the premium dollar flowing from the employer. Many of these IDS organizations are presently hospital-dominated, but physicians are increasingly asking why they should not take charge in the managed-care world because they have the most experience and the greatest ability to actually manage care and achieve cost savings. It is not clear whether the capital and organizational ability of the hospital or the patient-management ability of the physician will win or whether true partnerships will evolve.

ASSIGNMENTS

1. HMOs are a subset of alternative health insurance options. How does an HMO differ from a traditional indemnity health insurance plan?

2. You have been hired as a consultant to a major health insurance company to help identify ways to reduce payments for health care benefits. Please identify some possible methods that may be useful in cutting costs.

3. You represent a medical group that is considering joining a PHO whose sole objective is to negotiate with HMOs and employers for the provision of hospital and physician services on a capitated basis. If your state regards this PHO as a health insurance company and requires licensure, what possible effects might this have?

4. Your multispecialty group has been approached by an HMO that wishes to contract with you for the provision of all physician services for a fixed capitated rate on a PMPM basis. How would you decide what to do in this situation?

5. You represent an IDS that is in negotiations with an HMO for a capitated rate to cover all hospital and physician services for a defined population. The following utilization data have been given to you (Table 6–7), which details last year's usage rates. You included your expected costs for selected services in this table. Using the data presented below, calculate a required break-even rate for this contract, assuming that you need a 15 percent retention factor to cover administrative costs.

6. Memorial Hospital is trying to calculate its expected payments from a proposed fee structure with a local HMO. The HMO projects its hospital budget at 465 patient days per 1000 members, with a payment rate of $1,000 per patient day. The covered population is 25,000 members, which produces a hospital budget of $11,625,000 (465 × 25 × $1,000). The HMO proposes that a ten percent withhold be put into effect, which translates to an actual per diem payment of $900. The risk pool would be shared equally by the doctors (one half) and the hospital (one half). Any negative balance in the risk pool would be assumed by the HMO. Calculate the amount of payment to Memorial Hospital under two assumptions: 550 patient days per 1000 and 430 patient days per 1000.

Table 6–7 Hospital and Physician Services Rates and Usage Rates

Category	Annual Frequency per 1000	Unit Cost	PMPM	Copay Frequency per 1000	Copay Amount	Copay PMPM	Net PMPM
Hospital inpatient							
Medical-surgical	400	$1,000		0	$0		
Maternity	15	1,000		0	0		
Mental health	50	400		0	0		
Subtotal							
Hospital outpatient							
Surgery	100	$1,500		0	$0		
X-ray and lab	500	300		0	0		
Emergency dept	150	300		150	50		
Subtotal							

continues

Table 6–7 continued

Category	Annual Frequency per 1000	Unit Cost	PMPM	Copay Frequency per 1000	Copay Amount	Copay PMPM	Net PMPM
Physician							
Inpatient surgery	100	$2,000		0	$0		
Outpatient surgery	500	300		0	0		
Office visits	5000	100		5000	10		
Inpatient visits	250	150		0	0		
Mental health	400	150		400	20		
Subtotal							
Total							

SOLUTIONS AND ANSWERS

1. HMOs differ from traditional indemnity plans in several ways. First, HMOs usually provide a wider range of benefits, especially in the area of outpatient benefits. To offset the cost of wider benefits, most HMOs restrict the panel of providers, hospitals, and doctors that can be seen. HMO members wishing to see a doctor or hospital not in the network are required to pay for those benefits themselves. Sometimes an HMO may offer a POS option that does permit members to seek care from providers not in the HMO's network, but the member must pay a portion, sometimes a substantial portion, of the cost. HMOs may also pay their health care providers on a capitated basis. This is in contrast to indemnity plans, which usually pay providers on a fee-for-service basis.

2. Health care benefit cost can be expressed as the product of utilization and price. Possible methods for reducing prices paid to providers would include selective contracting with the providers on a discounted basis, use of copayment provisions and deductibles to shift some of the cost to the insured health plan member, and development of a fee schedule that limits payments to all providers. Utilization options for reducing costs would include methods that either reduced the frequency of procedures or used less-expensive procedures. For example, better utilization review and prior authorization for medical procedures could be implemented. Case management of chronic conditions might also cut utilization by reducing the use of expensive inpatient procedures. Incentive structures for physicians, such as capitation payments or risk pools might also be useful in decreasing utilization.

3. Aside from the legal filing requirements and increased government supervision of the PHO, it is also likely that certain reserve requirements must be maintained. These reserves may range from several hundred thousand dollars to several million dollars. This will create additional capital requirements for the PHO creation.

4. The critical issue to be resolved is the maximum amount of service that could be provided under the PMPM rate and still break even. In a fixed PMPM payment system, revenue is fixed, while costs vary with volume. The group needs to carefully consider the expected costs per unit. If total expected cost on a PMPM basis is less than the PMPM premium, it might make sense to accept the capitated rate.

5. Table 6–8 calculates a required net PMPM rate of $138.50. When that rate is increased 15 percent to cover retention, the required PMPM rate would be $159.28.

Table 6–8 PMPM Rate Calculations

Category	Annual Frequency per 1000	Unit Cost	PMPM	Copay Frequency per 1000	Copay Amount	Copay PMPM	Net PMPM
Hospital inpatient							
Medical-surgical	400	$1,000	$33.33	0	$0	$0.00	$33.33
Maternity	15	1,000	1.25	0	0	0.00	1.25
Mental health	50	400	1.67	0	0	0.00	1.67
Subtotal			$36.25			$0.00	$36.25

continues

Table 6–8 continued

Category	Annual Frequency per 1000	Unit Cost	PMPM	Copay Frequency per 1000	Copay Amount	Copay PMPM	Net PMPM
Hospital outpatient							
Surgery	100	$1,500	$12.50	0	$0	$0.00	$12.50
X-ray and lab	500	300	12.50	0	0	0.00	12.50
Emergency dept	150	300	3.75	150	50	0.63	3.12
Subtotal			$28.75			$0.63	$28.12
Physician							
Inpatient surgery	100	$2,000	$16.67	0	$0	$0.00	$16.67
Outpatient surgery	500	300	12.50	0	0	0.00	12.50
Office visits	5000	100	41.67	5000	10	4.17	37.50
Inpatient visits	250	150	3.13	0	0	0.00	3.13
Mental health	400	150	5.00	400	20	0.67	4.33
Subtotal			$78.97			$4.84	$74.13
Total			$143.97			$5.47	$138.50

6. Table 6–9 provides the calculations for hospital payment under the two assumptions.

Table 6–9 Hospital Payment by Patient-Day Level

Patient-Day Level	Hospital Payment @ $900 per Day	Risk Pool (Budget-Paid)	Hospital Share of Risk Pool	Total Hospital Payment
550 PD per 1000	$12,375,000	($750,000)	negative / 0 share	$12,375,000
430 PD per 1000	$9,675,000	$1,950,000	$975,000	$10,650,000

Chapter 7

General Principles of Accounting

LEARNING OBJECTIVES

After studying this chapter, you should be able to do the following:

1. Describe the differences between financial and managerial accounting.
2. Define the concept of an accounting entity.
3. Describe the duality principle and define the fundamental accounting equation.
4. Discuss the methods of valuation for assets and liabilities on a balance sheet.
5. Discuss the differences between the accrual- and cash-basis methods of accounting.
6. Describe some of the effects that inflation can have on revenues and expenses.
7. Discuss fund accounting and the three categories of net assets.
8. Discuss the accounting conventions that affect the application of accounting principles.

REAL-WORLD SCENARIO

Betty James was appointed recently to the Board of St. Mark's Convalescent Center, a religious nursing home in her community. Betty's first assignment was to join the Finance Committee because of her prior business experience; however, she has no understanding of accounting or financial issues because her career has been in the public relations area. She is currently reviewing St. Mark's quarterly financial statements in preparation for the Finance Committee's meeting. She is overwhelmed by the amount of detailed financial and operating data that is presented in the documents, but has noticed a dramatic decline in operating cash available. At the close of the most recent quarter, St. Mark's had consumed 50 percent of the beginning cash and currently had less than ten days of average operating expenses available. Mary Johnson, CFO at St. Mark's, indicated in her narrative accompanying the quarterly statements that the recently completed quarter was outstanding from a financial perspective. Net income was up over 50 percent from the prior quarter and 75 percent above the same quarter last year. Mary explained that the primary reason for the improvement was the negotiation of a contract with a health plan to treat rehabilitation patients who would be transferred from local hospitals. This arrangement has led to a substantial increase in revenue, far above initial budgetary expectations. The provision of care is expected to be very profitable to St. Mark's because the marginal cost of care provided to these patients is estimated to be less than 40 percent of the marginal revenue received. Patient accounting had difficulty, however, in implementing appropriate billing procedures and invoices only recently were sent to the health plan.

Mary Johnson made no mention of the erosion in cash position in her report to the Finance Committee, and Betty is wondering how cash can decline so dramatically when profits are supposedly so strong. Upon further review of the financial statements, she noted that St. Mark's accounts receivable were up over 30 percent from beginning values. The increase in receivables almost matches the decline in cash. Betty is puzzled by this and wants to know if there is some relationship between cash balances and accounts receivable. She remembers from an accounting course taken more than 20 years ago that there was a difference between cash accounting and accrual accounting. Perhaps this could be the explanation for the erosion in cash position, but Betty is still concerned about St. Mark's ability to pay near-term expenditures for payroll, supplies, and maturing debt.

Information does not happen by itself; it must be generated by an individual or a formally designed system. Financial information is no exception. The accounting system generates most financial information to provide quantitative data, primarily financial in nature, that are useful in making economic decisions about economic entities.

LEARNING OBJECTIVE 1

Describe the differences between financial and managerial accounting.

FINANCIAL ACCOUNTING

Financial accounting provides general-purpose financial statements or reports to aid many internal and external decision-making groups in making a variety of decisions. The primary outputs of financial accounting are four financial statements that are discussed in Chapter 8 (see Tables 8–1, 8–2, 8–3, and 8–4 and Exhibit 8–1). They are the following:

1. The balance sheet
2. The statement of operations (or statement of revenues and expenses)
3. The statement of cash flows
4. The statement of changes in net assets

The field of financial accounting is restricted in many ways regarding how certain events or business transactions may be accounted for. The term "generally accepted accounting principles" is often used to describe the body of rules and requirements that shape the preparation of the four primary financial statements. For example, an organization's financial statements that have been audited by an independent certified public accountant (CPA) would bear the following language in an unqualified opinion:

> We have audited the accompanying balance sheets of the XYZ Hospital (the Hospital) as of December 31, 20X3 and 20X2, and the related statements of operations, changes in net assets, and cash flows for the years then ended. These financial statements are the responsibility of the Hospital's management. Our responsibility is to express an opinion on these financial statements based on our audits.
>
> We conducted our audits in accordance with generally accepted auditing standards. Those standards require that we plan and perform the audit to obtain reasonable assurance about whether the financial statements are free of material misstatement. An audit includes examining, on a test basis, evidence supporting the amounts and disclosures in the financial statements.
>
> An audit also includes assessing the accounting principles used and significant estimates made by management, as well as evaluating the overall financial statement presentation. We believe that our audits provide a reasonable basis for our opinion.
>
> In our opinion, such financial statements present fairly, in all material respects, the financial position of the Hospital at December 31, 20X3 and 20X2, and the results of its operations and its cash flows for the years then ended are in conformity with generally accepted accounting principles.

Financial accounting is not limited to preparation of the four statements. An increasing number of additional financial reports are being required, especially for external users for specific decision-making purposes. This is particularly important in the health care industry. For example, hospitals submit cost reports to a number of third-party payers, such as Blue Cross Blue Shield, Medicare, and Medicaid. They also submit financial reports to a large number of regulatory agencies, such as planning agencies, rate review agencies, service associations, and many others. In addition, CPAs often prepare financial projections that are used by investors in capital financing. Although not usually audited by independent CPAs, these statements are, for the most part, prepared in accordance with the same generally accepted accounting principles that govern the preparation of the four basic financial statements.

MANAGERIAL ACCOUNTING

Managerial accounting is primarily concerned with the preparation of financial information for specific purposes, usually for internal users. Because this information is used within the organization, there is less need for a body of principles restricting its preparation. Presumably, the user and the preparer can meet to discuss questions of interpretation. Uniformity and comparability of information, which are desired goals for financial accountants, are clearly less important to management accountants.

PRINCIPLES OF ACCOUNTING

In addressing the principles of accounting, we are concerned with both sets of accounting information, financial and managerial. Although managerial accounting has no formally adopted set of principles, it relies strongly on financial accounting principles. Understanding the principles and basics of financial accounting is therefore critical to understanding both financial and managerial accounting information.

The case example in our discussion of the principles of financial accounting is based on a newly-formed, nonprofit health care organization, which we refer to as "Alpha HCO."

LEARNING OBJECTIVE 2

Define the concept of an accounting entity.

ACCOUNTING ENTITY

Obviously, in any accounting process there must be an entity for which the financial statements are being prepared. Specifying the entity on which the accounting will focus defines the information that is pertinent. Drawing these boundaries is the underlying concept behind the accounting entity principle.

Alpha HCO is the entity for which we will account and prepare financial statements. We are not interested in the individuals who may have incorporated Alpha HCO or other health care organizations in the community, but solely in Alpha HCO's financial transactions.

Defining the entity is not as clear-cut as one might expect. Significant problems arise, especially when the legal entity is different from the accounting entity. For example, if one physician owns a clinic through a sole proprietorship arrangement, the accounting entity may be the clinic operation, whereas the legal entity includes the physician and the physician's personal resources as well. A hospital may be part of a university or government agency, or it might be owned by a large corporation organized on a for profit or nonprofit basis. As a result of corporate restructuring, many hospitals now have become subsidiaries of holding companies. Careful attention must be paid to the definition of the accounting entity in these situations. If the entity is not properly defined, evaluation of its financial information may be useless at best and misleading at worst.

The common practice of municipalities directly paying the fringe benefits of municipal employees employed in the hospital illustrates this situation. Such expenses may never show up in the hospital's accounts, resulting in an understatement of the expenses associated with running the hospital. In many cases, this may produce a bias in the rate-setting process.

Money Measurement

Accounting in general, and financial accounting in particular, is concerned with measuring economic resources and obligations and their changing levels for the accounting entity under consideration. The accountant's yardstick is not intended to measure size, color, weight, or other attributes; it is limited exclusively to money. However, there are significant problems in money measurement, which will be discussed in the following text.

Economic resources are defined as scarce means, limited in supply, but essential to economic activity.

They include supplies, buildings, equipment, money, claims to receive money, and ownership interests in other enterprises. The terms "economic resources" and "assets" may be interchanged for most practical purposes. Economic obligations are responsibilities to transfer economic resources or provide services to other entities in the future, usually in return for economic resources received from other entities in the past through the purchase of assets, the receipt of services, or the acceptance of loans. For most practical purposes, the terms "economic obligations" and "liabilities" may be used interchangeably.

In most normal situations, assets exceed liabilities in money-measured value. Liabilities represent the claim of one entity on another's assets; any excess or remaining residual interest may be claimed by the owner. In fact, for entities with ownership interest, this residual interest is called "owner's equity."

For most nonprofit entities, including health care organizations, there is no residual ownership claim. Any assets remaining in a liquidated not-for-profit entity, after all liabilities have been dissolved, legally become the property of the state. Residual interest is referred to as "fund balance" or "net assets" for most nonprofit health care organizations.

In the Alpha HCO example, assume that the community donated $1,000,000 in cash to the health care organization at its formation, hypothetically assumed to be December 31, 20X2. At that time, a listing of its assets, liabilities, and net assets would be prepared in a balance sheet and read as presented in Exhibit 7-1.

LEARNING OBJECTIVE 3

Describe the duality principle and define the fundamental accounting equation.

Exhibit 7-1   Alpha HCO's Balance Sheet at Formation

Alpha HCO Balance Sheet
December 31, 20X2

Assets	Liabilities and Net Assets
Cash $1,000,000	Net assets $1,000,000

DUALITY

One of the fundamental premises of accounting is a simple arithmetic requirement: the value of assets must always equal the combined value of liabilities and residual interest, which we have called net assets. This basic accounting equation, the duality principle, may be stated as follows:

$$Assets = Liabilities + Net\ assets$$

This requirement means that a balance sheet will always balance: the value of the assets will always equal the value of claims, whether liabilities or net assets, on those assets.

Changes are always occurring in organizations that affect the value of assets, liabilities, and net assets. These changes are called transactions and represent the items that interest accountants. Examples of transactions are borrowing money, purchasing supplies, and constructing buildings. The important thing to remember is that cash transactions must be carefully analyzed under the duality principle to keep the basic accounting equation in balance.

To better understand how important this principle is, let us analyze several transactions in our Alpha HCO example:

- Transaction 1. On January 2, 20X3, Alpha HCO buys a piece of equipment for $100,000. The purchase is financed with a $ 100,000 note from the bank.
- Transaction 2. On January 3, 20X3, Alpha HCO buys a building for $2,000,000, using $500,000 cash and issuing $1,500,000 worth of 20-year bonds.
- Transaction 3. On January 4, 20X3, Alpha HCO purchases $200,000 worth of supplies from a supply firm on a credit basis.

If balance sheets were prepared after each of these three transactions, they would appear as presented in Exhibit 7-2.

In each of these three transactions, the change in asset value is matched by an identical change in liability value. Thus, the basic accounting equation remains in balance.

It should be noted that as the number of transactions increases, the number of individual asset and liability

Exhibit 7–2 Alpha HCO's Balance Sheet, Transactions 1 through 3

• *Transaction 1*

Alpha HCO Balance Sheet
January 2, 20X3

Assets		*Liabilities and Net Assets*	
Cash	$1,000,000	Notes payable	$ 100,000
Equipment	100,000	Net assets	1,000,000
Total	$1,100,000	Total	$1,100,000

Assets: Increase $100,000 (equipment increases by $100,000)
Liabilities: Increase $100,000 (notes payable increases by $100,000)

• *Transaction 2*

Alpha HCO Balance Sheet
January 3, 20X3

Assets		*Liabilities and Net Assets*	
Cash	$ 500,000	Notes payable	$ 100,000
Equipment	100,000	Bonds payable	1,500,000
Building	2,000,000	Net assets	1,000,000
Total	$2,600,000	Total	$2,600,000

Assets: Increase $1,500,000 (cash decreases by $500,000 and building increases by $2,000,000)
Liabilities: Increase $1,500,000 (bonds payable increases by $1,500,000)

• *Transaction 3*

Alpha HCO Balance Sheet
January 4, 20X3

Assets		*Liabilities and Net Assets*	
Cash	$ 500,000	Accounts payable	$ 200,000
Supplies	200,000	Notes payable	100,000
Equipment	100,000	Bonds payable	1,500,000
Building	2,000,000	Net assets	1,000,000
Total	$2,800,000	Total	$2,800,000

Assets: Increase $200,000 (supplies increase by $200,000)
Liabilities: Increase $200,000 (accounts payable increases by $200,000)

items also increases. In most organizations, there is a large number of these individual items, which are referred to as accounts. The listing of these accounts is often called a chart of accounts; it is a useful device for categorizing transactions related to a given health care organization. There is already significant uniformity among hospitals and other health care facilities in the chart of accounts used; however, there is also pressure, especially from external users of financial information, to move toward even more uniformity.

LEARNING OBJECTIVE 4

Discuss the methods of valuation for assets and liabilities on a balance sheet.

COST VALUATION

Many readers of financial statements make the mistake of assuming that reported balance sheet values represent the real worth of individual assets or liabilities. Asset and liability values reported in a balance sheet are based on their historical or acquisition cost. In most situations, asset values do not equal the amount of money that could be realized if the assets were sold. However, in many cases, the reported value of a liability in a balance sheet is a good approximation of the amount of money that would be required to extinguish the indebtedness.

Examining the alternatives to historical cost valuation helps clarify why the cost basis of valuation is used. The two primary alternatives to the historical cost valuation method of assets and liabilities are market value and replacement cost valuation methods.

Valuation of individual assets at their market value sounds simple enough and appeals to many users of financial statements. Creditors especially are often interested in what values assets would bring if liquidated. Current market values give decision makers an approximation of liquidation values.

The market value method's lack of objectivity, however, is a serious problem. In most normal situations, established markets dealing in second-hand merchandise do not exist. Decision makers must rely on individual appraisals. Given the current state of the art of appraisal, two appraisers are likely to produce different estimates of market value for identical assets. Accountants' insistence on objectivity in measurement thus eliminates market valuation of assets as a viable method.

Replacement cost valuation of assets measures assets by the money value required to replace them. This concept of valuation is extremely useful for many decision-making purposes. For example, management decisions to continue delivery of certain services should be affected by the replacement cost of resources, not their historical or acquisition cost—which is considered to be a sunk cost, irrelevant to future decisions. Planning agencies or other regulatory agencies also should consider estimates of replacement cost to avoid bias. Considering only historical cost may improperly make old facilities appear more efficient than new or proposed facilities and projects.

Replacement cost may be a useful concept of valuation; however, it too suffers from lack of objectivity in measurement. Replacement cost valuation depends on how an item is replaced. For example, given the rate of technologic change in the general economy, especially in the health care industry, few assets today would be replaced with like assets. Instead, more refined or ca-

pable assets probably would replace them. What is the replacement cost in this situation? Is it the cost of the new, improved asset, or the present cost of an identical asset that most likely would not be purchased? Compound this question by the large number of manufacturers selling roughly equivalent items and you have some idea of the inherent difficulty and subjectivity in replacement cost valuation.

Historical cost valuation, with all its faults, is thus the basis that the accounting profession has chosen to value assets and liabilities in most circumstances. Accountants use it rather than replacement cost largely because it is more objective. There is currently some fairly strong pressure from inside and outside the accounting profession to switch to replacement cost valuation, but it is still uncertain whether the profession as a whole will yield to such pressure.

One final, important point should be noted: At the time of initial asset valuation, the values assigned by historical cost valuation and replacement cost valuation are identical. The historical cost value is most often criticized for assets that have long, useful lives, such as building and equipment. Over a period of many years, the historical cost and replacement cost values tend to diverge dramatically, in part because general inflation in our economy erodes the dollar's purchasing power. A dollar of today is simply not as valuable as a dollar of ten years ago. This problem could be remedied, without sacrificing the objectivity of historical cost measurement, by selecting a unit of purchasing power as the unit of measure: Transactions then would not be accounted in dollars, but in dollars of purchasing power at a given point in time, usually the year for which the financial statements are being prepared. This issue is addressed later in this chapter, in the section entitled "Stable Monetary Unit."

REQUIRED RETURN ON INVESTMENT AND VALUATION ALTERNATIVES

Business firms, both voluntary nonprofit and investor-owned, must produce returns on their investment greater than the cost of capital used to finance their investment. For example, a business could not borrow money at ten percent and invest the proceeds in projects earning only five percent and expect to stay in business. Valuation of the investment at cost, market value, or replacement cost can have a significant effect on basic business decisions, such as expansion or closure. To illustrate this point, consider the following financial data of James Nursing Home, a fictitious voluntary nonprofit clinic.

James Nursing Home
Financial Data
20X4

Cash flow	$ 10,000
Cost of capital	12%
Investment cost	$ 80,000
Investment-replacement cost	$150,000
Investment-market value	$ 60,000

Return on investment (ROI) for James Nursing Home is 12.5 percent under a cost valuation ($10,000 ÷ $80,000), 6.7 percent under replacement-cost valuation ($10,000 ÷ $150,000), and 16.7 percent under a market-value valuation ($10,000 ÷ 60,000). What should the management and board of James Nursing Home do?

First, the ROI calculated under cost valuation is meaningless for future decisions. An ROI based upon historical cost tells you how well the investment has done, not how well it will do in the future. ROI calculated under replacement cost valuation will tell the decision maker the return using current replacement-cost values. In our example, the James Nursing Home is not profitable given current replacement cost values and is not viable in the future. Unless expectations about future cash flows change, the nursing home should not receive significant new investment. ROI calculated under market values shows the James Nursing Home to be viable in the short run. It is generating an ROI of 16.7 percent, which exceeds its cost of capital, 12 percent. Figure 7–1 illustrates the decision framework.

LEARNING OBJECTIVE 5

Discuss the differences between the accrual- and cash-basis methods of accounting.

ACCRUAL ACCOUNTING

Accrual accounting is a fundamental premise of accounting. It means that transactions of a business enterprise are recognized during the period to which they relate, not necessarily during the periods in which cash is received or paid.

It is common to hear people talk about an accrual-versus a cash-basis method of accounting. Most of us think in cash-basis terms. We measure our personal financial success during the year by the amount of cash we realized. Seldom do we consider such things as wear and tear on our cars and other personal items or the differences between earned and uncollected

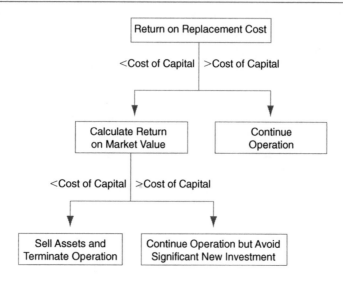

Figure 7–1 Return on Investment Relationships

income. Perhaps if we accrued expenses for items such as depreciation on heating systems, air conditioning systems, automobiles, and furniture, we might see a different picture of our financial well-being.

The accrual basis of accounting significantly affects the preparation of financial statements in general; however, its major impact is on the preparation of the statement of revenues and expenses. The following additional transactions for Alpha HCO illustrate the importance of the accrual principle:

- Transaction 4. Alpha HCO bills patients $100,000 on January 16, 20X3, for services provided to them.
- Transaction 5. Alpha HCO pays employees $60,000 for their wages and salaries on January 18, 20X3.
- Transaction 6. Alpha HCO receives $80,000 in cash on January 23, 20X3 from patients who were billed earlier in Transaction 4.
- Transaction 7. Alpha HCO pays the $200,000 of accounts payable on January 27, 20X3, for the purchase of supplies that took place on January 4, 20X3.

Balance sheets prepared after each of these transactions would appear as presented in Exhibit 7–3.

In Transactions 4 and 5, there is an effect on Alpha HCO's residual interest or its fund balance. In Transaction 4, an increase in net assets occurred because patients were billed for services previously rendered. Increases in net assets or owners' equity resulting from the sale of goods or delivery of services are called revenues. It should be noted that this increase occurred even though no cash was actually collected until January 23, 20X3, illustrating the accrual principle of accounting. Recognition of revenue occurs when the revenue is earned, not necessarily when it is collected.

In Transaction 5, a reduction in fund balance occurs. Costs incurred by a business enterprise to provide goods or services that reduce net assets or owners' equity are called expenses. Under the accrual principle, expenses are recognized when assets are used up or liabilities are incurred in the production and delivery of goods or services, not necessarily when cash is paid.

The difference between revenue and expense is often referred to as net income. In the hospital and health care industry, this term may be used interchangeably with the term "excess of revenues over expenses" or "revenues and gains in excess of expenses."

The income statement or statement of operations summarizes the revenues and expenses of a business enterprise over a defined period. If an income statement is prepared for the total life of an entity, that is, from inception to dissolution, the value for net income would be the same under both an accrual- and a cash-basis of accounting.

In most situations, frequent measurements of revenue and expense are demanded, creating some important measurement problems. Ideally, under the accrual accounting principle, expenses should be matched to the revenue that they helped create. For example, wage, salary, and supply costs usually can be easily associated with revenues of a given period. However, in certain circumstances, the association between revenue and expense is impossible to discover, necessitating the accountant's use of a systematic, rational method of allocating costs to a benefiting period. The best example of this type of method is the recording of depreciation. This process entails allocating costs, such as those associated with building and equipment, over the estimated useful life of the assets.

To complete the Alpha HCO example, assume that the financial statements must be prepared at the end of January. Before they are prepared, certain adjustments must be made to the accounts to adhere fully to the accrual principle of accounting. The following adjustments might be recorded:

- Adjustment 1. There are currently $100,000 of patient charges that have been incurred, but not yet billed.
- Adjustment 2. There are currently $50,000 worth of unpaid wages and salaries for which employees have performed services.
- Adjustment 3. A physical inventory count indicates that $50,000 worth of initial supplies have been used.
- Adjustment 4. The equipment of Alpha HCO has an estimated useful life of ten years, and the cost is being allocated over this period. On a monthly basis, this amounts to an allocation of $833 per month.
- Adjustment 5. The building has an estimated useful life of 40 years, and the cost of the building is being allocated equally over its estimated life. On a monthly basis, this amounts to $4,167.
- Adjustment 6. Although no payment has been made on either notes payable or bonds payable, there is an interest expense associated with using

Exhibit 7–3 Alpha HCO's Balance Sheet, Transactions 4 through 7

• *Transaction 4*

Alpha HCO Balance Sheet
January 16, 20X3

Assets		*Liabilities and Net Assets*	
Cash	$ 500,000	Accounts payable	$ 200,000
Accounts receivable	100,000	Notes payable	100,000
Supplies	200,000	Bonds payable	1,500,000
Equipment	100,000	Net assets	1,100,000
Building	2,000,000	Total	$2,900,000
Total	$2,900,000		

Assets: Increase $100,000 (accounts receivable increases by $100,000)
Net assets: Increase $100,000

• *Transaction 5*

Alpha HCO Balance Sheet
January 18, 20X3

Assets		*Liabilities and Net Assets*	
Cash	$ 440,000	Accounts payable	$ 200,000
Accounts receivable	100,000	Notes payable	100,000
Supplies	200,000	Bonds payable	1,500,000
Equipment	100,000	Net assets	1,040,000
Building	2,000,000	Total	$2,840,000
Total	$2,840,000		

Assets: Decrease by $60,000 (cash decreases by $60,000)
Net assets: Decrease $60,000

• *Transaction 6*

Alpha HCO Balance Sheet
January 23, 20X3

Assets		*Liabilities and Net Assets*	
Cash	$ 520,000	Accounts payable	$ 200,000
Accounts receivable	20,000	Notes payable	100,000
Supplies	200,000	Bonds payable	1,500,000
Equipment	100,000	Net assets	1,040,000
Building	2,000,000	Total	$2,840,000
Total	$2,840,000		

Assets: No change (cash increases by $80,000; accounts receivable decrease by $80,000)

• *Transaction 7*

Alpha HCO Balance Sheet
January 27, 20X3

Assets		*Liabilities and Net Assets*	
Cash	$ 320,000	Accounts payable	$ 0
Accounts receivable	20,000	Notes payable	100,000
Supplies	200,000	Bonds payable	1,500,000
Equipment	100,000	Net assets	1,040,000
Building	2,000,000	Total	$2,640,000
Total	$2,640,000		

Assets: Decrease by $200,000 (cash decreases by $200,000)
Liabilities: Decrease by $200,000 (accounts payable decreases by $200,000)

money for this one-month period. This interest expense will be paid later. Assume that the note payable carries an interest rate of eight percent and the bond payable carries an interest rate of six percent. The actual amount of interest expense incurred for the month of January would be $8,167 ($667 on the note and $7,500 on the bond payable).

The effects of these adjustments on the balance sheet of Alpha HCO and on the ending balance sheet are presented in Exhibit 7–4. It is also possible to prepare the statement of revenues and expenses presented in Exhibit 7–5.

Note that the difference between revenue and expenses during the month of January was $26,833, the exact amount by which the net assets of Alpha HCO changed during the month. The hospital began the month with $1,000,000 in its net asset account and ended with $1,026,833. This illustrates an important point to remember when reading financial statements: the individual financial statements are fundamentally related to one another.

Stable Monetary Unit

The money measurement principle of accounting discussed earlier restricted accounting measures to money. In accounting in the United States, the unit of measure is the dollar. At the present time, no adjustment to changes in the general purchasing power of that unit is required in financial reports; a 2000 dollar is assumed to be equal in value to a 2007 dollar. This permits arithmetic operations, such as addition and subtraction. If this assumption were not made, addition of the unadjusted historical cost values of assets acquired during different periods would be inappropriate, like adding apples and oranges. Current generally accepted accounting principles incorporate the stable monetary unit principle.

LEARNING OBJECTIVE 6

Describe some of the effects that inflation can have on revenues and expenses.

Exhibit 7–4 End-of-Period Adjusting Entries and End-of-Month Balance Sheet

Adjustment	Change	Account(s) Increased	Account(s) Decreased
1	$100,000	Net assets Accounts receivable	None None
2	$50,000	Wages and salaries payable	Net assets
3	$50,000	None	Net assets Supplies
4	$833	None	Net assets Equipment
5	$4,167	None	Net assets Building
6	$8,167	Interest payable	Net assets

Alpha HCO Balance Sheet
January 31, 20X3

Assets		Liabilities and Net Assets	
Cash	$320,000	Wages and salaries payable	$50,000
Accounts receivable	120,000	Interest payable	8,167
Supplies	150,000	Notes payable	100,000
Equipment	99,167	Bonds payable	1,500,000
Building	1,995,833	Net assets	1,026,833
Total	$2,685,000	Total	$2,685,000

Exhibit 7–5 Statement of Revenue and Expenses

Alpha HCO Statement of Revenue and Expenses For month ended January 31, 20X3	
Revenues	$200,000
Less expenses	
Wages and salaries	$110,000
Supplies	50,000
Depreciation	5,000
Interest	8,167
Total	$173,167
Excess of revenue over expenses	$ 26,833

The stable monetary unit principle may not seem to pose any great problems. However, even modest rates of inflation at around four percent per year can quickly compound to produce major financial distortions. For example, a dollar paid in the year 2017 would be equivalent to 67 cents paid in 2007 with a four percent annual inflation rate. Imagine that the inflation rate in the economy is currently 100 percent, compounded monthly. Consider a neighborhood health care center that has all its expenses, except payroll, covered by grants from governmental agencies. Its employees have a contract that automatically adjusts their wages to changes in the general price level. (With a monthly inflation rate of 100 percent, it is no wonder.) Assume that revenues from patients are collected on the first day of the month after the one in which they were billed, but that the employees are paid at the beginning of each month. Rates to patients are set so that the excess of revenues over expenses will be zero. With the first month's wages set equal to $100,000, Exhibit 7–6 shows the income and cash flow position results for the first six months of the year.

Note the tremendous difference between income and cash flow. Although the income statement would indicate a break-even operation, the cash balance at the end of June would be a negative $3,150,000. Obviously, the health care center's operations cannot continue indefinitely in light of the extreme cash hardship position imposed.

Fortunately, the rate of inflation in our economy is not 100 percent. However, smaller rates of inflation compounded over long periods could create similar problems. For example, setting rates equal to historical cost depreciation of fixed assets leaves the entity with a significant cash deficit when it is time to replace the asset. Many health care boards and management organizations of nonprofit firms do not adequately reflect increasing replacement costs in their pricing.

LEARNING OBJECTIVE 7

Discuss fund accounting and the three categories of net assets.

FUND ACCOUNTING

Fund accounting is a system in which an entity's assets and liabilities are segregated in the accounting

Exhibit 7–6 Sample Income and Cash Flows, 100 Percent Inflation

	Income flows			Cash flows		
	Expense	Revenue	Net income	Inflow	Outflow	Difference
January	$100,000	$100,000	0	$50,000	$100,000	($50,000)
February	200,000	200,000	0	100,000	200,000	(100,000)
March	400,000	400,000	0	200,000	400,000	(200,000)
April	800,000	800,000	0	400,000	800,000	(400,000)
May	1,600,000	1,600,000	0	800,000	1,600,000	(800,000)
June	3,200,000	3,200,000	0	1,600,000	3,200,000	(1,600,000)
	$6,300,000	$6,300,000	0	$3,150,000	$6,300,000	($3,150,000)

*$50,000 is equal to the revenue billed in December.

records. Each fund may be considered an independent entity with its own self-balancing set of accounts. The basic accounting equation discussed earlier must be satisfied for each fund: assets must equal liabilities plus net assets for the particular fund in question.

The Financial Accounting Statement Board (FASB) pronouncement #117 changed the nature of fund accounting for voluntary nonprofit health care organizations. It stipulated that only three classifications of net assets or net assets be used. They are as follows:

* Unrestricted net assets
* Temporarily-restricted net assets
* Permanently-restricted net assets

The last two categories of net assets, temporarily- and permanently-restricted net assets, are related to the existence of a donor-imposed restriction. The difference between the two is based upon the nature of the donor's restriction. Temporarily-restricted assets are funds that can be used for a specific purpose only, or may be released for a specific purpose only, or that may be released for general purposes after a passage of time. Permanently-restricted net assets are often of an endowment nature. Only the income of the fund can be used, and the principal cannot be used to fund any purpose. Generally, donor-restricted net assets can consist of the following three common types:

1. Specific-purpose funds
2. Plant replacement and expansion funds
3. Endowment funds

Specific-purpose funds are donated by individuals or organizations and restricted for purposes other than plant replacement and expansion or endowment. Monies received from government agencies to perform specific research or other work are examples of specific-purpose funds.

As one might guess, plant replacement and expansion funds are restricted for use in plant replacement and expansion. Assets purchased with these monies are not recorded in the fund. When the monies are used for plant purposes, the amounts are transferred to the unrestricted net assets. For example, if $200,000 in cash from the plant replacement and expansion fund were used to acquire a piece of equipment, equipment and unrestricted net assets would be increased.

Endowment funds are contributed to be held intact for generating income. The income may or may not be restricted for specific purposes. Some endowments are classified as "term" endowments. That is, after the expiration of some period, the restriction on use of the principal is lifted. The balance is then transferred to the general fund.

CONVENTIONS OF ACCOUNTING

The accounting principles discussed up to this point are important in the preparation of financial statements. However, several widely-accepted conventions modify the application of these principles in certain circumstances. Three of the more important conventions are discussed in the following text:

1. Conservatism
2. Materiality
3. Consistency

Conservatism affects the valuation of some assets. Specifically, accountants use a "lower of cost or market" rule for valuing inventories and marketable securities. The lower of cost or market rule means that the value of a stock of inventory or marketable securities would be the actual cost or market value, whichever is less. For these resources, there is a deviation from cost valuation to market valuation whenever market value is lower.

Materiality permits certain transactions to be treated out of accordance with generally accepted accounting principles. This might be permitted because the transaction does not materially affect the presentation of financial position. For example, theoretically, paper clips may have an estimated useful life greater than one year. However, the cost of capitalizing this item and systematically and rationally allocating it over its useful life is not justifiable; the difference in financial position that would be created by not using generally accepted accounting principles would be immaterial.

Consistency limits the accounting alternatives that can be used. In any given transaction, there is usually a variety of available, generally acceptable, accounting treatments. For example, generally accepted accounting principles permit the use of double-declining balance, sum-of-the-years' digits, or straight-line methods for allocating the costs of depreciable assets over their estimated useful life; but the consistency convention limits an entity's ability to change from one acceptable method to another.

SUMMARY

In this chapter, we discussed the importance of generally accepted accounting principles in deriving financial information. Although these principles are formally required only in the preparation of audited financial statements, they influence the derivation of most financial information. An understanding of some of the basic principles is critical to an understanding of financial information in general.

The following six specific principles of accounting were discussed in some detail:

1. Accounting entity
2. Money measurement
3. Duality
4. Cost valuation
5. Accrual accounting
6. Stable monetary unit

In addition to these, the general importance of fund accounting as it relates to the hospital and health care industry was discussed. The chapter concluded with a discussion of three conventions that may modify the application of generally accepted accounting principles in specific situations.

ASSIGNMENTS

1. ABC Medical Center has undergone a recent corporate reorganization. The structure presented in Figure 7-2 resulted. What difficulties might be experienced in preparing financial statements for the ABC Hospital?

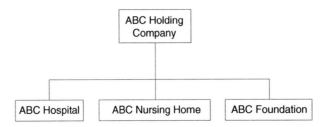

Figure 7–2 ABC Medical Center's Reorganization

2. Does the value of total assets represent the economic value of the entity?

3. What is the difference between stockholders' equity and net assets (or unrestricted net assets)?

4. A home health care firm has purchased five automobiles. Each automobile costs $24,000 and has an estimated useful life of three years. Each year, the replacement cost of the automobiles is expected to increase ten percent. At the end of the third year, the replacement cost would be $31,944 per vehicle. The firm anticipates that each automobile will be used to make 1500 patient visits per year. If the firm prices each visit to recover just the historical cost of the automobiles, it will include a capital cost of $5.33 per visit ($24,000 divided by 4500 total visits). Assuming the revenue generated from this capital charge is invested at ten percent, will the firm have enough funds available to meet its replacement cost? How would this situation change if price level depreciation were used to establish the capital charge?

5. A health maintenance organization (HMO) has just been formed. During its first year of operations, the organization reported an accounting loss of $500,000. Cash flow during the same period was a positive $500,000. How might this situation exist, and which measure better describes financial performance?

6. What is the difference between restricted and unrestricted net assets?

7. Why is consistency in financial reporting critical to fairness in financial representation?

SOLUTIONS AND ANSWERS

1. It may be difficult to associate specific assets and liabilities for the ABC Hospital. For example, debt may have been issued by the holding company to finance projects for both the hospital and the nursing home. In addition, commonly-used assets may be involved, such as a dietary department providing meals for both hospital and nursing home patients. Some expenses also may be difficult to trace to either the hospital or the nursing home. For example, how should expenses that are common to the hospital, the nursing home, and the foundation (such as administrative expenses of the holding company) be allocated? Thus, many problems of jointness may make preparation of the financial statements for the hospital difficult, but such statements are still likely to be a necessity for adequate planning and control.

2. Only coincidentally would the value of total assets equal the economic value of the entity. Total assets, as reported in the balance sheet, represent the undepreciated historical cost of assets acquired by the entity. Economic value of an entity is related to the discounted value of future earnings or the market value of the entity if sold.

3. Both stockholders' equity and net assets (or unrestricted net assets), represent the difference between total assets and total liabilities. Stockholders' equity is used in investor-owned corporations to designate the residual owners' claims. Net assets are used in not-for-profit corporations in which there is no residual ownership interest.

4. Exhibit 7–7 presents data relevant to the pricing decision of the home health care firm regarding the five automobiles. Funds available are shown with historical cost depreciation per automobile. Exhibit 7–8 presents funds available with price level depreciation per automobile. Thus, the prices should be set equal to expected replacement cost. Clearly, pricing services to recover capital costs is critical to long-term financial survival.

Exhibit 7–7 Historical Cost Depreciation for Home Health Care Firm's Automobiles

	Depreciation	*Years Invested (10%)*	*Value, End of Third Year*
Year 1	$8,800	2	$9,680
Year 2	8,000	1	8,800
Year 3	8,000	0	8,000
	$24,000		$26,480

Shortage = $31,944 − $26,480 = $5,464 per automobile

Exhibit 7–8 Price Level Depreciation for Home Health Care Firm's Automobiles

	Depreciation*	*Years Invested (10%)*	*Value, End of Third Year*
Year 1	$8,000	2	$10,648
Year 2	9,680	1	10,648
Year 3	10,648	0	10,648
	$29,128		$31,944

*Price level depreciation in year $t = [(\$24,000 \ (1.10)^t] \div 3$
Shortage = $31,944 − $31,944 = 0

5. The HMO could have received large payments in advance for providing health services to major employers. This would mean that a liability to provide future services exists. Both accounting loss and cash flow are important in assessing financial performance. The accounting loss is symbolic of a critical operational problem regarding revenue and expense relationships. The positive cash flow may be temporary unless revenue exceeds expenses in future periods.

6. A restricted fund has a third-party donor restriction placed on the utilization of the funds. An unrestricted fund has no such restriction.

7. Changes in financial reporting can impair the comparability of financial results between years for a given firm.

Chapter 8

Financial Statements

LEARNING OBJECTIVES

After studying this chapter, you should be able to do the following:

1. Explain why it is important to know the scope of business being reviewed when using financial statements.
2. Identify the four major types of financial statements and explain the type of information provided on each.
3. Explain the account structure usually found in a balance sheet.
4. Identify and distinguish between the types of allowances that affect health care organizations' receivables.
5. Discuss the major components of a statement of revenue and expenses (or a statement of operations).

REAL-WORLD SCENARIO

Tom Johnson, a 2004 graduate of a well-respected health administration graduate program, recently accepted a job offer to work as a financial analyst in the Controller's Office at Northern Healthcare Corporation (NHC), an investor-owned provider of outpatient and rehabilitative health care services. Tom, who will start his job next month, obtained the company's financial statements for the past several years so that he can better understand the company's recent financial position and performance.

Tom knows that Northern Healthcare owns nearly 2000 rehabilitation facilities and ambulatory surgery centers across the United States. In recent years, NHC has expanded rapidly through multiple acquisitions, construction of new facilities, and growth at existing facilities. Yet, even with all this rapid growth, Tom knows that the financial performance has been unsatisfactory in recent years and that management is feeling intense pressure by shareholders to improve performance.

Upon his first inspection of NHC's financial statements, Tom noticed that the financial statements from 1998 forward were in accordance with the provisions of Statement of Financial Accounting Standards (SFAS) No. 131, "Disclosures about Segments of an Enterprise and Related Information," which had been issued by the Financial Accounting Standards Board (FASB) in 1997. Tom learned in school that SFAS No. 131 requires an enterprise to report operating segments based upon the way its operations are managed. This approach defines operating segments along the lines used by management to assess performance and to make operating and resource allocation decisions. Among other requirements, Tom knows that segments must be segregated by product and service, by geographic area, by legal entity, and by type of customer. Based on its management and reporting structure, NHC's segment information was presented for inpatient and other clinical services and outpatient services.

Tom now looked closer at the company's balance sheet. He noticed that the company's cash balance had steadily declined in recent years, while inventories had risen. Given the company's rapid growth, Tom was not surprised to see that total assets had also risen substantially over the past few years; but he was concerned that the amount of long-term debt had just about doubled over a recent two-year period.

Tom then turned to the income statement. Despite the company's increased leverage, as reflected by the substantial rise in debt, the company's earnings per share had fallen by about 80 percent in recent years compared with reaching an all-time high just a few years ago. The declining income was all the more surprising because revenues had risen by one-third over the same period. At first, this seemed somewhat paradoxical to Tom. Then, he noticed that the company's discounts and allowances had risen by upwards of 500 percent over this period. Perhaps, he thought, this figure helped to explain the recent poor performance.

Tom sighed, realizing that trying to more fully understand the company's financial performance would require a lot of time and effort. He would have to study the company's four major financial statements in greater detail. Additionally, he would need to read the accompanying footnotes to the financial statements and would need to supplement that information with additional knowledge of economic, regulatory, and other factors to get a more accurate sense of why NHC's financial performance had deteriorated so much in recent years.

Understanding the principles of accounting is a critical first step in understanding financial statements. However, the average reader may not be able to understand the format and language of financial statements. In this chapter, we discuss in some detail the following four major general purpose financial statements:

1. Balance sheet
2. Statement of revenues and expenses or statement of operations
3. Statement of cash flows
4. Statement of changes in fund balances or net assets

In addition, we examine the footnotes to the financial statements.

The balance sheet and statement of revenues and expenses are more widely published and used than the other two statements. Understanding them enables a reader to use the other two financial statements and financial information in general. Therefore, in the following discussion, we pay major attention to the balance sheet and statement of revenues and expenses. Omega Health Foundation (OHF) is the entity in our example.

LEARNING OBJECTIVE 1

Explain why it is important to know the scope of business being reviewed when using financial statements.

ORGANIZATIONAL STRUCTURE

When reviewing the financial position of any firm, a useful first step is to clearly define the scope of the business being reviewed. Figure 8–1 provides an organizational chart for OHF. The basis for this chart is contained in Item 1 in Exhibit 8–1.

Omega Health Foundation is a complex business with two hospitals, Omega and Able Memorial, plus a number of related medical-service providers. All of the

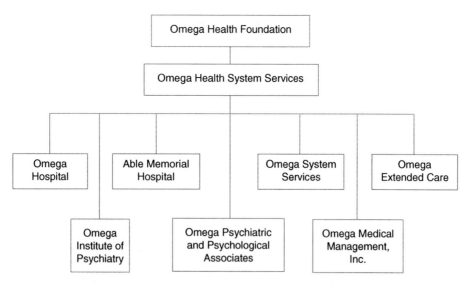

Figure 8-1 Omega Health Foundation Organization Structure

related entities are nonprofit, with the exception of Omega Medical Management, Inc. (OMMI). OMMI is a wholly-owned taxable subsidiary that is involved in a variety of business ventures, among them the operation of family medicine centers where physicians are directly employed. To create incentive programs for employed doctors, many nonprofit health care firms have created taxable subsidiaries, such as OMMI, which permit them more latitude in structuring compensation programs that are not subject to the same issues of inurement examined by the Internal Revenue Service in nonprofit firms.

LEARNING OBJECTIVE 2

Identify the four major types of financial statements and explain the type of information provided on each.

LEARNING OBJECTIVE 3

Explain the account structure usually found in a balance sheet.

BALANCE SHEET

Current Assets

Assets that are expected to be exchanged for cash or consumed during the operating cycle of the entity (or one year, whichever is longer) are classified as current assets on the balance sheet. The operating cycle is the length of time between acquisition of materials and services and collection of revenue generated by them. Because the operating cycle for most health care organizations is significantly less than one year (perhaps three months or fewer), current assets are predominantly those that may be expected to be converted into cash or used to reduce expenditures of cash within one year.

Cash and Cash Equivalents

Cash consists of coin, currency, and available deposited funds at banks. Negotiable instruments such as money orders, certified checks, cashier's checks, personal checks, or bank drafts are also viewed as cash. Cash equivalents include savings accounts, certificates of deposit, and other temporary marketable securities. Categorization as a cash equivalent requires that two criteria be met. First, management must intend to convert the investment into cash within one year or during the operating cycle, whichever is longer. Second, the investment must be readily marketable and capable of being transformed into cash easily.

In Table 8-1, OHF has $7,929,000 in cash and cash equivalents plus $1,763,000 in short-term investments for a total of $9,692,000 at the end of 2009. These monies are readily available to meet normal daily demands for cash such as wages and salaries, federal and state withholding, and supplier invoices. OHF also has $990,000 held by a trustee for payment of the current

Exhibit 8–1   Notes to Combined Financial Statements for Omega Health Foundation

1. Basis of Presentation

The combined financial statements of Omega Health Foundation (OHF) and its controlled entity, Omega Health System Services (OHSS), include the accounts of the following:

- Omega Health Foundation (Foundation), a tax-exempt, nonprofit corporation, engaged in investment and fundraising activities for the benefit of its controlled entities
- Omega Health System Services (OHSS), a tax-exempt, nonprofit entity engaged in providing management services to its controlled entities and subsidiary

The following are the controlled entities and subsidiary of OHSS:

- Omega Hospital (Hospital), a tax-exempt, nonprofit acute-care hospital
- Able Memorial Hospital (Able), a tax-exempt entity whose principal operations include an acute-care and long-term care hospital and a home health care agency
- Omega System Services (OSS), a tax-exempt, nonprofit entity engaged in providing physician and management services to the Hospital and OMMI
- Omega Institute of Psychiatry (OIP), a tax-exempt, nonprofit entity organized to provide outpatient mental health services
- Omega Psychiatric and Psychological Associates (OPPA), a tax-exempt, nonprofit entity, organized to provide mental health services to the public, other organizations, and institutions serving the public
- Omega Extended Care (OEC), a tax-exempt, nonprofit entity, whose principal operations include providing health and wellness services to the public and other organizations and operating an assisted-living personal residence community for the elderly
- Omega Medical Management, Inc., and subsidiaries (OMMI), a wholly owned, taxable subsidiary of OHSS, whose principal operations include rental of durable medical equipment, operation of family medicine center, and various joint venture operations

2. Summary of Significant Accounting Policies

The significant accounting policies OHF follows in the accompanying combined financial statement are as follows:

Principles of Combination

The combined financial statements include the accounts of OHF. All significant intercompany accounts and transactions have been eliminated in combination.

Net Patient Service Revenue

Net patient service revenue is reported at the estimated net realizable amounts from patients, third-party payers, and others for services rendered, including estimated retroactive adjustments under reimbursement agreements with third-party payers. Retroactive adjustments are accrued on an estimated basis during the period the related services are rendered and will be adjusted in future periods for tentative and final settlements.

Charity Care

OHF provides care without charge or at amounts less than its established rates to patients who meet certain criteria under its charity care policy. Because OHF does not pursue collection of amounts qualifying as charity care, they are not reported as revenue.

Statements of Revenues and Expenses of General Funds

For purposes of display, transactions deemed by management to be ongoing, major, or central to the provision of health care services are reported as revenue and expenses. Transactions management deems incidental to operations are reported as nonoperating gains and losses.

Cash and Cash Equivalents

Cash and cash equivalents include cash management funds and repurchase agreements, excluding amounts designated for limited use per the board of directors.

OHF typically maintains cash and cash equivalents in local banks.

Short-Term Investments

Short-term investments, which consist of combined investment trust funds, are carried at the lower of cost or market value. Realized gains and losses on sales of investments are based on cost.

Investments

Investments in cash management funds, real estate, U.S. government obligations, and other interest-bearing accounts are carried at cost. Investments in the combined investment trust, mutual funds, bonds, and common stock funds are carried at the lower of cost or market value. Realized gains and losses on sales of investments are based on cost (specific identification method). The combined investment trust includes a variety of financial instruments, such as preferred and common stocks, U.S. government obligations, and mutual funds.

Inventories

Inventories of pharmaceutical and medical supplies are stated at lower of cost (first-in, first-out method) or market. Inventories of durable medical equipment, owned for lease to others, are valued at the lower of cost, net of depreciation, or net realizable sales value.

continues

Exhibit 8–1 continued

Assets That Have Limited Use

Assets that have limited use include self-insurance trust funds, board-designated funds, funded depreciation, and the portion of funds held by a trustee that has not been reflected as a current asset to meet the current portion of long-term debt. Self-insurance trust funds represent monies designated to fund current and future liabilities for payment of professional liability, workers' compensation, and employee health care benefit claims. Board-designated funds and funded depreciation represent amounts designated by the board of directors of the Hospital for capital acquisition and debt retirement.

Omega Health Foundation has a Workers' Compensation Security Trust (Security Trust). The Security Trust was established under agreement with the State of New York to meet the state's statutory requirements for self-insured workers' compensation arrangements.

Property, Plant, and Equipment

Property, plant, and equipment are stated as cost. Depreciation is computed using the straight-line method over the estimated useful lives of the assets. Gains and losses resulting from the sale of property, plant, and equipment are included in nonoperating gains, net.

Investments in Partnerships and Advances to Partnerships

Omega Health System Services, through its controlled entities and subsidiary, maintains an ownership interest in several partnerships that provide various clinical and nonclinical services. Under the terms of the partnership agreements, OHSS may be required to occasionally make additional cash contributions and provide working capital advances to the partnerships. The investments in partnerships are accounted for by the equity method.

Deferred Financing Costs

Deferred financing costs represent the costs incurred in connection with the issuance of the 1999 hospital revenue refunding bonds and the series of 1997 revenue bonds. These costs are being amortized over the life of the bonds based on the interest method.

Deferred Third-Party Reimbursement

Deferred third-party reimbursement consists of the reimbursement effect arising from the timing differences in recognizing the loss on the advanced refunding of the 1995 hospital revenue refunding bonds, the funding of self-insurance trust funds, and the funding of pension and other postretirement benefits for financial accounting and third-party purposes. The Hospital accounts for deferred reimbursement are based on existing definitive legislation, management's estimate of future utilization, and management's estimate of future recoverability.

Accrued Insurance Costs

Accrued insurance costs consist of reserves for incurred, but not reported claims related to medical malpractice incidents and workers' compensation incidents.

Retirement Programs

Omega Health Foundation has a noncontributory defined benefit pension plan covering most of its employees. It also has a supplemental noncontributory defined benefit pension plan covering certain executives of OHF.

There is a defined contribution tax-sheltered annuity thrift plan covering most OHF employees, except those employed by OMMI. OMMI sponsors a 401(k) tax-deferred savings plan covering most of its employees. Both plans allow participating employees to contribute up to 20 percent of their annual salaries. Employee contributions are matched at a rate of fifty cents per dollar up to the first six percent of the employee's annual earnings.

Taxes (Income Taxes)

All entities, except OMMI, are exempt from federal income tax under section 501(c)(3) of the Internal Revenue code. On such basis, these entities will not incur any liability for federal income taxes, except for possible unrelated business income. As of June 30, 2009, OMMI had net operating loss carryforwards of approximately $4,775,000, expiring in various years through 2019.

Fair Value of Financial Instruments

Statement of Financial Accounting Standards No. 107, "Disclosures about Fair Value of Financial Instruments" (SFAS No. 107), requires that OHF disclose the estimated fair values for certain of its financial instruments. Financial instruments include cash and cash equivalents, accounts receivable, accounts payable, and long-term debt. The carrying amounts reported in the balance sheets for accounts receivable and accounts payable approximate their fair values as of June 30, 2009, and 2008.

3. Third-Party Agreements

Payments to Omega Hospital and Able Hospital from the Medicare and New York Medical Assistance programs for inpatient hospital services were made on a prospective basis. Under these programs, specific, predetermined payments are made for each discharge based on the patient's diagnosis. Blue Cross Blue Shield reimburses the Hospital for inpatient services on a reasonable cost basis. Medicaid pays the Hospital and Able for capital costs on a prospective basis. Medicare makes additional payments for the cost of approved graduate medical education programs and for cases that involve an extremely long hospital stay or unusually high costs compared to national or statewide averages.

continues

Exhibit 8–1 continued

Medicare reimburses the Hospital for outpatient services on a reasonable cost basis, except for clinical lab services, of which reimbursement is based upon a fee schedule, and ambulatory surgery and diagnostic radiology services, of which reimbursement is based upon the lower of cost or blended rate.

Revenue received under agreements with third-party payers is subject to audit and retroactive adjustment. Included in net patient service revenue for 2009 and 2008 are favorable (unfavorable) expense adjustments related to the settlements of prior year cost reports of approximately $334,000 and $43,000, respectively. Adjustments related to final settlements with third-party payers are included in the determination of revenue and gains in excess of expenses and losses during the year in which such adjustments become known.

Capital Cost Payment by Medicare

The Health Care Financing Administration (HCFA) promulgated regulations changing the method by which the Medicare program reimburses hospitals for inpatient capital costs effective beginning fiscal year 1996.

For fully prospective hospitals, these regulations set forth a prospective payment based on rates using a blend of the June 30, 1995, hospital-specific, base-period capital cost per Medicare discharge and the national average Medicare cost per discharge. Annually, the proportion of the hospital-specific rate and the national rate (ten percent for the hospital-specific rate and 90 percent for the national rate as of June 30, 1996) will be adjusted ten percent over a ten-year implementation period until the prospective payments based on 100 percent of the national rate are made.

4. Charity Care, Community Expense, and Bad Debt

Omega Health Foundation provides services without charge or at amounts less than the established rates to patients who meet the criteria of its charity care policy. Criteria for charity care consideration include: family income levels, household size, and ability to pay. Federal poverty guidelines are used as a means to determine the patient's ability to pay. Individuals who qualify for charity care do not have insurance or other coverage.

Charges foregone for providing charity care to individuals as determined in accordance with the AICPA Audit guide will be approximately $1,843,000 and $2,033,000 in 2009 and 2008, respectively. Such amounts have been excluded from net patient service revenue.

5. Property, Plant, and Equipment and Accumulated Depreciation and Amortization

Property, plant, and equipment as of June 30, 2009, and 2008 consist of:

	2009	2008
Land	$ 3,845,050	$ 3,599,917
Land improvements	1,315,653	860,188
Building and building improvements	84,015,323	79,866,619
Equipment, including capitalized leases of $260,007	57,532,494	52,768,949
	146,708,520	137,095,673
Accumulated depreciation, including amortization on capital leases	(70,803,892)	(63,252,010)
	75,904,628	73,843,663
Construction-in-progress	55,478	965,386
	$75,960,106	$74,809,049

6. Long-Term Debt

Long-term debt as of June 30, 2009, and 2008 consists of (data in thousands):

	2009	2008
Omega Hospital revenue refunding bonds, series 2004	$48,480	$49,405
Variable rate Hospital revenue bonds	6,143	6,286
Term loan payable in monthly installments of $16,600 including interest, collateralized by certain equipment of OPPA (7.25 percent and 6 percent at June 30, 2014, and 2013, respectively)	852	998
Various mortgages, loans, and capitalized leases, at various interest rates	707	806
	56,182	57,495
Less current portion:		
Long-term debt and capitalized leases	411	581
Revenue bonds (included in payable from funds held by trustee)	990	925
	$54,781	$55,989

Maturity requirements on long-term debt, including capitalized leases, during the next five years and thereafter are as follows (data in thousands):

2010	$ 1,401
2011	1,488
2012	1,566
2013	1,806
2014	1,715
Thereafter	48,204
	$ 56,180

continues

Exhibit 8–1 continued

7. Funds Held by Trustee

Funds held by trustee as of June 30, 2009, and 2008 consist of (data in thousands):

	2009	2008
Able Mastersite project fund		$ 386
Debt service and revenue funds	$1,011	947
Debt service reserve fund	317	317
	1,328	1,650
Less current portion	990	925
	$ 338	$ 725

8. Retirement Programs

Omega Health Foundation sponsors a noncontributory defined benefit pension plan (Plan) covering most employees. Plan benefits are generally based on the employee's highest average rate of earnings for any five consecutive years during the last ten years of employment. OHF's policy is to annually fund at least the minimum amount required by the Employee Retirement Income Security Act of 1974.

The Plan's aggregate funded status and amounts recognized in the combined balance sheets as of June 30, 2009, and 2008 follow.

	2009	2008
Accumulated present value of benefit obligation:		
Vested	$ 33,387,862	$ 29,117,999
Nonvested	642,769	745,054
	$ 34,030,631	$ 29,863,053
Projected benefit obligation	(49,675,796)	(43,584,435)
Plan assets at fair value	42,726,273	40,718,368
Plan assets in excess of (less than) projected benefit obligation	(6,949,523)	(2,866,067)
Unrecognized net assets	(1,055,892)	(1,187,878)
Unrecognized prior service cost	109,195	130,356
Unrecognized net loss	5,957,690	3,650,026
Contributions during fourth quarter	699,999	500,001
(Accrued) prepaid pension cost	$ (1,238,531)	$ 226,438

Plan assets consist principally of listed stocks and U.S. government obligations.

Aggregate pension costs were $3,864,969 and $2,571,502 for the years ending June 30, 2009, and 2008, respectively. In addition, OHF offered early retirement to certain individuals in 2009, resulting in special termination benefits of $951,303.

Net periodic pension costs for 2009 and 2008 consisted of the following components:

	2009	2008
Service cost benefits earned during the period	$ 2,623,847	$ 2,242,670
Interest cost on projected benefit obligation	3,219,007	2,835,990
Actual return on plan assets	(973,906)	(3,809,141)
Net amortization and deferral	(1,955,282)	1,301,983
Special termination benefits	951,303	
Net periodic pension costs charged to operations	$ 3,864,969	$ 2,571,502

Assumptions used in determining the actuarial value of the projected benefit obligation for 2009 and 2008 were:

	2009	2008
Discount rate	7.25%	7.25%
Rate of increase in compensation levels	6.00%	6.00%
Expected long-term rate of return on assets	7.00%	7.00%

9. Insurance Coverage

Omega Health Foundation maintains self-insurance trust funds for workers' compensation and excess professional liability claims. OHF's contributions to its professional liability self-insurance trust fund are based on actuarial assumptions from independent actuaries; OHF's contributions to its workers' compensation trust fund are based on estimated claims and statutory funding limits.

Directors' and officers' liability coverage is underwritten through Aetna. Coverages are provided under a guaranteed cost agreement on a claims-made policy.

Omega Health Foundation is insured under a comprehensive liability policy provided by ABC Insurance Company. Coverages are provided under a retrospectively rated agreement on a claims-made policy. Before April 2008, coverages were provided under a guaranteed cost agreement on a claims-made policy. Coverages included in this contract are general liability, institutional professional liability, and physician professional liability.

As of June 30, 2009, OHF's professional liability limits were $200,000 for each occurrence and $1,000,000 in the aggregate, and physicians' liability limits were $200,000 for each occurrence and $600,000 in the aggregate. Additionally, OHF participates in a catastrophic loss fund with limits of $1,000,000 for each occurrence and $3,000,000 in the aggregate. An excess liability policy covers individual and aggregate claim liability between $1,200,000 and $11,200,000. OHF maintains excess general liability coverage under an umbrella policy with a limit of $10,000,000. OHF purchases directors' and officers' liability coverage with limits of $5,000,000 and excess workers' compensation insurance with statutory limits over a self-insured retention of $400,000 per occurrence.

continues

Exhibit 8–1 continued

10. Restructuring Costs

During fiscal 2009, OHF underwent a comprehensive restructuring process to optimize work flow and contain operating costs, which resulted in a charge to expenses for restructuring costs of approximately $5,110,000 for severance and termination benefits and consulting fees. The remaining liability as of June 30, 2009, is approximately $2,100,000.

portion of long-term debt as Item 6 in Exhibit 8–1 suggests. OHF also has an additional $2,264,000 held in a self-insurance trust fund. Item 9 explains the current insurance arrangements of OHF, which self-insures for both workers' compensation and professional liability. OHF is estimating that actual claims paid the next year, 2010, will amount to $2,264,000.

Accounts Receivable

Accounts receivable represent legally enforceable claims on customers for prior services or goods. OHF has net accounts receivable of $24,324,000 at the end of 2009. This value represents the amount of money that OHF expects to collect in the next year (2010) from services provided to patients and other customers in 2009 that as of yet have not been paid. There are several other accounts in the current asset and current liability section of the balance sheet that need to be considered when calculating the amount of outstanding receivables. The following schedule recasts accounts receivable as of 2009:

	2009 Value
Accounts receivable	$24,324,000
Add: Due from third-party payers	280,000
Subtract: Due to third-party payers	11,571,000
Net accounts receivable due at 6/30/09	$13,033,000

Omega Health Foundation has a substantial "due to third-party payers," a current liability account, in both 2009 and 2008. The values for both due to and from third-party payers usually reflect differences between interim payments for medical services in the preceding year and estimated final payments. For example, a large payer such as Blue Cross Blue Shield may agree to make biweekly payments of $1,000,000 for services to its beneficiaries. At year-end, a final accounting will be made to determine the actual amounts that should have been paid based on actual utilization and cost. In the case of OHF, a large balance is due to the payers, which may be offset against future payments from the payer. OHF has reduced its investment in accounts receivable substantially by getting its payers to pay for medical services before these services are rendered, enabling OHF to benefit from an interest-free loan.

Omega Health Foundation also has an "advance from third-party payers" listed in its current liability section of $1,205,000 in 2009. This amount is usually associated with a working capital advance by a third-party payer. These advances are usually made to provide funding for medical providers to account for expenses the providers must incur before payments for those services are made. Few third-party payers have such an arrangement in today's economic climate.

LEARNING OBJECTIVE 4

Identify and distinguish between the types of allowances that affect health care organizations' receivables.

What makes health care industry accounts receivable charges different from most other organizations' is that the charges actually billed to patients are often settled for substantially smaller amounts. The differences also are known as allowances. The following four major categories of allowances are used to restate accounts receivable to expected, realizable value:

1. Charity allowances
2. Courtesy allowances
3. Doubtful account allowances
4. Contractual allowances

A charity allowance is the difference between established service rates and amounts actually charged to indigent patients. Many health care facilities, especially clinics and other ambulatory care settings, have a policy of scaling the normal charge by some factor based on income. A courtesy allowance is the difference between established rates for services and rates billed to special patients, such as employees, physi-

Table 8-1 Balance Sheet for Omega Health Foundation as of June 30, 2009 and 2008 (Data in Thousands)

Assets

	2009	2008
Current		
Cash and cash equivalents	$7,929	$7,287
Short-term investments	1,763	1,629
Accounts receivable, less uncollectible accounts of		
$8,532 in 2009 and $8,372 in 2008	24,324	25,597
Due from third-party payers	280	63
Due from donor-restricted funds		179
Inventories	1,763	2,251
Prepaid expenses and other assets	1,135	1,316
Current portion of funds held by trustee	990	925
Current portion of self-insurance trust funds	2,264	3,021
Total current assets	40,448	42,268
Assets that have limited use		
Self-insurance trust funds, net of current portion	9,321	9,013
Board-designated funds	4,959	4,609
Funded depreciation	50,835	37,717
Funds held by trustee, net of current portion	338	726
	65,453	52,065
Property, plant, and equipment, net	75,990	74,829
Investments in and advances to partnerships	2,497	2,226
Deferred financing costs, net	1,139	1,306
Deferred third-party reimbursement		674
Other assets	1,067	654
Total	$186,594	$174,022

Liabilities

	2009	2008
Current		
Current portion of long-term debt	$411	$581
Notes payable		250
Accounts payable and accrued expenses	11,087	7,215
Accrued salaries, wages, and fees	4,342	4,238
Accrued restructuring costs	2,078	
Accrued vacation	3,288	3,331
Accrued insurance costs	2,234	2,284
Advance from third-party payer	1,205	1,142
Due to third-party payers	11,571	10,688
Total current liabilities	36,216	29,729
Accrued retirement costs	8,846	1,736
Accrued insurance costs, net of current portion	4,636	3,450
Deferred third-party reimbursement	3,489	3,488
Long-term debt, net of current portion	54,781	55,989
Other liabilities	1,228	927
Total liabilities	109,196	95,319
Unrestricted net assets	77,398	78,703
Total	$186,594	$174,022

cians, and clergy. A doubtful account allowance is the difference between rates billed and amounts expected to be recovered. For example, a medically indigent patient might actually receive services that have an established rate of $100, but be billed only $50. If it is anticipated that the patient will not pay even the $50, then that $50 will show up as a doubtful account allowance.

In most situations, contractual allowances represent the largest deduction from accounts receivable. A contractual allowance is the difference between rates billed to a third-party payer, such as Medicare, and the amount that actually will be paid by that third-party payer. For example, a Medicare patient may receive hospital services priced at $55,000 but actually pay the hospital only $28,000 for those services, based on the patient's diagnosis-related group classification. If this account is unpaid at the fiscal year end, the financial statements would include the net amount of cash expected to be received, not the gross prices charged. Accounts receivable represent the amount of cash expected to be received, not the gross prices charged. Because most major payers, such as Medicare, Medicaid, and Blue Cross Blue Shield, have a contractual relationship that permits payment on a basis other than charges, contractual allowances can be, and usually are, very large.

The allowances are estimates and will, in all probability, differ from the actual value of accounts receivable that eventually will be written off. For example, OHF shows an expected value of accounts receivable to be collected as $24,324,000 in 2009, but it actually has $32,856,000 of outstanding accounts receivable.

Net accounts receivable	$24,324,000
Allowances	8,532,000
Accounts receivable gross	$32,856,000

Because estimation of allowances is so critical to the reported value of accounts receivable, the methodology should be scrutinized. Just how was the estimate developed? Has the estimating method been used in the past with any degree of reliability? An external audit performed by an independent certified public accountant can usually provide the required degree of reliability and assurance.

Inventories/Supplies

Inventories in a health care facility represent items that are to be used in the delivery of health care ser-

vices. They may range from normal business office supplies to highly-specialized chemicals used in a laboratory.

Prepaid Expenses

Prepaid expenses represent expenditures already made for future service. In the case of OHF, they may represent prepayment of insurance premiums for the year, rents on leased equipment, or other similar items. For example, an insurance premium for a professional liability insurance policy may be $600,000 per year, due one year in advance. If this amount was paid on January 1, then on June 30, $300,000 (one-half of the total) would be shown as a prepaid expense.

Property and Equipment

Property and equipment are sometimes called fixed assets or listed more descriptively as plant, property, and equipment. Items in this category represent investment in tangible, permanent assets; they are sometimes referred to as the capital assets of the organization. These items are shown at the historical cost or acquisition cost, reduced by allowances for depreciation.

Land and Improvements

Land and improvements represent the historical cost of land owned by the health care facility and the historical cost of any improvements erected on it. Such improvements might include water and sewer systems, roadways, fences, sidewalks, shrubbery, and parking lots. Although land may not be depreciated, land improvements may be depreciated. Land held for investment purposes is not shown in this category, but appears as an investment in the other assets section.

Buildings and Equipment

Buildings and equipment represent all buildings and equipment owned by the entity and used during the normal course of its operations. These items are also stated at historical cost. Buildings and equipment not used in the normal course of operations should be reported separately. For example, real estate investments would not be shown in the fixed asset or property, plant, and equipment sections, but in the other assets section. Equipment in many situations is classified into three categories: (1) fixed equipment—affixed to the building in which it is located, including items such as elevators, boilers, and generators; (2) major movable equipment—usually stationary, but capable of being moved, including reasonably expensive items such as automobiles, laboratory equipment, and x-ray apparatuses; and (3) minor equipment—usually low in cost with short estimated useful lives, including such items as wastebaskets, glassware, and sheets.

Construction-in-Progress

Construction-in-progress represents the amount of money that has been expended on projects that are still not complete when the financial statement is published. OHF currently has $55,478 of construction in progress (Item 5 in Exhibit 8–1). When these projects are completed, the values will be charged to property and equipment.

Allowance for Depreciation

Allowance for depreciation represents the accumulated depreciation taken on the asset as of the date of the financial statement. The concept of depreciation is important and useful regarding a wide variety of decisions. The following example illustrates the depreciation concept: A $500 desk is purchased and depreciated over a five-year life. The balance sheet values are presented in the following:

	Year				
	1	2	3	4	5
Historical equipment cost	$500	$500	$500	$500	$500
Allowance for depreciation	100	200	300	400	500
Net	$400	$300	$200	$100	$ 0

In the case of OHF, there is $70,803,892 of accumulated depreciation as of June 30, 2009. The historical cost base for this amount is $146,708,520 (Item 5 in Exhibit 8–1), the historical cost value of buildings and equipment. This means that 48.3 percent of the historical cost of present facilities has been depreciated in prior years. As the ratio of allowance for depreciation to building and equipment increases, it usually signifies that a physical plant will need to be replaced in the near future. OHF appears to be in such a situation, which may partially explain the current construction.

Assets That Have Limited Use

Most organizations will have some amounts listed under "Assets That Have Limited Use." In Table 8–1, OHF has $65,453,000 at the end of 2009. The nature of the asset limitation is usually derived in one of two ways. First, the board may restrict certain funds to be used in designated ways. For example, the board has restricted $9,321,000 for paying insurance costs and $50,835,000 for funded depreciation. These monies have been set aside and restricted by the board for these designated purposes. They could not be spent for any other purpose without the formal approval of the board.

Aside from a board restriction, funds also may be restricted by a third party. These restrictions are not from a third-party donor. If they were, there would be a balance shown as either temporarily or permanently restricted net assets. OHF has only unrestricted net assets presently. A common third-party nondonor restriction is an indenture agreement. OHF has $338,000 of funds restricted under bond indenture. These are funds held by the bond trustee, usually for one or more purposes. Item 7 to OHF's financial statements (Exhibit 8–1) describes the nature of the restrictions under bond indenture.

Other Assets

Other assets are assets that are neither current nor involve property and equipment. Typically, they are either investments or intangible assets. OHF has several categories of investments. It has some investment in partnership through its Ohio Medical Management subsidiary. OHF also has some deferred financing costs. Deferred financing costs are costs incurred initially by a borrower to issue bonds. Such costs include legal fees, accounting fees, and underwriter's costs. The costs are amortized over the life of the bonds, much like depreciation.

Two other intangible asset items that may be included in some health care facility balance sheets are goodwill and organization costs. Goodwill represents the difference between the price paid to acquire another entity and the fair market value of the acquired entity's assets, less any related obligations or liabilities. Goodwill is included mainly in balance sheets of proprietary facilities, although increasingly, it is also being seen in balance sheets of voluntary not-for-profit organizations as they acquire other health care entities, especially physician practices. Organization costs are expended for legal and accounting fees and other items incurred at the formation of the entity. The cost of these items is usually amortized over some allowable life.

Current Liabilities

Current liabilities are obligations that are expected to require payment in cash during the coming year or operating cycle, whichever is longer. Like current assets, they are generally expected to be paid in one year.

Accounts Payable

Accounts payable may be thought of as the counterpart of accounts receivable. They represent the entity's promise to pay money for goods or services it has received.

Accrued Liabilities

Accrued liabilities are obligations that result from prior operations. They are thus a legal obligation to make future payment. The expense of accruing interest, discussed in Chapter 7, is an example. Other examples of accrued expenses are payroll, vacation pay, tax deductions, rent, and insurance. In some cases, especially payroll, accrued liabilities are desegregated to show material categories. OHF classifies accrued liabilities into the following four categories: (1) salaries and wages, (2) vacation, (3) insurance, and (4) restructuring. Accrued restructuring costs represent costs incurred in a "reengineering" program that is explained in Item 10 of Exhibit 8–1.

Current Portion of Long-Term Debt

Current portion of long-term debt represents the amount of principal that will be repaid on the indebtedness within the coming year. It does not equal the total amount of the payments that will be made during that year. Total payments include both interest and principal; current portion of long-term debt includes just the principal portion. For example, if at the June 30 fiscal year close, a total of $360,000 ($30,000 per month) will be paid on long-term indebtedness during the coming year, and of this amount only $120,000 is principal payment, then $120,000 would be shown as a current portion of the long-term debt.

Noncurrent Liabilities

Noncurrent liabilities include obligations that will not require payment in cash for at least one year or more. Omega Health Foundation shows five types of noncurrent liabilities: accrued retirement costs, accrued insurance costs, deferred third-party reimbursement, long-term debt (net of current portion), and other liabilities.

Accrued Insurance Costs

Omega Health Foundation has recorded $4,636,000 of estimated noncurrent insurance costs at the close of 2009. In Exhibit 8–1, item 9 describes this account and its derivation in more detail. The amount reported for estimated insurance costs represents the present value of expected or "estimated" claims that the organization will be responsible for paying. In the case of OHF, there are $4,636,000 of estimated claims that company will be responsible for paying that are not covered by their insurer. OHF has sufficient reserves to cover the expected present value of professional liability and workers' compensation claims at the present time. The asset side of the balance sheet shows $9,321,000 of long-term reserves, far in excess of the current estimated future costs.

Long-Term Debt, Net of Current Portion

Long-term debt, net of current portion represents the amount of long-term indebtedness that is not due in the next year. OHF reported $54,781,000 in 2009. When the current portion of long-term debt ($411,000) is added to the long-term portion, the total amount of debt is determined. The footnotes to financial statements (Item 6, Exhibit 8–1, for OHF) usually provide additional information on maturities, interest rates, and types of outstanding debt.

Unrestricted Net Assets

Unrestricted net assets, as discussed earlier, represent the difference between assets and the claim to those assets by third parties or liabilities. Increases in this account balance usually arise from one of two sources: (1) contributions or (2) earnings.

In the nonprofit health care industry, there is usually no separation in the fund balance account to recognize these two sources. Thus, there is no indication of how much of OHF's unrestricted net assets of $77,398,000 was earned and how much was contributed. Financial statements prepared for proprietary entities do show this breakdown. Earnings of prior years, reduced by dividend payments to stockholders, are shown in an account labeled "retained earnings."

In any given year, however, it is possible to determine the sources of change in unrestricted net assets by examining the statement of changes in fund balance. Table 8–2 shows that OHF's increase in its unrestricted net assets did not result totally from the excess of revenues over expenses in either 2008 or 2009.

The value of the unrestricted net assets account at any point is often confused with the cash position of the entity. However, cash and unrestricted net assets rarely will be equal. In most situations, the cash bal-

Table 8–2 Statements of Changes in Unrestricted Net Assets for Omega Health Foundation as of June 30, 2009 and 2008 (Data in thousands)

	2009	2008
Balance, beginning of year	$78,703	$71,003
Excess of revenues over expenses	(904)	5,706
Change in net unrealized gains and losses on other than trading securities	(498)	1,963
Decrease in unrecognized net periodic pension cost	97	31
Balance, end of year	$77,398	$78,703

ance will be much less than the fund balance. For example, in Table 8–1, OHF has $77,398,000 in unrestricted net assets as of December 31, 2009, but only $7,929,000 in cash at the same date. Thus, the assumption that the $77,398,000 reported as unrestricted net assets can be converted into cash is false.

LEARNING OBJECTIVE 5

Discuss the major components of a statement of revenues and expenses (or a statement of operations).

STATEMENT OF REVENUES AND EXPENSES

The statement of revenues and expenses, otherwise known as an income statement, has become increasingly important in both the proprietary and nonproprietary sectors. It represents operations in a given period better than a balance sheet does. A balance sheet summarizes the wealth position of an entity at a given point by delineating its assets, liabilities, and unrestricted net assets. An income statement provides information concerning how that wealth position was changed through operations.

An entity's ability to earn an excess of revenue over expenses is an important variable in many external and internal decisions. A series of income statements indicates this ability well. Creditors use income statements to determine the entity's ability to pay future and present debts; management and rate regulating agencies use them to assess whether current and proposed rate structures are adequate.

The entity principle is an important factor in analyzing and interpreting the statement of revenue and expense. Income, the excess of revenue over expenses, comes from a large number of individual operations within a health care entity and is aggregated in the statement of revenues and expenses. For example, in Table 8–3, OHF has aggregated the revenues and expenses from its subsidiaries to create a consolidated statement of revenues and expenses. Individuals interested in details about any of the individual entities that constitute OHF would need to see income statements for those organizations. Information about revenues and expenses by product line also are often needed when making managerial decisions. Here, however, our focus is on the general-purpose statement of revenues and expenses, which is an aggregate of individual product lines.

Revenue

Generally speaking, health care facility revenue comes from three sources:

1. Patient services revenue
2. Other revenue
3. Nonoperating gains (losses)

Patient Services Revenue

Patient services revenue represents the amount of revenue that results from the provision of health care services to patients. It is often shown on a net basis in the statement of revenues and expenses, with additional detail in the footnotes. OHF reported net patient services revenue of $160,574,000 in fiscal year 2009. This value is the amount that OHF expects to collect from the patient services it has provided. Actual charges for these services would have been much higher, but are reduced for contractual allowances and charity care.

As discussed earlier in this chapter, charity care represents services provided for which payment was never expected. Most health care organizations have some stated policy regarding charity care. There is no charge generated for a charity patient because payment is not pursued; but it is sometimes useful to identify

Table 8–3 Statements of Revenues and Expenses for Omega Health Foundation as of June 30, 2009 and 2008 (Data in thousands)

	2009	2008
Revenues		
Net patient service revenue	$160,574	$162,323
Equity in net income from partnership	732	1,135
Gifts and bequests	258	435
Other	8,760	8,742
Total revenues	170,324	172,635
Expenses		
Salaries and wages	81,032	81,476
Fringe benefits	18,627	19,876
Professional fees	8,980	12,743
Supplies and other	39,607	38,539
Interest	4,364	4,369
Bad-debt expense	4,551	6,419
Depreciation and amortization	8,545	7,861
Restructuring costs	5,110	
Total expenses	170,816	171,283
Income (loss) from operations	(492)	1,352
Nonoperating gains (losses):		
Income on investments, including net realized gains on sale of investments of approximately $1,150 in 2009 and $1,367 in 2008	4,717	4,658
Gifts and bequests	41	297
Loss on disposal of assets	(84)	(601)
Nonoperating gains, net	4,674	4,354
Excess of revenue over expenses before cumulative effect of change in accounting principle	4,182	5,706
Cumulative effect of change in accounting principle	(5,086)	
Excess of revenues over expenses	($904)	($5,706)

the amount of charges or costs incurred to provide charity care. Item 4 in Exhibit 8–1 shows that OHF provided $1,843,000 in charges to charity patients.

It should be emphasized that bad debts are different from charity care. Bad debts are incurred on patients for whom services were provided and payment was expected, but from whom no payment was received. Bad debts are not reported as a deduction from gross patient services revenue. Instead, bad debts are reported as an expense. As shown in Table 8–3, OHF had $4,551,000 of bad debt expense in 2009. This value represents the amount of charges to patients who are not expected to pay. Much of the bad debt expense in many health care firms is related to uninsured patients. Sometimes a portion of the total charges for a patient encounter are charged to charity fare. For example, a $5,000 charge to an uninsured patient may be reduced to $2,000 with the

$3,000 reduction charged to charity care because the patient met defined charity care guidelines of the firm. The remaining $2,000 charged to the patient is often not paid. If no payment was received, then the remaining $2,000 balance would be charged to bad debts. There is a current debate in the health care industry regarding inclusion of any bad debt in the computation of total charity care provided by a healthcare firm.

The value that is reported for net patient services revenue is part fact and part estimate. At the close of the fiscal year, someone must estimate what amounts actually will be paid by third-party payers under existing contracts. This is not an easy task in most situations, and there is likely to be some error. This is important to recognize when revenue figures are examined for periods shorter than one year (for example, monthly) and when those statements are not audited by an independent auditor. This does not mean that the data are not valid, only that some caution should be exercised in using them.

Usually, it is important to get some information about major third-party payers, such as how they pay and what their relative volume is. Oftentimes, the footnotes can be helpful in this regard. Item 3 in Exhibit 8–1 also explains how Medicare, Blue Cross Blue Shield, and Medicaid make payments to the hospitals.

Other Revenue

Other revenue is generated from normal day-to-day operations not directly related to patient care. In Table 8–3, Omega Hospital reports $8,760,000 of other revenue for 2009. There is no indication regarding the source of this revenue in the financial statements, but the usual sources include revenue from the following:

* Educational programs
* Research and grants
* Rentals of space or equipment
* Sales of medical and pharmacy items to nonpatients
* Cafeteria sales
* Gift shop sales
* Parking lot fees
* Investment income on borrowed funds held by a trustee
* Investment income on malpractice trust funds

It is not entirely clear in all cases whether an item should be categorized as other revenue or as a nonoperating gain or loss. The general rule is that items are categorized as nonoperating gains or losses when they are peripheral or incidental to the activities of the health care provider. For example, donations could be classified as a gain to some organizations and as other revenue to other organizations.

Operating Expenses

In these days of increasing concern regarding health care costs, decision makers are paying more attention to health care facilities' operating expenses. Generally speaking, there are two ways that expenses may be categorized: (1) by cost or responsibility center, or (2) by object or type of expenditure.

In most general-purpose financial statements, costs are reported by cost object. OHF breaks down expenses into the following categories:

1. Salaries and wages
2. Fringe benefits
3. Professional fees
4. Supplies
5. Interest
6. Bad debt expense
7. Depreciation and amortization
8. Restructuring costs

Fringe-benefit costs represent amounts for employee benefits and tax payments. Among items included are social security, unemployment tax, workers' compensation, retirement costs, health insurance, and other fringe-benefit programs.

Bad-debt provisions recognize the amount of gross charges that will not be collected from patients from whom payment was expected. For example, if a patient had commercial insurance coverage that paid 80 percent of the patient's bill of $10,000, the hospital would bill the patient for $2,000. If the patient refused to pay the $2,000 and no payment was expected, the $2,000 charge would be written off as a bad debt. OHF had $4,551,000 of bad-debt expense in 2009.

Depreciation and interest are two special accounts that have great importance in financial analysis and are discussed in Chapter 9.

It should be noted that expense and expenditure (or payment of cash) may not be equivalent in any given period. For example, a health care facility may incur an expenditure of $1,000,000 to buy a piece of equipment, but may charge only $200,000 as depreciation expense in a given year. In general, expenditure reflects the payment of cash, whereas expense recognizes a prior expenditure that has produced revenue. The following three major categories of expenditures usually are not treated as expenses:

1. Retirement or repayment of debt
2. Investment in new fixed assets
3. Increases in working capital or current assets

One major category of expense—depreciation of fixed assets—does not involve a cash expenditure. In addition, other normal accruals, such as vacation and sick leave benefits, may be recognized as expense, but involve no immediate cash outlay.

Nonoperating Gains (Losses)

Gains and losses result from peripheral or incidental transactions. The definitions of peripheral and incidental transactions are not exactly clear, and the terms could be treated inconsistently. For example, OHF reports $4,717,000 of investment income in 2009 (Table 8–3). Most likely, these earnings resulted from funds restricted by the board for funded depreciation. Is the investment of funded depreciation or capital replacement reserves incidental to OHF? OHF must believe that it is, but another organization with exactly the same situation might choose to categorize it differently.

In general, the following items are often categorized as nonoperating gains or losses:

- Contributions or donations that are unrestricted income from endowments
- Income from the investment of unrestricted funds
- Net rentals of facilities not used in the operation of the facility

STATEMENT OF CASH FLOWS

The statement of cash flows is designed to give additional information on the flow of funds within an entity. As we have noted, the concept of expense does not necessarily give decision makers information on funds flow. The statement of cash flows is designed to give information on the flow of funds within an entity, and to summarize the sources that make funds available and the uses for those funds during a given period.

Omega Health Foundation reports its statement of cash flows in Table 8–4. In general, there are three activities that generate or use cash flows for an organization: (1) operating activities, (2) investing activities, and (3) financing activities. OHF derived $23,878,000 of cash flow from operating activities during 2009. It then spent $22,305,000 on investments, primarily property, equipment, and funded depreciation. It also spent $1,473,000 for financing activities during 2009. The difference is the net increase in cash and cash equivalents during the year, or $102,000. A statement of cash flows can be thought of simply as a statement that explains the sources for changes in the cash accounts during the year.

The amount of cash flow generated from operating activities can be thought of as the amount of excess of revenues over expenses subject to several adjustments: The first adjustment is for expenses that did not involve an actual outlay of cash. The biggest items here are depreciation and provision for bad debts. Provision for bad debts is added back because the expense did not involve an outlay of cash, merely a write-off of a receivable.

Another major use of cash flow involves working capital items, the difference between current assets and current liabilities. OHF experienced an increase of $3,278,000 in its patient accounts receivable. In general, the following equation will define the amount of cash flow used to increase patient accounts receivable:

[Ending accounts receivable − Beginning accounts receivable + Provision for bad debts] = Cash change in accounts receivable

[$24,324 − $25,597 + $4,551] = $3,278

Other working capital items, such as a decrease in accounts payable can use cash and reduce cash flow.

STATEMENT OF CHANGES IN UNRESTRICTED NET ASSETS

The statement of changes in unrestricted net assets merely accounts for the changes in unrestricted net assets during the year. Table 8–2 shows that the majority of the change in unrestricted net assets is attributed to excess of revenues over expenses, or net income. OHF does, however, show sizable values for changes in net unrealized gains and losses on other than trading securities. In 2009, OHF experienced a $498,000 reduction compared to an increase of $1,963,000 in 2008. These changes represent valuation adjustments for nontrading securities, usually equity investments, with objective market values, such as publicly traded values. For example, in 2009, the market value of OHF's stock investments may have decreased $498,000 from their beginning market value. When the securities are finally sold, the difference between the sales price and acquisition cost will be recognized as a realizable gain.

SUMMARY

In this chapter, we have discussed the contents of the following four general-purpose financial statements:

1. Balance sheet
2. Statement of revenues and expenses
3. Statement of cash flows
4. Statement of changes in unrestricted net assets

Table 8–4 Statements of Cash Flows of General Funds for Omega Health Foundation Foundation as of June 30, 2009 and 2008 (Data in thousands)

	2009	*2008*
Cash flows from operating activities and gains and losses		
Revenue and gains in excess of (less than) expenses and losses	($904)	$5,706
Adjustments to reconcile revenue and gains in excess of expenses and losses to net cash provided by operating activities and gains and losses:		
Gain on investments	(1,150)	(1,367)
Provision for bad debts	4,551	6,419
Depreciation and amortization	8,545	7,861
Loss on disposal of assets	84	346
Equity in earnings of partnerships	(732)	(1,135)
Amortization of deferred financing costs	167	87
Change in assets and liabilities:		
Increase in patient accounts receivable	(3,278)	(8,482)
Increase in due from donor-restricted funds, net	(100)	(132)
Decrease in inventories	487	1,610
Decrease (increase) in prepaid expenses and other assets	181	(836)
Increase in accounts payable and accrued expenses	3,871	256
Increase in accrued salaries and vacation	61	601
Increase in accrued insurance	1,135	693
Decrease in amounts due from third-party payers	730	
Increase in accrued restructuring costs	2,078	
Increase in advance from third parties	63	200
Increase in amounts due to third-party payers	883	1,859
Increase in accrued retirement costs	7,206	160
Net cash provided by operating activities	23,878	13,846
Cash flows from investing activities		
Purchase of property, plant, and equipment	(10,307)	(14,843)
Cash invested in self-insurance trust funds	258	1,581
Cash invested in and advance to partnerships	(358)	(209)
Distributions and payments received from partnerships	519	832
Cash acquired in acquisitions		66
Cash paid for acquisitions		(596)
Change in minority interest	(3)	(4)
Cash invested in short-term investments	(133)	(164)
Cash invested in board-designated funds, funds held by trustee and funded depreciation	(12,281)	(3,128)
Net cash used by investing activities	(22,305)	(16,465)
Cash flows from financing activities		
Repayments of long-term debt	(1,312)	(1,411)
Issuance (repayments) of notes payable	(249)	21
Issuance of equity in OMMI	88	1,957
Net cash provided by (used by) financing activities	(1,473)	567
Net (decrease) increase in cash and cash equivalents	102	(2,049)
Cash and cash equivalents at beginning of year	$7,827	$9,876
Cash and cash equivalents at end of year	$7,929	$7,827

Primary attention was directed at the first two, the balance sheet and the statement of revenues and expenses, which provide a basis for most financial information.

This chapter focused on understanding the basic information available in these four financial statements. Later chapters describe how that information can be interpreted and used in actual decision making.

ASSIGNMENTS

1. Determine the amount of net operating income that would result for a hospital whose payer mix and expected volume (100 cases) is as follows:

30 Medicare cases	pay $2,000 per case
30 Blue Cross Blue Shield cases	pay $2,200 per case
20 commercial cases	pay 100 percent of charges
10 Medicaid cases	pay average cost
8 self-pay cases	pay 100 percent of charges
2 charity cases	pay nothing

Average cost per case is expected to be $2,200, and the average charge per case is $2,500.

2. How does one determine the amount of debt principal that will be retired during the next year through an examination of the financial statements?

3. What are the titles of the four financial statements that are usually included in an audited financial report?

4. Shady Rest nursing home has just acquired a home health firm for $850,000 in cash. The balance sheet of the home health firm looked as follows just before the acquisition:

Current assets	$200,000
Net fixed assets	100,000
Total	$300,000
Current liabilities	$100,000
Shareholder's equity	200,000
Total	$300,000

Assume that the fair market value of the net fixed assets is $300,000 and fair market value of current assets is $200,000. Describe how this acquisition might be reflected on the balance sheet of Shady Rest.

5. Describe several items that are treated as expenses in the income statement, but that do not require any expenditure of cash in the present period.

6. A major medical supplier has donated $45,000 worth of medical supply items to your firm. These items are then used in the treatment of patients. Explain how this transaction would be recorded in your firm's financial statements.

7. Your HMO is experiencing a critical shortage of funds. Using the statement of cash flows as a framework for discussion, explain how you might attempt to reduce the need for additional funds?

8. Your hospital has experienced negative levels of net income for the last five years. The total amount of accumulated deficits is $5 million, but you have noticed that unrestricted net assets have increased $2 million during the same period. How might this situation be explained?

9. You have been reading the notes to your hospital's financial statements and were surprised to see that the actuarial present value of accumulated pension plan benefits is $4,500,000. A footnote cites a fund of $8,500,000 that has been established to pay these benefits. However, you can find no mention of either the liability or the fund in the balance sheet. What might explain this situation?

1. The calculations to determine the hospital's net operating income would be as follows:

Gross patient revenue	
Medicare (30 × $2,500)	$ 75,000
Blue Cross Blue Shield (30 × $2,500)	75,000
Commercial (20 × $2,500)	50,000
Medicaid (10 × $2,500)	25,000
Self-pay (8 × $2,500)	20,000
Charity (2 × $2,500)	5,000
Total	$ 250,000
Deductions from gross patient revenue	
Medicare [30 × ($2,500 − $2,000)]	$ 15,000
BCBS [30 × ($2,500 − $2,200)]	9,000
Commercial [20 × ($2,500 − $2,500)]	0
Medicaid [10 × ($2,500 − $2,200)]	3,000
Self-pay [8 × ($2,500 − $2,500)]	0
Charity [2 × ($2,500 − 0)]	5,000
Total deductions	$ 32,000
Net patient revenue	$ 218,000
Total expenses (100 × $2,200)	$ 220,000
Excess of revenues over expenses	$ (2,000)

2. The value reported for current maturities of long-term debt in the balance sheet should represent the value of debt principal that will be retired during the next fiscal year.

3. The four financial statements are the following:

   1. Balance sheet
   2. Statement of revenues and expenses or statements of operations or income statement
   3. Statement of cash flows
   4. Statement of changes in unrestricted net assets

4. First, fair market value of the assets acquired by Shady Rest would be determined. In this example, we will assume that the current asset value would not change, but that the fixed assets would be restated to $300,000 at fair market value. Shady Rest is thus acquiring total assets worth $500,000 and assuming liabilities of $100,000 for a net book value of $400,000. Because Shady Rest is paying $850,000 for these assets, there would be a goodwill account of $450,000 created for the residual. The following account changes would occur:

   * Cash—decrease of $850,000
   * Current assets—increase of $200,000
   * Net fixed assets—increase of $300,000
   * Goodwill—increase of $450,000
   * Current liabilities—increase of $100,000

   The goodwill value would be charged to expense in future periods.

5. Pension expense would not require an actual expenditure of cash at the present time, although a payment may be made to a trustee for investment. Other accruals—such as vacation benefits, sick-leave benefits, and FICA (Federal Insurance Contributions Act) accruals—may not require immediate cash expenditures.

6. The fair market value of the items donated would be treated as other revenue. In this case, if $45,000 is the fair market value, that amount would be shown as other revenue.

7. Major categories of fund usage in the statement of cash flows are the following:

   * Repayment of debt
   * Purchase of fixed assets
   * Increase in working-capital items such as accounts receivable

   Conservation of funds could occur in any one of these three areas. For example, the HMO could postpone or delay new fixed asset acquisitions. It also could try to restructure its debt, especially in situations when a large proportion of the debt is short-term. Finally, it could attempt to reduce the amount of funds necessary for working-capital increases. This could be accomplished through a reduction in the HMO's receivable cycle or through an increase in its payable cycle.

8. In this example, the hospital has increased its total equity by $7 million through sources other than income. The most likely sources of these funds are transfers from restricted net assets, such as from plant replacement, or from direct equity transfers from related parties, such as a holding company. It is important to note that the funds were not derived from unrestricted contributions. Unrestricted contributions would have been shown as revenue and thus included in the computation of excess of revenues over expenses. It is also possible that unrealized gains on other than trading securities could have taken place.

9. Pension funds in a defined benefit plan are often held by a trustee and are not shown on the firm's financial statements. This is most likely the situation here. It is important to examine periodically the relationship between the pension fund and the actuarial present value of the pension fund liability. Changes in actuarial assumptions—for example, in mortality, investment yield, or inflation rates—can have a dramatic influence over the size of the liability. The relevant information can be found in the notes to the financial statements.

Chapter 9

Accounting for Inflation

LEARNING OBJECTIVES

After studying this chapter, you should be able to do the following:

1. Discuss the major types of asset valuation.
2. Describe the alternative units of measurement in financial reporting.
3. Describe the uses of financial report information.
4. Describe the difference between monetary and nonmonetary accounts.

REAL-WORLD SCENARIO

Melissa Wynn has been the chief financial officer at Bayside Medical Center for the last five years. She is now in the annual process of reviewing the profitability of all of Bayside's contracts. Her analysis indicates that Bayside's profitability on the Coastal HMO contract is steadily declining over time. Melissa is surprised at this result because she had helped to negotiate a long-term contract with Coastal shortly after she joined Bayside. She recalled from her graduate studies that she needed to be aware of medical price inflation when pricing the contract, especially in a long-term contract. Consequently, Melissa had insisted on rate increases that were tied to the Bureau of Labor Statistics' Medical Consumer Price Index (MCPI). In doing so, she felt she had protected Bayside from profit erosion due to increasing prices. Her analysis does not reveal any substantial changes in unit costs for any major component of Bayside's costs.

As she investigates further, she notices that there have been substantial changes over the years in the mix of services provided to Bayside's patients. Pharmaceutical prices are representing an increasing portion of the hospital's costs of treating patients. She wonders if this fact might be related to the declining profitability. She further investigates how the MCPI is constructed and learns that the weights applied to the inputs (such as pharmaceuticals) that constitute the market basket of goods and services used to construct the MCPI, are based on historical data and can be anywhere from five to fifteen years out of date. She begins to realize that medical price inflation is more complex than she had originally thought and wondered whether this new information might help explain Bayside's eroding profitability on the Coastal contract.

Over the last thirty-five years, the Financial Accounting Standards Board (FASB) has issued a number of pronouncements to adjust for the effects of changing price levels. In September 1979, the FASB issued Statement 33, which required large public enterprises to provide supplemental information on the effects of changing price levels in their annual financial reports. In particular, Statement 33 required firms to disclose the following in notes to the financial statements: current cost and constant dollar earnings; certain other income statement items; and current cost of inventory, property, plant, and equipment. This was a major step for the FASB and marked the first time that firms were required to report price-level effects in their financial reports.

In 1986, when the inflation rate had subsided to less than five percent, the FASB substantially modified its initial position set forth in Statement 33 with the publication of Statement 89. This pronouncement left much of Statement 33 intact, except that it designated the reporting as voluntary. Consequently, most publicly-traded companies stopped disclosing inflation-adjusted earnings. Statement 89 encouraged, but did not require business enterprises to report supplementary information on the effects of changing prices in the following areas for the most recent five years:

* Net sales and operating revenues, using constant purchasing power
* Income from continuing operations on a current cost basis
* Purchasing power gains or losses from holding monetary items
* Increases in specific prices of net plant, property, and equipment net of inflation
* Foreign currency translation adjustments on a current cost basis
* Net assets (assets less liabilities) on a current cost basis
* Income per common share from continuing operations on a current cost basis
* Cash dividends per common share
* Market price per common share at year end

The rationale for these changes in financial reporting stems from the inaccuracy and inability of present, unadjusted, and historical cost reports to measure financial position accurately in an inflation-riddled economy. Although the U.S. inflation rate has been low in recent years, inflationary pressures can increase at any time and will never be removed entirely. Many countries around the world still experience high inflation. Mexico and Brazil have required some accounting inflationary adjustments for over 20 years. Furthermore, some analysts expect a worldwide shortage of energy sources by 2010 or 2020, which might lead to a long-term increase in inflation rates. Thus, inflation accounting will continue to be relevant.

Since inflationary pressures in the economy cannot be removed entirely, it seems logical to assume that alternative financial reporting systems that can account for the effects of changing price levels might be adopted at some point. It also seems logical to expect that the accounting profession eventually will extend alternative reporting requirements to all business organizations. Hospitals and other health care organizations will, in all probability, be included.

Presently, the effect of these financial-reporting changes has not been clearly demonstrated. Thus, many individuals have formed beliefs and expectations about financial-reporting changes that may not be accurate.

The major purpose of this chapter is to discuss and describe the major alternatives for reflecting the effects of inflation in financial statements. Specific methods are described and the adjustments that need to be made to convert historical cost statements are illustrated. This discussion will provide a basis for understanding and using financial statements that have been adjusted for inflation.

REPORTING ALTERNATIVES

Methods of financial reporting can be categorized using two dimensions: (1) the method of asset valuation and (2) the unit of measurement. Two major methods of asset valuation are (1) acquisition (or historical) cost and (2) current (or replacement) value.

LEARNING OBJECTIVE 1

Discuss the major types of asset valuation.

Asset valuation at acquisition cost means that the value of the asset is not changed over time to reflect changing market values. Amortization of the value may take place, but the basis is the acquisition cost. Depreciation is recorded using the acquisition (historical) cost of the asset. Use of an acquisition cost valuation method postpones the recognition of gains or losses from holding assets until the point of sale or retirement.

Current valuation of assets revalues the assets in each reporting period. The assets are stated at their current value rather than their acquisition cost. Likewise, depreciation expense is based on the current value, not the historical cost. Current valuation recognizes gains or losses from holding assets before sale or retirement.

LEARNING OBJECTIVE 2

Describe the alternative units of measurement in financial reporting.

There are also two major alternative units of measurement in financial reporting: (1) nominal (unadjusted) dollars and (2) constant dollars measured in units of general purchasing power. Use of a nominal dollar unit of measurement simply means that the attribute being measured is the number of dollars. From an accounting perspective, a dollar of one year is no different from a dollar of another year. No recognition is given to changes in the purchasing power of the dollar because the attribute is not measured. The major outcome associated with the use of this measure unit is that gains or losses, regardless of when they are recognized, are not adjusted for changes in purchasing power. For example, if a piece of land acquired in 1987 for $1 million were sold for $5 million in 2007, it would generate a $4 million gain, regardless of changes in the purchasing power of the dollar during the twenty-year period.

A constant dollar measuring unit reports the effects of all financial transactions in terms of constant purchasing power. The unit that is usually used is the purchasing power of the dollar at the end of the reporting period or the average during the fiscal year. The calculation for converting nominal dollars to a measure of constant purchasing power consists of the multiplication of the unadjusted, or nominal, dollars by a price index. During periods of inflation, when using a constant dollar measuring unit, gains from holding assets are reduced, whereas losses are increased. Thus, in the previous land sale example, the initial acquisition cost would be restated to 2007 dollars, and as result reduce the gain from the sale (Exhibit 9–1).

Exhibit 9–1 Constant Dollar Measurement

Sale price of land (2007 dollars)	$5,000,000
Less acquisition cost restated	
(2007 dollars)	2,038,504
Gain on sale	$2,961,496

Constant dollar measurement has a further significant effect on financial reporting. The gains or losses created by holding monetary liabilities or assets during periods of purchasing power changes are recognized in the financial reporting. For example, an entity that owed $25 million during a year when the purchasing power of the dollar decreased by ten percent would report a $2.5 million (0.10 × $25 million) purchasing power gain. All gains or losses would be recognized, regardless of the valuation basis used.

Monetary assets and liabilities are defined as those items that reflect cash or claims to cash that are fixed in terms of the number of dollars, regardless of changes in prices. Almost all liabilities are monetary items, whereas monetary assets consist primarily of cash, marketable securities, and receivables. Purchasing power gains or losses are recognized on monetary items because there is an assumption that the gains or losses are already realized, because repayments or receipts are fixed.

The interfacing of the valuation basis and the unit of measurement basis produces four alternative financial reporting methods (Table 9–1). Each of the four methods is a possible basis for financial reporting. The unadjusted historical cost (HC) method represents the present method used by accountants; the other three methods are alternatives that would provide some degree of inflationary adjustment not present in the HC method. The HC-general price level adjusted (HC-GPL) method is referred to as historical cost/constant dollar accounting, whereas the current value-general price level adjusted (CV-GPL) method is referred to as current cost accounting.

Table 9–2 summarizes the effects the four reporting methods would have on the following three major income statement items: (1) depreciation expense, (2) purchasing power gains or losses, and (3) unrealized gains in replacement value. However, the net effect of the changes in these items on net income for an individual institution cannot be predicted; the composition and age of the assets, as well as the prior patterns of financing, will determine whether the net effect will be positive or negative and to what degree.

Table 9–1 Alternative Financial Reporting Bases

Unit of Measurement	Asset Valuation Method	
	Acquisition cost	Current Value
Nominal dollars	Unadjusted historical cost (HC)	Current value (CV)
Constant dollars	Historical cost-general price level adjusted (HC–GPL) Constant dollar accounting	Current value-general price level adjusted (CV–GPL) Current cost accounting

LEARNING OBJECTIVE 3

Describe the uses of financial report information.

USES OF FINANCIAL REPORT INFORMATION

The measurement of financial position is an important function, and its results are useful to a great variety of decision makers, both internal and external to the organization. Changes in financial reporting methods unquestionably will alter the resulting measures of financial position reported in financial statements. These changes are likely to produce changes in the de-

cisions that are based on the financial reports (Figure 9–1).

Lenders represent an important category of financial statement users who may change their decisions on the basis of a new financial reporting method. A lender's major concern is the relative financial position of both the individual firm and the industry. A decrease in the relative financial position of the industry could seriously affect both the availability and the cost of credit. If, for a variety of reasons, new measurements of financial position make the health care industry appear weaker than other industries, financing terms could change. Particularly for the health care industry, which is increasingly dependent on debt financing, the importance of changes in financial reporting methods cannot be overstated. Research on the results of changing to an HC–GPL method has shown that the relative

Table 9–2 Major Effect of Alternative Reporting Methods on Net Income Measurement

Reporting Methods	Impact Variables		
	Depreciation Expense	Purchasing Power Gains/Losses	Unrealized Gains in Replacement Value
HC	No change recognized	No change/not recognized	No change/not recognized
HC–GPL	Increase/GPL depreciation recognized	Gain or loss/depends on the net monetary asset position	No change/not recognized
CV	Increase/will recognize replacement cost	No change/not recognized	Gain/will recognize increase in replacement cost
CV–GPL	Increase/will recognize current replacement cost	Gain or loss/depends on the net monetary asset position	Gain/will recognize increase in replacement cost but will reduce amount by changes in the GPL

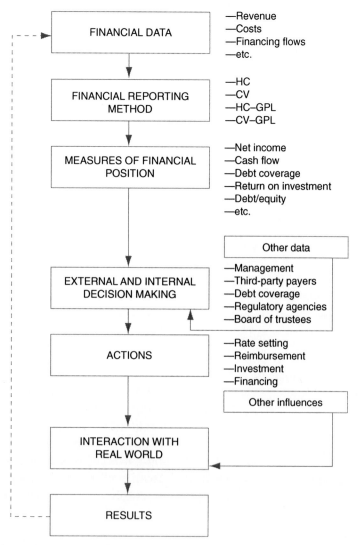

Figure 9–1 Financial Data in Decision Making

---

financial positions of individual firms and industries are also likely to change.

Changes in financial reporting methods also could have an effect on decisions reached by regulatory and rate-setting organizations. As a result of such changes, comparisons of costs across institutions may be more meaningful than they were previously. For example, depreciation in firms that operate in relatively new physical plants cannot be compared with the unadjusted historical depreciation costs of older facilities. Without financial reporting adjustments, new facilities may appear to have higher costs and thus be less efficient, whereas, in fact, the opposite may be true.

The actions of interested community leaders who have access to, and make decisions based on financial statements also might be affected by reporting method changes. For example, suppose that individual-, corporate-, and public agency-giving is in part affected by reported income. Many, in fact, regard reported income as a basic index of need, and the relationship between income and giving seems logical. Thus, because each of the alternative financial reporting methods we have discussed will produce a different measure of income, total giving in each case could be affected.

Internal management decisions also might change with a new financial reporting method. Perhaps the most obvious example of such a change would be rate-setting. Organizations that have control over pricing decisions and are not reacting to market-determined prices should set prices at levels at least high enough

Table 9–3 Statement of Income for Williams Convalescent Center (000s Omitted)

	HC 20Y4	Constant Dollar (HC–GPL) 20Y4	Current cost (CV–GPL) 20Y4
Operating revenue	$3,556	$3,625	$3,625
Operating expenses	3,253	3,316	3,316
Depreciation	74	177	185
Interest	102	104	104
Net income	$127	$28	$20
Purchasing power gain from holding net monetary liabilities during the year	–	43	43
Increase in specific prices of property, plant, and equipment during the year	–	–	136
Less effect of increase in general price level	–	–	144
Increase in specific prices over (under) increase in the general price level	–	–	(8)
Change in equity due to income transactions	$127	$71	$55

to recover their costs. The use of any of the three alternative methods of reporting will increase reported cost levels and therefore increase rates.

CASE EXAMPLE: WILLIAMS CONVALESCENT CENTER

In the remainder of this chapter, we show how adjustments to take into account the effects of inflation are made in the income statement and balance sheet of Williams Convalescent Center, a 120-bed skilled and intermediate care facility. The center's two financial statements are shown in Tables 9–3 and 9–4. You will note that values are reported for each of the following three reporting methods: (1) HC, (2) HC–GPL, and (3) CV–GPL. In this discussion, we do not describe or apply the CV method. The accounting profession presently is not seriously considering this method, and it is not likely to be considered in the future. The CV method suffers from a serious flaw: it does not recognize the effects of changing price levels on equity. In short, the CV method would treat increases in the replacement cost of assets as a gain and not restate them for changes in purchasing power.

Table 9–5 presents values for the consumer price index (CPI). The CPI is the price index that is presently used by the accounting profession to adjust financial statements for the effects of inflation.

Price Index Conversion

Both of the two methods we have selected to adjust the financial statements of the Williams Convalescent Center (CV–GPL and HC–GPL) use a constant dollar as the unit of measurement. This means that purchasing power, not the dollar, is the unit of measurement. That is, all reported values in the financial statements are expressed in dollars of a specified purchasing power. Usually, the purchasing power used is the period end value. In our case example, Williams Convalescent Center uses purchasing power as of December 31, 20Y4, as its unit of measurement.

Restatement of nominal or unadjusted dollars to constant dollars is a relatively simple process, at least conceptually. All that is required are the following three pieces of information:

1. The unadjusted value of the account in historical or nominal dollars
2. A price index that reflects the purchasing power in which the unadjusted value is currently expressed
3. A price index that reflects the purchasing power at the date the account is to be restated

For example, Williams Convalescent Center's long-term debt at December 31, 20Y3, is $1,203 (see Table 9–4). To express that amount in constant dollars as of

Table 9–4 Balance Sheet for Williams Convalescent Center (000s Omitted)

| | HC | | Constant Dollar (HC–GPL) | Current Cost (CV–GPL) |
	20Y3	20Y4	20Y4	20Y4
Current assets				
Cash	$98	$21	$21	$21
Accounts receivable	217	249	249	249
Supplies	22	27	27	27
Prepaid expenses	36	36	36	36
Total current assets	$373	$333	$333	$333
Property and equipment				
Land	200	200	530	525
Building and equipment	2,102	2,228	5,333	5,570
	2,302	2,428	5,863	6,095
Less accumulated depreciation	783	844	2,020	2,186
Net property and equipment	1,519	1,584	3,843	3,909
Investments	161	596	596	596
Total assets	$2,053	$2,513	$4,772	$4,838
Current liabilities	412	493	493	493
Long-term debt	1,203	1,478	1,478	1,478
Partner's equity	438	542	2,801	2,867
	$2,053	$2,513	$4,772	$4,838

December 31, 20Y4, the following adjustment would be made:

$$\text{Unadjusted amount} \times$$

$$\frac{\text{Price index converting to}}{\text{Price index converting from}} =$$

$$\text{Constant dollar value}$$

or

$$\$1,203 \times \frac{315.5}{303.5} = \$1,251$$

The value of the beginning long-term debt for the center would be $1,251, expressed in purchasing power as of December 31, 20Y4. The previously described adjusted method can be used for all other accounts. The price index to which the conversion is made is usually the price index at the ending balance sheet date (December 31, 20Y4, in our example). The price index from which the conversion is made represents the purchasing power in which the account is currently expressed. This value will vary depending on

the classification of the account as either monetary or nonmonetary.

Describe the difference between monetary and nonmonetary accounts.

MONETARY VERSUS NONMONETARY ACCOUNTS

When restating financial statements from one based on an HC method to one based on a constant dollar method, it is critical to distinguish between monetary accounts and nonmonetary accounts. Monetary accounts are automatically stated in current dollars and therefore require no price level adjustments. Monetary items, discussed earlier in this chapter, consist of cash, claims to cash, or promises to pay cash that are fixed in terms of dollars, regardless of price-level changes. Nonmonetary accounts require price-level adjustments to be stated in current dollars.

Table 9–5 Consumer Price Index, Year-End Values

Year	CPI
19X0	119.1
19X1	123.1
19X2	127.3
19X3	138.5
19X4	155.4
19X5	166.3
19X6	174.3
19X7	186.1
19X8	202.9
19X9	229.9
20Y0	258.4
20Y1	283.4
20Y2	292.4
20Y3	303.5
20Y4	315.5

Because of the fixed nature of monetary items, holding them during a period of changing price levels creates a gain or loss. This can be seen in Table 9–6, which includes data from the Williams Convalescent Center.

The data in Table 9–6 assume that a repayment and new issue occurred at the midpoint of the year, June 30, 20Y4. The price index at that point would have been approximately 309.5. This resulted from taking the average of the beginning and ending values (303.5 + 315.5) ÷ 2. In constant dollars, the Williams Convalescent Center would have reported $1,531 of long-term debt as of December 31, 20Y4. However, the actual value of the long-term debt at that date was $1,478. The difference of $53 represents a purchasing power gain to the center during the year. Because the price level increased during 20Y4, the value of the

long-term debt actually owed by the center declined when measured in constant purchasing power.

Nonmonetary asset accounts always must be restated to purchasing power as of the current date. The price index at the time of acquisition represents the price index from which the conversion is made. The price index at the current date represents the index to which the conversion is made. To illustrate the adjustment, assume that the building and equipment account of the Williams Convalescent Center has the age distribution presented in Table 9–7.

The data in Table 9–7 show that assets with a historical cost of $2,228 represent $4,948 of cost when stated in dollars as of December 31, 20Y4. The latter value is much more meaningful than the former as a measure of actual asset cost in 20Y4. It provides the center with a measure of cost that is expressed in dollars as of the current date, and thus better represents its actual investment. Depreciation expense also should be restated in 20Y4 dollars to accurately portray the center's actual cost of using its building and equipment in the generation of current revenues. (Please note that the value reported for building and equipment cost in Table 9–4 does not match the $4,948 calculated because a different method was used to estimate cost.)

Adjusting the Income Statement

Operating Revenues

If one assumes that revenues are realized equally throughout the year, the restatement is significantly simplified. If the assumption is valid—and in most cases it is—it means that the revenues can be considered realized at the midpoint of the year, which in our case is June 30, 20Y4. As already noted, the price

Table 9–6 Computation Purchasing Power Gains and Losses data in thousands

	Unadjusted	Conversion Factor	Constant Dollars
Beginning long-term debt (12/31/Y3)	$1,203	315.5/303.5	$1,251
– Repayment (6/30/Y4)	152	315.5/309.5	155
+ New debt (6/30/Y4)	427	315.5/309.5	435
Ending long-term debt (12/31/Y4)	$1,478		$1,531
– Actual ending long-term debt (12/31/Y4)			$1,478
Purchasing power gain			$53

Table 9–7 Restatement of Nonmonetary Assets (data in thousands)

Year Acquired	Cost	Conversion Factor	Constant Dollar Cost (12/31/Y4)
19X0	$1,500	315.5/119.1	$3,974
19X8	401	315.5/202.9	624
20Y1	201	315.5/283.4	224
20Y4	<u>126</u>	315.5/315.5	<u>126</u>
	$2,228		$4,948

index at June 30, 20Y4 can be assumed to be the average of the beginning and ending price index, or 309.5. The restated operating revenue would be calculated as follows:

$$\$3,556 \times 315.5 \div 309.5 = \$3,625$$

Operating Expenses

Based on the same assumption that we used with operating revenues, the adjustment for operating expenses would be as follows:

$$\$3,253 \times 315.5 \div 309.5 = \$3,316$$

Operating expenses do not include depreciation or interest. Separate adjustments for these two items may be required.

Depreciation

The depreciation expense adjustment is different from the earlier adjustments in two ways. First, depreciation expense represents an amortization of assets purchased over a long period, usually many years. This means that the midpoint conversion method used for operating revenues and operating expenses is clearly not appropriate. Second, the adjustment methods for the constant dollar and current cost methods diverge. Depreciation expense may vary considerably because the current cost of the assets may differ dramatically from the constant dollar cost. Remember, a price index represents price changes for a large number of goods and services; specific price changes of individual assets may vary significantly from that index.

Constant Dollar Adjustment. Two methods can be used to adjust depreciation expense to a constant dollar amount. The most accurate method is to perform an adjustment for each asset. This can be a time-consuming process, however, and may not be worth the effort. Alternatively, the average acquisition date can be estimated by first determining the average age of the assets as follows:

$$\text{Average age} = \frac{\text{Accumulated depreciation}}{\text{Depreciation expense}}$$

$$\frac{\$844}{\$74} = 11.4 \text{ years}$$

Straight-line depreciation, which estimates average age, is reasonably reliable. For Williams Convalescent Center, an average of 11.4 years would imply that the assets were purchased sometime in 19X3. Interpolation would yield a price index of 131.8 = (127.3 + .4*(185.5 − 127.3)). Thus, depreciation expense in 20Y4, expressed in constant dollars, would be the following:

$$\$74 \times 315.5 \div 131.8 = \$177$$

Current Cost Adjustment. The identification of the current cost of existing physical assets is a subjective and complex process. To many individuals, the current cost method provides little additional value compared with the constant dollar method. Whether it will be eliminated eventually and replaced by the constant dollar method is not clear at this time.

The first issue to address in the adjustment is the definition of current cost. By and large, current cost can be equated to the replacement cost of the assets. In short, we must determine what the cost of replacing assets in today's dollars would be. This could be estimated through a variety of techniques using, for example, insurance appraisals or specific price indexes. In the case of Williams Convalescent Center, we will assume that a recent insurance appraisal indicated a replacement cost of $5,570 for buildings and equipment. With this estimate, depreciation expense could be adjusted as follows:

$$\frac{\text{Appraisal cost}}{\text{Historical cost}} \times \text{Depreciation expense} =$$

Restated depreciation expense

or

$$\frac{\$5,570}{\$2,228} \times \$74 = \$185$$

Interest Expense

We will again assume that interest expense is paid equally throughout the year. This assumption would produce the following interest expense adjustment:

$$\$102 \times 315.5 \div 309.5 = \$104$$

Purchasing Power Gains or Losses

A purchasing power gain results if one is a net debtor during a period of increasing prices, whereas a purchasing power loss results if one is a net creditor during such a period. In most health care firms, purchasing power gains result because liabilities exceed monetary assets. A firm is thus paying its debts with dollars that are of less value than the ones it received at the time of the initial loan.

To calculate purchasing power gains or losses, net monetary asset positions must first be calculated. The net monetary position for Williams Convalescent Center is presented in Table 9–8. The actual calculation of the purchasing power gain for Williams Convalescent Center is presented in Table 9–9.

Because the center was in a net monetary liability position during the year, it experienced a purchasing power gain of $43. This value is not an element of net income; rather, it is shown below the net income line in Table 9–3. It thus affects the change in equity.

Increase in Specific Prices Over General Prices

The adjustment to consider—an increase in specific prices over general prices—is made only in the current cost method. The constant dollar method does not recognize any increases (or reductions) in prices that are different from the general price level. In short, no gains or losses from holding assets are permitted in the constant dollar method.

Table 9–8 Net Monetary Asset Schedule (data in thousands)

	Beginning (12/31/Y3)	Ending (12/31/Y4)
Monetary assets		
Cash	$98	$21
Accounts receivable	217	249
Prepaid expenses	36	36
Investments	161	596
Total monetary assets	$512	$902
Monetary liabilities		
Current liabilities	$412	$493
Long-term	1,203	1,478
Total monetary liabilities	$1,615	$1,971
Net monetary assets	($1,103)	($1,069)

The calculations involved in this adjustment can be complex. In our Williams Convalescent Center example, we will make some assumptions to simplify the arithmetic without impairing the reader's conceptual understanding of the adjustment. We will assume the following data (data in thousands):

Insurance appraisal of buildings and equipment, 12/31/Y3	$5,015
Insurance appraisal of buildings and equipment, 12/31/Y4	$5,570
Appraised value of land, 12/31/Y3	$500
Appraised value of land, 12/31/Y4	$525
New equipment bought on 12/31/Y4	$126

Table 9–10 shows the increase in specific prices over general prices. These data show that, during 20Y4, the value of physical assets held by Williams Convalescent Center did not increase more than the general price level. This may be a positive sign for the center if it is not contemplating a sale. The replacement cost for its assets is increasing less than the general price level. Therefore, revenues could increase less than the general price level and replacement could still be ensured.

Adjusting the Balance Sheet

Monetary Items

None of the monetary items—cash, accounts receivable, prepaid expenses, investments, current liabilities,

Table 9–9 Purchasing Power Gain (Loss) Schedule (data in thousands)

	Actual Dollars	*Conversion Factor*	*Constant Dollars*
Beginning net monetary liabilities	$1,103	315.5/303.5	$1,147
− Decrease	34	315.5/309.5	35
Ending net monetary liabilities	$1,069		$1,112
− Actual			$1,069
Purchasing power gain			$43

or long-term debt—require adjustment. The values of these items already reflect current dollars.

Land

In our discussion of the increase in specific prices over the general price level in the Williams Convalescent Center's income statement, we assumed an appraisal value for land of $525. That value will be used here with the current cost method. With the constant dollar method, we will assume that the land was acquired in 19X0 for $200. To restate that amount to purchasing power as of December 31, 20Y4, the following calculation would be made:

$$\$200 \times 315.5 \div 119.1 = \$530$$

Buildings and Equipment

Values for the center's buildings and equipment and the related accumulated depreciation already have been cited for the current cost method. We will assume those same values here. This produces a value for buildings and equipment of $5,570 (000s omitted) based on an appraisal. The value for accumulated depreciation was derived as follows:

Adjusted accumulated depreciation =

Unadjusted accumulated depreciation ×

$$\frac{\text{Appraised value} - \text{Current year acquisitions}}{\text{Historical cost} - \text{Current year acquisitions}} =$$

or

$$\$2,186 = \$844 \times \frac{(\$5,570 - \$126)}{(\$2,228 - \$126)}$$

The constant dollar method values can be derived by using the estimated average age of the plant. In earlier discussions relating to depreciation expense, we computed the average age to be 11.4 years and the related

price index at acquisition to be 131.8. With this information, the following values result:

Buildings and equipment =
$$\$2,228 \times 315.5 \div 131.8 = \$5,333$$

Accumulated depreciation =
$$\$844 \times 315.5 \div 131.8 = \$2,020$$

Equity

Equity calculations are not discussed in any detail here. It is enough for our purposes to recognize that equity is a derived figure. Equity must equal total assets less liabilities. In our Williams Convalescent Center example, this generates values of $2,801 for the constant dollar method and $2,867 for the current cost method.

SUMMARY

Financial reporting suffers from its current reliance on the HC valuation concept. Inflation has made many of the reported values in current financial reports meaningless to decision makers. The example used in this chapter illustrates this point. The total asset investment of Williams Convalescent Center is approximately 100 percent larger when adjusted for inflation under the current cost or constant dollar method. Net income, however, decreased. The result is a dramatic deterioration in return on investment—the single most important test of business success.

Table 9–11 summarizes return on assets and return on equity for Williams Convalescent Center. These reductions are so drastic that they would prompt an investor to seriously question the continuation of the present investment, let alone replacement. More profitable avenues of investment very likely may be available.

To the extent that our Williams Convalescent Center example is representative of many health care firms—and it probably is—decisions regarding health care

Table 9-10 Increase in Specific over General Prices Schedule (data in thousands)

	Building and Equipment	Land	Total
Ending appraised value less acquisitions	$5,444	$525	$5,969
− Accumulated depreciation on appraised value	2,186	0	2,186
Ending net appraised value	$3,258	$525	$3,783
Beginning appraised value	$5,015	$500	$5,515
− Accumulated depreciation on appraised value	1,868	−	1,868
Beginning net appraised value	$3,147	$500	$3,647
Increase in specific prices during the year			$136
Effect of increase in general price level	$3,647 × [(315.5/303.5) − 1.0]		$144
Increase in specific prices over general price level			($8)

business continuation must be evaluated seriously. It is imperative that health care companies, like all other businesses, adjust their financial reports to reflect inflation. Whether the method used is current cost or constant dollar is not the issue. The important point is that ignoring the effects of inflation is unwise at best.

Table 9-11 Effect of Alternative Reporting Methods on Financial Measures

	Historical Cost	Constant Dollar	Current Cost
Return on assets (ROA)			
Net income/Total assets	5.1%	0.6%	0.4%
Revised ROA			
Change in equity due to income transaction/Total assets	5.1	1.5	1.1
Return on equity (ROE)			
Net income equity	23.4	10.0	0.7
Revised ROE			
Change in equity due to income transactions/Equity	23.4	2.5	1.9

ASSIGNMENTS

Use the data and information presented in Exhibit 9–2 to answer the following questions:

1. What index was used to restate to constant dollars?

2. What method was used to determine current cost values?

3. Is the American Medical Firm (AMF) a net debtor or a net creditor?

4. In 2001, AMF showed a minus $24 million value for the increase in specific prices over general prices. What does this mean?

5. Why are AMF's net operating revenues in 2004 identical for the HC, constant dollar, and current cost methods of reporting?

6. Why is depreciation expense greater in the current cost method than in the constant dollar method?

Exhibit 9–2 Supplementary Financial Information for American Medical Firm (AMF)

EFFECTS OF CHANGING PRICES	The company's financial statements have been prepared in accordance with generally accepted accounting principles and reflect historical cost. The goal of the supplemental information that follows is to reflect the decline in the purchasing power of the dollar resulting from inflation. This information should be viewed only as an indication, however, and not as a specific measure of the inflationary impact.

The constant dollars were calculated by adjusting historical cost amounts by the CPI. Current costs, however, reflect the changes in specific prices of land, buildings, and equipment from the date acquired to the present; they differ from constant dollar amounts to the extent that prices in general have increased more or less rapidly than specific prices. The current cost of buildings and equipment was determined by applying published indices to the historical cost.

Net income has been adjusted only for the change in depreciation expense. Other operating expenses, which are the result of current transactions, are, in effect, recorded in amounts approximating purchasing power on the primary financial statements. Depreciation index was determined by applying primary financial statement depreciation rates to restated building and equipment amounts. Because only historical costs are deductible for income tax purposes, the income tax expense in the primary financial statements was not adjusted.

During a period of inflation, the holding of monetary assets (cash, receivables, etc.) results in a purchasing power loss, whereas owing monetary liabilities (current liabilities, long-term debt, deferred credits, etc.) results in a gain. Net monetary gains or losses are not included in the adjusted net income amounts reported.

continues

Exhibit 9–2 continued

CONSOLIDATED STATEMENT OF INCOME ADJUSTED FOR CHANGING PRICES ($ IN MILLIONS)

For the Year Ended December 31, 2004

	As reported in Primary Statements (Historical Cost)	Adjusted for General Inflation (Constant $)	Adjusted for Changes in Specific Prices (Current Costs)
Net operating revenue	$2,065	$2,065	$2,065
Operating and administrative expenses	$1,698	$1,698	$1,698
Depreciation and amortization	84	98	111
Interest	91	91	91
Total cost and expenses	$1,873	$1,887	$1,900
Income from operations	$192	$178	$165
Investment earnings	$24	$24	$24
Income before taxes on income	$216	$202	$189
Taxes on income	$95	$95	$95
Net income	$121	$107	$94
Effective income tax rate	44%	47%	50%
Changing price gains not included in adjusted income:			
Increase in specific prices (current cost) of property, plant, and equipment held during the year*			$139
Less effect of increase in general price level			68
Excess of increase in specific prices over increase in the general price level			$71

FINANCIAL DATA ADJUSTED FOR EFFECTS ON CHANGING PRICES ($ IN MILLIONS)

	2004	2003	2002	2001	2000
Net operating revenues					
Adjusted for general inflation	$2,065	$1,852	$1,271	$1,070	$832
Net income					
Adjusted for general inflation	107	85	73	54	36
Adjusted for changes in specific prices	94	73	64	46	27
Earnings per share					
Adjusted for general inflation	1.54	1.29	1.18	.95	.82
Adjusted for changes in specific prices	1.35	1.12	1.04	.82	.61
Purchasing power gain from holding net monetary liabilities during the year	28	15	16	22	32
Increase in specific prices of property, plant, and equipment over (under) increase in the general price level	71	85	16	(24)	.77
Net assets at year end (total assets less total liabilities)					
Adjusted for general inflation	1,095	972	756	657	413
Adjusted for changes in specific prices	1,332	1,162	894	809	470
Cash dividends declared per common share					
Adjusted for general inflation	$0.43	$0.39	$0.34	$0.28	$0.21
Market price per common share at year end:					
adjusted for general inflation	$20.24	$29.41	$12.39	$24.30	$11.66
Average CPI—all urban consumers	303.9	293.4	280.3	257.5	230.0

*As of December 31, 2004, current cost of property, plant, and equipment, net of accumulated depreciation, was $1,915 (historical cost $1,349). "Property, plant, and equipment" in both the previous and following data includes land held for expansion.

SOLUTIONS AND ANSWERS

1. AMF used the CPI, which is required by Financial Accounting Standards Board Statement 33, to restate historical costs to constant dollars.

2. AMF used specific price indexes to restate historical costs to current costs. This method contrasts with the use of appraisals discussed in the chapter example.

3. AMF is a net debtor. It has experienced a purchasing power gain in each year from 2000 to 2004. Because prices were increasing during that period, AMF must have had a net monetary liability position in each year.

4. In 2001, the specific prices of AMF's fixed assets must have increased less than the general price level as determined by using the CPI.

5. AMF does not restate revenues or expenses to the fiscal year end, December 31. Instead, they restate to the midpoint of the fiscal year, June 30. Because it is usually assumed that revenues are received equally throughout the year, the midpoint (June 30) would represent the index from which the conversion is made. Because AMF is converting to the midpoint index, the adjustment is 1.0.

6. Depreciation expense under the current cost method exceeds depreciation expense under the constant dollar method because the current cost value of depreciable assets exceeds the constant dollar value of depreciable assets.

Chapter 10

Analyzing Financial Statements

LEARNING OBJECTIVES

After studying this chapter, you should be able to do the following:

1. Describe the balanced scorecard and dashboard reporting.
2. Describe the four key elements of dashboard reporting.
3. Explain what the most important measure of financial success is.
4. Explain what a health care firm's primary financial objective should be.
5. Describe the critical drivers of financial performance.
6. Discuss relevant healthcare financial performance measures.
7. Describe the hospital cost-index measure.

REAL-WORLD SCENARIO

Michael Dean has been recently appointed to the Board of Kenyon Medical Center, a 300-bed nonprofit community hospital. Mike is an attorney who specializes in labor law and is the firm's primary litigation expert in this area. He is reviewing the financial information that was sent to him this morning in preparation for his first board meeting this evening. His total financial package includes 28 pages of financial information consisting of current monthly income statements, a balance sheet, and other monthly actual-to-budget comparisons of performance with some selected financial ratios. Tonight's meeting is a critical one because the board's major item for discussion is related to a proposed bond issue to finance a major hospital renovation. Mike recognizes that he has a fiduciary responsibility to protect the assets of the hospital and to ensure its continued financial viability, but he does not know how to determine if the hospital can afford to take on this additional debt. There is so much information and no apparent pattern as to what really is important. He is also concerned about assessing how the proposed financing would impact the hospital's financial performance and thus, its ability to repay both interest and principal on the debt. He recently read a report on "Dashboard Reporting" and wonders if some structure like this would help him and other board members to get a better appreciation for the financial performance of the hospital.

The major purpose of this chapter is to introduce some analytical tools for evaluating the financial condition of health care entities. Think for a moment how confusing and difficult it would be, without a key, to reach any conclusions about financial position from any of the financial statements presented in Chapter 8. Unless your training is in business or finance, the statements may look like a mass of endless numbers with little meaning. In short, there may be too much information in most financial statements to be digested easily by a general-purpose user.

During the last 25 years, there has been an explosion in the adoption and integration of information technology for financial reporting. Financial data are collected, analyzed, and distributed to decision makers in a more accurate and timely manner, and in greater quantity than ever before. However, many people believe that the technology has not had a positive impact upon performance. While we have made important strides in the technology of information collection and distribution, we have failed to realize significant improvements in the decision-making value of that information.

What accounts for the failure to take advantage of information-technology advances? We think the answer is very clear and is one that most executives would readily acknowledge. We have been using the technology to rapidly deliver data (and more of it) to decision-makers, but we have ignored the issue of information relevance. As a result, we have in many cases simply used technology to deliver irrelevant or inappropriate data more quickly. Bad data delivered more quickly is not likely to improve performance in either the short run or the long run.

LEARNING OBJECTIVE 1

Describe the balanced scorecard and dashboard reporting.

The concept of "Balanced Scorecards" developed by Robert Kaplan and David Norton represents an attempt to enhance the value of information and exploit the capability of information technology to deliver true value to decision makers. Balanced scorecards, in their stripped-down version, simply state that reporting should be available on those key attributes affecting perfor-

mance. More data are of little value if they do not provide information to a decision maker that can be used to improve the performance of the firm. "Dashboard" reporting is a natural subset of balanced scorecards and is being increasingly used in almost all sectors of the economy to keep managers focused on critical areas that will affect overall firm performance.

In 1988, one major company won a Vision Award issued by Business Finance for its dashboard reporting system. The company's present dashboard system is intranet-based and replaced the company's monthly 200-page binder system that was sent to managers. The mix of 16 financial, operating, and human resource measures is available online in a drill-down format into which managers can dig deeper if they desire. The system is extremely easy to use and focuses on critical performance drivers.

WHAT IS REQUIRED TO DEVELOP AN EFFECTIVE FINANCIAL REPORTING SYSTEM?

LEARNING OBJECTIVE 2

Describe the four key elements of dashboard reporting.

Assuming that many health care providers are interested in developing a dashboard reporting system for key executives and board members, what needs to be done? In general, four critical questions must be answered:

* What is most important to the firm's success?
* What are the critical drivers that influence performance attainment?
* What are the most relevant measures that reflect critical driver relationships?
* What relevant benchmarking data are available to assess performance?

In the remainder of this chapter, we will answer the four questions above with respect to financial performance. We will then examine a specific hospital example to illustrate the definition and utilization of financial indicators to assess financial performance and to identify critical opportunities for management intervention.

WHAT IS MOST IMPORTANT: SUSTAINABLE GROWTH

Understanding financial performance in any business requires some global or summary measure of financial success. For many health care organization executives, this measure is often the operating margin (operating income divided by revenues). We believe that this measure is wrong and can be misleading in many situations. For example, low operating margins may not always be bad and high operating margins may not always be good.

LEARNING OBJECTIVE 3

Explain what the most important measure of financial success is.

What should be the primary criterion for financial success in health care organizations? We believe that a financially successful organization is capable of generating the resources needed to meet its mission. This creates two immediate questions. First, what are resources? Second, what level of resources is needed to fulfill the mission? Economic resources that are owned or controlled by a business firm are referred to as assets and would include such items as supplies, equipment, buildings, and other factors of production that must be present to produce health services. Human resources are not usually shown as assets because the firm does not own an individual, but human resources also are required in the production of products or services. Resources or assets owned by a health care organization are shown in its balance sheet, which provides a listing of its assets and the pattern of financing used to acquire those assets. The level of resources required by a health care organization depends largely on the range and quantity of health services envisioned in the mission statement. In situations when there is no scientific standard for resource requirements, benchmarking against other health care organizations may be used to partially address the issue of resource need. A hospital or health care firm can find itself in a situation where it may have too little investment in assets to meet the production needs for services, or it may have excessive investment in assets of a certain category.

Resources can be financed with either debt or equity funds, as any balance sheet clearly shows. A financially successful organization must therefore be capable of generating the amount of funds through debt and/or equity that is needed to finance the required level of resources. Figure 10–1 depicts a simple balance sheet illustrating these concepts. In this example, our health care organization needs to increase its investment in assets, or resources, by $100 million over the next seven years to fulfill its mission. This level of future investment should be a by-product of the firm's strategic plan. A strategic plan should provide some information about projected service levels, which in turn should drive expected investment. Strategic financial planning will be the topic of a later chapter. The rate of annual compounded asset growth for the example in Figure 10–1 is approximately ten percent per year. This rate equals the average rate of asset growth in many voluntary nonprofit hospitals during the last five years. Although this growth rate may seem high, remember that this rate incorporates replacement of assets at higher prices, acquisition of new technology, entry into new product lines requiring new investment, and increases in working capital such as accounts receivable. The health care organization depicted in Figure 10–1 has chosen a financing mix of 50 percent equity and 50 percent debt. This means that seven years later, the target financing mix will be $100 million of debt and $100 million of equity to finance the $200 million investment in assets.

The principle of sustainable growth states that no business entity can generate a growth rate in assets (ten percent in our example) that is greater than its growth rate in equity (also ten percent in our example) for a prolonged period. It may be possible to generate new asset growth of 15 percent for several years, when equity growth is only five percent, by changing the percentages of equity and debt financing. There is no mystery in the principle of sustainable growth; it is not some esoteric finance concept that bears no relationship on reality. Any business will have its asset growth rates limited by its ability to generate new equity growth. To not believe in the validity of this concept would imply that a firm could always increase its percentage of debt financing to any level. There are no exceptions to this theorem. It is not something that represents a nice target; it is a fundamental principle of business from which no one is exempt. Some governmental health care organizations

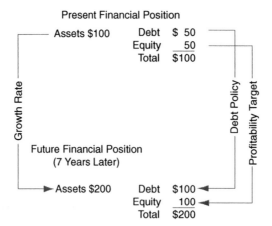

Figure 10–1 Sustainable Growth (figures in millions)

may argue that they always generate growth rates in equity less than their asset growth because they receive capital funds directly from their governmental sponsors. Those transfers represent a transfer of equity and are a part of equity growth.

Explain what a health care firm's primary financial objective should be.

There is no other financial objective that is more important than equity growth for measuring long-term financial success in any business entity. Health care organizations that expect low rates of equity growth in the future most likely will not be able to provide the level of resources sufficient to meet their mission. If your health care organization anticipates growth rates in equity of only five percent over the next decade, it is almost certain that your asset growth potential will be no greater than five percent. Although the objective is not to add assets or investments for the sake of growth, health care organizations that remain viable must add new investments. Health care organizations with low rates of growth in equity most likely will experience most of their asset growth in working-capital areas, such as accounts receivable and supplies. These firms will invest very little in renovation and replacement of existing plant and equipment, and very little in new capital required for entry into new markets. If they are surrounded by firms that are not also experiencing low equity growth rates, their market share will decrease as their relative delivery capability deteriorates.

Growth rate in equity (GRIE) can be expressed as follows:

$$\frac{\text{Change in equity}}{\text{Equity}} = \frac{\text{Net income}}{\text{Equity}} \times \frac{\text{Change in equity}}{\text{Net income}}$$

Most voluntary nonprofit health care organizations do not have a source of equity other than net income. This means that no transfers of funds from government or large restricted endowments exist to increase the firm's equity from the level of reported net income. In these situations, the term change in equity/net income equals one; therefore, GRIE can be defined as net income divided by equity, or return on equity (ROE). ROE is therefore the primary financial criterion that should be used to evaluate and target financial performance for voluntary nonprofit health care organizations when transfers of new equity are not likely. ROE is also the primary financial criterion that should be used to evaluate and target financial performance for taxable for-profit firms.

Return on equity can be factored into a number of components that help executives analyze and improve their ROE values. The following equation defines ROE:

$$\text{ROE} = \frac{\text{Operating income} + \text{Non-operating income}}{\text{Revenue}}$$

$$\times \frac{\text{Revenue}}{\text{Assets}}$$

$$\times \frac{\text{Assets}}{\text{Equity}}$$

LEARNING OBJECTIVE 5

Describe the critical drivers of financial performance.

LEARNING OBJECTIVE 6

Discuss relevant healthcare financial performance measures

WHAT ARE THE CRITICAL DRIVERS OF PERFORMANCE?

The previous formula for ROE tells us that there are a variety of ways that an organization can improve its ROE. First, it can improve its operating margins (operating income divided by revenue). Second, it can increase its non-operating gain ratio (non-operating income divided by revenue). Third, it can increase its total asset turnover (revenue divided by assets). Fourth, it can reduce its equity-financing ratio (equity divided by assets). Operating margin improvement is an important strategy for improving ROE, but it is not the only way that ROE can be increased and sustainable growth achieved. Figure 10–2 depicts the critical relationships affecting financial performance in most health care firms.

If we assume that return on equity, or business unit value, is the primary measure of financial performance success, the schematic in Figure 10–2 provides a roadmap of the critical drivers of performance. The schematic shows that the three primary determinants of value are profit, investment, and cost of capital. These three primary determinants of value can be related to a set of macro drivers, and then ultimately to a number of micro value drivers that will enable measurement and modeling for effective dashboard reporting.

It is important that every health care firm interested in developing a set of measures to monitor and evaluate performance start with a model similar to the one defined in Figure 10–2. Without this type of framework, many executives simply try to define a set of measures from those that currently exist or could be created. Defining measures without understanding key relationships can be dangerous. For example, reporting man-hours-per-discharge without adjusting for case-mix intensity can lead to erroneous conclusions and potentially bad decisions. Know your business before you determine how best to capture the essence of its performance.

MEASUREMENT OF CRITICAL VARIABLES

Understanding the relationships that drive performance permits one to define performance measures that focus management attention on areas that need correction. There is always a dilemma encountered in the definition of the measures that will be used for reporting. First, the absolute number of measures used must be limited. The selected measures should have a high probability of problem/opportunity detection. For example, in our sample hospital's dashboard report, we assess the probability of a supply or drug cost problem by examining costs for four high-profile DRGs. Second, the measures should be naturally related to the key driver map developed earlier (Figure 10–2). In the case of our dashboard report, we identify 13 critical performance driver categories:

1. Market factors
2. Pricing
3. Coding
4. Contract negotiation
5. Overall cost
6. Labor costs
7. Supply costs
8. Departmental costs
9. Service intensity
10. Non-operating income
11. Investment efficiency
12. Plant obsolescence
13. Capital position

Third, the selected measures should be capable of external validation or benchmarking. Measuring current performance with past performance may be helpful in some cases, but ideally comparative industry benchmarks should be available.

Our "Hospital Dashboard" report contains 51 measures that are related to the 13 critical performance driver categories. Each of these measures can be related to external comparative data, as well as compared with individual market area competitors. Benchmarking

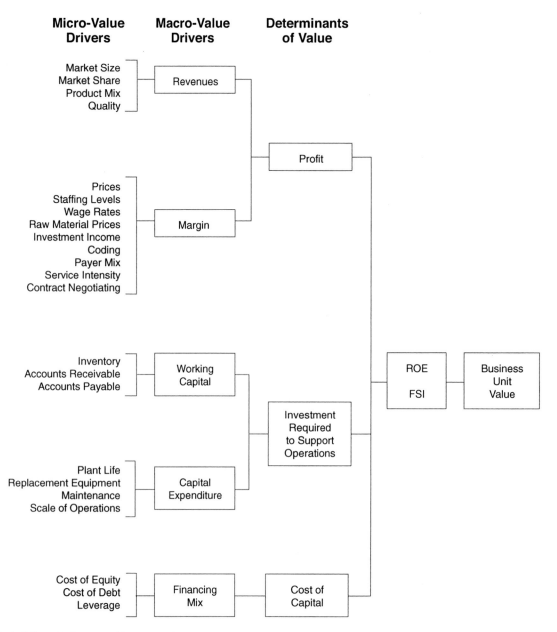

Figure 10–2 Micro-Drivers and Macro-Drivers

data from competitors is extremely valuable. We will be discussing the measures used for each of the 13 performance drivers when we begin our case discussion.

RELEVANT BENCHMARKING DATA

Comparative benchmarking data are crucial ingredients to the success of any dashboard reporting system. Ideally, a business needs some comparative reference points so it can ask itself questions like: How am I doing with respect to similar firms in my industry? How am I doing relative to my primary competitors?

Identifying measures that capture the nuances of revenue or cost drivers is nice, but they may be of little or no value if external comparative benchmarks can be found. For example, most hospitals would like to measure and compare nursing costs on an acuity-adjusted basis, but uniform benchmarks are not currently available. In this situation, direct nursing cost per patient day may be the best that one can do.

The measures that are used in our case example allow external comparisons and competitor comparisons because the databases employed in the measure definition are publicly available in the following sources:

* Medicare cost reports
* Standard analytical outpatient file
* MedPAR file

CASE EXAMPLE: ALPHA HEALTH CARE SYSTEM

For the remainder of this chapter, we will illustrate the use of financial analysis techniques through a case example based on the fictitious Alpha Health Care System (AHCS). AHCS is a 170-bed acute-care facility with a 20-bed skilled-nursing facility. Balance sheet and income statement data are presented in Tables 10–1 and 10–2. Performance measures for AHCS, its closest competitor, and the U.S. median are presented in Table 10–3.

Overall Performance

Three measures of overall performance are identified in Table 10–3:

1. Return on equity (ROE)
2. Financial strength index (FSI)
3. Total margin (TM)

High values are desirable for all three of these measures. A quick review of the data in Table 10–3 reveals a strong position for AHCS when compared to U.S. medians. There may be some financial and operating issues that need to be addressed if AHCS is to continue as a financially strong health care provider. Before we discuss these measures, we will define them and compute values for 2007.

$$ROE = \frac{\text{Excess of Revenue over Expenses}}{\text{Net Assets}}$$

$$= \frac{15,793}{160,559} = 9.8\%$$

$$TM = \frac{\text{Excess of Revenues over Expenses}}{\text{Operating Revenue + Non-operating Gains}}$$

$$= \frac{15,793}{118,292 + 8,017} = 12.5\%$$

$$FSI = \left[\frac{Total\ Margin - 4.0}{4.0}\right] = \frac{12.5 - 4.0}{4.0} = 2.13$$

$$+ \qquad +$$

$$\left[\frac{\text{Days Cash on Hand} - 50}{50}\right] = \frac{318 - 50}{50} = 5.36$$

$$+ \qquad +$$

$$\left[\frac{50 - \text{Debt Financing \%}}{50}\right] = \frac{50.0 - 24.7}{50.0} = 0.51$$

$$+ \qquad +$$

$$\left[\frac{9.0 - \text{Average Age of Plant}}{9.0}\right] = \frac{9.0 - 7.2}{9.0} = 0.20$$

$$= 2.13 + 5.36 + 0.51 + 0.20 = 8.20$$

AHCS's value for ROE is 9.8 percent, which indicates that the firm has a positive bottom line. A review of the data in Table 10–2 shows that AHCS has reported sizable balances of both operating and non-operating income in 2007 and 2006. Also note in Table 10–2 the sizable increases in equity that resulted from unrealized gains on investments ($2,171,000 in 2007 and $8,354,000 in 2006). While these gains will not impact net income until the securities are sold, they did raise the level of total equity at AHCS.

Total margin measures the return on revenue from both operating and non-operating sources. AHCS is realizing positive returns in both areas, but non-operating returns in 2007 were lower than those in 2006.

The final overall measure is the financial strength index (FSI). FSI attempts to measure the four areas of financial position that collectively determine a firm's financial strength:

* Profits – measured by total margin
* Liquidity – measured by days' cash-on-hand
* Debt expense – measured by debt financing percentage
* Age of physical facilities – measured by average age of plant

Simply stated, firms that have high profits, lots of cash, little debt, and new plants, have great financial strength. Firms with losses, little cash, lots of debt, and old physical facilities will not be in business long. Each of the four measures is "normalized" around a

Table 10–1 AHCS Balance Sheet, December 31, 2007 and 2006 (Data in Thousands)

	2007	2006
Assets		
Current assets		
Cash and investments	$ 3,124	$ 4,394
Patient accounts receivable	21,447	16,094
Inventory	2,122	3,254
Other current assets	480	345
Total current assets	$ 27,173	$ 24,087
Assets for which use is limited		
Capital improvements	$ 87,608	$ 93,185
Trustee-held funds	20,448	0
Donor restricted	9,056	8,290
Total assets for which use is limited	$117,112	$101,475
Property, plant, and equipment		
Property, plant, and equipment	$113,416	$ 96,256
Less accumulated depreciation	45,322	46,842
Net property, plant, and equipment	$ 68,094	$ 49,414
Other assets	$792	$336
Total assets	$213,171	$175,312
Liabilities and net assets		
Liabilities		
Current liabilities		
Accounts payable	$6,093	$ 5,531
Accrued expenses	5,040	4,587
Current installment of long-term debt	515	725
Due to third-party payers	4,078	4,741
Total current liabilities	$ 15,726	$ 15,584
Long-term debt	36,068	15,047
Other long-term liabilities	818	2,566
Total liabilities	$52,612	$ 33,197
Net Assets		
Unrestricted	$151,849	$134,271
Restricted	8,710	7,844
Total net assets	$160,559	$142,115
Total liabilities and net assets	$213,171	$175,312

predefined average for the measure. This permits us to add the four measures to create a composite indicator of total financial strength. AHCS has a very strong overall financial strength index (FSI) due primarily to its favorable total margin position and its strong cash position. AHCS's strong cash position is also a factor that impacts total margin. In 2007, more than 50 percent of AHCS's total net income was derived from investment income. Debt levels at AHCS are also below normative values, which further enhances its overall financial strength.

A critical objective for AHCS in coming years will be to maintain its current financial position. We will now focus our attention on reviewing the 13 critical drivers of performance listed earlier to identify possible areas of opportunity for AHCS.

Market Factors

There are many factors which influence the financial performance of a health care provider, as the schematic in Figure 10–2 shows. Market factors play an important role in the final financial performance of any business. There are six measures of market factors identified in Table 10–3 which are defined below:

Table 10-2 AHCS Statements of Operations, Years Ended December 31, 2007 and 2006 (Data in Thousands)

	2007	*2006*
Operating revenue		
Gross patient revenue		
Gross inpatient revenue	$122,908	$106,108
Gross outpatient revenue	85,543	74,538
Total gross patient revenue	$208,451	$189,646
Less contractual allowances	93,639	80,080
Net patient revenue	$114,812	$100,566
Other operating revenue	3,480	3,377
Total operating revenue	$118,292	$103,943
Operating expenses		
Wages, salaries, and benefits	$ 58,132	$ 51,418
Supplies	23,489	21,447
Professional fees	3,855	4,176
Depreciation and amortization	6,307	4,941
Interest	337	786
Provision for bad debts	3,488	2,825
Other	14,916	11,032
Total operating expenses	$110,515	$ 96,625
Excess (deficit) of revenues over expenses from operations	7,777	7,318
Non-operating gains—investment income	$ 8,016	$ 8,549
Excess (deficit) of revenues over expenses	$ 15,793	$ 15,867
Unrealized gains (losses) on investments	2,171	8,354
Net assets released from restrictions	298	282
Transfer to affiliate	(694)	0
Increase (decrease) in unrestricted net assets	$ 17,578	$ 24,503

$$\text{Inpatient Revenue \%} = \frac{\text{Gross IP Revenue}}{\text{Gross Patient Revenue}} = \frac{122,908}{208,451} = 60.0\%$$

$$\text{Surgical Cases \%} = \frac{\text{Medicare Surgical Discharges}}{\text{Medicare Total Discharges}} = 28.5\%$$

$$\text{Market Share \%} = \frac{\text{Net patient Revenue}}{\text{Sum of Net Patient Revenue in County}} = 39.2\%$$

$$\text{Medicaid Days \%} = \frac{\text{Medicaid Patient Days}}{\text{Total Patient Days}} = 16.5\%$$

$$\text{Medicare Days \%} = \frac{\text{Medicaid Patient Days}}{\text{Total Patient Days}} = 53.8\%$$

$$\text{Revenue Growth (Last Year) \%} = \frac{\text{Operating Revenue Current Year}}{\text{Operating Revenue Prior Year}} - 1$$

$$= \frac{118,292}{103,943} - 1 = 13.8\%$$

Inpatient revenue at AHCS is 60.0 percent compared to 57.0 percent at its competitor and 55.6 percent nationwide. In most situations, a higher percentage of inpatient revenue is desirable because profit margins are usually higher on inpatient product lines. For example, many U.S. hospitals make positive margins on Medicare inpatients, but most hospitals lose money on Medicare outpatients.

AHCS performs more surgeries compared to the U.S. median, but fewer than its competitor does. Usually, surgical inpatient cases are more profitable than medical cases.

Market share is perhaps the most critical measure of performance in the market factor category. High market share often leads to higher realized prices and lower cost per unit. If a health care provider had no competitors and operated as a monopoly, it could conceivably dictate price to all payer groups except Medicare and Medicaid. The market share position of AHCS is lower than that of its competitor. AHCS's competitor enjoys greater market share, which may give it a better contract negotiation position. Since this market is dominated by only two providers, both hospitals should, however, be able to demand and receive

Table 10–3 AHCS's Critical Financial Measures of Performance, 2007

	AHCS	Competitor	U.S. Median*
Overall measures			
Return on equity %	9.8	22.4	7.3
Financial strength index	8.2	4.1	0.1
Total margin %	12.5	17.4	3
Market factors			
Inpatient revenue %	60.0	57.0	55.6
Surgical cases %	28.5	37.6	20.1
Market share %	39.2	53.3	38.6
Medicaid days %	16.5	5.2	10.2
Medicare days %	53.8	57.7	54.6
Revenue growth last year (%)	13.8	4.0	7.5
Pricing factors			
Medicare charge per discharge (CMI=1.0)	$12,754	$11,183	$12,513
Medicare charge per visit (Relative Wt.=1.0)	$215	$176	$217
Routine room rate	$501	$492	$660
Chest x-ray (71020)	$163	$84	$166
Coding factors			
Two year change in Medicare CMI %	−3.1	6.0	0.4
Medicare CMI	1.3466	1.6995	1.2469
DRG 079/-(DRG 079 + DRG 089)	14.0	22.0	21.0
DRG 475/-(DRG 475 + DRG 127)	6.0	16.0	12.0
Injectable drugs without injection procedure %	94.9	31.5	34.8
Contract negotiation factors			
Mark-up %	189.0	200.0	220.0
Nongovernment payer %	29.7	37.1	32.4
Deduction %	44.9	41.2	54.5
Overall cost factors			
Hospital cost index	109.60	89.20	102.30
Medicare cost per discharge (CMI=1.0)	$6,666	$5,134	$5,586
Medicare cost per visit (Relative Wt.=1.0)	$67	$60	$71
Labor cost factors			
Net patient revenue per FTE	$116,418	$129,756	$107,397
FTE's per adjusted patient day	5.7	4.8	5.1
Salary & benefits per FTE	$58,936	$47,625	$43,252
Supply and drug cost factors			
DRG 209 supply cost	$5,721	$4,106	$4,493
DRG 116 supply cost	$6,418	$4,718	$5,780
DRG 89 pharmacy cost	$1,253	$611	$725
DRG 79 pharmacy cost	$2,682	$878	$1,179
Non-operating income factors			
Days' cash-on-hand	318	85	36
Investment yield %	11.2	4.3	3.3
Portfolio in equity %	47.8	n/a	n/a
Service intensity factors			
Medicare LOS (CMI=1.0)	4.4	2.6	4.0
Medicare ancillary cost per discharge (CMI=1.0)	$4,031	$3,271	$2,798
Departmental cost factors			
Direct cost per routine day	$295	$265	$273
Direct cost per ICU/CCU day	$782	$628	$649

continues

Table 10–3 continued

	AHCS	Competitor	U.S. Median*
Departmental cost factors			
Direct administrative cost per adjusted patient day	$313	$198	$201
Direct capital cost per adjusted patient day	$102	$94	$100
Overhead cost %	35.1	23.9	33.0
Investment efficiency factors			
Days in accounts receivable	68	57	59
Inventory to net patient revenue %	1.8	2.9	1.9
Revenue to net fixed assets	1.74	1.91	2.49
Plant obsolescence factors			
Average age of plant	7.2	8.3	9.3
Two-year capital expenditure growth %	62.7	4.1	2.9
Capital position factors			
Debt financing %	24.7	13.4	47.3
Long-term debt to equity %	22.5	5.2	34.0
Average cost of equity %	8.7	8.2	9.4
Cash flow to total debt %	42.0	192.5	21.1
Debt service coverage	21.1	n/a	n/a

*U.S. Median dollar values are stated in a wage index of 0.9304; U.S. averages are for 2004.

favorable contract terms because neither hospital has the capacity to service the entire market.

Market share increases also can provide significant improvements in profits because of lower cost per unit. Table 10–3 shows an average cost per Medicare discharge at a case mix equal to 1.0 of $6,666. For the same discharge, Medicare pays AHCS $5,623. The payment number is not shown in Table 10–3, but was derived elsewhere, producing an average loss of $1,043 ($5,623 − $6,666). The data suggest that little or no profit might be realized from an increase in Medicare volume, given AHCS's relatively high cost structure. While cost is clearly a problem, which we will address shortly, market share increases for Medicare patients may still be profitable. The critical question to be raised is: What would the variable cost of increased volume be? Usually a figure of 60 percent is assumed, but for this case, let us assume variable cost would be 80 percent, or $5,333 (.80 × $6,666). This assumption, if accurate, would mean a marginal profit of $290 ($5,623 − $5,333) per additional Medicare case with a case weight of 1.0. AHCS's primary competitor currently treats 4500 Medicare inpatients compared to 3800 at AHCS. Assuming an average case weight of 1.35 (AHCS's current Medicare case-mix index), a transfer of ten percent of its competitor's Medicare inpatient cases to AHCS would result in a small increase in profit:

Medicare Cases	CMI	Marginal Profit/Case	Marginal Profit
450	× 1.35	× $290	= $176,175

Medicare and Medicaid percentages provide an indication of payer segment importance. Usually, Medicaid is perceived as a less desirable payer, while Medicare in many hospitals is a desirable payer, especially for acute inpatient care. AHCS appears to have an unfavorable relationship here. It has much higher Medicaid volume compared to its competitor and the U.S. median, while it has similar percentages of Medicare. AHSC's geographical location has placed it closer to the Medicaid population than is its primary competitor. Losses on Medicaid patients are substantial and when combined with Medicare losses, a need is created for higher payments from the limited private-payer base.

Revenue growth at AHCS is above both its competitor and the U.S. median. This is most likely a result of AHCS's greater growth in Medicaid volume. While revenue growth is desirable, revenue growth in profitable product lines is critical. AHCS has experienced growth in some less profitable lines such as Medicaid, and this has hurt overall profitability.

Conclusions reached from our review of market factors are:

- AHCS must concentrate growth strategies in product lines that are profitable, especially inpatient surgical areas.
- If market share enhancement is not feasible, cost cutting must be pursued or unprofitable product lines must be eliminated.
- Reduced reliance on Medicaid business would be desirable.

Pricing Factors

Pricing can still have a sizable influence on a health care firm's profitability, even considering that many payers have fixed-fee reimbursement schedules. Of concern to many is the price elasticity of health care services. In simple terms, will volume drop if I raise prices? This is a difficult question to answer, but in many cases price elasticity is believed to be negligible for many health care services. If a health care firm's prices are lower than those of its competitors', the issue of price elasticity becomes of less importance. The first objective is, therefore, to determine if your prices are above or below those of your competitors'. The four pricing measures are all developed from public data sets and are presented in Table 10–3. The data show that AHCS has prices well above those of its competitor's, but similar to the U.S. median.

Average charge per Medicare discharge (CMI = 1.0) defines the average price for a Medicare discharge with a case-mix weight of 1.0. Table 10–4 provides a simple example to illustrate how this measure is developed. Adjusting charges or cost to a case weight of 1.0 permits meaningful comparisons across firms. Table 10–3 also indicates that this measure for the U.S. median is stated in the hospital's wage index of .9304. This removes potential cost-of-living issues that might impair comparability. Charges for a specific discharge or an outpatient encounter are the product of two factors:

- Intensity of service
- Charges for specific procedures

An inpatient discharge has a large number of services provided, such as routine nursing, laboratory procedures, surgical procedures, drugs, and many others. Total charges may be high not because of high procedure prices, but because of high utilization of services,

for example, a long length of stay. A high total charge can also result from high procedure-level prices, even in situations of low service intensity. AHCS's inpatient charge per case is similar to the U.S. median on a case- and wage-index-adjusted basis, but it is higher than its competitor's. Most likely, AHCS's higher charges can be attributed to its higher cost structure and its high Medicaid volume. High percentages of Medicaid are often associated with large indigent populations, which often increase prices to the private-payer base.

Average charge per Medicare visit adjusted for relative weight is a concept similar to the average charge per Medicare discharge case-mix-adjusted measure just described. It uses the weights assigned by Medicare to pay for outpatient procedures to case-mix adjust individual claims. We will discuss this measure further when we review cost measures. Data for the outpatient charge measure are similar to the inpatient measure just discussed. AHCS has a charge structure similar to that of the U.S. median, but well above its local competitor.

The last two measures, routine room rate and chest x-ray (CPT code 71020) represent two high-volume specific procedures. AHCS again has high prices in both areas relative to its competitor.

Even though prices at AHCS are high compared to those of its competitor, a rate increase might be initiated with little or no damage to its competitive position. A rate increase of eight percent would most likely keep AHCS in the same relative market position, but how much profit would result? The answer depends upon the percentage of patients who pay for services on a charge or discounted charge basis. Table 10–5 provides some results for alternative charge-payer percentages. The possible improvement in profit from a price increase is large and could maintain AHCS's profitability. Most hospitals have charge-payer percentages that are between 10 and 20 percent, so the range is realistic. In fact, many managed care contracts provide for fixed case or per-diem inpatient payments for inpatient care, but percentage-of-charges payments for outpatient care.

Conclusions reached from our pricing review are:

- AHCS should consider a rate increase or approximately eight percent even though its current prices are high.
- An increase of this size could generate close to $3 million in profit.

Table 10–4 Illustration of Case-Mix Weighting

DRG	Case Weight	Number of Cases	Aggregate Case Weight	Total Charges
1	.80	10	8.00	$ 64,000
2	1.20	10	12.00	96,000
3	1.60	10	16.00	128,000
		30	36.00	$288,000

$$\text{Average charge per case} = \frac{\$288,000}{30} = \$9,600$$

$$\text{Average charge per case (CMI} = 1.0) = \frac{\$9,600}{1.2} = \$8,000$$

$$\text{Average case weight} = \frac{36}{30} = 1.2$$

Coding Factors

Coding can have a significant effect on the actual payment received in almost every health care sector—from physician services to hospitals—and for almost every type of payer—from self-pay to Medicare. Coding can also be a double-edged sword. Code too aggressively or fraudulently, and you may be prosecuted. Under-code patient services, and you will lose sizable legitimate payments.

In our hospital dashboard of Table 10–3, we identify five primary coding measures that assess Medicare inpatient coding. Data for these measures are again provided from publicly available sources.

Medicare case-mix index (CMI) indicates the average complexity of Medicare inpatients seen. Table 10–4 provides a simple example to illustrate the computation of a case-mix index. In that example, the average case-mix index for the 30 patients was 1.2. AHCS

has a Medicare CMI of 1.3466, which is below its competitor's value (1.6995) but above the U.S. median (1.2469). Of special interest is the two-year decline in AHCS's Medicare case mix. This decline compares to a 6.0 percent increase at its primary competitor and 0.4 percent increase nationally.

A more specific way to assess coding reasonableness is to review so-called DRG dyads. These are pairs of DRGs in which possible missed information in the medical records could affect DRG assignment. We have provided two DRG dyad measures in Table 10–3. The actual DRG measures and their relative weights are presented in Table 10–6. Actual values from Table 10–3 for both DRG dyads suggest that AHCS may be incorrectly coding its inpatient DRGs. The data show that AHCS had reported lower frequencies of the higher-weighted DRG than its primary competitor; they were also lower than the U.S. median. This could be further corroboration of coding issues at AHCS. Of special interest is the DRG 475 and DRG 127 dyad. In many cases, a patient may be admitted with a heart attack, but also be experiencing respiratory problems and be put on a ventilator. The case weight values in Table 10–6 show a significant difference in payment for DRG 127 when compared to DRG 475. Table 10–7 shows the potential difference in payment if AHCS had a coding pattern similar to that of the U.S. AHCS may be losing $139,032 ($1,190,493 − $1,051,461) on this one DRG dyad.

The last measure of coding is the percentage of Medicare outpatient claims with an injectable drug present, but with no drug-administration code (injection

Table 10–5 Profit Resulting from Pricing Increase

	Percentage of Charge Payers	
	10%	20%
Present gross charges	$208,451,000	208,451,000
× Charge payer %	10	20
Charge-driven revenue	$20,845,100	$41,690,200
× Rate increase %	8	8
Profit Change	$ 1,667,608	$ 3,335,216

Table 10–6 DRG Dyads

DRG	Definition	2006 Relative Weight
079	Respiratory infections with cc	1.6238
089	Simple pneumonia with cc	1.0320
096	Bronchitis and asthma with cc	3.6091
097	Bronchitis and asthma without cc	1.0345
475	Respiratory system diagnosis with ventilator support	3.6091
127	Heart failure and shock	1.0345

procedure) present. At AHCS, this situation was present 94.9 percent of the times. Assuming Medicare pays $90 per injection procedure, AHCS lost more than $40,000 in this one area alone from Medicare-only patients.

The conclusion reached from our coding review is:

- AHCS appears to have coding problems. A review of current coding and billing procedures should be undertaken.

Contract Negotiation Factors

A popular saying in many management circles is, "You don't get what you deserve, but rather what you negotiate." The same appears to be true in the large number of managed care contracts that health care providers negotiate with health plans. The contract terms are especially important to most health care providers because favorable terms often spell the difference between financial success or failure. For most health care providers, there is no opportunity to negotiate terms for Medicare and Medicaid payment. The terms are fixed and are made on a take-it-or-leave-it basis. The magnitude of patient volume in these two payer categories makes it a must for most providers.

The real opportunity comes in negotiation of non-government-payer terms.

We have provided three measures for contract negotiation assessment. Collectively, these measures help assess any possible weakness in current contract terms. The first measure is nongovernment-payers' percentage and represents the percentage of revenues not derived from Medicare or Medicaid patients. A high number indicates greater relative importance of effective contract negotiation. AHCS has a relatively low percentage of nongovernment payers (29.7 percent) relative to the U.S. median (32.4 percent) and much less than its competitor (37.1 percent).

The second measure reviewed is mark-up:

$$\text{Markup} = \frac{\text{Gross Patient Revenue}}{\text{Total Expenses}} = \frac{\$208,451}{110,515} = 1.89$$

AHCS has relatively low mark-up ratios relative to both its competitor and the U.S. median. Because prices at AHCS are above those of its competitor, the lower mark-up ratio signals higher costs at AHCS relative to its competitor. Given this information, we would expect the deduction percent measure to be high:

$$\text{Deduction \%} = \frac{\text{Contractual Allowances}}{\text{Gross Patient Revenue}} = \frac{\$93,639}{\$208,451} = 44.9$$

The three contract negotiation measures suggest that AHCS has contracts more favorable than does the average U.S. hospital, but not as favorable as its primary competitor. In fact, most of AHCS's contracts are discount from billed charges, which explains how AHCS has realized operating profitability with a high mix of Medicaid patients and high costs. Charges at AHCS are currently 15 to 20 percent higher than those of its primary competitor, but deduction percentages at both hospitals are similar (44.9 and 41.2, respectively). We believe current contracts for both AHCS and its competitor must have similar rates of payment. AHCS's

Table 10–7 Possible Payment Change Due to Coding

DRG	Cases	Expected Cases	Case Payment	Present Payment	Expected Payment
127	138	129	$6,207	$856,566	$800,703
475	9	18	21,655	194,895	389,790
				$1,051,461	$1,190,493

competitor is realizing greater profit, primarily through its lower cost structure.

Conclusions reached from our review of contract negotiation factors are:

- AHCS and its competitor are most likely receiving similar payment from managed care plans.
- Renegotiation of these contracts at similar rates could be a problem, given AHCS's competitor's greater market share and lower prices.

LEARNING OBJECTIVE 7

Describe the hospital cost-index measure.

COST POSITION – A NEW APPROACH

We indicated previously that we believe AHCS's primary area of opportunity is cost reduction. To better assess relative cost positions, we will introduce a new construct for reviewing total hospital cost. This construct is further described in a July 2002 article published in Healthcare Financial Management, "The Hospital Cost Index: A New Way to Assess Hospital Efficiency." Figure 10–3 provides a schematic of the methodology. Most hospitals currently use an adjusted-discharge or adjusted-patient-day output measure, which we believe to be flawed.

Problems with Adjusted-Discharge Measures of Cost

Most U.S. hospitals can divide their patient operations into inpatient and outpatient areas. Gross patient revenue is often subdivided along these lines. In the last 20 years, outpatient activity has gone from under 20 percent in most hospitals to close to 40 percent in 2004. This dramatic increase in outpatient revenue has caused more individuals to question the validity of incorporating outpatient activity into a consolidated measure of cost by using adjusted discharges or adjusted patient days.

The critical measurement concept in an adjusted discharge or day measure is the weighting for outpatient revenue. The usual methodology for defining adjusted discharges or days is expressed as a formula:

$$\text{Adjusted Discharges (days)} = \text{Inpatient Discharges (days)} \times \left[1 + \frac{\text{Gross Outpatient Revenue}}{\text{Gross Inpatient Revenue}} \right]$$

Procedure Pricing

The computation of adjusted discharges is heavily influenced by specific procedure prices in the hospital's Charge Description Master (CDM). Some hospitals may price procedures with high outpatient utilization at higher levels to take advantage of the greater presence of "percentage of billed charges" payment arrangements.

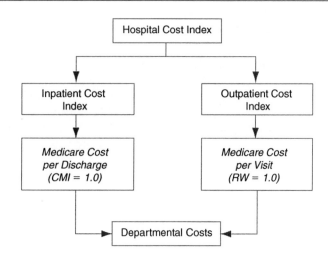

Figure 10–3 Analysis of Overall Cost

Other hospitals may keep high outpatient procedures at lower levels because of a large self-pay presence, implying greater price elasticity. Some data suggest that the majority of hospitals overstate outpatient costs because of higher procedure prices. If this is so, hospitals with heavier percentages of outpatient activity or higher outpatient prices would have larger values for adjusted discharges and, therefore, lower costs per adjusted discharge. This may partially explain why smaller hospitals, which often have greater percentages of outpatient revenue, have lower costs per adjusted discharge.

Output Differences

Another major factor that affects the comparability of cost measures using an adjusted-discharge basis is output differences. Even if there were only inpatient discharges and no outpatient activity, discharges would not be an ideal measure to make comparisons of cost across hospitals because of case-mix differences. Many cost-per-adjusted-discharge measures are further adjusted by dividing by the case-mix index of the hospital for the time period. There are two alternative case-mix indexes that are often used:

- All-payer case-mix index
- Medicare case-mix index

Obviously, the all-payer case-mix index will do a better job of reflecting output differences than will a Medicare-only case-mix index. However, there is one major issue with the utilization of all-payer case-mix-index adjustments. You may be able to adjust your cost for case-mix effects, but will the external comparative cost measures be adjusted in similar fashion? Competitor data extracted from public files, such as Medicare Cost Reports, will not have all-payer case-mix-index values. For controlled subscriber-based benchmarking services, the all-payer case-mix-index adjustments may be accurate, but the comparisons will be limited to other subscribing hospitals and will exclude specific competitor comparisons.

For the above reasons, Medicare case-mix-index adjustments are often utilized in a number of comparative reports. In many cases, the Medicare case-mix index can remove cost variance and better isolate possible problems. The Medicare case-mix-index adjustment will be an issue, however, when the non-Medicare patient population differs dramatically from the Medicare patient population. For example, a hospital that specialized in orthopedics and obstetrics would present problems.

Using the Medicare case-mix index would grossly overstate case-mix complexity because all of the obstetric cases, which would be lower-case weighted, however not applicable to Medicare claims.

Geographical Cost-of-Living Differences

The final area affecting the comparability of cost-per-adjusted-discharge measures is geographic cost-of-living differences. Hospitals in Oakland, California, have higher operating costs than do hospitals in rural North Dakota. The usual method of adjustment is to divide the unadjusted cost measure by the local area cost-of-living index. This division would restate costs into a cost-of-living index equal to 1.0. The wage index used by Medicare is the most often-used index and may be applied to total cost or some percentage of total cost. The rationale for a percentage is that some portion of hospital costs, e.g., supplies, may not be affected by cost-of-living differences. Medicare assumes that the wage index affects 71 percent of total cost. The remaining 29 percent is presumed not to be affected by wage variation.

Cost-of-living differences are important and the adjustments can be easily handled. Of the three problems affecting cost comparability (procedure pricing, output differences, and geographical cost-of-living differences), cost-of-living differences can be resolved. The problems with procedure pricing and output differences are still present in a CPAD measure, even after case-mix indexes have been applied.

HOSPITAL COST INDEX (HCI)

We believe that a better measure of facility-wide hospital costliness can be constructed by weighting two measures:

1. Medicare cost per discharge, case-mix, and wage-index adjusted (MCPD)
2. Medicare cost per outpatient visit, relative value unit and wage-index adjusted (MCPV)

The HCI is then constructed as follows:

$$HCI = \% \text{ Inpatient Revenue} \times \frac{MCPD}{\text{U.S. Median}}$$

$$+ \% \text{ Outpatient Revenue} \times \frac{MCPD}{\text{U.S. Median}}$$

Medicare Cost per Discharge (MCPD)

Medicare cost per discharge is a good reflection of inpatient cost. Data for computing this measure can be derived from the following public-use files: Medpar and Medicare Cost Reports. Each Medicare inpatient claim is costed by using the relevant departmental ratio of cost-to-charge (DRCC) values derived from the Medicare Cost Report and applying them to charges from the inpatient claim. The DRCC values are mapped to specific revenue codes in the claims file. Finally, a Medicare-assigned wage index is used to re-state costs to an index of 1.0. This process results in a unique publicly available number for most hospitals in the U.S.

The MCPD is not a perfect measure of relative inpatient costs, but we believe it is better than any other publicly available measure of cost or inpatient cost at the facility level for several reasons. The output unit is more comparable than any other. There is no application of outpatient-equivalent discharges to distort output similarity. The case-mix index used to adjust it is specific to those patients and is not extended to non-Medicare patients. The cost measures are adjusted using department-specific cost-to-charge ratios, not facility-wide cost-to-charge ratios. Finally, the costs are adjusted for cost-of-living differences.

The major problem with MCPD is its comprehensiveness. In short, the measure may or may not be reflective of costs in other non-Medicare areas. We believe that this is not a major issue for the following reasons. First, Medicare represents the largest payer for most hospitals: approximately 53 percent of all inpatient days and 44 percent of discharges. Second, with a fixed payment per DRG, there is an incentive to keep costs low. If costs are high in the Medicare area, they will most likely be high in other non-Medicare areas.

Medicare Cost per Outpatient Visit (MCPV)

We use MCPV to assess costliness on the outpatient side of hospital operations. We can construct this measure from public data—Medicare Outpatient Claims and Medicare Cost Reports—which make its availability a reality for most U.S. hospitals. To derive the measure, we divide the cost per claim defined through the DRCC extensions by the relative value units of the claim. We estimate RVUs based on the following taxonomy:

Line-Item Type	RVU Assignment
APC	APC weight
Fee schedule	Fee schedule/nat'l price per APC = 1.0
Pass-through drug and biologicals	Avg. wholesale price/nat'l price per APC = 1.0
Pass-through device	Estimate payment/nat'l price per APC = 1.0

We believe the introduction of the Outpatient Prospective Payment System (OPPS) has provided an opportunity to adjust outpatient costs for relative-value unit differences in a manner similar to case-mix-index adjustment on the inpatient side. We do not know of any other measure of facility-wide outpatient cost that incorporates relative-value unit adjustment to this degree. Medical groups have used resource-based relative value scales (RBRVS) measure, but these were not applicable to hospital outpatient operations.

The MCPV is not a perfect measure of outpatient costliness. Like the MCPD, the MCPV does not necessarily reflect cost for non-Medicare patients. Medicare patients are, however, a significant percentage of total outpatient business (21 percent in 1999). Medicare also pays on a fixed-fee basis now, so that is a strong incentive to keep costs low. If costs are high for Medicare outpatients, it seems reasonable to conclude that they would be high for other categories.

Merging the MCPD and the MCPV

The final step in the development of the HCI is to combine the MCPD and MCPV. To combine these two measures, we must weight them by the percentage of business activity. The MCPD is, therefore, multiplied by the percentage of inpatient revenue, and the MCPV is multiplied by the percentage of outpatient revenue. The sum of inpatient revenue and outpatient revenue percentages should equal 1.0. Data for these values will be taken from Medicare Cost Reports.

The final step is to "normalize" the MCPD and MCPV around some central value. We use the current U.S. median values for both measures.

OVERALL COST FACTORS

Using the three measures just described (HCI, MCPD, and MCPV), we can see from Table 10–3 that AHCS is a high-cost hospital with respect to both its primary competitor and the U.S. median. AHCS's HCI is currently at 109.6, which is 7.1 percent above the U.S. median (102.3) and 22.9 percent above its primary competitor. The data also show us that AHCS has a greater opportunity for cost reduction in the inpatient arena where its cost per discharge on a case-mix basis is significantly above both that of its competitor and the U.S. median.

Labor Cost Factors

Health care providers, in general, and hospitals in particular are labor-intensive operations. More than 50 percent of their costs are connected to staffing. To analyze labor costs, we have selected two measures of productivity and one measure of compensation.

Net Patient Revenue per FTE

$$= \frac{\text{Net Patient Revenue}}{\text{FTEs}} = \frac{114{,}812{,}000}{986.2} = \$116{,}418$$

FTEs per Adjusted Patient Day

$$= \frac{\text{FTE} \times 365}{\text{Adjusted Patient Days}}$$

$$= 986.2 \times \frac{365}{63{,}037} = 5.7$$

Salary and Benefits per FTE

$$= \frac{\text{Salaries \& Benefits}}{\text{FTEs}} = \frac{58{,}123{,}000}{986.2} = \$58{,}936$$

Collectively, the labor cost measures suggest a problem. Salary and fringe benefit costs are very high compared to the U.S. median and also high relative to those of its competitor. Fringe benefit costs do appear excessive. Much of this cost is directly related to a very expensive "defined benefit" retirement plan, as well as a very liberal educational benefit program.

Labor productivity at AHCS is also worse on both measures when compared to its competitor. Part of the issue at AHCS may be related to a very generous sick leave and vacation policy. Further in-depth analysis needs to be directed to department-specific benchmarks.

Conclusions reached from our review of labor cost factors are:

- Compensation costs appear out of line with the U.S. median and costs of ACHS's competitor. Fringe benefit costs appear out of line when compared to any reasonable benchmark. AHCS should explore the termination of its present retirement program and explore one that is of a comparable cost relative to other employers' programs, especially the program of its competitor.
- Labor productivity appears to be worse than competitor values. Comparative analysis at departmental levels should be initiated to determine where specific problems exist.

Supply and Drug Costs

Supply and drug costs can be significant factors for a large number of medical and surgical procedures. The magnitude of total supply and drug costs is complicated because of the underlying factors that influence cost. These particular costs are a product of the quantity used and the price paid. Lower costs can be realized by either reducing the intensity of usage or reducing the price paid. Lower prices can be realized through better purchasing contracts or using lower priced supplies or drugs. The issue is often complicated by physician preferences. Health care executives can attempt to influence physician behavior in supply or drug selection, but ultimately, the physician will determine which drug or supply item will be used and in what quantity.

We provide four measures of inpatient supply and drug costs. Two of these measures define supply costs for DRGs whose supply costs are usually sizable:

- DRG 209 – Major joint and limb attachment procedures—lower extremity
- DRG 116 – Other permanent cardiac pacemaker, implant, or Automatic Implantable Cardioverter Defibrillators (AICD).

Both measures indicate that AHCS has costs much larger than the U.S. median and also much larger than competitor values. While the variance exists, the explanation is not clear without further review. Possible explanations could be:

- Poorly-negotiated purchase contracts, which result in higher prices
- Usage of more expensive supply items by physicians

Further review suggests that physician preference for higher-priced supply items is the primary cause. This results in a medical decision-making dilemma. Should physicians use less costly supply items to improve the hospital's bottom line, and would these lower-cost supply items adversely affect patient care?

Two DRG drug cost measures are also reviewed:

* DRG 089 – Simple pneumonia and pleurisy
* DRG 079 – Respiratory infections and inflammations

AHCS also appears to have higher drug costs than do the other two players in this analysis. Similar issues for supply costs also appear present with respect to drug usage.

Conclusions reached from our review of drug and supply costs are:

* Supply and drug costs appear to be very high and result primarily from physician preferences.
* Review of supply and drug costs with selected physicians should be undertaken with the desired outcome of supply and drug standardization.

Non-Operating Income

Many nonprofit health care providers, especially hospitals, derive a large percentage of their total net income from non-operating sources. The usual source of non-operating income for most hospitals is investment income. Data from Table 10–2 show this to be especially true for AHCS.

We have defined three measures to assess performance in the non-operating income area:

$$\text{Days Cash on Hand} = \frac{\text{Unrestricted Cash and Investments}}{(\text{Total Expenses} - \text{Depreciation}) / 365}$$

$$= \frac{3,124 + 87,608}{(110,515 - 6,307) / 365} = 318$$

$$\text{Investment Yield} = \frac{\text{Investment Income} + \text{Unrealized Gains (Losses)}}{\text{Unrestricted Cash and Investments}}$$

$$= \frac{\$8016 + 2,171}{3,124 + 87,608} = 11.2\%$$

$$\text{Portfolio in Equity} = \frac{\text{Equity Investment}}{\text{Unrestricted Cash and Investments}}$$

$$= \frac{43,412}{3,124 + 87,608} = 47.8\%$$

AHCS has a very sizable investment in securities, as seen from its days' cash-on-hand value of 318 days. Only investments that are not restricted by donors or third parties are included. This explains why trustee-held funds ($20,448) and donor-restricted funds ($9,056) are excluded.

In addition, AHCS has a very sizable percentage of its investment in equities: 47.8 percent. This high percentage of equity investment can increase yields, but

risk is also increased. Investment income includes both interest and dividend income, as well as realized gains or losses on securities sold during the period.

Conclusions for AHCS with respect to its investment portfolio are:

* Review current investment strategy and perhaps place equity investment in funds that replicate broad market segments, such as the Standard and Poor's 500 or the Wilshire 5000.
* Determine if AHCS is willing to assume the relatively high risk of equity investments or whether a reduced reliance on equity funds is more consistent with projected needs for these funds.

Service Intensity

Service intensity is a critical driver of health care cost. Cost per encounter of service can be defined as:

$$\frac{\text{Services}}{\text{Encounters}} \times \frac{\text{Inputs}}{\text{Services}} \times \text{Prices of Resources}$$

Each of these three factors will drive total health care costs. The first term (services/encounters) is referred to as service intensity. The two major drivers of service intensity for inpatient care are length of stay (LOS) and ancillary service usage. We have, therefore, included two measures to help assess service intensity:

* Medicare length of stay, case-mix-index adjusted
* Medicare ancillary cost per discharge, case-mix-index adjusted

Both of these measures are taken from Medicare data and are case-mix adjusted to 1.0. The use of these measures assures that there will be comparability across hospitals because the measures are "apple-to-apple" comparisons.

AHCS has a high LOS on a case-mix-adjusted basis when compared to the U.S. median. Its value is also above that of its primary competitor's. Its high length of stay is a reason its cost per discharge is so high. Please note that AHCS's Medicare LOS unadjusted is actually 5.92, but its Medicare case-mix index was 1.3466, which deflates the LOS to 4.4 on a case mix-adjusted basis. Significant opportunity exists for cost reduction from further LOS declines.

Ancillary costs are also above the U.S. median and warrant review. Prior discussion has already disclosed high prices paid for supply and drug items. This is most likely the cause for the variance. It should also be noted that a higher length of stay may not affect ancillary costs. Most of these services are not necessarily related to LOS.

Table 10–8 documents the potential savings for one DRG and illustrates the potential from LOS reduction and reduced drug usage.

Conclusions reached from our service intensity review are:

- AHCS has significant opportunity for major savings in this area.
- Low levels of efficiency, especially LOS management, exist.

Departmental Cost Factors

We have included five measures of departmental cost:

- *Nursing Cost Measures*
  1. Direct cost per routine day
  2. Direct cost per ICU/CCU day
- *Overhead Measures / Adjusted Patient Day*
  3. Administrative cost per adjusted patient day

4. Capital-related cost per adjusted patient day
5. Overhead cost percentage

Direct costs of nursing for both routine care and ICU/CCU care are high relative to the U.S. median and the costs of ACHS's competitor. These cost measures include only the direct cost of the department and do not include overhead allocations. The cost data are extracted from filed Medicare Cost Reports. The high nursing cost values are somewhat surprising, given the high LOS at AHCS. Usually, nursing intensity is highest in the early days of care; and it would be reasonable to expect higher costs per day of care in low-LOS situations.

The three overhead measures of cost also suggest some inefficiency. AHCS appears to have higher administrative and capital costs than the U.S. median reflects and should be reviewed.

Conclusions reached from the review of departmental cost factors are:

- AHCS has high direct nursing costs per day. This is a result of both a higher RN mix and higher salaries.

Table 10–8 DRG Savings Opportunities

DRG 478 (Other Vascular Proc w cc)	AHCS	Competitor	U.S. Median
Discharges	38	46	43
Medicare LOS	8.89	5.59	7.01
Avg Routine LOS	7.13	4.59	4.93
Avg ICU/CCU LOS	1.76	1.00	2.08
Routine care costs	3,996	3,515	2,813
ICU/CCU costs	2,035	1,408	2,291
Subtotal	6,031	4,923	5,104
Medical/surgical supplies	2,009	2,035	2,161
Laboratory	1,288	889	636
Operating room	6,227	4,674	2,555
Radiology	1,011	1,494	797
MRI	123	41	37
Pharmacy	2,411	1,202	1,162
Emergency room	102	53	86
Cardiology	248	483	244
Blood	145	313	183
Physical/occupational therapy	564	103	139
Inhalation therapy	211	91	134
Other	943	766	522
Subtotal	15,282	12,144	8,656
Grand Total	21,313	17,067	13,760

* Overhead costs at AHCS are high, especially in the administration area. Reductions in administrative costs should be pursued.

Investment Efficiency Factors

As discussed earlier in this chapter, it is not the amount of profit realized that is of prime concern, but rather the amount of profit in relation to investment. For most health care providers, the three critical areas of control are plant, property, and equipment; accounts receivable; and inventory. To assess performance in these three areas, we have defined three measures that assess the productivity of investment.

$$\text{Days in Accounts Receivable} = \frac{\text{Net Accounts Receivable}}{(\text{Net Patient Revenue} / 365)}$$
$$= \frac{21,447}{114,812 / 365} = 68.2$$

$$\text{Inventory to Net Patient Revenue} = \frac{\text{Inventory}}{\text{Net Patient Revenue}}$$
$$= \frac{2,122}{114,812} = 1.8\%$$

$$\text{Revenue to Net Fixed Assets} = \frac{\text{Operating Revenue}}{\text{Net Fixed Assets}} = \frac{118,292}{68,094} = 1.74$$

AHCS has poor investment productivity with respect to both accounts receivable and fixed assets. Reductions in both categories could enhance the financial performance of the firm significantly.

High values for receivables can be the result of many factors, but in general result from three primary causes:

* Payment delays by payers, especially commercial health plans
* Large balances of old accounts whose collection is suspect
* Billing delays that prevent prompt invoicing of provided care

A review of AHCS's billing and collection systems indicates that poor coding and documentation delays are preventing the hospital from sending out bills promptly. The hospital also has large balances of old receivables from self-pay patients that need more aggressive collection efforts. Table 10–9 provides an estimate of potential flow savings realizable if current balances in receivables could be reduced. Almost $230,000 per year in additional investment income could be realized if AHCS could bring its accounts receivable down to the U.S. median of 59 days.

Table 10–9 Cash Flow Impact of Accounts Receivable Reduction

Present AR balance	$21,447,000
Present days in AR	68.2
U.S. median days in AR	59.0
Potential day savings	9.2
Average net patient revenue per day*	$314,533
Potential dollar reduction in AR	$2,893,892
Annual investment income on reduction (8% yield)	$231,511

Calculation: *$114,812,000/365 = $314,553

Alpha Health Care System also appears to have excess investment in net fixed assets. It currently generates 1.74 of operating revenue per dollar of investment in net fixed assets compared to a U.S. median of 2.49 and a competitor value of 1.91. Determining the desired level of investment in fixed assets is not an easy decision and is heavily influenced by a large number of stakeholders in the firm, including doctors, board members, employees, and the community. Long-term investment levels in property and equipment are often a part of the firm's strategic plan and reflect perceived community needs, as well as financial and marketing objectives. Oftentimes many nonprofit health care executives forget that capital has a real cost and excessive fixed asset investment can impair the firm's long-term financial viability.

What is the potential cost of AHCS's excessive investment in fixed assets? There are several ways that this could be measured. First, we could isolate the direct costs of the excessive investment in terms of depreciation and interest expenses. Second, we could impute some opportunity cost of the excess investment, using the expected yield on alternative investments. Third, we could multiply the firm's estimated cost of capital times the excess investment.

To determine the amount of excess investment in fixed assets, we need a target revenue to fixed assets standard. For this purpose, let's use the U.S. median of 2.49. The desired level of investment in fixed assets would be:

$$\frac{\text{Operating Revenue}}{\text{Target Revenue to Fixed Assets}} = \frac{\$114,812}{2.49} = \$46,109$$

AHCS has $21,985,000 in excess investment ($68,094,000 − $46,109,000). This surplus investment represents 32.2 percent of AHCS's present investment in net fixed assets. Assuming that 32.2 percent of the firm's depreciation and interest is not necessary produces one estimate of annual cost:

$$.322 \times (\$6,307,000 + \$337,000) = \$2,139,368$$

Alternatively, we could assume a possible yield on risk-free investment of 6.0 percent as our opportunity cost. This would produce an annual savings of $1,319,100 (.06 × $21,985,000).

No matter what method of cost savings is used, AHCS has a heavy cost associated with its excess investment in fixed assets. Much of this surplus is a direct result of intense physician pressure to finance new investment in clinic facilities to support the integrated network of services provided by AHCS.

Conclusions reached from our investment efficiency review are:

- Receivables are very high at AHCS, primarily due to poor coding and documentation. Reductions to U.S. medians could produce $231,511 in annual cash flow.
- Fixed asset investment at AHCS is $22 million above the U.S. median. This surplus investment could cost AHCS somewhere between $1.3 million and $2.1 million annually. Tighter capital-expenditure review policies need to be implemented to prevent this problem from getting worse.

Plant Obsolescence Factors

While excessive investment in fixed assets can impair the realization of reasonable return on investment, investment in old facilities and outdated technology can be fatal. If a health care firm, especially a hospital, has old and outdated facilities, it will likely affect the quality of care rendered to its patients. It may also lead medical staff to practice at facilities where they believe the welfare of their patients may be better served. We have defined two measures to assess the issue of plant obsolescence:

$$\text{Average Age of Plant} = \frac{\text{Accumulated Depreciation}}{\text{Depreciation Expense}} = \frac{45,322}{6,307} = 7.2$$

$$\text{2-Year Capital Expenditure Growth Rate} = \frac{\text{Capital Expenditures in Last 2 Years}}{\text{Gross Fixed Assets Two Years Ago}} = \frac{48,124}{76,714} = 62.7\%$$

AHCS has spent more on fixed assets than the U.S. median in the last two years, resulting in more state-of-the-art facilities. The data suggest that AHCS has a newer physical facility than does its competitor, which may give it a competitive advantage.

The conclusion regarding plant obsolescence is:

- AHCS has kept up with current technology and has been replacing its current physical facilities and investing in new areas.

Capital Position

The last area of performance factors to be reviewed is capital position. Successful firms have profitable operations with reasonable levels of investment. They also keep their cost of financing at a reasonable level. Capital funds in any firm are provided from either debt or equity; and each has a cost. Debt has an explicit cost that can be easily determined by either examining current financing documents or obtaining present bond market yields. Debt also affects the cost of equity capital. Higher levels of debt or financial leverage increase the risk of business failure and lead to higher required returns for invested equity capital, irrespective of its source. A religious, government, community, or investor-owned firm must obtain higher returns on its equity as it raises the level of risk through increased borrowing. We have identified five measures of capital position:

$$\text{Debt Financing \%} = \frac{\text{Total Liabilities}}{\text{Total Assets}} = \frac{52,612}{213,171} = 24.7\%$$

$$\text{Long-Term Debt-to-Equity \%} = \frac{\text{Long-Term Debt}}{\text{Equity}} = \frac{36,068}{160,559} = 22.5\%$$

$$\text{Average Cost of Equity} = \left(\begin{array}{c} \text{Risk Free} \\ \text{Return on} \\ \text{US Govt} \\ \text{Obligations} \end{array} \right) + (\text{Beta of Firm} \times \text{Market-Risk Premium}) = \% \ 8.7\%$$

$$\text{Cash Flow to Debt \%} = \frac{\text{Net Income} + \text{Depreciation}}{\text{Total Liability}} = \frac{15,793 + 6,307}{52,612} = 42.0\%$$

$$\text{Debt Service Coverage} = \frac{\text{Net Income} + \text{Depreciation} + \text{Interest}}{\text{Principal Payment} + \text{Interest}}$$

$$= \frac{15,793 + 6,307 + 337}{725 + 337} = 21.1$$

AHCS has less financial leverage when compared to U.S. median values. It has borrowed extensively to finance its capital investment program, but has also used its extensive capital reserves. This increased debt has raised the cost-of-equity capital. AHCS's cost-of-equity capital is explained in Figure 10–4. The cost of a firm's equity increases as debt financing rises, but the firm's weighted cost of capital may not increase. Weighted cost of capital is defined as:

$$
\begin{bmatrix}
\text{\% of Long-Term} \\
\text{Debt to Equity} \\
\text{plus Long-Term Debt}
\end{bmatrix}
\times
\begin{bmatrix}
\text{Interest} \\
\text{Rate on} \\
\text{Debt}
\end{bmatrix}
+
\begin{bmatrix}
\text{\% of Equity to} \\
\text{Equity plus} \\
\text{Long-Term Debt}
\end{bmatrix}
\times
\begin{bmatrix}
\text{Cost} \\
\text{of} \\
\text{Equity}
\end{bmatrix}
$$

$$[18\% \times 5.1\%] + [82\% \; 3 \; 8.7\%] = 8.1\%$$

AHCS has minimal debt at the present, even after its additional borrowing in 2007. Most of its debt is vari-

able rate, with average rates running less than one percent. We have chosen to use a 5.1 percent rate on debt, which better reflects what AHCS would pay on non-variable-rate debt.

The conclusion regarding the capital position of AHCS is:

- AHCS has minimal levels of debt, and its ability to meet debt-service obligations is excellent.

SUMMARY

Our financial review of AHCS suggests possible improvements in profitability. Most of the opportunity for profit enhancement at AHCS is related to both revenue

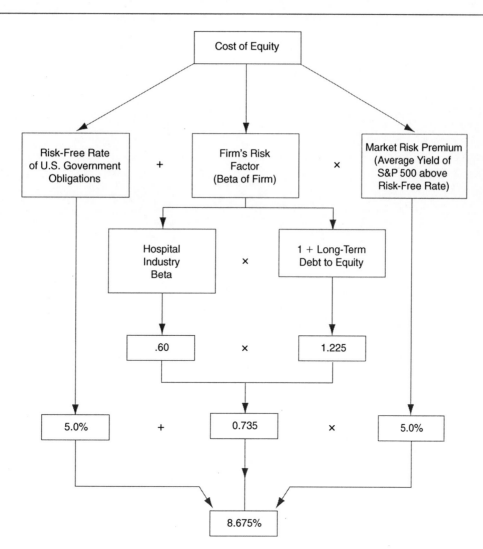

Figure 10–4 AHCS's Cost of Equity

and cost issues. Areas identified for improvement include the following:

Action	Annual Profit Improvement Range
Increase market share	$200,000 to $1,000,000
Increase prices	$1,000,000 to $4,000,000
Coding reviews	$2,000,000 to $4,000,000
Renegotiate managed care contracts	$0
Review compensation structure	$0 to $5,000,000
Standardize medical and drug supply items	$1,000,000 to $3,000,000
Review investment portfolio management	$0
Reduce accounts receivable	$100,000 to $200,000
Implement capital-expenditure contracts	$0 to $2,000,000
Total	$4,300,000 to $19,200,000

The dashboard approach used in this case can be very helpful in focusing management attention on either potential problems or areas of opportunity. Ultimately, management must, however, make changes. The best dashboard design, combined with accurate and timely reporting, will accomplish nothing without actual management intervention.

REFERENCES

Robert S. Kaplan and David P. Norton, The Balanced Scorecard, Harvard Business School Press, 1996.

ASSIGNMENTS

1. Operating margins in your hospital have been consistently below national norms for the past three years. Discuss the factors that might have created this situation and the ways in which you might determine specific causes.

2. Your firm reported net income of $5,000,000, but the change in equity was only $3,000,000. What could account for this difference?

3. Determine the amount of incremental profit that would be realized with a ten percent across-the-board rate increase at Thunderbird Hospital. Thunderbird's present payment composition is 80 percent fixed-fee and 20 percent charges or discounted charges. Present operating income is defined below:

Gross patient revenue	$100,000,000
less Contractual allowances	40,000,000
Net patient revenue	$60,000,000
less Expenses	59,000,000
Operating income	$1,000,000

4. You have been reviewing documentation in your medical records department for the last week and have discovered a potential issue with respect to documentation for DRG 127 (heart failure and shock) and DRG 475 (respiratory system diagnosis with ventilator support). You have discovered 20 cases that were coded as DRG 127, when in fact these patients had been put on a ventilator. These patients also had a respiratory system diagnosis. If the respiratory system diagnosis had been the principal diagnosis, these patients would have been coded as DRG 475. If the hospital's base payment rate for a case weight of 1.000 is $5,000, determine the incremental payment the hospital would have received. Assume the case weight for DRG 127 is 1.000 and 3.700 for DRG 475.

5. Your firm's investment portfolio was valued at $100,000,000 at the beginning of the year. Approximately 60 percent of the portfolio was invested in fixed-income securities, primarily U.S. government bonds. The remaining 40 percent was invested in mutual funds selected by your firm's portfolio manager. During the year, the U.S. government bonds yielded 6.0 percent, and the change in the Standard and Poor's 500 index was 10.0 percent. Reported investment income during the year was $6,000,000, including realized gains. The firm also reported an unrealized loss of $1,000,000. Total yield on the portfolio was thus $5,000,000. What value would you have expected given the facts above?

6. Your present length of stay on Medicare patients is 6.3 days for 2000 Medicare admissions. This value is unadjusted for case-mix effects. You have discovered that a normal length of stay should have been 5.0 days. If this level had been realized, you would have had 2600 fewer days of care for Medicare patients. You are trying to determine the amount of actual savings that would be realized if the shorter length of stay could be affected. You have been told that a shorter length of stay would affect only direct costs of nursing. Your present direct cost of nursing per day is $300. Some of this cost is considered fixed and would not be changed. If 60 percent of the nursing cost were considered variable, how much savings would be realized through the length-of-stay reduction?

7. Charles S. Lewis has just been named the CEO of Community Hospital, a 230-bed hospital located in an agricultural community of approximately 150,000 people. There is one

other similar-sized hospital in the community. C.S. Lewis has been told by his CFO, J.R.R. Tolkein, that the hospital is in excellent financial condition, but Mr. Lewis is not convinced. He has requested and received the summary financial statements presented in Table 10–10.

You have been asked to help Mr. Lewis identify the trends in financial position for the hospital over the last five years. Please compute the values for the financial ratios described in Chapter 10 and provide Mr. Lewis with your assessment of Community Hospital's financial position.

Table 10–10 Summary Financial Information of Community Hospital* (2003–2007) (Data in Thousands)

	2003	2004	2005	2006	2007
Balance sheet accounts					
Cash & cash equivalents	$ 34,402	$ 30,444	$ 45,848	$ 46,010	$ 73,711
Patient accounts receivable	39,506	38,878	35,444	38,853	35,647
Inventory	2,133	2,318	2,398	3,197	3,279
Gross fixed assets	187,278	221,548	240,988	256,652	276,458
Accumulated depreciation	73,227	79,523	89,324	101,007	113,851
Net fixed assets	114,051	142,025	151,664	155,645	162,607
Unrestricted capital funds	10,720	13,625	20,160	25,615	17,716
Total assets	$ 238,365	$ 265,784	$ 276,965	$ 287,193	$ 311,140
Current maturities of LTD	111	1,794	1,431	2,211	1,143
Current liabilities	$ 37,426	$ 38,492	$ 33,240	$ 31,699	$ 35,862
Long-term debt	2,032	12,821	11,720	9,578	9,570
Net assets	$ 188,743	$ 204,262	$ 222,606	$ 237,022	$ 251,241
Income statement accounts					
Net patient revenue	$208,861	$ 225,950	$ 244,976	$ 257,784	$ 282,461
Other revenue	1,569	1,756	1,929	2,170	1,757
Total operating revenue	$ 210,430	$ 227,706	$ 246,905	$ 259,954	$ 284,218
Total operating expenses	$ 203,043	$ 219,768	$ 233,867	$ 254,382	$ 278,629
Operating income	7,387	7,938	13,038	5,572	5,589
plus Non-operating revenue	6,806	7,579	8,971	8,430	8,696
Excess of revenue over expenses	$ 14,193	$ 15,517	$ 22,009	$ 14,002	$ 14,285
Depreciation	$ 10,588	$ 11,161	$ 11,659	$ 12,184	$ 12,524
Interest	115	611	471	419	392

*Please note that not all asset and liability items are shown. The totals do not, therefore, foot to the individual account values.

SOLUTIONS AND ANSWERS

1. Low operating margins are the result of either low prices or high costs. Low prices may be difficult to change in either competitive markets or situations involving high percentages of fixed-price payers, such as Medicare. High costs may result from excessive length of stay, poor productivity, or high salaries.

2. A transfer of funds from the entity may have taken place. This is often the case in investor-owned companies, because of the payment of dividends. It also may occur in a voluntary entity because of corporate restructuring. Unrealized losses on the firm's investment portfolio may have occurred.

3. The amount of incremental profit is equal to the percent of charge patients x price increase $\times$ present gross patient revenue, or $2,000,000. The increase in charges is $10,000,000, or 10 percent times $100,000,000. Of that amount, 20 percent, or $2,000,000, will be to charge or discounted-charge payers.

4. The difference in payment would be 20 patients $\times$ $5,000 $\times$ (3.700 − 1.000), or $270,000.

5. The expected yield should have been $7,600,000:

$$\text{Expected fixed-income yield} = \$60,000,000 \times 6.0\% = \$3,600,000$$

$$\text{Expected equity yield} = \$40,000,000 \times 10\% = \$4,000,000$$

6. The estimated savings would be days saved $\times$ direct cost of nursing $\times$ variable cost percentage (2,600 $\times$ $300 $\times$ 60%), or $468,000.

7. Only selected financial ratios for Community Hospital can be calculated for the period 2003 through 2007. These values are shown in Table 10–11, Major observations that would result include the following:

   • Present financial position at Community Hospital is strong. Current financial strength is a result of two primary factors: minimal levels of long-term debt and above-average total margins.

   • The trend in margins is downward, however. The primary cause is an erosion of operating-income levels. Expenses have been growing more rapidly than revenues since 2005.

Table 10–11 Selected Financial Ratios

	2003	2004	2005	2006	2007
Overall					
Return on equity %	7.5	7.6	9.9	5.9	5.7
Total margin %	6.5	6.6	8.6	5.2	4.9
Financial strength index	2.2	1.9	3.1	2.2	2.3
Non-operating income					
Days' cash-on-hand	86	77	108	108	125
Investment efficiency					
Days in accounts receivable	69	63	53	55	46
Revenue to net fixed assets	1.9	1.7	1.7	1.7	1.8
Plant obsolescence					
Average age of plant	6.9	7.1	7.7	8.3	9.1
Capital position					
Debt financing %	20.8	23.1	19.6	17.5	19.3
Cash flow to debt %	49.9	43.4	61.9	52.2	44.8

Chapter 11

Financial Analysis of Alternative Health Care Firms

LEARNING OBJECTIVES

After studying this chapter, you should be able to do the following:

1. List some of the major non-hospital and non-physician sectors of the health care industry.
2. Discuss the sources of revenue for the nursing home industry.
3. Discuss the major sources of revenue and expenses of medical groups.
4. List and describe the major organizational types of physicians groups.
5. Describe alternative HMO organizational arrangements.

REAL-WORLD SCENARIO

Laura Rose was appointed recently to the Board of ElderCare, a large, for-profit operator of skilled nursing facilities (SNFs) around the country. Laura's first committee assignment is to the Treasury Committee because of her prior business experience. Although Laura has extensive experience as a hospital administrator, she has relatively little familiarity with the SNF industry. Upon reviewing ElderCare's recent financial statements, she is concerned about the dramatically declining financial position. She notices that revenues are declining on per-facility and per-patient bases. Meanwhile, the company's debt has been downgraded and its borrowing costs have risen substantially.

She is aware that in recent years Medicare implemented a skilled nursing facility (SNF) prospective payment system (PPS) as part of the Balanced Budget Act of 1997. Payment increases by Medicare and Medicaid have not kept pace with increases in costs in recent years. She wonders whether this might be a factor in the company's financing issues. In general, profitability in the long-term care industry has declined significantly in recent years, and several industry leaders have filed for bankruptcy protection. While some believe that SNF PPS is largely to blame, other factors, such as ill-advised acquisitions, excessive long-term debt, and poor balance sheets, probably contributed as well. In essence, she is unsure whether ElderCare's financing difficulties are unique to management issues at ElderCare or whether they reflect more general market conditions and economic and reimbursement trends.

To understand the issue better, Laura needs to be able to estimate the direct financial impact of SNF reimbursement. She asked the ElderCare treasury and controller's office staff to prepare an analysis of the financial performance of selected long-term care facilities for the period 2005 to 2007. In particular, she wants to know how SNF bond ratings have been affected by PPS and what other factors might have contributed to the industry's deteriorating financial performance.

In the last chapter, we discussed the measures and concepts of financial analysis in some detail, but most of the examples and industry standards were from the hospital sector. The hospital industry is by far the largest sector in the health care industry, but it is not the only sector; its rate of growth in recent years has been slower than in other areas. This chapter will provide some additional information about alternative health care firms.

List some of the major non-hospital and non-physician sectors of the health care industry.

First, we will discuss the financial characteristics of the following three specific alternative sectors:

1. Nursing homes
2. Medical groups
3. Health plans

It is impossible to describe all of the specific operating characteristics of these three sectors in one chapter, but we will try to highlight the important differences that affect financial measures. It is important to remember that the financial measures and concepts discussed in the previous chapter are still applicable. For example, the concept and measurement of liquidity is the same for a hospital as it would be for a health plan. However, operating differences between health plans and hospitals will produce different values and standards. Health plans have much lower days in receivables than do hospitals, and are required to carry much higher cash balances to meet transaction needs, namely claims payments.

It is not just the higher relative growth rates of non-hospital sectors that cause us to separately examine the topic of financial analysis for alternative health care firms. Many of the alternative health care firms have been consolidating through both horizontal and vertical mergers and have now become major corporations

in our nation's economy. For example, UnitedHealth Group, Aetna, and Wellpoint are among the largest corporations in the country, employing large numbers of people and absorbing significant amounts of capital to finance their continued growth. Much financial analysis and discussion are now devoted to these firms because of their almost continuous needs for financing. Major brokerage houses now have analysts who devote their time to narrow sectors of the health care industry, such as home health firms or medical groups.

Table 11–1 presents financial ratio medians for the three sectors, along with comparative values for the investor-owned hospital industry sector. We have calculated ratio averages by computing the ratio average for three large publicly traded firms in each industrial group. Table 11–2 shows the composition for each of the three groups.

LONG-TERM CARE FACILITIES AND NURSING HOMES

It is not always clear what types of firms individuals are referring to when they talk about the long-term care industry. For our purposes, we will be referring primarily to nursing homes, both skilled and intermediate-care facilities. The nursing home industry has experienced significant growth during the last decade, and expectations about the aging of America have led many analysts to project even more rapid growth in the future. Growth in the nursing home industry is inextricably linked to government payment and regulatory policy.

As of 2004, there were over 15,000 nursing homes in the United States, and of those, more than 65 percent were investor-owned. Investor-owned presence in the nursing home industry is much larger than it is in the hospital industry, where only 15 percent of hospital capacity is investor-owned. Many of the investor-owned nursing homes are part of large national chains, such as Beverly Enterprises, Kindred Healthcare, and Manor Care. However, there still are many investors that may own as few as one or two nursing homes to

Table 11–1 Financial Ratio Medians

Financial Ratio	Nursing Homes	Medical Groups	Health Insurer	Hospitals
Liquidity				
Current	1.11	1.54	1.59	1.75
Days in receivables	48.0	64.5	21.3	50.8
Days-cash-on-hand	26.2	9.5	224.0	35.0
Capital Structure				
Debt financing percentage	64.3	49.8	45.6	66.2
Long-term debt to capital	35.7	35.8	19.1	54.9
Cash flow to debt percentage	18.3	33.7	35.7	18.3
Times interest earned	4.39	30.1	17.1	2.91
Activity				
Total asset turnover	1.67	1.01	1.20	1.00
Fixed asset turnover	4.09	10.90	29.50	2.00
Current asset turnover	7.52	3.95	2.60	1.75
Profitability				
Total margin percentage	2.9	10.9	4.7	4.8
Return on equity percentage	12.4	22.0	17.9	18.2

Source: Cleverley & Associates, Columbus, Ohio.

as many as twenty. Most of the large investor-owned chains became involved in the industry when the government started to finance a sizable percentage of nursing home care through the Medicaid program. Heavy government financing provided a stable source of payment that was not present before Medicaid.

LEARNING OBJECTIVE 2

Discuss the sources of revenue for the nursing home industry.

Financing of nursing home care is a critical driver of nursing home supply, as it is for most other health care sectors. Table 11–3 summarizes sources of financing for nursing homes as of 2004.

The data in Table 11–3 reflect the dramatic increase in the percentage of nursing home financing that is derived from public sources, and a corresponding reduction in private financing. The percentage of Medicare financing increased sharply in the first half of the 1990s as hospitals discharged more patients into nursing home settings to cut their costs per case and to maximize their profit per Medicare case. Much of this shift probably was related to the financial incentives created by the Medicare program when the government shifted to a per-case payment system in 1983.

Although the federal government pays more than 50 percent of Medicaid nursing home costs, actual nursing home payments for Medicaid patients are set by the states. There is wide variation among the states between retrospective and prospective systems. In many states, there may be a mix of both systems. For example, capital costs may be paid on a retrospective basis, whereas all other costs may be paid on a prospective basis. Many states also use a case-mix-adjustment methodology to provide higher payments for nursing homes treating more severely ill patients.

Medicaid payments from states are usually the second largest state expenditure and, as a result, are subject to dramatic changes based upon the economic condition in the state. When economic times are bad and states have a difficult time meeting their budgets, one of the areas usually affected is nursing home payments.

The level of nursing home beds by state varies dramatically. Many states have used the supply of nursing home beds as a means to control state expenditures for nursing home care. The number of nursing home beds per 1000 people older than 85 years ranges from 184.8 in West Virginia to 504.4 in Indiana (Center for Medicare and Medicaid Services. Division of Payment Systems,

Table 11–2 Industry Composition

Industry/Firms		Most Recent Revenue (millions)
Health insurance		
United Healthcare Group	(UNH)	$44,000
Wellpoint, Inc.	(WLP)	41,000
Aetna	(AET)	22,000
Nursing homes		
Manor Care	(HCR)	$3,400
Kindred Healthcare	(KND)	3,900
Beverly Enterprises	(BEV)	2,300
Medical group/Physicians		
Pediatrix Medical Group	(PDX)	$680
Apria Healthcare Group	(AHG)	1,500
Renal Care Group	(RCI)	1,500
Hospital		
HCA, Inc	(HCA)	$24,200
Tenet Healthcare	(TNT)	9,700
Triad Hospitals	(TRI)	4,700

Table 11–3 Financing Percentages for Nursing Home Expenditures

	1985	1990	1995	2004
Private financing	49	51	40	41
Insurance	3	6	7	8
Out-of-pocket	39	37	27	28
All other	7	8	6	5
Public financing	51	49	60	59
Medicare	1	3	10	12
Medicaid	47	44	48	45
All other	3	4	2	2

Source: Reprinted from the Center for Medicare and Medicaid Services.

1999). Licensure laws and Certificate of Need (CON) have been the primary means for controlling nursing home beds in most states. Rates of payment for Medicaid patients also serve as an indirect method of controlling nursing home capacity. As rates are held down, less capital becomes available for expansion and renovation. Major national nursing home chains have been known to sell all of their nursing homes in certain states where they believed that reasonable profits would be difficult to obtain because of restrictive state payment policies.

It is expected that demand for nursing home care will increase dramatically in the next thirty years as the baby boomers reach the age of 75 plus, which is the age at which nursing home demand peaks. Nursing homes are also diversifying and expanding their product lines. For example, many nursing homes are becoming continuing care retirement communities (CCRCs). In a CCRC, there is a continuum of care that runs the gamut from independent living, to assisted living, to skilled care.

Continuing care retirement communities also have discovered that their resident populations are desirable targets for HMOs that are seeking to expand their Medicare risk contracts. The CCRC is in a strong position to market itself to a managed care group be-

cause of the economies of scale provided from its continuum of care and its personal relationship with the Medicare population. At the same time, hospitals are looking for ways to expand their revenue base and have begun to develop skilled-care units and other subacute units that can expand their business along the continuum of care and compete with existing nursing homes. In many respects, some of the historical distinctions among health care industry segments are becoming blurred as vertical integration accelerates.

The financial statements in Tables 11–4 and 11–5 reflect the operations of Friendly Village, a church-owned CCRC. A review of these financial statements will give the reader some idea of the nature of business operations in this type of health care organization. A CCRC usually provides three levels of care: nursing home care, assisted living, and independent living. Often, residents progress through these three levels of care. An elderly person may enter the CCRC with independent-living status and occupy one of the independent-living apartments. These apartments often are similar to apartments in other settings except that the residents are all retired and there are usually a variety of social activities to keep the residents active and united. As the health of a resident erodes, that resident may move to an assisted-living environment. In an assisted-living environment, there will be some health care services provided to enable the resident to maintain daily activities. For example, medication administration, medical monitoring, or some help with daily living functions such as bathing, toileting, and cooking may be required. Many residents

Table 11–4 Friendly Village and Subsidiary Consolidated Balance Sheets

	June	
	2007	*2006*
Assets		
General Funds		
Current assets:		
Cash and cash equivalents	$222,032	$168,091
Investments (at cost-approximate market value of $293,000 in 2007 and $530,000 in 2006)	193,991	397,469
Cash and investments that have limited use	616,425	301,582
Receivable—Friendly Church entrance fee fund (Note 3)	2,089,315	2,106,442
Resident and patient accounts receivable, less allowance for doubtful accounts (2007—$195,000; 2006—$115,000)	780,227	432,321
Mortgage escrow deposits	29,991	79,574
Inventories, prepaid expenses and other assets	115,112	139,896
Total current assets	**$4,047,093**	**$3,625,375**
Assets that have limited use:		
Cash and investments (at cost, which approximates market value)		
Under bond indenture agreement—held by trustee (Note 4)	$4,954,756	$642,929
Repair and replacement—held by trustee	274,931	345,041
Resident deposits	284,235	276,455
	$5,513,922	$1,264,425
less cash and investments required for current liabilities	(616,425)	(301,582)
	$4,897,497	$962,843
Receivable—Friendly Church entrance-fee fund, *less* portion classified as current assets (Notes 3 and 5)	5,691,916	4,992,891
	$10,589,413	$5,955,734
Property and equipment, less allowances for depreciation (Notes 4 and 6)	$12,925,048	$10,433,986
Unamortized debt financing costs	535,631	219,515
Total general funds	**$28,097,185**	**$20,234,610**
Donor-restricted funds		
Cash and investments (at cost-approximate market value of $1,121,000 in 2007 and $1,210,000 in 2006)	$1,171,460	$1,043,820
Receivable—Friendly Foundation	192,635	184,085
Due from general funds	190,868	183,085
Due from nurse scholarship recipients	13,939	5,887
Due from employee hardship recipients	3,171	
Total donor-restricted funds	**$1,572,073**	**$1,416,877**
Liabilities and fund balances		
General Funds		
Current liabilities:		
Accounts payable	$862,611	$674,165
Interest payable	330,544	169,475
Salaries, wages and related liabilities	737,374	676,173
Funds held for others	29,672	29,201
Due to donor-restricted funds	190,868	183,104

continues

Table 11–4 continued

	June	
	2007	2006
Estimated third-party settlement (Note 2)	44,507	428
Current portion of deferred entrance fees	800,000	958,496
Current portion of note payable to Friendly Church entrance-fee fund (Note 5)	27,467	39,698
Current portion of long-term liabilities (Note 5)	413,750	363,750
Total current liabilities	**$3,436,793**	**$3,094,490**
Deferred entrance fees, less current portion (Notes 1 and 5)	2,888,683	4,159,368
Deposits—residents	279,650	266,581
Note payable to the entrance-fee fund, less current portion (Note 5)	617,258	647,135
Long-term liabilities, less current portion (Note 4)	15,507,312	8,025,153
Refundable entrance fees	27,291	29,036
Obligation to provide future services and use of facilities	185,000	185,000
General fund balance	5,155,198	3,827,847
Total general funds	**$28,097,185**	**$20,234,610**
Donor-restricted funds		
Fund balances		
Sustaining fund	$729,814	$672,155
Foundation fund	192,634	184,085
Medical-memorial fund	334,618	326,378
Specific-purpose fund	190,869	183,104
Nurse-scholarship fund	46,069	44,295
Employee-hardship fund	11,871	6,860
Pooled-income fund	66,198	
Total donor-restricted funds	**$1,572,073**	**$1,416,877**

are prolonging admission into an assisted-living center, and assisted-living residents are becoming similar to the nursing home residents of ten years ago. The last level of care is nursing home services, either intermediate or skilled. Many CCRCs also may have specialized units to treat patients with Alzheimer's disease or who have experienced a stroke.

The income statement of Table 11–5 reports revenues from a variety of sources. The largest share is from the nursing home and is referred to as routine health care center services ($6,033,751 in 2007). The second largest source of revenue is fees generated from care and services provided to residents of the assisted-living center or the independent-living apartments ($3,922,230 in 2007). Some other revenue is generated from entrance fees and consists of $1,049,160 from an amortization of entrance fees and $2,111,079 from investment income earned on the

entrance fee fund. Some residents pay entrance fees upon entrance into the independent-living or assisted-living center. These deposits guarantee that a nursing home bed will be available if needed and that the rate for that nursing home bed will be less than the nursing home's current rates. For example, the CCRC may guarantee that the resident would have to pay only 50 percent of the posted rate for a nursing home bed if needed.

The amount of the entrance fee may be based upon age at entrance. The fund is then amortized or recognized as income as the patient ages or dies. There is also income earned on the deposits that is recognized as income each year. The entrance fee fund is listed several times in the balance sheet depicted in Table 11–4. On the asset side, there is a receivable from the church, which holds the entrance fees, in both the current asset and assets that have limited-use sections. On

Table 11–5 Friendly Village and Subsidiary Consolidated Statements of Revenue and Expenses of General Funds

	Year Ended June 30	
	2007	*2006*
Revenues		
Routine health care center services, net	$6,033,751	$5,692,688
Care and service fees, net	3,922,230	3,685,316
Amortization of entrance fees	1,049,160	958,497
Other medical services	670,479	656,520
Applicant fees	6,200	5,900
Investment income on restricted funds	278,894	94,432
Other	276,467	203,349
Total revenues	$12,237,181	$11,296,702
Expenses		
Salaries and wages	$5,731,524	$5,418,725
Employee benefits	1,022,276	935,969
Purchased services	994,078	948,193
Other medical services	757,452	741,082
Supplies	1,044,831	925,812
Repairs and maintenance	133,882	105,871
Utilities	582,935	519,091
Equipment rental	7,531	4,739
Interest and amortization	1,274,492	770,507
Provision for doubtful accounts	63,804	24,675
Taxes	376,858	359,522
Insurance–property, liability and general	76,534	91,050
Other	81,649	85,066
Total expenses	$12,147,846	$10,930,302
Gain from operations before depreciation and other operating revenues	$89,335	$366,400
Other operating revenues and expenses		
Unrestricted contributions	$ 19,230	$ 65,538
Investment income on entrance fee fund, net	2,111,079	752,331
Gain from operations before depreciation	$2,219,644	$1,184,269
Provision for depreciation	(895,632)	(801,185)
Gain from operations	$1,324,012	$383,084
Nonoperating loss		
Loss on disposal of property and equipment	(49,594)	(9,802)
Excess of revenues over expenses and nonoperating loss	$1,274,418	$373,282

the liability side, there are accounts in both the current and non-current sections that represent deferred entrance fees. We will discuss shortly what these accounts represent because they are one of the most confusing accounting aspects of CCRCs.

The expense structure of a CCRC or nursing home is similar to other health care providers and is labor intensive. At Friendly Village, salaries and wages plus benefits constitute slightly more than 50 percent of total

expenses. Also, notice that depreciation is not shown in the expense section, but is separately shown as other expense. This is not uncommon for not-for-profit CCRCs that oftentimes regard capital as a gift and do not regard replacement of the existing assets as an operating expense.

Perhaps the most unusual feature of a CCRC's financial statement relates to the entrance fee fund and the deferred revenue that results from the receipt of those moneys upon admission to the retirement community. To understand the concepts of entrance fees and their amortization and deferred-revenue recognition, we will use a simple example and then relate those concepts to the data for Friendly Village. Let's assume that a resident enters the CCRC at the beginning of the year and contributes $35,000 to the entrance fee fund. This amount will be amortized over the expected life of the resident, which we will assume to be seven years. During the year, the resident spends twenty days in the skilled nursing facility and is required to pay only 60 percent of the $150 per-day charge, or $90 per day. This means that a payment of $60 per day for twenty days, or $1,200, will be paid to the skilled nursing facility for 40 percent of the residents' charges by the entrance fee fund. Finally, assume that the $35,000 entrance fee fund earned investment income during the year in the amount of $2,000. The following entries would be made:

Entry No. 1. Record receipt of the $35,000 entrance fee
Increase entrance fee fund by $35,000
Increase deferred revenue by $35,000

Entry No. 2. Record transfer of money to skilled nursing facility
Increase unrestricted cash by $1,200
Decrease entrance fee fund by $1,200

Entry No. 3. Record annual amortization of entrance fee fund
Increase revenue account amortization of entrance fees by $5,000
Decrease deferred revenue by $5,000

Entry No. 4. Record the investment income earned during the year
Increase entrance fee fund by $2,000
Increase investment income on entrance fee fund by $2,000

These are the accounting entries that would be made to reflect activities related to the entrance fee fund and the deferred revenue account relating to the entrance fee fund. The entrance fee fund is an asset account that represents the funds available to meet contractual commitments to provide future health care services to residents. The deferred revenue account is a liability account that represents the estimated present value of

future contractual obligations to provide health care services to residents.

Discuss the major sources of revenue and expenses of medical groups.

MEDICAL GROUPS

Expenditures for physician and clinical services amount to approximately $400 billion in 2004 and are second only to hospital expenditures. Physician expenditures have been increasing more rapidly than expenditures of most other sectors of the health care industry, which has increased the relative importance of physicians. However, it is not just the absolute level of expenditures made to physicians that make doctors an important element in our health care industry. It is widely believed that doctors directly or indirectly control up to 85 percent of all health care expenditures. Doctors admit and discharge patients to hospitals; they prescribe drugs, order expensive diagnostic imaging services, and schedule rehabilitative services. The stroke of a doctor's pen directs a massive amount of health care resources to or away from an individual patient. Managed care plans realized the demand-influencing behavior of physicians early and have attempted to incorporate incentives for cost control in physician payment plans.

Although few would debate the importance of physicians in controlling health care costs, physicians have yet to realize their importance in the medical marketplace because of their lack of organization. Of the 700,000 physicians in the United States, two-thirds operate in one- or two- person practices. It is difficult for physicians to realize their central role in cost and quality decision making in health care negotiations. This is because most of them are part of delivery organizations that are too small to exert much, if any, bargaining leverage in health care negotiations. Physicians are slowly realizing this weakness and are now becoming part of larger organizations that are being developed by hospitals, health plans, large practice management companies, and large physician-controlled medical groups.

Table 11–6 presents some data on sources of financing for the physician sector of the health care industry.

Table 11-6 Financing Percentages for Physician Expenditures

	1985	1990	1995	2004
Private financing	<u>71</u>	<u>69</u>	<u>69</u>	<u>67</u>
Insurance	37	43	49	50
Out-of-pocket	27	19	12	10
All other	7	7	8	7
Public financing	<u>29</u>	<u>31</u>	<u>31</u>	<u>33</u>
Medicare	19	19	19	19
Medicaid	4	5	7	7
All other	6	7	5	7

Source: Reprinted from the Center for Medicare and Medicaid Services.

Perhaps the most significant trend is the dramatic reduction in the percentage of physician expenditures financed by out-of-pocket payments from patients. In the period from 1985 to 2004, the percentage dropped from 27 to 10. It is not exactly clear what has caused this decrease, but the decline of indemnity coverage and the corresponding increase in HMO and PPO plans may be possible causes. Many HMO plans require a low copayment or no copayment for routine office visits, whereas most traditional indemnity programs have a coinsurance and deductible provision. For example, indemnity programs may require a subscriber to make all routine physician payments until some deductible is met, for example $500. This might change in the years ahead if consumer-driven health plans with large deductibles become more pervasive.

Physicians do receive a much larger percentage of their total revenue from the private sector than do most other major health care sectors. In 2004, physicians received 67 percent of their total revenues from the private sector, whereas hospitals received only 41 percent. Medicare covers nearly 100 percent of hospital service charges for the elderly, but is subject to a 20 percent coinsurance payment for most physician services. Most Medicare beneficiaries will finance this payment with supplemental insurance, which creates a shift from public to private financing.

Physician expenditures are increasing because there is increased usage of physician services. Table 11-7 documents the increasing number of health care visits per year as people get older. The number of visits within age groups also is increasing (not shown). As the population ages, demand for physician services is expected to increase sharply. The substitution of ambulatory care for inpatient care also will further accelerate demand for physicians.

As we discussed earlier, physicians are beginning to align themselves with larger groups and are moving quickly from one- or two-person practices to these larger groups. Some of this movement is a reflection of personal tastes. Physicians who practice in larger groups can make arrangements for weekend or evening coverage. Large group practices often provide their doctors with better consultative services and also reduce administrative burden, permitting greater patient-contact time. Lifestyle considerations may be an important cause of physicians joining larger groups, but the primary cause is related to economics. Physicians have seen hospitals and health plans merge and become more and more dominant in the local health care marketplace. Prior to increasing physician organization to counterbalance these large bargaining entities, physicians perceived themselves as being at a disadvantage.

LEARNING OBJECTIVE 4

List and describe the major organizational types of physician groups.

Table 11-7 Health Care Visits Per Year, 1998: Percent Distribution by Age Group[1]

Age Group	None	1–3	4–9	10 or More
Under 18 years	11.7	54.5	25.6	8.2
18–44	21.6	47.7	18.6	12.2
45–64	15.9	43.6	24.3	16.2
65–74	8.4	36.6	34.3	20.8
Older than 74 years	6.0	30.8	36.5	26.7

[1]*Source:* National Center for Health Statistics. Based on a summary measure that combines information about visits to doctors' offices or clinics, emergency departments, and home visits.

Physicians can choose whether to align with other physicians or to remain independent. If they choose to align with other physicians, there are four primary organizational alternatives for them to consider. They are the following:

- Alignment with other medical groups
- Alignment with hospitals
- Alignment with health plans
- Alignment with physician practice-management firms

Alignment with physicians is, in some respects, most appealing to physicians because their control is maximized in this type of organizational setting. Oftentimes, the critical limitation is capital. To achieve large-scale integration and development of new information systems and administrative structures, massive amounts of both financial and human capital are required. Only recently have outside investors come forward to provide this external capital. For integration with other physicians to be successful, a physician activist is needed who will not only arrange the financing of capital needs, but who will also provide the administrative leadership.

Hospitals have the financial capital to create large groups, but in some cases their administrative experiences with physician-practice management are limited. This limitation, coupled with differing incentives, can lead to organizational conflict. In a managed-care environment, the objective is to empty hospital beds, not fill them, and this oftentimes leads to conflict between hospitals and doctors. Hospitals also have been dominated by specialists, but primary care physicians are the key in managed-care markets. Primary care physicians often believe that hospitals do not understand them or their needs.

Health plans also have the capital to put together large medical groups, but a conflict may arise between the incentives of health plans and its employee doctors. The health plan has a strong incentive to reduce fees or salaries of its doctors, while also controlling utilization. Physicians do not react favorably to lower income and also object to mandates or controls over their practice patterns.

Physician practice management firms are a relatively recent development that has evolved to meet the needs of both the physicians and the marketplace. Some of these firms are publicly traded and can have capital and management pools to draw upon to develop large, integrated organizations. Physician practice management

firms usually offer physicians some type of profit sharing and also provide for an equity stake in the firm. This equity participation can make the attraction of merger or acquisition by a physician practice management firm hard to resist. In short, physician practice management firms often can afford to pay large sums of money to acquire physician practices and they also promise physicians a strong degree of autonomy.

The financial statements in Tables 11–8 and 11–9 provide financial information for Waverly Health Clinic (WHC), a hospital-owned network of eight primary care clinics with 24 full-time physicians and 122 non-physician employees. The clinic recorded 101,542 patient encounters during the past year with an average resource-based relative value scale relative value unit (RBRVS RVU) of 1.5 per patient encounter. WHC is a separately incorporated for-profit subsidiary of the hospital, and all of its physicians are salaried with profit and productivity incentives.

The financial statements of WHC provide some interesting information about physician practices, espe-

Table 11–8 Balance Sheet Waverly Health Clinic, December 31, 2007

Assets

Current assets

Cash	$364,631
Net accounts receivable	$1,411,013
Prepaid expenses	$143,481
Other current assets	$731,550
Total current assets	$2,650,675
Net property, plant, and equipment	$1,855,869
Intangible assets	$188,941
Total assets	**$4,695,485**

Liabilities and equity

Current liabilities

Accounts payable	$168,131
Withheld taxes	$84,694
Employee benefits withheld	$3,281
Accrued salaries and wages	$335,513
Other current liabilities	$98,482
Total current liabilities	$690,101

Equity

Contributed capital	$8,234,890
Retained earnings	($4,229,506)
Total equity	$4,005,384
Total liabilities and equity	**$4,695,485**

Table 11–9 Income Statement Waverly Health Care, December 31, 2007

Revenue

Gross physician charges	$13,292,570
Other revenue	2,866,090
Adjustments and write-offs	(3,078,500)
Net revenue	**$13,080,160**

Operating Expenses

Personnel expense	$5,999,400
Supplies expense	525,200
Occupancy expense	2,456,500
Purchased services	267,400
General and administrative expense	1,154,400
Total operating expense	**$10,402,900**
Physician expense	**4,449,800**
Total expense	**$14,852,700**
Net profit	**($1,772,540)**

cially those owned by hospitals. We can see that the practice lost $1,772,540 in the current year. It is not unusual for hospital-owned physician practices to lose money. Revenues from the practice are oftentimes less than expenses. Many hospital executives argue that although the direct revenues and expenses of the practice may show a loss, there are substantial benefits realized from operating the practice. These benefits result from the admitting and referral patterns of the acquired physician practices, which raise volume at the hospital. Greater integration with the physicians themselves also may result in better cost control, which is important for managed care contracts. Although all of this may be true, in many cases, it is simply poor management that creates the financial loss. Most of these acquired practices were profitable before hospital acquisition, yet once they become hospital-owned and operated, they suddenly become unprofitable. A review of the finan-

cial information for WHC can help shed some light on the most common reasons for lack of profitability. Table 11–10 shows values for WHC expressed on a per-physician full-time equivalent (FTE) basis, compared to national values for primary care medical group practices derived from a study by the Medical Group Management Association (MGMA) in 2004.

The Waverly Health Clinic has many more operating expenses than does a typical medical group. Some of this is due to staffing. WHC has 5.08 support staff persons per physician FTE, whereas the national norm is close to 4.71. The bottom line is that WHC spends $43,818 ($433,454 − $389,636) per physician FTE above what a typical medical group would spend for operating expenses. WHC also generates $37,300 less revenue per physician FTE than the national norm. Some of this problem is directly related to lower physician productivity. WHC physicians generated lower RBRVS RVUs than expected when compared to national averages—9850 vs. 10,179.

The Waverly Health Clinic is losing money because its physicians see fewer patients and have significantly larger overhead associated with their practice. It is doubtful that these same physicians practiced in this manner when they were in private practice. The critical factor for the long-term success of owning physician practices is directly related to the incentive structures used for physicians. Ideally, incentives should promote and not destroy physician entrepreneurial spirit.

LEARNING OBJECTIVE 5

Describe alternative HMO organizational arrangements

Table 11–10 Comparative Operating Norms for Waverly Health Care

Indicator	WHC Value	MGMA Median*
Operating expense per physician FTE	$433,454	$389,636
Revenue per physician FTE	$545,007	$582,307
Physician compensation per physician FTE	$185,408	$229,638
Support staff per physician FTE	5.08	4.71
Operating expenses to net revenue percent	79	63
RBRVS RVUs per physician FTE	9,850	10,791

*Source: Cost Survey for Multispecialty Practices, Medical Group Management Association, 2005.

HEALTH PLANS

Most individuals in the United States are covered by either public or private health insurance. In some cases, both public and private coverage may be combined. For example, many Medicare beneficiaries have obtained private health insurance to pay for health expenses not covered by Medicare. At the end of 2003, most of the 40 million Medicare beneficiaries had obtained Medicare supplemental insurance from private insurance companies. Although the vast majority of Americans have health insurance of some type, many Americans do not have either public or private health insurance. The Bureau of the Census estimated that approximately 45.8 million Americans were uninsured in 2004. This large pool of non-covered Americans creates costs of treatment that must be paid by someone. To date, it is not clear who will be responsible for paying for this group of people. Will it be the government, the health plans, or the providers?

The cost of private health insurance has been rapidly increasing during the last 20 years, as Table 11–11 shows. Health insurance companies always have been big business, but the amount of money spent in selling, administration, reserve retention, and profit has increased greatly. In 2004, $128.2 billion was spent by private health insurance firms for either administrative costs, reserve retention, or profit. Actual claims paid to providers amounted to $646.9 billion in 2004. Adding the $128.2 billion cost of private health insurance to actual $646.9 billion claims paid, produces total premiums paid to private health insurance firms of $775.1 billion. Table 11–11 shows that the cost of private health insurance in relation to claims paid has been increasing sharply. It is this administrative cost that has

caused much discussion among policy analysts. They have argued that most of these moneys spent for administration and profit are not necessary and add to the cost of health care in the United States. It seems unreasonable to pay 19.8 cents per dollar of claims paid.

The costs of private health insurance may not, however, be wasteful. The nature of risk and regulation in the industry may require these levels of expenditures. Insurance companies agree to provide a benefits package of services for some specified sum of money. If costs of services exceed this amount, the insurance company loses money. This is often referred to as underwriting risk. In addition, insurance companies are regulated and are required to maintain certain reserve balances to protect policyholders in the event of a financial catastrophe. The only alternative to private health insurance would be some type of government-financed and government-managed program. Government costs might be just as high or higher.

Health care insurance companies come in many different forms. The Health Insurance Association of America (HIAA) categorizes health care insurance firms as commercial, Blue Cross Blue Shield, and health maintenance organizations (HMOs). The trend toward managed care has blurred some of these distinctions. Commercial insurance companies often provide an HMO option, as do most Blue Cross Blue Shield plans. HMOs have broadened their coverage plans to include more traditional indemnity programs, and most provide some point-of-service (POS) option whereby enrollees can go outside the HMO network for care if they are willing to pay higher copayments or deductibles.

In their 1995 *Source Book of Health Insurance Data*, the HIAA defined managed care as a system that integrates the financing and delivery of appropriate

Table 11–11 Private Insurance Trends

Year	All Personal Exenditures (Billions)	Private Payments (Billions)	Cost of Private Insurance (Billions)	Cost of Private Health Insurance to Insurance Payments
2004	$1,549.0	$646.9	$128.2	19.80%
1990	614.7	201.8	30.6	15.20%
1980	217.0	62.0	7.7	12.40%

Table 11-12 Hospital HMO Balance Sheet

	2007	2006
Assets		
Current assets		
Cash and cash equivalents	$1,324,206	$1,669,372
Short-term investments	1,659,278	1,451,923
Premiums receivable	789,735	1,198,034
Investment income receivables	28,208	44,018
Amounts due from affiliates	7,502	2,513
Total current assets	$3,808,929	$4,365,860
Other assets		
Restricted cash and other assets	$172,783	$135,009
Long-term investments	688,292	929,423
Total other assets	$861,075	$1,064,432
Property and equipment		
Total property and equipment	386,254	239,851
Total assets	$5,056,258	$5,670,143
Liabilities and net worth		
Current liabilities		
Accounts payable	$394,333	$523,907
Claims payable (reported and unreported)	1,032,715	1,174,091
Unearned premiums	98,113	156,619
Aggregate write-ins for current liabilities	10,000	13,000
Total current liabilities	1,535,161	1,867,617
Other liabilities		
Amounts due to affiliates (Schedule J)	1,628,923	2,217,411
Total liabilities	3,164,084	4,085,028
Net worth		
Total net worth	1,892,174	1,585,115
Total liabilities and net worth	$5,056,258	$5,670,143

health care services to covered individuals. The most common examples of managed-care organizations are HMOs and PPOs (preferred provider organizations). A PPO typically offers more flexibility than does an HMO by allowing more provider choice, but it attempts to direct patients to providers with whom it has negotiated special contracts.

Usually, there are five types of HMOs that are defined in the literature:

1. *Staff model.* Physicians practice as employees of the HMO and are usually paid a salary.
2. *Group model.* The HMO pays the physician group a per-capita rate, which the physician group then distributes among its members.
3. *Network model.* The HMO contracts with two or more groups and pays them on a per-capita rate, which the groups then distribute to individual physicians.
4. *Independent practice association (IPA) model.* The HMO contracts with individual physicians or with associations of independent physicians and pays them a per-capita rate or a negotiated fee-for-service rate.
5. *Mixed model.* This model combines two or more of the previous options.

The information in Tables 11-12 and 11-13 present financial statements for a small hospital-owned HMO. It is important to point out that financial and operating information on any HMO is usually available publicly by contacting the Department of Insurance in the state where the HMO operates. In fact, this is the source of the financial information used in our example.

The data in Tables 11–12 and 11–13 reveal a lot about the structure of an HMO. First, you will note that a small percentage of the total assets of the HMO is invested in property, plant, and equipment—less than eight percent. HMOs are not fixed-asset intensive; the bulk of their investment is in cash and investments. Our HMO has $1,892,174 in equity at the end of 2007, which represented about 37 percent of the total assets. This gives the appearance of a debt-laden organization relative to the financial standards listed in Table 11–1, but it should be noted that a loan due to an affiliate in the amount of $1,628,923 also exists. The sponsoring hospital granted this loan and, in some ways, it reflects equity. A large portion of this loan was paid off during 2007, which can be seen from the decline in the loan balance from $2,217,411 in 2006 to $1,628,923 at the end of 2007.

The income statement in Table 11–13 depicts a large decrease in net income, from $784,649 in 2006 to $202,399 in 2007. One of the reasons for this decline is the drop in member months, from 191,465 in 2006 to 174,967 in 2007. Table 11–14 analyzes the expenses on a per-member per-month (PMPM) basis.

The decline in net income for our HMO example is the direct result of premiums on a PMPM basis increasing less than expenses. Although not the largest increase, administration expenses increased sharply on both an absolute basis and a PMPM basis. Much of the cost in this area is fixed and cannot be reduced when volume declines. Inpatient expenses also sharply increased. It is not clear from this information whether the cause is higher rates per hospital visit or higher utilization. Additional information in the insurance filing which is not produced in our tables show that inpatient days in 2007 were 4187, or 287 days per 1000 members. In 2006, inpatient days per 1000 members were 278, or 4447 total days. The average price per inpatient day paid in 2007 was

Table 11–13 Hospital HMO Statement of Revenue, Expenses, and Net Worth

	2007	2006
Member months	174,967	191,465
Revenues		
Premium	$20,882,715	$21,367,747
Fee-for-service	0	0
Title XVIII—Medicare	0	0
Investment	59,014	26,623
Aggregate write-ins for other revenues	45,668	74,308
Total revenues	$20,987,397	$21,468,678
Expenses		
Medical and hospital		
Physician services	$1,535,928	$1,640,367
Other professional services	1,781,773	1,736,742
Outside referrals	4,175,302	4,217,545
Emergency room and out-of-area	935,322	1,384,142
Inpatient	7,635,927	7,245,575
Aggregate write-ins for other medical and hospital expenses	2,729,462	2,713,019
Subtotal	$18,793,714	$18,937,390
Reinsurance expenses net of recoveries	365,574	359,954
Total medical and hospital	$19,159,288	$19,297,344
Administration		
Compensation	$876,327	$758,889
Occupancy, depreciation, and amortization	81,368	102,917
Aggregate write-ins for other administration expenses	668,015	524,879
Total administration	$1,625,710	$1,386,685
Total expenses	20,784,998	20,684,029
Net income (loss)	$202,399	$784,649

$1,824 ($7,635,927/4,187) compared to $1,629 ($7,245,575/4,447) in 2006. Therefore, both increased use and higher per diems paid to the hospitals contributed to the inpatient expense increase.

Table 11–14 Per Member Per Month (PMPM) Profitability

	2007	2006
Premiums	$119.35	$111.66
Expenses:		
Physicians services	$8.78	$8.57
Other professional services	10.18	9.07
Outside referrals	23.86	22.02
ER and out-of-area	5.35	7.23
Inpatient	43.64	37.84
Other medical and hospital	15.60	14.17
Reinsurance net of recoveries	2.09	1.88
Total medical and hospital	$109.50	$100.78
Administration	9.29	7.24
Total expenses	$118.79	$108.02
Net income	$0.56	$3.64

The American Association of Health Plans publishes The HMO Industry Profile, which provides numerous financial, operating, and utilization statistics. For example, the 1996 edition of this book provides utilization information for enrollers under 65 years of age (Table 11–15).

SUMMARY

This chapter briefly examined the financial and operating characteristics of alternative health care firms. Although the concepts of financial analysis are the same across all firms, there are some industry specifics that will alter the interpretation of financial results. It is important to become familiar with the industry sector being analyzed before reaching general conclusions regarding the performance of any given firm.

Table 11–15 Inpatient HMO Use Rates

Utilization Measure	Use Rate per 1000 Members
Acute inpatient discharges	68.7
Acute inpatient days	258.8
Ambulatory encounters	4.3

ASSIGNMENTS

1. Using the information provided in Table 11–16 for UnitedHealthcare Group, a major HMO, discuss some of the primary observations that you would conclude regarding the financial performance of the firm. Relate your discussion to the values presented in Table 11–1.

Table 11–16 UnitedHealthcare Group, Inc., 2004 (Data in Millions)

Balance Sheet Data

Current assets

Cash and short-term investments	$4,505
Net accounts receivable	906
Inventory	
Other current assets	2,830
Total current assets	$8,241
Net fixed assets	1,139
Long-term investments	7,748
Other assets	10,751
Total assets	$27,879

Liabilities and equity

Total current liabilities	$11,329
Long-term debt	3,350
Other liabilities	2,483
Equity	10,717
Total liabilities and equity	$27,879

Income Statement Data

Total revenue	$37,218
Expenses	
Depreciation and amortization	$374
Interest expense	128
Other operating expense	32,743
Total operating expense	$33,245
Net income before taxes	$3,973
Income tax	1,386
Discontinued operation loss	0
Net income after tax	$2,587

2. Using the information in Table 11–17 for Manor Care, a major nursing home firm, discuss some of the primary observations that you would conclude regarding the financial performance of the firm.

Table 11–17 Manor Care Financial Data (Data in Thousands)

Balance Sheet

	12/31/2004	12/31/2003	12/31/2002
Assets			
Current Assets			
Cash and cash equivalents	$32,915	$86,251	$30,554
Net receivables	482,690	471,664	456,289
Other current assets	24,762	27,484	23,974
Total current assets	$540,367	$585,399	$510,817
Property, plant, and equipment	1,495,152	1,514,250	1,534,339
Goodwill	92,672	87,906	85,814
Intangible assets	9,099	9,397	10,457
Other assets	203,408	199,759	165,505
Total Assets	$2,340,698	$2,396,711	$2,306,932
Liabilities			
Total current liabilities	$402,254	$387,502	$641,864
Long-term debt	555,275	659,181	373,112
Other liabilities	264,492	237,723	196,836
Deferred long-term liability charges	134,518	137,200	79,073
Total liabilities	$1,356,539	$1,421,606	$1,290,885
Total stockholder equity	$984,159	$975,105	$1,016,047

Income Statement

	12/31/2004	12/31/2003	12/31/2002
Total revenue	$3,208,867	$3,029,441	$2,905,448
Cost of revenue	2,647,849	2,523,534	2,401,636
Gross profit	$561,018	$505,907	$503,812
Operating expenses			
Selling, general, and administrative expenses	140,587	157,566	131,628
Non-recurring expenses	—	—	33,574
Depreciation	127,821	128,810	124,895
Operating income or loss	$292,610	$219,531	$213,715
Total other income	4,689	12,808	36,620
Earnings before interest and taxes	$297,299	$232,339	$250,335
Interest expense	42,420	41,927	37,651
Income before taxes	$254,879	$190,412	$212,684
Income tax expense	86,657	71,405	80,820
Net income from continuing operations	$168,222	$119,007	$131,864
Effect of accounting changes	—	—	(1,314)
Net income	$168,222	$119,007	$130,550

3. Using the information in Table 11–18 for Pediatrix Medical Group, a major medical group, discuss some of the primary observations that you would conclude regarding the financial performance of the firm.

Table 11–18 Pediatrix Medical Group Financial Data (Data in Thousands)

Balance Sheet

	12/31/2004	12/31/2003	12/31/2002
Assets			
Current Assets			
Cash and cash equivalents	$16,972	$27,896	$73,195
Net receivables	128,026	113,567	80,871
Other current assets	7,236	4,094	7,289
Total current assets	$152,234	$145,557	$161,355
Property, plant, and equipment	26,621	27,194	16,820
Goodwill	588,874	527,422	463,032
Intangible assets	8,940	7,761	996
Other assets	12,220	9,660	6,476
Total Assets	$788,889	$717,594	$648,679
Liabilities			
Total current liabilities	$131,054	$121,045	$81,800
Long-term debt	54,693	1,178	1,985
Deferred long-term liability charges	32,111	22,993	16,896
Total liabilities	$217,858	$145,216	$100,681
Total stockholder equity	$571,031	$572,378	$547,998

Income Statement

	12/31/2004	12/31/2003	12/31/2002
Total revenue	**$619,929**	**$551,197**	**$465,481**
Cost of revenue	350,354	329,366	278,956
Gross profit	$269,275	$221,831	$186,525
Operating expenses			
Selling, general, and administrative expenses	103,699	76,537	68,315
Depreciation	9,353	8,405	6,135
Operating income or loss	$156,223	$136,889	$112,075
Total other income	893	482	818
Earnings before interest and taxes	$157,116	$137,371	$112,893
Interest expense	1,295	1,372	1,156
Income before taxes	$155,821	$135,999	$111,737
Income tax expense	57,542	51,671	42,961
Net income	$98,279	$84,328	$68,776

SOLUTIONS AND ANSWERS

1. Table 11–19 provides financial ratio values for UnitedHealthcare for 2004. United Healthcare is achieving values of profitability that are above industry averages at the present. Its higher return on equity results from higher margins and the use of more debt in its capital structure. Current liquidity appears fine, but cash reserves are below industry averages. The large value of other assets ($10.7 billion) is largely goodwill that has resulted from prior acquisitions.

Table 11–19 Financial Ratios UnitedHealthcare Group, Inc., 2004

Financial Ratio	2004	Average Medical Group
Liquidity		
Current ratio	0.73	1.59
Days in receivables	8.90	21.29
Days' cash-on-hand	136.10	224.03
Capital structure		
Debt financing %	61.56	45.26
Long-term debt to *capital* %	23.81	19.11
Cash flow to debt %	20.17	35.69
Times interest earned %*	32.00	17.13
Activity		
Current asset turnover	4.52	8.79
Fixed asset turnover	32.68	29.53
Total asset turnover	1.33	1.18
Profitability		
Return on equity %	24.14	17.92
Total margin %	6.95	4.72

*Time's interest earned is net income before interest and taxes divided by interest.

2. Table 11–20 provides financial ratios for Manor Care for the last three years. Manor Care has experienced rates of profitability that are above industry averages. Return on equity at Manor Care is being positively impacted by higher margins. Coverage of existing debt obligations appears adequate when compared to industry averages. Short-term liquidity at Manor Care may be a problem, given low levels for cash reserves. Manor Care also appears to have lower relative asset efficiency. Much of this is due to low fixed asset efficiency. The low values for fixed-asset turnover may be a reflection of a newer plant and equipment base.

Table 11–20 Financial Ratios Manor Care

Financial Ratio	2004	2003	2002	Nursing Home Average
Liquidity				
Current ratio	1.34	1.51	0.80	1.11
Days in receivables	54.9	56.8	57.3	48.0
Days' cash-on-hand	4.1	11.3	4.2	26.3
Capital structure				
Debt financing %	58.0	59.3	56.0	64.3
Long-term debt to *capital* %	36.1	40.3	12.3	35.7
Cash flow to total debt %	21.8	17.4	19.8	18.3
Times interest earned %*	7.01	5.54	6.65	4.39
Activity				
Total asset turnover	1.37	1.26	1.26	1.67
Fixed asset turnover	2.15	2.00	1.89	4.09
Current asset turnover	5.94	5.18	5.69	7.52
Profitability				
Return on equity %	17.1	12.2	12.8	12.4
Total margin %	5.2	3.9	4.5	2.9

*Times interest earned is net income before interest and taxes divided by interest.

3. Table 11–21 provides financial ratio values for Pediatrix for the last three years. Pediatrix appears to be a very profitable firm with margins above the industry average. Return-on-equity values are below industry averages because Pediatrix has not used much debt financing relative to the industry average. The reason for low-debt usage may be related to low levels of investment in plant, property, and equipment, which can be seen from its very high fixed-asset-turnover ratios. Usually, long-term debt is associated with fixed assets, and Pediatrix has low levels of fixed-asset investment. Pediatrix has experienced a sizable growth in revenue during the last few years and has used much of its cash reserves to finance its growth. A major concern is a very large percentage of total investment in goodwill. This investment, which has arisen from prior acquisitions, will become a drain on earnings as these values are amortized in the future.

Table 11–21 Financial Ratios Pediatrix

Financial Ratio	2004	2003	2002	Average Medical Group
Liquidity				
Current ratio	1.16	1.20	1.97	1.54
Days in receivables	75.4	75.2	63.4	64.5
Days' cash-on-hand	12.1	22.2	68.4	9.51
Capital structure				
Debt financing %	27.6	20.2	15.5	49.8
Long-term debt to *capital* %	8.7	0.2	0.4	35.8
Cash flow to total debt %	49.4	63.8	74.4	33.7
Times interest earned %*	121.3	100.1	97.7	30.1
Activity				
Total asset turnover	0.79	0.77	0.72	1.01
Fixed asset turnover	23.30	20.27	27.67	10.93
Current asset turnover	4.07	3.79	2.88	3.95
Profitability				
Return on equity %	17.20	14.73	12.55	21.95
Total margin%	15.86	15.30	14.78	10.92

*Times interest earned is net income before interest and taxes divided by interest.

Chapter 12

Strategic Financial Planning

After studying this chapter, you should be able to do the following:

1. Describe the relationship between financial planning and strategic planning.
2. List and describe the key financial policy targets for which the board is responsible.
3. List and describe the ten requirements for effective financial planning and policy-making.
4. Explain the four steps involved in the development of a financial plan.
5. Explain how management control is used in conjunction with the financial plan.

REAL-WORLD SCENARIO

Joanna Eyre is the CEO of Golden Village, a large religious continuing care retirement community (CCRC), located in an East Coast metropolitan area. She is preparing materials for the upcoming board retreat that will establish a clear direction for her firm in the years ahead. Her board is actively considering a number of strategies, which they believe are necessary to maintain the competitive position of the firm, as well as meet the needs of their constituency. All of the ideas for growth that board members currently support involve significant capital outlays, followed by dramatic expansions in operating expenses.

One of the most controversial strategies calls for the complete relocation of the CCRC to a more suburban location. Many board members feel that Golden must make major renovations to its plant to remain a competitive alternative to the large number of new CCRCs that have sprung up in suburban areas. The expected capital cost for this move is $50 million with a potential recovery of $12 million from the sale of the existing facility. It is not clear, however, if the sponsoring religious group would allow Golden to retain any of the $12 million from the expected sale of the land on which the present facility is located. Without any proceeds from the $12 million sale, Golden would be faced with a debt burden that may put the firm in default, which in turn could lead to bankruptcy.

Margins at Golden Village have been dropping in the past few years for a variety of reasons. The increasing excess capacity in Golden's market has resulted in lower prices for both assisted living and independent housing units. This has hit Golden Village hard because while their facility has exceptional services for residents (which are very costly to provide), the actual units themselves are looking more and more dated. The nursing facility has also experienced a dramatic reduction in realized revenue as both Medicare and Medicaid have begun to ratchet back reimbursement levels.

Joanna believes that current financial projections show that Golden would find it very hard to pay for only modest capital renovations at the present site. Relocation would require a debt burden that simply could not be repaid without a change in current reimbursement trends. On the other hand, most board members believe that Golden Village is doomed if it stays at its present site. Most elderly people seeking CCRC accommodations want modern facilities in suburban locations and the present marketplace provides ample low cost alternatives. Joanna does not know which strategy to recommend to the board at their retreat and is becoming more confused as she examines more data.

Is there a need to define corporate financial policy in a health care firm? If so, who should be responsible—the board of trustees, the chief executive officer, the chief financial officer, or some combination of these? How should the definition of 'financial policy' be accomplished? What are the steps required?

These kinds of questions are only now beginning to surface in the health care industry. Finance and financial management have long been areas of concern, but their orientation has recently shifted. Reimbursement and payment system management have given way to financial planning. Survival tomorrow is no longer guaranteed. Health care firms must establish realistic and achievable financial plans that are consistent with their strategic plans. The primary purpose of this chapter is to help provide a basis for the crucial task of forming financial policies in health care firms.

LEARNING OBJECTIVE 1

Describe the relationship between financial planning and strategic planning.

THE STRATEGIC PLANNING PROCESS

Most observers probably would agree that financial policy and financial planning should be closely integrated within the strategic planning process. Thus, understanding the strategic planning process is a first step in defining and developing financial policy and financial planning. It would be ideal if there was agreement among leading experts regarding the definition of strategic planning, but this is not the case. The literature on

strategic planning is fairly recent; initial publications appeared starting about 1965. The application of strategic planning principles to the health care industry is even more recent; the bulk of the literature on such applications has been published since 1980.

One trend in health care strategic planning does appear clear, however: there is a definite movement away from "facilities planning" to a more market-oriented approach. Health care firms can no longer decide which services they want to deliver without assessing the economics of demand. This requirement appears consistent with the concept of strategic planning as it is used in general industry. Indeed, as the business environments of the health care industry and general industry become more alike, strategic planning in the two areas should become increasingly similar.

Much of the literature that deals with the strategic-planning process in business organizations appears to be concerned with two basic decision outcomes: first, a statement of mission or goals (or both) is required to provide guidance to the organization. Second, a set of programs or activities to which the organization will commit resources during the planning period is defined.

Figure 12–1 shows the integration of the financial-planning process with the strategic-planning process. Financial planning is fashioned by defining programs and services and then assessing their financial feasibility. In many cases, a desired set of programs and services may not be financially feasible. This may cause a redefinition of the organization's mission and its desired programs and services. For example, a hospital may decide to change from a full-scale hospital to a specialty hospital, or it may decide to eliminate specific clinical programs, such as pediatrics or obstetrics.

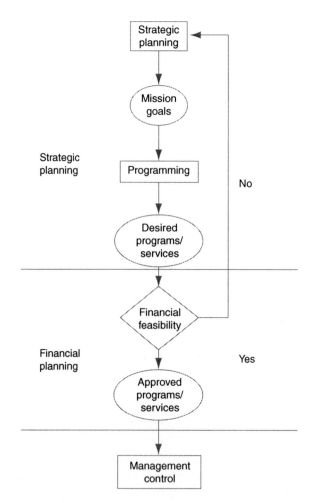

Figure 12–1 Integration of Strategic and Financial Planning

Three points concerning the integration of strategic and financial planning should be emphasized. First, both strategic planning and financial planning are the primary responsibility of the board of trustees. This does not exclude top management from the process because they should be active and participating members of the board. Second, strategic planning should precede financial planning. In some situations, the board may make strategic decisions based on the availability of funding. Although this may be fiscally conservative, it often can inhibit creative thinking. Third, the board should play an active, not passive, role in the financial-planning process. The board should not await word concerning the financial feasibility of its desired programs and services; it should actively provide guidelines for management or its consultants (or both) to use in developing the financial

plan. Specifically, the board should establish key financial policy targets in the following three major areas:

1. Growth rate in assets
2. Debt policy
3. Profitability objective (return on equity)

LEARNING OBJECTIVE 2

List and describe the key financial policy targets for which the board is responsible.

FINANCIAL POLICY TARGETS

The term "financial feasibility" is often associated with an expensive study performed by a consulting firm in conjunction with the issue of debt. In such cases, the financial projections are so incredibly complex that few people admit to understanding them, and even fewer actually comprehend them. In many people's minds, financial planning consists of a large number of mathematical relationships that can simulate future financial results, given certain key inputs. The validity of the projections is dependent on the reliability of the mathematical relationships, or model, and on the accuracy of the assumptions. Most financial feasibility studies developed in this way are never reviewed and never updated.

But conditions are changing and changing rapidly. A large number of health care firms are now beginning to develop formal strategic plans. They are beginning to redefine, or at least reconsider, their basic mission and to identify future market areas. It is increasingly clear that their financial plans and financial strategies must be integral parts of their overall strategic plan.

Granted that health care board members and health care executives have an urgent need to understand financial policy and financial planning, can the requisite body of knowledge be conveyed in a manner that is understandable? Must board members and executives remain passive observers in financial planning, or can they be given the means to establish key policy directives?

Figure 12–2 identifies the critical financial-planning relationships, and also the sequencing of the financial-planning process. The premise on which the financial plan is built rests on some projection of services or levels of activity, which is the first step in the financial planning process. The strategic plan usually provides this information by indicating which product lines the firm expects to provide during the next five years, and at what level of expected activity. The first line in Figure 12–2 is from the income statement and shows present and projected revenues. The projection of revenues can be directly related to the strategic plan. After all, revenue is merely the product of price multiplied by quantity. If the strategic plan specifies volume of services, then multiplying those volumes by expected price yields revenues.

Projected revenue serves as the basis for projecting the required level of investment or assets, which is the second step in the financial-planning process set forth in Figure 12–2. In any business firm, there are usually some specific relationships between investment required and production. For example, a health care firm with no existing clinic capacity that expected to provide 50,000 clinic visits per year five years from now would be required to invest heavily in physician practices to acquire this capacity. In the simple illustration of Figure 12–2, there appears to be a one-to-one relationship between revenue and investment: one dollar of investment in assets is required for every dollar of revenue.

The third step is for the board to establish a debt policy for the organization. Stated simply, what percentage of the firm's investment will the board permit to be financed with debt? In Figure 12–2, the debt policy appears to be set at 50 percent. Fifty percent of the $2,000 investment in year 5 is financed with debt, which leaves the remaining 50 percent to be financed with equity.

The fourth and final step would appear to be the easiest stage in the planning process. If balance sheets balance, and they always do, the firm illustrated in Figure 12–2 will need to have $1,000 in equity at the end of year 5. A $1,000 equity balance when combined with the board-approved debt target of $1,000 will exactly finance the $2,000 required investment in assets.

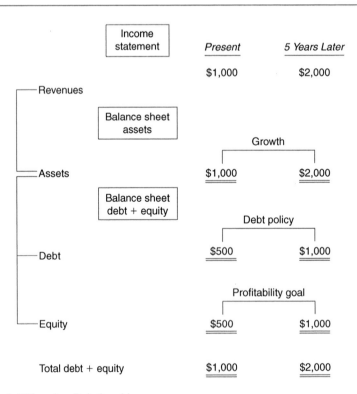

Figure 12–2 Critical Financial Planning Relationships

The critical question, however, is can the firm generate $500 in new equity during the next five years? Because most, if not all, of this equity must be generated from profits of the firm, the feasibility of this increase in equity relates directly to the reasonableness of forecasted profitability targets or goals. If the firm is not able to generate $500 in new equity, what will happen? First, a balance sheet must always balance, so the firm is faced with one of two decisions. It must either reduce its level of investment, which of course translates into fewer services, or it must increase its risk exposure through the addition of higher debt limits. This process is most likely iterative and can be related to Figure 12–1. When the financial plan is feasible, an approved set of programs and services is in place and resources are allocated to accomplish the firm's goals. The financial plan then serves as the basis for management control.

It is essential to understand the key financial ratio targets that determine the success or failure of a financial plan. The most important relationship is the firm's growth rate in equity (GRIE). A firm that requires a ten percent annual GRIE to meets its stated asset growth and debt policy goals, must manage the critical drivers that define GRIE. GRIE can be defined as:

$$\text{GRIE} = \text{Return on Equity(ROE)}/\text{Reported Income Index(RII)}$$

The RII is simply current net income divided by current change in equity. In most situations, net income for the period will equal the change in equity and therefore the RII will be 1.0. This makes ROE the primary measure of financial performance as was discussed in Chapter 10. ROE can be expressed as follows.

$$\text{Return on equity} = \frac{[\text{OM} + \text{NOR}] \times \text{TAT}}{\text{EF}}$$

where

OM = Operating Margin = Operating Income/ Total Revenue

NOR = Nonoperating Revenue = Nonoperating Income/Total Revenue

TAT = Total Asset Turnover = Total Revenue/ Total Assets

EF = Equity Financing = Equity/Total Assets

List and describe the ten requirements for effective financial planning and policy-making.

REQUIREMENTS FOR EFFECTIVE POLICY-MAKING

The preceding discussion of the elements of financial planning and the three major target areas of financial policy suggest certain requirements for effective financial planning and policy-making. The following ten requirements are of special importance.

1. The accounting system should be capable of providing data on cost, revenue, and investment along program lines.

Programs, or "strategic business units," are the basic building blocks of any strategic plan. The financial plan must be developed on a basis consistent with the strategic plan. Unfortunately, present accounting systems are geared to provide data along responsibility center or departmental lines. For example, psychiatry may represent a program in the strategic plan, but the financial data on costs, investments, and revenues for the program may be intertwined with those of many departments, such as dietary, housekeeping, occupational therapy, and pharmacy. Still, this problem is not unique to health care firms. Many organizations have programs that cut across departmental lines. In such cases, the financial data can be accumulated along programmatic lines, but some adjustments in cost and revenue assignments will be necessary.

With the advent of the diagnosis-related group (DRG) payment system, the hospital industry has been making major advancements in the accumulation of financial data in terms of DRG categories. It is now possible to define major programs or product lines in a hospital as consisting of a specific set of DRGs. For example, if obstetrics was a program, it might be defined as DRG #370 (Cesarean section with CC) to DRG #391 (normal newborns).

It is important to note that although problems exist in obtaining financial data along program lines, they are not insurmountable. The health care industry is, of course, different from the automotive industry, but the differences do not necessarily imply greater difficulties in costing.

2. *No growth does not imply a zero-growth rate in assets.*

The fact that no growth does not necessarily imply zero growth in assets is so obvious that it is often overlooked by many planning committees. Inflation will create investment needs that exceed present levels, even though the organization's strategic plan may call for program stabilization or an actual retrenchment. An annual rate of inflation equal to four percent means a doubling of investment values every 18 years. For example, a nursing home with assets of $25 million today should plan on being a $50-million-asset firm 18 years from now. Just because the investment involved may not represent an increase in productive capacity does not negate the need for a financial plan that will generate $25 million in new equity and debt financing over the next 18 years.

Over time, of course, expectations about future rates of inflation may change. The financial plan should reflect the best current thinking in this area. This may necessitate periodic changes in the financial plan (Requirement 9). It is also important to recognize that there may be differences in investment inflation rates across programs. In some programs, such as oncology, in which dramatic technologic changes are likely to occur, a greater relative inflation rate may have to be assigned.

3. *Working capital is a major element in computing total future asset needs.*

In computing future investment needs, it is not uncommon to omit the working capital category. Most investment in any strategic plan is usually in bricks, mortar, and equipment. However, working capital can still be a rather sizable component, accounting for 20 to 30 percent of total investment in many health care firms.

The term "net working capital" is often used to describe the amount of permanent financing required to finance working capital or current assets. Net working capital is defined as current assets less current liabilities. It is important to remember this, because some current liability financing is automatic or unnegotiated. Just as inflation increases the dollar value of outstanding accounts receivable, it also increases wages or salaries payable and accounts payable. It is the net amount of working capital that must be financed.

As an example, let's consider again the nursing home with $25 million in assets introduced in Requirement 2.

Assume 30 percent of its assets are current assets, or $7.5 million ($25 million × 30 percent). If the firm has a prudent current ratio of 2.0, then the firm has $3.75 million in current liabilities (7.5 million ÷ 3.75 million = 2.0). Its net working capital then is $3.75 million ($7.5 million of current assets less $3.75 million of current liabilities). As the nursing home grows its total assets to $50 million over the next 18 years, its current assets will also grow at a four percent rate and will reach a value of $15 million. Assuming a stable current ratio of 2.0 implies that current liabilities would be $7.5 million. Thus, the firm's new net working capital will be $7.5 million, an increase in net working capital of $3.75 million.

Working capital requirements vary by program. New programs usually have significant working capital requirements, whereas existing programs may experience only modest increases resulting from inflation. One of the primary causes for failure in new business ventures is often an inadequate amount of available working capital. New programs also may have significantly different working-capital requirements. For example, a home-health program may require little fixed investment in plant and equipment, but significant amounts of working capital may be required to finance a long collection cycle and initial development costs. Many firms that rushed into the development of home-health agency programs have become acutely aware of this problem.

If inadequate amounts of working capital are projected in the financial plan, the entire plan may be jeopardized. For example, an unanticipated $2 million increase in receivables requires an immediate source of funding, such as the liquidation of investments. If those investments are essential to provide needed equity in a larger financing program, certain key investments may be delayed or canceled in the future. A number of firms have had to reduce the scope of their strategic plans because of unanticipated demands for working capital.

4. *There should be some accumulation of funds for future investments critical to long-term solvency.*

Saving for a rainy day has not been a policy practiced by many health care firms to any significant degree. As of 2004, the average hospital had approximately 40 days of cash-on-hand. Assuming that at least 20 days are needed to meet day-to-day transaction needs, only 20 days remain to meet capital replacement needs. This implies that the average hospital would need to borrow a sizable percentage of its replacement needs. This level of debt financing may no longer be feasible in the hospital industry as lenders reassess the relative degree of risk involved. When composite weighted averages are used, the average days' cash-on-hand increases to 90 days. Larger hospitals clearly carry larger proportionate balances of cash and reserves, but even with 90 days of cash in larger hospitals, a significant percentage of future capital expenditures will need to be debt financed.

It is critical that health care boards and management establish formal policies for retention of funds for future investment. Health care firms can no longer expect to finance all of their investment needs with debt. They must set aside funds for investment to meet future needs in the same manner that pension plans are funded.

An actuarially-determined pension funding requirement is analogous to a board policy of replacement reserve funding. Yet, few health care firms set aside sufficient replacement funds for future investment needs, which partially explains the dramatic growth in debt in the hospital industry.

5. A formally-defined debt capacity ceiling should be established.

Few health care firms have formally defined their debt capacity or debt policy. This is in sharp contrast to most other industries. Without such a formally-established debt policy, one of two unfavorable outcomes may result. First, debt may be viewed as the balancing variable in the financial plan. If a firm expects a $25 million increase in its investment and a $5 million increase in equity, $20 million of debt is required to make the strategic plan financially feasible. The firm will then try to arrange for $20 million of new debt financing. This is a situation in which many health care firms have found themselves.

Second, the balancing variable in the financial plan may shift to the investment side, but on an ex post facto basis. An approved financial plan may be unrealistic because the level of indebtedness required to finance the strategic plan exposes the firm to excessive risks. Management may not realize this until the actual financing is needed. At that point, it may be required to scale down the programs specified in the strategic plan. If a realistic debt-capacity ceiling had been established earlier, existing funded programs might have been canceled or cut back to make funds available for more desirable programs.

Debt capacity can be defined in a number of ways. It can be expressed as a ratio, such as a long-term debt to equity ratio, or it can be defined in terms of demonstrated debt-service coverage. Whatever the method used, some limit on debt financing should be established. That limit should represent a balance between the organization's desire to avoid financial risk exposure and the investment needs of its strategic plan. Debt policy should be clearly and concisely established before the fact; it should not be an ad hoc result.

6. Return on investment (ROI) by program area should be an important criterion in program selection.

The principle that ROI by program area should govern program selection is related to the need for accounting data along product lines, as discussed previously. These ROI analyses by product line already are done outside the health care industry and need to be implemented in health care as well. To calculate ROI along program lines, financial data on revenues, expenses, and investment must be available along program lines. ROI should be used as part of an overall system of program evaluation and selection.

Portfolio analysis is a buzz word that has been used lately to categorize programs in terms of market share and growth rate. Health care writers have applied the concept to the literature on health care planning and marketing. However, one difficulty with the application of portfolio analysis to the health care industry is the selection of the dimensions for developing the portfolio matrix. In most portfolio matrices, the dimensions used are market share and growth. Market share and growth are assumed to have an explicit relationship to cash flow. High market share is associated with high profitability and, thus, with good cash flow. High market growth is assumed to require cash flow for investment. For example, a program with a high market share and low growth is regarded as a "cash cow." It produces high cash flow, but requires little cash flow for reinvestment because of its low-growth needs.

Here we will use a slight modification of the portfolio analysis paradigm, incorporating the dimension of profitability. Figure 12–3 illustrates the revised portfolio analysis matrix. Its two dimensions are (1) return on investment and (2) community need. ROI is used as the measure of profitability because it is most directly related to strategic and financial planning. Profit is merely new equity that can be used to finance new investment. Absolute levels of profit or cash flow mean little unless they are related to the underlying investment. For example, if Program A has a profit of $100,000 and an investment of $2,000,000, whereas Program B has a profit of $50,000 and an investment of $100,000, which program is a better cash cow if both programs have low community need? In this example, Program B is clearly the better cash cow because it generates a much better return on its investment (ROIA = 5% and ROIB = 50%).

In our revised portfolio analysis matrix, community need replaces the traditional marketing dimensions of growth and market share. Community need may be difficult to measure quantitatively, but the concept appears closely aligned to the missions of most voluntary health care firms—firms that usually were formed to provide health care services to some reasonably well-defined market.

Figure 12–3 categorizes programs as "dogs," "cash cows," "stars," and "Samaritans." With the exception of Samaritans, these terms are identical to those used in the existing literature. An example of a Samaritan program is one with a small or negative ROI, but a high community need. For example, a hospital may provide a drug-abuse program that loses money, but meets a community need not met by any other health care provider. The program can continue if—and only if—the hospital has some stars or cash cows to subsidize the program's poor profitability. Dogs, that is, programs with low community need and low profit, should be considered in light of the resources they draw from potential Samaritans. The new payment environment makes this kind of analysis mandatory.

7. Nonoperating sources of equity should be included in the financial plan.

In the preceding discussion of ROI, we were concerned primarily with operating profitability. However, in many voluntary health care firms, nonoperating income also can be extremely important. In fact, in 2004, nonoperating revenue accounted for 21 percent of total reported net income in the hospital industry (Cleverley and Associates, 2005). If nonoperating income can be improved, a significant new source of funding will be available to help finance the strategic plan. This could mean either that a greater percentage of desired programs can be undertaken or that reduced levels of indebtedness are possible. The primary source of nonoperating income for most health care firms is investment income and gains.

The investment portfolio of many health care firms is large. Funds are available for retirement plans, professional liability self-insurance plans, funded depreciation, bond funds, endowments, and other purposes. Thus, small increases in investment yields can create sizable increases in income. For example, a one percent improvement in the yield on invested pension funds may reduce annual pension expense by as much as ten percent. Clearly, management should formally establish and incorporate target investment yields in its financial plans.

New equity also can come from sources other than operating and nonoperating income. Corporate restructuring arrangements can create proprietary subsidiaries that can issue stock. Joint-venture relationships with medical staff and others can be used to finance plant assets. It is important that both board members and executives have a clear understanding of the possible alternatives available for raising new equity to finance the strategic plan. Raising new equity through stock or partnerships is no longer the exclusive domain of investor-owned firms.

8. The financial plan must be integrated with the management control system.

The integration of the financial plan with the management control system is an obvious requirement, but it is often overlooked. Frequently, a large fee is paid to a consultant or enormous amounts of internal staff time are used to develop a financial plan that is never used.

Ideally, the financial plan should be the basis for the annual budget. The key link between the budget and the financial plan should be the ROI targets specified in the financial plan. These ROI targets are critical to the long-term fulfillment of the strategic plan. Failure to achieve the targeted levels of profit will require revisions in the strategic plan.

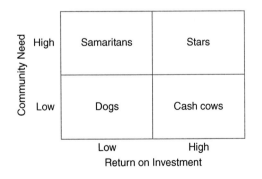

Figure 12–3 Revised Portfolio Analysis Matrix

Health care board members would not have to be involved in pricing debates if approved financial plans were available. In such situations, the profitability targets by program already would have been approved in the plans. The primary issues in the budgeting process should be the translation of profit targets by program lines to departmental lines via pricing allocations and the assessment of departmental operating efficiencies. Long, involved discussions about whether budgeted profit is too much or not enough should not be necessary.

9. The financial plan should be updated at least annually.

Management should have the most recent financial "road map" available at all times. Few people would plan a drive to San Francisco from Boston with a five-year-old road map, yet many organizations operate either with no long-range financial plan or with an outdated one. This can be especially dangerous for health care firms at the present time, as the business environment is changing rapidly. Today, financial plans based on yesterday's financial environment may be useless, or even misleading. In all financial plans, a careful reassessment of relative program profitability is periodically required, possibly prompting major revisions of the strategic plan. Knowing both where you are going and how you expect to get there is critical to survival in a competitive environment.

10. The financial plan is a board document and should be formally approved by the board.

In many firms, the financial plan, if it exists, is regarded as a management document. The board may be only mildly interested in reviewing it and not interested at all in relating it to the strategic plan. This is rather strange behavior. Most boards would never dream of letting management operate without a board-approved annual budget for fear of failing to fulfill their board responsibilities. Yet planning for periods longer than one year is not regarded as important.

A recent hospital board meeting that followed a two-day strategic planning retreat illustrates this traditional perspective. During the retreat, strategic discussions about the future were held. The board and management agreed on a plan for the future that called for significant expansion into new market areas, such as long term care. At the subsequent board meeting, the chief executive officer and the chief finance officer presented the strategic plan and the related financial plan. The board members regarded approval of the financial plan as a waste of time. They did approve it, but in body only, not in spirit. Their rationale for apathy was clear. They could not foresee any problem with the financing. Most of them had been board members for a long time. Whenever money was needed in the past, they raised rates or borrowed and they could not see any reason to change this policy in the future. This type of behavior in today's market is not only unwise, but also suicidal.

Fortunately, this kind of reaction is becoming less common. Board members today are beginning to realize that the financial plan and the strategic plan are integrally related. It is impossible to develop one without the other, and both are ultimately the responsibility of the board.

LEARNING OBJECTIVE 4

Explain the four steps involved in the development of a financial plan.

DEVELOPING THE FINANCIAL PLAN

In this section, we describe in some detail the steps involved in preparing a financial plan and then apply the steps to an actual case example. For our purposes, a financial plan may be defined as the bridge between two balance sheets. It is the income statement that provides the major connection between two balance sheets, and so we will describe both balance sheet and income statement projection.

The Developmental Process

Four steps are involved in the development of a financial plan:

1. Assessment of the present financial position and prior growth patterns
2. Definition of growth needs in total assets for the planning period
3. Definition of the acceptable level of debt for both current and long-term categories
4. Assessment of the reasonableness of required growth rate in equity

Assessment of Present Financial Position

The first step in the development of a financial plan is the assessment of present financial position. It is extremely important to determine the present financial health and position of the firm. Without such information, projections about future growth can be dangerous at best. In most situations, past performance is usually a good basis for projecting future performance. For example, a financial plan may call for a future growth rate in equity of 15 percent per year. If, however, the prior five-year period showed an average annual growth rate in equity of only five percent, there may be some doubt about the validity of the assumption of 15 percent and thus the reasonableness of the financial plan.

The following two categories of financial information need to be assembled to assess a firm's present financial position:

1. Financial statements for the past three to five years
2. Financial evaluation of the firm, using ratio analysis

The balance sheets presented in Table 12–1 are used to illustrate the application of this information in financial planning. These balance sheets provide historical information for Omega Health Foundation (OHF) for the years 2004 through 2006.

Tables 12–1, 12–2, and 12–3 present some useful historical data that will be helpful in assessing the present financial position and projecting asset growth rates. After a review of the three tables, the following summary may help to organize one's thinking about OHF's 2006 financial position.

- Omega Health Foundation has good levels of investment reserves. The present funded depreciation account has $55,794,000 in it and also has created a sizable amount of investment income. This value can be compared to the ending 2006 accumulated depreciation value of $70,804,000. OHF has 78.8 percent of its accumulated depreciation in funded depreciation. This is a large percentage and implies that OHF could finance approximately 78.8 of its present replacement needs with existing funds. The actual percentage may be lower when the effects of inflation are considered.

- Present operating profitability at OHF is not good and an operating loss of $492,000 was experienced in 2006. The primary cause for this poor operating position is an excessive cost structure. OHF took a restructuring charge of $5,110,000 in 2006, which reflects its commitment to further cost reduction.
- Age of plant at OHF is below the national average and might suggest lower levels of capital expenditures in the future. The board has, however, approved capital expenditures of $10,000,000 per year during the next five years.
- Omega Health Foundation has a capital structure that reflects more debt than national norms, but it has not issued any new debt in the last three years. The board's policy for future financing calls for no new long-term debt. Repayment of existing debt will continue using the existing debt principal schedule.
- Present days in accounts receivable are 55.3 and it is expected that this present situation will continue.

Defining Growth Rate in Assets

Table 12–4 defines the assumptions that will be used to develop the five-year financial plan for OHF. As discussed earlier, it is impossible to forecast asset investment without first forecasting revenues and also expenses. Revenue forecasts are an integral part of asset forecasts because the level of service drives the underlying required investment. For example, growth in property, plant, and equipment is directly related to the range and level of services expected to be provided in the planning period. Even items as mundane as accounts receivable are directly related to revenue forecasts. Projecting revenues leads to a forecast of expenses. When a firm defines its expected production levels, requirements for staffing, supplies, and other expenses, these items are often directly tied to these forecasts. In addition, certain areas of asset investment are often directly related to expense levels. For example, short-term cash is often directly related to expense levels, and inventory investment is often tied to expected annual supplies expense.

In the remainder of this section, we will discuss some of the more significant assumptions used in the financial plan developed for OHF. The projected balance sheet, income statement, and financial ratios are

Table 12–1 Balance Sheet for Omega Health Foundation as of June 30, 2006, 2005, and 2004 (Data in Thousands)

GENERAL FUNDS

Assets

	2006	2005	2004
Current			
Cash and short-term investments	$9,692	$9,456	$11,388
Accounts receivable	24,324	25,597	23,381
Due from third-party payers	0	56	185
Due from donor-restricted funds	280	179	47
Inventories	1,763	2,251	2,252
Prepaid expenses and other assets	1,135	1,520	1,963
Current portion of funds held by trustee	990	925	1,580
Current portion of self-insurance trust funds	2,264	2,284	2,917
Total current assets	$40,448	$42,268	$43,713
Assets that have limited use			
Self-insurance trust funds, net of current portion	$9,321	$9,013	$9,962
Board-designated funds and fund depreciation	55,794	42,326	37,520
Funds held by trustee, net of current portion	338	726	1,037
	$65,453	$52,065	$48,519
Gross property, plant, and equipment	$146,794	$137,631	$130,404
Less accumulated depreciation	70,804	62,802	64,087
Property, plant, and equipment, net	$75,990	$74,829	$66,317
Investments in and advances to partnerships	2,497	2,226	1,759
Deferred financing costs, net	1,139	1,306	1,394
Deferred third-party reimbursement	—	674	983
Other assets	1,067	654	575
Total	$186,594	$174,022	$163,260
Current			
Current portion of long-term debt	$1,401	$1,506	$1,784
Notes payable	—	250	—
Accounts payable and accrued expenses	11,087	7,215	6,791
Accrued salaries, wages, and fees	4,342	4,238	3,724
Accrued restructuring costs	2,078	—	—
Accrued vacation	3,288	3,331	3,223
Accrued insurance costs	2,234	2,284	2,917
Advance from third-party payer	1,205	1,142	941
Due to third-party payers	11,571	10,688	9,150
Total current liabilities	$37,206	$30,654	$28,530
Accrued retirement costs	$ 8,846	$ 1,736	$ 1,576
Accrued insurance costs, net of current position	4,636	3,450	2,124
Deferred third-party reimbursement	3,489	3,488	3,604
Long-term debt, net of current position	54,781	55,989	56,369
Other liabilities	238	2	—
Total liabilities	$109,196	$95,319	$92,203
Unrestricted net assets	77,398	78,703	71,057
Total	$186,594	$174,022	$163,260

Table 12-2 Statements of Revenue and Expenses of General Funds for Omega Health Foundation (Data in Thousands)

	2006	2005	2004
Revenues			
Net patient service revenue	$160,574	$162,323	$147,596
Equity in net income from partnership	732	1,135	1,216
Gifts and bequests	258	435	296
Other	8,760	8,742	7,655
Total revenues	$170,324	$172,635	$156,763
Expenses			
Salaries and wages	$81,032	$81,476	$75,942
Fringe benefits	18,627	19,876	16,391
Professional fees	8,980	12,743	13,541
Supplies and other	39,607	38,539	30,658
Interest	4,364	4,369	4,421
Bad debt expense	4,551	6,419	8,026
Depreciation and amortization	8,545	7,861	7,167
Restructuring costs	5,110	—	—
Total expenses	$170,816	$171,283	$156,146
Income (loss) from operations	$(492)	$1,352	$617
Nonoperating gains (losses)			
Income on investments	$4,717	$4,658	$3,837
Gifts and bequests	41	297	—
Loss on disposal of assets	(84)	(601)	(150)
Nonoperating gains, net	$4,674	$4,354	$3,687
Excess of revenues over expenses before cumulative effect of change in accounting principle	$4,182	$5,706	$4,304
Cumulative effect of change in account principle	(5,086)	—	—
Excess of revenues over expenses	$(904)	$5,706	$4,304

presented in Tables 12–5, 12–6, and 12–7. The forecast methodology used is described below:

- *Net patient revenues.* Net patient revenues were projected at an annual two percent growth rate. Net patient revenue actually decreased slightly in 2006, but increased 9.4 percent in 2005. What should we forecast? Clearly, revenues should be set equal to volumes of services expected multiplied by expected net prices. At first, two percent might seem like a relatively small growth rate, but OHF presently has a very high price structure, which it may not be able to maintain. A two percent growth rate is predicated on zero growth in net prices, but a two percent growth in volume of services. A two per-

cent growth in services seems reasonable given previous growth in outpatient and clinic services. The assumptions made about revenue growth (volume and price) are the most important variables in terms of impact upon the financial plan. Small changes in these assumptions can have a sizable influence on projected financial results.

- *Salaries and wages.* In the labor-intensive health care industry, the second most important assumption in any financial forecast is the cost of salaries and wages. Salary and wage cost are the product of three factors:

Salary and wage costs = Volume of services × Staffing ratios × Wage rates

Table 12–3 Historical Financial Ratios for Omega Health Foundation

	2004	2005	2006	U.S. Weighted Average*
Profitability				
Total margin percentage	2.7	3.2	−0.5	4.2
Operating margin percentage	0.4	0.8	−0.3	3.3
Nonoperating revenue percentage	2.3	2.5	2.7	0.9
Return on equity percentage	6.1	7.3	−1.2	7.3
Liquidity				
Current	1.53	1.38	1.09	1.89
Days in accounts receivable	57.8	57.6	55.3	67.4
Days' cash-on-hand	119.8	115.7	147.3	93.6
Capital structure				
Equity financing percentage	43.5	45.2	41.5	53.7
Long-term debt to equity percentage	79.4	71.1	70.8	56.3
Cash flow to debt percentage	13.5	15.7	8.3	14.9
Times interest earned	1.97	2.31	0.79	5.27
Activity				
Total asset turnover	0.98	1.02	0.94	0.92
Fixed asset turnover	2.42	2.37	2.30	2.24
Current asset turnover	3.67	4.18	4.32	3.02
Other ratios				
Average age of plant	7.5	8.0	8.3	9.4

Source: State of Hospital Industry—2005 Edition, Cleverley and Associates.

OHF has poor productivity and has undergone massive restructuring to try to reduce current staff levels and become more efficient. These staff reductions showed up as one-time restructuring costs in 2006, and finally will be written off in 2007. It is expected that future labor force reductions will be accomplished through attrition. It is, therefore, expected that salary and wages will increase only one percent per year over the next five years. Wage rates are expected to increase anywhere between three to five percent per year, but the reduction in staffing ratios resulting from attrition will keep the total increase to one percent. Any change in this assumption will also have a dramatic effect upon projected financial results.

* *Fringe benefits.* Fringe benefits on average have constituted between 20 to 24 percent of salaries and wages. It is expected that future fringe benefit costs will constitute approximately 23 percent of salary and wage costs.
* *Interest expense.* Projected average interest on existing long-term debt is expected to be 7.5 percent. This interest rate is applied to the beginning total of long-term debt plus current maturities of long-term debt.
* *Restructuring costs.* Restructuring costs were $5,110,000 in 2006, due in large part to costs associated with early retirement and layoffs. There are $2,078,000 of these costs still remaining as a current liability at the end of 2006. These costs will be expensed in 2007, and will be zero thereafter.
* *Depreciation expense.* Depreciation expense was 5.8 percent of gross property, plant, and equipment in 2006. This value is consistent with national averages and was used to forecast future depreciation.

Table 12–4 Financial Planning Assumptions for Omega Health Foundation, Years 2003 to 2007

Account	Assumptions
Revenues	
Net patient revenue	2% growth per year
Equity in partnerships	5% growth per year
Gifts and bequests	5% growth per year
Other	5% growth per year
Expenses	
Interest expense	7.5% of prior year long-term debt + current maturities of long-term debt
Salaries and wages	1% growth per year
Fringe benefits	23% of salaries and wages
Professional fees	5% growth per year
Supplies	5% growth per year
Restructuring costs	$2,078,000 in 2007; zero thereafter
Depreciation expense	5.8% of gross property and equipment
Bad debt expense	2.8% of net patient revenue
Nonoperating gains	
Investment income	8.3% of beginning balance in board-designated and board-funded depreciation
Gifts and bequests	$50,000 per year
Loss on disposals	$100,000 per year
Assets	
Cash and short-term investments	20 days' cash-on-hand
Accounts receivable	15% of net patient revenue
Due from donor-restricted funds	$300,000 per year
Inventories	Schedule $1,830,000 in 2007, increasing 5% per year thereafter
Prepaid expenses and other assets	5% growth per year
Current portion held by trustee	Schedule $1,055,000 in 2007, increasing by $65,000 per year
Current portion self insurance	5% growth per year
Total current assets	Subtotal of previous items
Gross property and equipment	Net new capital expenditures of $10,000,000 per year
Accumulated depreciation expense	Beginning balance + depreciation expense
Self-insurance trust	5% growth per year
Board-designated and board-funded depreciation	Balancing account, all surplus cash flow will be invested here
Funds held by trustee	$338,000 per year
Investments in partnerships	5% growth per year
Deferred financing costs	Schedule: $972,000 in 2007, decreasing by $167,000 per year
Other assets	10% growth per year
Liabilities	
Current maturities of long-term debt	Schedule based upon debt principal due
Accounts payable	5% growth per year
Accrued salaries and wages	5.3% of salaries and wages expense
Accrued restructuring costs	Value goes to zero in 2007 and remains at zero
Accrued vacation	Stable at $3,288,000
Accrued insurance costs	5% growth per year
Advances from third-party payers	0.75% of net patient revenue
Due to third-party payers	7.2% of net patient revenue

continues

Table 12–4 continued

Account	Assumptions
Liabilities	
Total current liabilities	Subtotal of previous items
Long-term debt	Schedule based upon payment of debt principal
Accrued retirement costs	5% growth per year
Accrued insurance costs	5% growth per year
Deferred third-party reimbursement	Stable at $3,489,000
Other liabilities	5% growth per year
Unrestricted net assets	Addition of net income to prior balance

Table 12–5 Forecasted Balance Sheet for Omega Health Foundation as of June 30, 2007, 2008, 2009, 2010, and 2011 (Data in Thousands)

GENERAL FUNDS

	2006	2007	2008	2009	2010	2011
Assets						
Current						
Cash and cash equivalents	$9,692	$8,907	$8,988	$9,190	$9,400	$9,616
Accounts receivable	24,324	24,568	25,059	25,560	26,072	26,593
Due from third-party payers	0	0	0	0	0	0
Due from donor-restricted funds	280	300	300	300	300	300
Inventories	1,763	1,830	1,921	2,017	2,118	2,224
Prepaid expenses and other assets	1,135	1,192	1,251	1,314	1,380	1,449
Current portion of funds held by trustee	990	1,055	1,120	1,185	1,250	1,315
Current portion of self-insurance trust funds	2,264	2,377	2,496	2,621	2,752	2,890
Total current assets	$40,448	$40,229	$41,135	$42,187	$43,272	$44,387
Other assets						
Gross property, plant, and equipment	$146,794	$156,794	$166,794	$176,794	$186,794	$196,794
Less total accumulated depreciation	70,804	79,898	89,572	99,826	110,660	122,074
Net property, plant, and equipment	$75,990	$76,896	$77,222	$76,968	$76,134	$74,720
Self-insurance trust funds, net of current portion	$9,321	$9,787	$10,276	$10,790	$11,330	$11,896
Board-designated funds & funded depreciation	55,794	59,726	67,246	75,561	84,131	93,538
Funds held by trustee, net of current position	337	338	338	338	338	338
Investments in and advances to partnerships	2,497	2,622	2,753	2,891	3,035	3,187
Deferred financing costs, net	1,139	972	805	638	471	304

continues

Table 12–5 continued

GENERAL FUNDS

	2006	2007	2008	2009	2010	2011
Other assets						
Deferred third-party reimbursement	0	0	0	0	0	0
Other assets	1,067	1,174	1,292	1,420	1,562	1,718
Total other assets	$70,155	$74,619	$82,710	$91,638	$100,867	$110,981
Total assets	$186,594	$191,745	$201,067	$210,793	$220,273	$230,088
Liabilities						
Current						
Current portion of long-term debt	$1,401	$1,488	$1,566	$1,806	$1,715	$1,525
Accounts payable and accrued expenses	11,087	11,641	12,223	12,835	13,476	14,150
Accrued salaries, wages, and fees	4,342	4,338	4,381	4,425	4,469	4,514
Accrued restructuring costs	2,078	0	0	0	0	0
Accrued vacation	3,288	3,288	3,288	3,288	3,288	3,288
Accrued insurance costs	2,234	2,346	2,463	2,586	2,715	2,851
Advance from third-party payer	1,205	1,228	1,253	1,278	1,304	1,330
Due to third-party payers	11,571	11,793	12,028	12,269	12,514	12,765
Total current liabilities	$37,206	$36,122	$37,202	$38,487	$39,481	$40,423
Accrued retirement costs	$8,846	$9,288	$9,753	$10,240	$10,752	$11,290
Accrued insurance costs, net of current position	4,636	4,868	5,111	5,367	5,635	5,917
Deferred third-party reimbursement	3,489	3,489	3,489	3,489	3,489	3,489
Long-term debt, net of current position	54,781	53,380	51,892	50,326	48,520	46,805
Other liabilities	238	250	262	276	289	304
Total liabilities	$109,196	$107,397	$107,709	$108,185	$108,166	$108,228
Unrestricted net assets	77,398	84,348	93,358	102,608	112,107	121,860
Total liabilities and unrestricted net assets	$186,594	$199,745	$201,067	$210,793	$220,273	$230,088

- *Bad debt expense.* Bad debt expense has been declining in recent years. In 2006, bad debt expense was 2.8 percent of net patient revenue. It is expected that future declines will be difficult to achieve and that present relationships will stabilize.
- *Cash and short-term investments.* Cash balances in this account are needed to meet normal transaction needs for cash, such as salary, wages, and accounts payable. A typical transaction balance is approximately twenty days.
- *Accounts receivable.* Accounts receivable have been approximately 15 percent of net patient revenue, or 55 days. It is expected that the present pattern of receivables will remain stable over the next five years.
- *Gross property and equipment.* Gross property and equipment will increase each year by the amount of capital expenditures less any assets that are sold or disposed. Table 12–8 shows the board-approved capital expenditure plan.

Table 12–6 Forecasted Income Statement for Omega Health Foundation (Data in Thousands)

	2006	2007	2008	2009	2010	2011
Revenues						
Net patient service revenue	$160,574	$163,785	$167,061	$170,402	$173,810	$177,287
Equity in net income from partnership	732	769	807	847	890	934
Gifts and bequests	258	271	284	299	314	329
Other	8,760	9,198	9,658	10,141	10,648	11,180
Total revenues	$170,324	$174,023	$177,810	$181,689	$185,662	$189,730
Expenses						
Salaries and wages	$81,032	$81,842	$82,661	$83,488	$84,322	$85,165
Fringe benefits	18,627	18,824	19,012	19,202	19,394	19,588
Professional fees	8,980	9,429	9,900	10,395	10,915	11,461
Supplies and other expenses	39,607	41,587	43,667	45,851	48,143	50,550
Interest	4,364	4,214	4,115	4,009	3,910	3,768
Bad debt expense	4,551	4,586	4,678	4,771	4,867	4,964
Depreciation and amortization	8,545	9,094	9,674	10,254	10,834	11,414
Restructuring costs	5,110	2,078	0	0	0	0
Total expenses	$170,816	$171,654	$173,707	$177,970	$182,385	$186,910
Income (loss) from operations	$(492)	$2,369	$4,103	$3,719	$3,277	$2,820
Nonoperating gains (losses)						
Income on investments	$4,717	$4,631	$4,957	$5,581	$6,272	$6,983
Gifts and bequests	41	50	50	50	50	50
Loss on disposal of assets	(84)	(100)	(100)	(100)	(100)	(100)
Nonoperating gains, net	$4,674	$4,581	$4,907	$5,531	$6,222	$6,933
Excess of revenues over expenses	$4,182	$6,950	$9,010	$9,250	$9,499	$9,753

Definition of Debt Policy

Having defined the desired levels of investment for OHF, the next step is to define the debt policy for the five-year forecast period. Debt should not be viewed as the balancing variable in the financial plan. That is, the financial plan should not project assets and equity and then balance the equation with debt. Sound financial policy requires that the board and management define in advance what their position is regarding the assumption of debt. Table 12–9 presents OHF's management and board policy on debt for the next five years. The forecast methodology used for OHF's liabilities is presented below:

* *Long-term debt.* OHF board members have determined that they do not wish to borrow any additional moneys on a long-term basis over the next five years. They believe that their present capital structure has too much long-term debt as evidenced by a high long-term debt to equity ratio. The present debt will, therefore, be repaid in accordance with existing debt amortization schedules. Table 12–9 summarizes OHF's long-term debt position over the next five years.
* *Accrued salaries and wages.* Although it may not be thought of as a form of debt, all current liabilities represent a form of financing. Accrued salaries and wages represent a form of financing from the firm's employees. The employees have contributed their labor before receiving their wages. Accrued salaries and wages, on average, have constituted about 5 percent of salaries and wages and constituted 5.3 percent in 2006. This value is used in the forecast.
* *Due to third-party payers.* This current liability account represents overpayment by third-party payers during the course of the year and is a

Table 12-7 Forecasted Financial Ratios for Omega Health Foundation

	2007	2008	2009	2010	2011
Profitability					
Total margin percentage	3.9	4.9	4.9	5.0	5.0
Operating margin percentage	1.3	2.3	2.0	1.7	1.4
Nonoperating revenue %	2.6	2.9	3.0	3.2	3.5
Return on equity percentage	8.2	9.7	8.8	8.5	8.0
Liquidity					
Current	1.11	1.11	1.09	1.09	1.09
Days in accounts receivable	54.8	54.8	54.8	54.8	54.8
Days' cash-on-hand (short term)	20.0	20.0	20.0	20.0	20.0
Capital structure					
Equity financing percentage	44.1	46.4	48.7	50.9	53.0
Long-term debt to equity percentage	63.3	55.6	49.1	43.2	38.4
Cash flow to debt percentage	14.9	17.4	18.0	18.8	19.6
Times interest earned	2.65	3.19	3.31	3.43	3.59
Activity					
Total asset turnover	0.93	0.91	0.89	0.87	0.85
Fixed asset turnover	2.32	2.37	2.43	2.52	2.63
Current asset turnover	4.44	4.44	4.44	4.44	4.44
Other ratios					
Average age of plant	8.8	9.3	9.7	10.2	10.7

sizable account for OHF. In 2006, the account balance was $11,571,000. OHF has consistently reported sizable values for this account and this overpayment situation is expected to continue into the future. It is expected that the present relationship between net patient revenue and due to third-party payers will stabilize at approximately 7.2 percent. This is a critical relationship and represents interest-free financing that is currently being provided by OHF's third-party payers. Any change in this relationship would have a significant influence on OHF's financial projections.

Assessing the Reasonableness of Required Equity Growth

At this stage in the development of the financial plan, we have projected balance sheets (Table 12–5), income statements (Table 12–6), and financial ratios (Table 12–7). The following two questions must be answered before our financial plan can be accepted:

1. Can we actually achieve the results currently projected; are our assumptions realistic?
2. Are the projected financial results acceptable; are we satisfied with the current projected financial performance?

Regarding the first question about the realistic nature of our assumptions, we already have discussed these assumptions and the basis for them. This does not mean that they are attainable and we should review again the critical assumptions on which the forecast is based. Especially important are the assumptions regarding revenue and expense growth.

One useful way to review the validity of a financial plan is to compare the projected financial ratios with historical values. Comparing the financial ratio values found in Table 12–3 and 12–7 seems to indicate that the plan may be reasonable. The only major significant change appears in the area of profitability, especially margins. Operating income is projected to increase sharply from 2006 levels. The basis for this increase is

Table 12–8 Forecasted Property and Equipment for Omega Health Foundation

	2007	2008	2009	2010	2011
Beginning gross property and equipment	$146,794	$156,794	$166,794	$176,794	$186,794
Net capital expenditures	10,000	10,000	10,000	10,000	10,000
Ending gross property and equipment	$156,794	$166,794	$176,794	$186,794	$196,794

directly related to a modest one percent growth in salaries and wages. If we remain convinced that this goal is achievable because of scheduled productivity improvements, our initial forecast appears to be attainable.

Regarding the second question of acceptability, a comparison of historical and projected financial ratios will prove useful. In the initial forecast, there was no target set for board-designated and board-funded depreciation reserves. Surplus cash generated in the forecast was added to this balance, and any cash deficits would be subtracted from beginning balances. During the five-year forecast, OHF has added almost $38 million in new board-designated and board-funded depreciation reserves. The ending balance in 2011 is projected to be $93,538,000. On the surface, this seems like a healthy increase. But how does this compare to our replacement cost needs? In 2011, our projected accumulated depreciation will be $122,074,000. The percentage of our projected funded depreciation to projected accumulated depreciation is 76.6 percent. This value is almost identical to the present 78.8 percent relationship and we appear not to have compromised our replacement reserve integrity over the five year plan.

A further review of the financial ratios suggests only one area that may need some revision. The net plant and equipment actually declines during the five-year financial planning period. Furthermore, OHF's average age of plant increases from 8.3 to 10.6 years. This may signal under-investment in plant and equipment. For the present time, however, we will assume that the projected level of capital expenditures is adequate, given the current surplus investment in inpatient facil-

ities that will not require replacement. Most of the new capital will be deployed to fast-growing outpatient and clinic operations.

LEARNING OBJECTIVE 5

Explain how management control is used in conjunction with the financial plan.

INTEGRATION OF THE FINANCIAL PLAN WITH MANAGEMENT CONTROL

The development of a financial plan is a useless exercise unless that plan is integrated into the management control process. Management needs to know whether the plan is being realized and, if it is not, what corrective action can be taken. In some cases, there may be little that management can do. For example, assume that the entity has experienced an unusually large reduction in its operating margins as a result of declining prices due to increased competition. In this case, perhaps the only course of action open to management is to revise its plan to more accurately reflect the current situation or to cut expenses if possible. Indeed, it is important for management to assess the accuracy of its financial plan annually and to make appropriate changes as needed.

Some structure is needed to integrate the financial plan with the management control process. Financial ratios provide that structure. The chart in Figure 12–4 depicts detailed targets for OHF, reflecting its financial

Table 12–9 Forecasted Long-Term Debt for Omega Health Foundation

	2007	2008	2009	2010	2011	2012
Beginning long-term debt (LTD)	$54,781	$53,380	$51,892	$50,326	$48,520	$46,805
Less beginning current maturities of LTD	(1,401)	(1,488)	(1,566)	(1,806)	(1,715)	(1,525)
Ending long-term debt	$53,380	$51,892	$50,326	$48,520	$46,805	$45,280

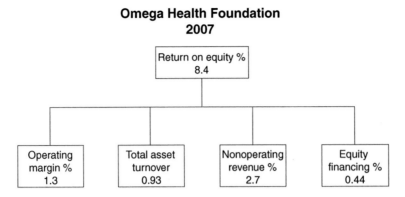

**Omega Health Foundation
2007**

Figure 12–4 Financial Ratio Targets for Omega Health Foundation

plan. In the chart, specific ratio values are delineated. The primary targets involve the four major ratios that together determine the hospital's return on equity. The secondary targets are concerned with additional data that can be used to monitor actual performance and detect possible problems.

To understand how the chart in Figure 12–4 might be used in management control, let us assume that the year 2007 has just ended and the financial data essential to the calculation of the ratios are now available. OHF's actual return on equity for 2007 is assumed to be 7.6 percent, which represents an unfavorable variance from the required value of 8.4 percent.

Actual values for the primary indicators are the following:

	2007 Values
Operating margin ratio percent	1.0
Total asset turnover ratio	.93
Equity financing ratio percent	44.0
Nonoperating revenue percent	2.6

The major cause of the unfavorable variance in return on equity deviates from the expected operating margin of 1.3 percent to 1.0 percent. In addition, the nonoperating revenue ratio also was below expectations, with an actual value of 2.6 percent compared with an expected value of 2.7 percent. All other ratio targets that determine equity growth were met. This would narrow any corrective actions to the two areas of operating margins and nonoperating gains.

It is extremely important to remember the concept of "sustainable growth" introduced in Chapter 10: sustainable growth simply means that no organization can

generate a growth rate in assets that exceeds its growth rate in equity for a prolonged period. Ultimately, an organization is limited by the rate at which it can generate new equity.

Return on equity can be defined as follows:

$$\text{Return on equity} = \frac{[OM + NOR] \times TAT}{EF}$$

where:

OM = operating margin ratio
NOR = nonoperating revenue ratio
TAT = total asset turnover ratio
EF = equity financing ratio

If top management and board members concentrate on this simple formula and the key relationships represented by it, financial focus and direction will improve dramatically.

SUMMARY

In the process of identifying the requirements for effective financial policy formulation in health care firms, it is especially important to relate the strategic plan to the financial plan. Neither should be developed in isolation. The plans need to be developed together, reflecting similar individual requirements and assumptions. A strategic plan is not valid if it is not financially feasible, and a financial plan is of little value if it does not reflect the strategic decisions reached by management and the board.

A financial plan should be updated at least annually, projecting a forecast period of three to five years. Financial plans that are not updated stand a good chance of becoming invalid. The environment of health care delivery is changing, and a health care entity's financial plan must reflect the changes. In fact, a failure to update its financial plan can have disastrous consequences for an entity, leading perhaps to market share retrenchment or even financial failure.

Finally, financial plans should be integrated into the management control process. Financial ratios can be useful in this regard. In particular, specific ratios can be usefully related to the key financial planning target of growth rate in equity.

REFERENCES

Cleverley and Associates. (2005). State of Hospital Industry. 2005 Edition, Worthington, OH, Cleverley & Associates.

ASSIGNMENTS

1. A financial plan may be thought of as a bridge between two balance sheets. What are the major categories of assumptions that must be specified to project a future balance sheet, given a current balance sheet?

2. What problems result from the present responsibility center or departmental orientation of most accounting systems in providing data for financial planning?

3. Your director of marketing is urging you to develop a new drug-abuse program. She has argued that there is no capital investment involved in the development of the new service. Do you believe this is an accurate statement?

4. Your hospital has a current funded depreciation to accumulated depreciation ratio of 0.20. What are the implications of this indicator for your hospital's financial planning?

5. Your controller has just provided you with ROI figures for your firm's major product lines. You have noticed that obstetrics has a very low ROI. What factors should be considered before you eliminate this service?

6. You are in the process of developing your firm's financial plan for the next five years. As an initial step, you are analyzing financial ratios for the last five years. You notice that, over the five-year period, the average age of plant ratio has increased from 8.5 years to 12.2 years. What are the implications of this for your financial plan?

7. If current assets are expected to increase by $4 million over the next five years and you wish to increase your current ratio from 1.5 to 2.0, what additional amount of new equity must be generated to finance the increase in the current ratio on the incremental $4.0?

8. Beginning equity is $50 million and equity in five years is projected to be $100 million. What is the annual rate of growth implied by these values?

9. You are assessing the financial plan developed for you by a prestigious "Big 5" accounting firm. You are especially interested in the attainability of the projected growth rate in equity. You know that if that growth rate is not realistic, the financial plan is not valid and you may have to scale back your projected increase in assets. Table 12–10 summarizes your findings. Does the accounting firm's plan appear to be reasonable?

Table 12–10 Financial Plan Summary Values

	Historical Average	Five-Year Projections
Reported income index ratio	1.000	.900
Operating margin ratio	.025	.027
Total asset turnover ratio	1.100	1.200
Nonoperating revenue ratio	.011	.011
Equity financing ratio	.500	.500
Equity growth rate	7.86%	10.29%

10. Using the data presented for Omega Health Foundation in this chapter, revise the existing financial plan. Assume that salaries and wages will increase two percent per year, not the original one percent used in the forecast. Prepare a revised forecasted balance sheet, income statement, and ratios for OHF.

1. Projection of a future balance sheet requires assumptions in the following three categories:

   * Rates of growth for individual asset accounts
   * Debt-financing policy for both current and long-term debt
   * Realizable rate of growth in equity that is factored into five ratio areas:
     –operating margins
     –nonoperating revenue
     –equity financing
     –total asset turnover
     –reported income index (defined as net income divided by the change in equity)

2. Strategic financial planning is usually done along program or product lines, not responsibility centers or departments. This requires the financial planner to transfer revenue, cost, and investment assignments from responsibility centers to product lines. This can be a difficult process.

3. Although some new investment in fixed assets may be required to start a drug-abuse program, the investment in working capital may be sizable. For example, there may be sizable staffing costs that are required before the program is underway and there may also be legal costs associated with obtaining approval to start the program. Some projection of the investment should be made to assess the potential return on investment that is likely to result.

4. A funded depreciation to accumulated depreciation ratio of 0.20 implies that your hospital will need to borrow 80 percent of its replacement needs in the future. The percentage of debt financing is derived by the following formula:

   Debt financing = 100 percent − Funded Depreciation to Accumulated Depreciation Ratio

   This directly affects the debt policy assumptions that will be used in the financial plan. It also will have an impact on the firm's operating margins because of the potentially large increase in debt and the resulting increase in interest expense.

5. Eliminating a product line solely on the basis of an inadequate ROI may not be consistent with the firm's goals and objectives. Specifically, obstetrics may meet a community need and may be essential to the firm's mission; it may, in fact, be classified as a Samaritan (see Figure 12–3). Alternatively, a low ROI can sometimes be deceiving. The product line may have important externalities. For example, obstetrics may lose money, but gynecology may be very profitable. Eliminating obstetrics may mean that the firm's gynecology line, and its profits, would be reduced.

6. The current average age of plant ratio implies that the firm has a very old plant relative to industry norms. This will almost certainly mean that significant new investment will be required in the planning period.

7. Use of a current ratio of 2.0 implies that the incremental investment of $4 million in current assets would be financed with $2 million of current liabilities. Use of a current ratio of 1.5 would imply current liability financing of $2.67 million. Therefore, the change in the current ratio implies that an additional equity requirement of $670,000 would be required.

8. The implied annual rate of growth is 14.86 percent.

9. The accounting firm's plan specifies a 30 percent increase in the annual growth rate in equity, compared with the historical five-year average (7.86 percent versus 10.29 percent). The major changes are in the reported income index and total asset turnover ratios. In the past five years, the firm has had no unreported income because the value for the reported income index is 1.0. It is important to determine the expected source of the new equity. The increase in total asset turnover, although not large, does play an important role in the higher projected growth rate in equity. Reasons for this increase should be verified.

10. Tables 12–11 through 12–13 list the revised forecasts for Omega Health Foundation. Note the dramatic reduction in profit from such a small change in one item. Also, OHF now will have $76,109,000 in board-designated funded depreciation in 2011, not the original amount of $93,538,000. To understand the impact on board-designated funds, recognize that the increase in salary expense plus the associated increase in fringe benefits will reduce net income and therefore reduce the balance of cash available for investment. There is one other effect however, and that is an increased requirement for holding nonincome-yielding cash and cash equivalents to meet the 20-day working capital requirement. For example, in 2007 the increase in salary costs was $811,000 ($82,653,000 less $81,842,000) and the increased fringe benefits on this salary expense were 23 percent or $186,000 ($19,010,000 less $18,824,000). The total increased expense is $997,000 which creates a demand to raise short-term cash balances by $55,000 (($997,000/365) times 20 days). The 2007 balance sheet value for cash and cash equivalents in Table 12–5 was $8,907,000 and the same value in Table 12–11 is $8,962,000, a $55,000 difference that is attributed to the increase in salary and fringe benefit costs. The reduction in the ending invested balance also cost the hospital in reduced investment income, which will affect future year's investment and investment income levels. There is also a small financing advantage that results from the increased values for accrued salaries and wages. As the dollar amount of salaries and wages increases, there will be some benefit from the increased accrual.

Table 12–11 Revised Forecasted Balance Sheet for Omega Health Foundation as of June 2007, 2008, 2009, 2010, and 2011 (Data in Thousands)

GENERAL FUNDS

	2007	2008	2009	2010	2011
Assets					
Current					
Cash and cash equivalents	$8,962	$9,099	$9,359	$9,628	$9,906
Accounts receivable	24,568	25,059	25,560	26,072	26,593
Due from third-party payers	0	0	0	0	0
Due from donor-restricted funds	300	300	300	300	300
Inventories	1,830	1,921	2,017	2,118	2,224
Prepaid expenses and other assets	1,192	1,251	1,314	1,380	1,449
Current portion of funds held by trustee	1,055	1,120	1,185	1,250	1,315
Current portion of self-insurance trust funds	2,377	2,496	2,621	2,752	2,890
Total current assets	$40,284	$41,246	$42,356	$43,500	$44,677
Other assets					
Gross property, plant, and equipment	$156,794	$166,794	$176,794	$186,794	$196,794
Less total accumulated depreciation	79,898	89,572	99,826	110,660	122,074
Net property, plant, and equipment	$76,896	$77,222	$76,968	$76,134	$74,720
Self-insurance trust funds, net of current portion	$9,787	$10,276	$10,790	$11,330	$11,896
Board-designated funds	58,718	64,121	69,083	72,936	76,109
Funds held by trustee, net of current position	338	338	338	338	338
Investments in and advances to partnerships	2,622	2,753	2,891	3,035	3,187
Deferred financing costs, net	972	805	638	471	304
Deferred third-party reimbursement	0	0	0	0	0
Other assets	1,174	1,291	1,420	1,562	1,718
Total other assets	$73,611	$79,584	$85,160	$89,672	$93,552
Total assets	$190,791	$198,052	$204,484	$209,306	$212,949
Liabilities					
Current					
Current portion of long-term debt	$1,488	$1,566	$1,806	$1,715	$1,525
Accounts payable and accrued expenses	11,641	12,223	12,835	13,476	14,150
Accrued salaries, wages, and fees	4,381	4,468	4,557	4,650	4,741
Accrued restructuring costs	0	0	0	0	0
Accrued vacation	3,288	3,288	3,288	3,288	3,288
Accrued insurance costs	2,346	2,463	2,586	2,715	2,851
Advance from third-party payer	1,228	1,253	1,278	1,304	1,330
Due to third-party payers	11,793	12,028	12,269	12,514	12,765
Total current liabilities	$36,165	$37,289	$38,619	$39,662	$40,650
Accrued retirement costs	$9,288	$9,753	$10,240	$10,752	$11,290
Accrued insurance costs, net of current position	4,868	5,111	5,367	5,635	5,917
Deferred third-party reimbursement	3,489	3,489	3,489	3,489	3,489
Long-term debt, net of current position	53,380	51,892	50,326	48,520	46,805
Other liabilities	250	262	276	289	304
Total liabilities	$107,440	$107,796	$108,317	$108,347	$108,455
Unrestricted net assets	83,351	90,256	96,167	100,959	104,494
Total liabilities and unrestricted net assets	$190,791	$198,052	$204,484	$209,306	$212,949

Table 12–12 Revised Forecasted Income Statement for Omega Health Foundation (Data in Thousands)

	2007	2008	2009	2010	2011
Revenues					
Net patient service revenue	$163,785	$167,061	$170,402	$173,810	$177,287
Equity in net income from partnership	769	807	847	890	934
Gifts and bequests	271	284	299	314	329
Other	9,198	9,658	10,141	10,648	11,180
Total revenues	$174,023	$177,810	$181,689	$185,662	$189,730
Expenses					
Salaries and wages	$82,653	$84,306	$85,992	$87,712	$89,466
Fringe benefits	19,010	19,390	19,779	20,174	20,577
Professional fees	9,429	9,900	10,395	10,915	11,461
Supplies and other expenses	41,587	43,667	45,850	48,143	50,550
Interest	4,214	4,115	4,009	3,910	3,768
Bad debt expense	4,586	4,678	4,771	4,867	4,964
Depreciation and amortization	9,094	9,674	10,254	10,834	11,414
Restructuring costs	2,078	0	0	0	0
Total expenses	$172,651	$175,730	$181,050	$186,555	$192,200
Income (loss) from operations	$1,372	$2,080	$639	$(893)	$(2,470)
Nonoperating gains (losses)					
Income on investments	$4,631	$4,874	$5,322	$5,734	$6,054
Gifts and bequests	50	50	50	50	50
Loss on disposal of assets	(100)	(100)	(100)	(100)	(100)
Nonoperating gains, net	$4,581	$4,824	$5,272	$5,684	$6,004
Excess of revenues over expenses	$5,953	$6,904	$5,911	$4,791	$3,534

Table 12–13 Revised Forecasted Financial Ratios for Omega Health Foundation

	2007	2008	2009	2010	2011
Profitability					
Total margin percentage	3.5	4.0	3.4	2.7	1.9
Operating margin percentage	0.8	1.2	0.4	−0.5	−1.4
Nonoperating revenue %	2.7	2.8	3.0	3.2	3.3
Return on equity percentage	7.1	7.7	6.2	4.8	3.4
Liquidity					
Current	1.11	1.10	1.10	1.10	1.10
Days in accounts receivable	54.8	54.8	54.8	54.8	54.8
Days' cash-on-hand (short term)	20.0	20.0	20.0	20.0	20.0
Capital structure					
Equity financing percentage	43.7	45.6	47.0	48.2	49.1
Long-term debt to equity percentage	64.0	57.5	52.3	48.1	44.8
Cash flow to debt percentage	14.0	15.4	14.9	14.4	13.8
Times interest earned	2.41	2.67	2.47	2.23	1.94
Activity					
Total asset turnover	0.88	0.87	0.86	0.86	0.86
Fixed asset turnover	2.19	2.23	2.25	2.36	2.40
Current asset turnover	4.18	4.17	4.15	4.13	4.10
Other ratios					
Average age of plant	8.8	9.3	9.7	10.2	10.7

Chapter 13

Cost Concepts and Decision Making

After studying this chapter, you should be able to do the following:

1. Discuss some of the ways to classify costs.
2. Discuss the four major categories of costs.
3. Explain what is meant by cost behavior, and differentiate between the five general types of cost behavior.
4. Explain the difference between controllable and noncontrollable costs.
5. Discuss the four types of costs that might be relevant when considering alternative projects.
6. Explain the role of direct and indirect costs in the costing process.
7. Describe the three methods of cost allocation.
8. Establish the importance of the semi-variable cost function.
9. Calculate estimated fixed and variable costs using one of the described methods.
10. Calculate break-even volume and the volume necessary to achieve a desired net income.

REAL-WORLD SCENARIO

Dr. Tim Martyn, the chief executive officer of Colonial Hospital, asked Stephen Carey, the chief financial officer of the hospital, to come to his office. Dr. Martyn wanted to talk to Mr. Carey about the hospital's maintenance expenses. Dr. Martyn, who generally had not paid much attention to such expenses, recently noticed that they varied considerably from month to month and wanted to know why.

As Stephen sat down, Tim mentioned that the maintenance expense report showed that over the last six months the maintenance expenses had been as low as $72,000 and as high as $96,000 per month. Not surprised, Stephen responded that this amount of variation actually is quite normal; but Tim knew that the hospital budgeted a constant $82,000 per month for those expenses. Why, he wondered, couldn't they do a better job of projecting those expenses? "With these kinds of fluctuations, how does management know if it has spent too much on maintenance expenses in a given month?" he said. He added, "What explains these fluctuations?"

Stephen responded that his staff was in the process of trying to answer exactly those questions, in order to improve their budgeting for and control of maintenance expenses. He explained that the first step is to break all of the maintenance costs down into fixed and variable components. He elaborated by explaining that some costs are fixed and shouldn't change much. Other costs go up and down depending on how much patient volume the hospital has. The key is to figure out what is driving the variable component of the costs.

Tim asked why the patient volume has such an impact on maintenance costs. Stephen explained that he thinks that when Colonial treats more patients, the equipment is used more intensively, which leads to more maintenance expense. That information further begs the question: what measure to use for the overall activity level? Patient days seemed a logical choice, since each day a patient is in the hospital counts as one patient day. The greater the number of patient days in a month, the busier the hospital is.

Stephen explained that once the maintenance costs are broken down into fixed and variable components, they then would be able to predict what maintenance costs should be as a function of the number of patient days. This information could be used for budgeting purposes and for benchmarking. Tim was pleased to hear about the analysis being done by Stephen's group and asked him to report when the analysis was complete.

In the last five chapters, we have focused on understanding and interpreting the financial information prepared through the financial accounting system and presented in general-purpose financial statements. This chapter focuses more on the use of cost information in decision making. Cost information is produced through an entity's cost accounting system. In most situations, cost information is shaped by the financial accounting system and the generally accepted principles of financial accounting on which financial accounting is based. However, cost information must be flexible because it usually provides information for identifiable and specific decision-making groups, such as budgetary cost variance reports to department managers, cost reports to third-party payers, and forecasted project cost reports to planning agencies.

Cost is a noun that never really stands alone. In most situations, two additional pieces of information are added that enhance the meaning and relevance of the cost statistic. First, the object being costed is defined. For example, we might state that the cost of a clinic visit is $85. Objects of costing are usually of two types: (1) products (outputs or services) or (2) responsibility centers (departments or larger units). Often, we oversimplify this classification system and refer to cost information about products as planning information, and cost information about responsibility centers as control information.

Second, usually an adjective is added to modify cost. For example, we might state that the direct cost of routine nursing care in a hospital is $400 per day. A number of major categories of modifiers refine the concept of cost; they are all used to improve the decision-making process by precisely defining cost to make it more relevant to decisions.

This chapter discusses some of the basic concepts of cost used in cost analysis. It is important to explain this jargon if decision makers are to use cost information correctly. Different concepts of cost are required for different decision purposes. In most situations, these concepts require specific, unique methodologies of cost measurement.

LEARNING OBJECTIVE 1

Discuss some of the ways to classify costs.

CONCEPTS OF COST

Cost may be categorized in a variety of ways to meet decision makers' specific needs. See Table 13–1 for examples of some of the ways to classify costs.

The far-left column lists the classification categories. Different ways to describe costs within these categories

Table 13-1 Some of the Ways to Classify Costs

Cost Classifications	Category 1	Category 2	Category 3
Traceability	Direct costs	Indirect costs	—
Management control	Controllable costs	Non-controllable costs	—
Relation to budget	Budgeted costs	Actual costs	—
Relation to time	Avoidable and sunk costs	Incremental costs	Opportunity costs
Relation to activity	Fixed costs	Variable costs	Mixed costs

are shown in columns two, three, and, if applicable, four. For example, "direct" and "indirect costs" are different because of their traceability. Direct costs are directly linked and assigned to products or services. Direct costs would include, for example, direct labor and materials. Indirect costs such as administrative overhead are not easily traceable to a product or service. Indirect costs are traced to a product or service using some arbitrary allocation method.

Many of these classification systems will be covered in greater detail throughout this chapter. Regardless of the classification system, however, in most situations the total value of the costs is the same. Using one cost concept in place of another simply slices the total cost pie differently. For example, in Table 13–2, the total cost of a laboratory for June 2007 is $21,360. Of that

Table 13-2 Cost Report, Laboratory, June 2007

Classification	Amount
Direct costs	
Salaries	$10,000
Supplies	5,000
Other	5,000
Total direct costs	$20,000
Allocated costs	
Employee benefits	$150
Administration	500
Maintenance	250
Housekeeping	200
Laundry	100
Depreciation	160
Total indirect costs	$1,360
Total costs	$21,360
Relative value units (RVUs)	10,000

amount, $20,000 could be classified as direct cost and $1,360 as indirect cost. However, classifying costs by controllability might determine that $15,000 of the laboratory cost was controllable and $6,360 was not controllable, if the laboratory manager had no control over the $5,000 in the "Other" direct cost. The total cost, however, is the same in both cases.

This brings us to another important point. In most cases, because different concepts of cost simply slice total cost in different ways, there may be underlying relationships among the various concepts of costs. For example, direct costs and controllable costs may be related. In many situations, there are standard "rules of thumb" that may be used to relate cost measures.

The difference between cost and expense is another crucial definitional point. Accountants have traditionally defined cost in a way that leads one to think of cost as an expenditure. However, most people who are not accountants use the term "cost" to refer to expense. For example, in Table 13–2, depreciation is listed as a cost. However, depreciation is not an actual expenditure of cash, but an amortization of prior cost. In the present context, unless otherwise indicated, when we are discussing cost statistics, the terms "costs" and "expenses" may be used interchangeably.

LEARNING OBJECTIVE 2

Discuss the four major categories of costs.

For purposes of discussion, we examine the following four major categories of costs:

1. Traceability to the object being costed
2. Behavior of cost to output or activity
3. Management responsibility for control
4. Future costs versus historical costs

TRACEABILITY

Of all cost classifications, traceability is the most basic. Two major categories of costs classified by traceability are (1) direct costs and (2) indirect costs. A direct cost is specifically traceable to a given cost object. A cost object is a:

* product,
* process,
* department, or
* activity

for which the organization wishes to estimate the cost, such as a test, a visit, a patient or a patient day.

For example, the salaries, supplies, and other costs in Table 13–2 are classified as direct costs of the laboratory. Indirect costs cannot be traced to a given cost object without resorting to some arbitrary method of assignment. In Table 13–2, depreciation, employee benefits, and costs of other departments would be classified as indirect costs.

Not all costs classified as indirect may actually be indirect, however. In some situations, they could be redefined as direct costs. For example, it might be possible to calculate employee benefits for specific employees; these costs then could be charged to the departments in which the employees work and thus become direct costs. However, the actual costs of performing these calculations might be prohibitive.

The classification of a cost as either direct or indirect depends on the given cost object. This is a simple observation, but one that is forgotten by many users of cost information. For example, the $20,000 of direct cost identified in Table 13–2 is a direct cost only regarding the laboratory department. If another cost object is specified, the cost may no longer be direct. For example, dividing the $20,000 of direct costs by the number of relative value units (RVUs), 10,000, yields a direct cost per RVU of $2, but this is not a true figure. The direct cost of any given RVU may be higher or lower than the $2 calculated, which is the average value for all RVUs and not necessarily the cost for any specific unit.

Incorrect classification is a common problem in cost accounting. Costs are accumulated on a department or responsibility-center basis and may be direct or indirect regarding that department. However, it can be misleading to state that the same set of direct costs is also direct regarding the outputs of that department.

The major direct cost categories of most departments would include the following:

* Salaries
* Supplies
* Other (usually fees and purchased services such as dues, travel, and rent)

Indirect cost categories usually include the following:

* Depreciation
* Employee benefits
* Allocated costs of other departments

The concept of direct versus indirect cost may not seem to have much specific relevance to decision makers. To some extent, this is true; however, the concept of direct versus indirect costs is pervasive. It influences both the definition and measurement of other alternative cost concepts that do have specific relevance.

LEARNING OBJECTIVE 3

Explain what is meant by cost behavior, and differentiate between the five general types of cost behavior.

COST BEHAVIOR

Cost is also classified by the degree of variability in relation to output. The actual measurement of cost behavior is influenced by a department's classification of cost, which provides the basis for categorizing costs as direct or indirect.

For our purposes, we can identify five major categories of costs that are classified according to their relationship to output:

1. Variable
2. Fixed
3. Semifixed (or step fixed)
4. Semivariable
5. Curvilinear

Categories three, four and five sometimes are referred to generally as mixed cost behavior. All three general cost behavior patterns—variable, fixed, and mixed—are found in most organizations. The relative proportion of each type of cost present in a firm is known as the firm's cost structure. For example, a firm might have many fixed costs, but few variable or mixed costs. Alternatively, it might have many variable costs, but few fixed or mixed costs. A firm's cost structure can have a significant impact on decisions.

Variable costs change as output or volume (or some other activity level) changes in a constant, proportional manner. That is, if output increases by ten percent, costs also should increase by ten percent; that is, there is some constant cost increment per unit of output. Figure 13–1 illustrates, graphically and mathematically, the concept of variable cost for the laboratory example of Table 13–2. It is assumed that all supply costs in this case are variable. For each unit increase in RVUs, supply costs will increase by $0.50.

An activity is a measure of whatever causes the incurrence of variable cost. For this reason an activity base is sometimes referred to as a cost driver. Examples of common activity bases are direct labor hours, discharges, and patient visits. Other activity bases (cost drivers) might include the number of pounds of laundry processed by the laundry department, the number of letters typed by a secretary, or the number of occupied beds in a hospital or nursing home.

Fixed costs do not change in response to changes in volume. They are a function of the passage of time, not output. Figure 13–2 illustrates fixed-cost behavior patterns for the depreciation costs of the laboratory ex-

ample. Each month, irrespective of output levels, depreciation cost will be $160.

Semifixed (also called step fixed) costs do change with changes in output, but they are not proportional. A semifixed cost might be considered variable or fixed, depending on the size of the steps relative to the range of volume under consideration. For example, in Figure 13–3, it is assumed that the salary cost of the laboratory is semifixed. If the volume of output under consideration were between 6000 and 8000 RVUs, salary costs could be considered fixed at $9,000. Some semifixed costs may be considered variable for cost analysis purposes. For example, if people could be employed other than as full-time equivalents (FTEs), by using overtime or part-time pools, the size of the steps might be significantly smaller than the 2000 RVUs in our laboratory example. Presently, it is assumed that one additional FTE must be employed for every increment of 2000 RVUs. Treating salary costs as variable in this situation might not be a bad practice.

Semivariable costs include elements of both fixed and variable costs. Utility costs are good examples. There may be some basic, fixed requirement per unit of time (e.g., month or year), regardless of volume—such as normal heating and lighting requirements. But there is also likely to be a direct, proportional relationship between volume and the amount of the utility

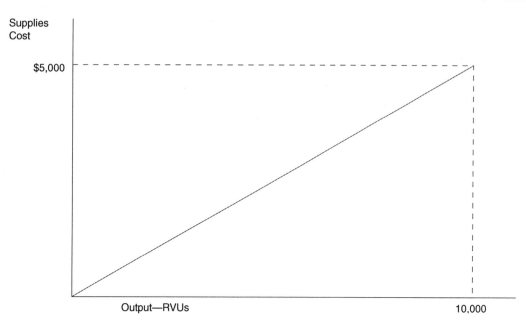

Figure 13–1 Cost Behavior of Supplies Cost, Variable
Note: Supplies cost = $.50 × number of RVUs.

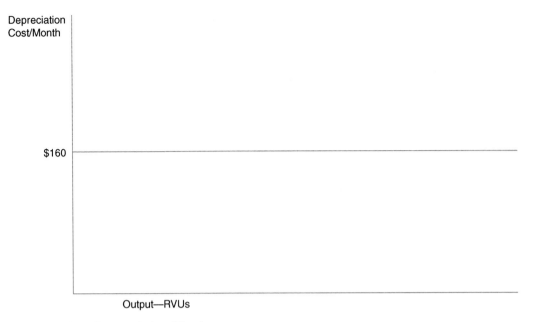

Figure 13–2 Cost Behavior of Depreciation, Fixed
Note: Depreciation cost = $160 per month.

cost. As volume increases, costs go up. Figure 13–4 illustrates semivariable costs in our laboratory example.

Many costs that often are classified as variable actually behave in a curvilinear fashion. The behavior of a curvilinear cost is shown in Figure 13–5. Although many costs are not strictly linear when plotted as a function of volume, a curvilinear cost can be satisfactorily approximated with a straight line within a narrow band of activity known as the relevant range. The relevant range is that range of activity within which the assumptions made by the manager about cost behavior are valid. For example, note that the dashed line in

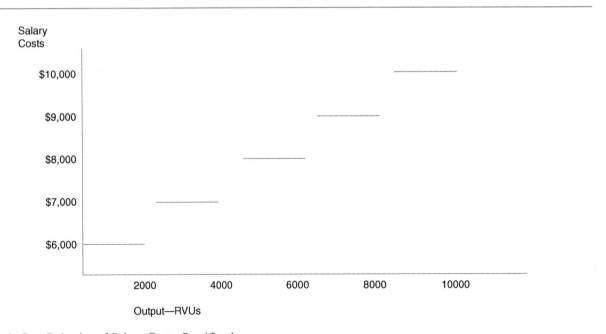

Figure 13–3 Cost Behavior of Salary Costs, Semifixed
Note: Salary costs = $6,000 if RVUs are less than 2000; $7,000 if RVUs are between 2001 and 4000; $8,000 if RVUs are between 4001 and 6000; $9,000 if RVUs are between 6001 and 8000; and $10,000 if RVUs are between 8001 and 10000.

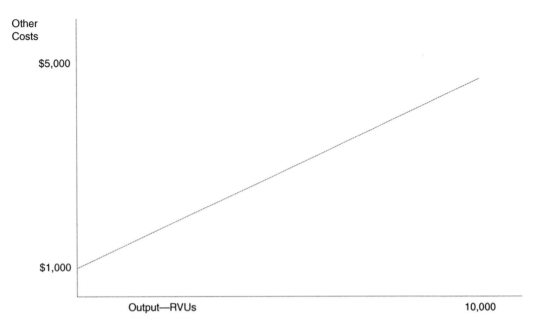

Figure 13–4 Cost Behavior of Other Costs, Semivariable
Note: Other costs = \$1,000 per month + \$.40 × RVUs.

Figure 13–5 can be used as an approximation to the curvilinear cost with very little loss of accuracy within the shaded relevant range. However, outside of the relevant range this particular straight line is a poor approximation of the curvilinear cost relationship as seen in Figure 13-5. Managers should always keep in mind that a particular assumption made about cost behavior

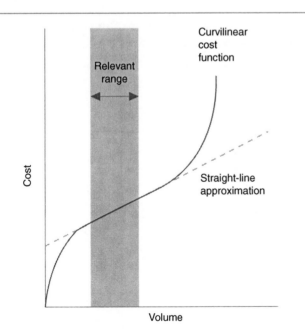

Figure 13–5 Curvilinear Costs and the Relevant Range

may be very inappropriate if activity falls outside of the relevant range.

In many situations, we do not focus on specific cost elements, but aggregate several cost categories of interest. It is interesting to see what type of cost behavior pattern emerges when we do this. Figure 13–6 aggregates four of the cost categories discussed earlier: variable, fixed, semifixed, and semivariable. A semivariable cost behavior pattern closely approximates the actual aggregated cost behavior pattern; this is true for many types of operations. In the next section, we discuss some simple but useful methods for approximating this cost function.

LEARNING OBJECTIVE 4

Explain the difference between controllable and noncontrollable costs.

CONTROLLABILITY

One of the primary purposes of gathering cost information is to aid the management control process. To facilitate evaluation of the management control process, costs must be assigned to individual responsibility centers, usually departments, where a designated

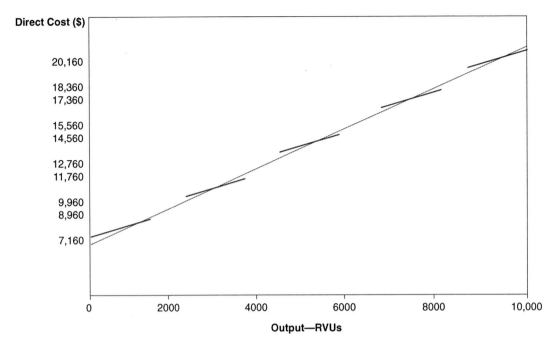

Figure 13–6 Cost Behavior of Aggregated Costs

manager is responsible for cost control. A natural question that arises is, for what proportion of the total costs charged to a department is the manager responsible? The answer to this question requires costs to be separated into two categories: controllable and noncontrollable costs.

Controllable costs can be influenced by a designated responsibility center or departmental manager within a defined control period. It has been stated that all costs are controllable by someone at some time. For example, the chief executive officer of a health care facility,

through the authority granted by the governing board, is ultimately responsible for all costs.

The matrix of costs shown in Figure 13–7 categorizes the laboratory cost report data of Table 13–2. All costs must fall into one of the six cells of the matrix; however, it may be possible to categorize a cost that falls into several different categories into more than one cell of the matrix. In the laboratory example, "Other" cost was viewed as semivariable, implying that part of the cost would be described as a direct variable cost ($4,000) and part as a direct fixed cost ($1,000).

Cost Behavior

Traceables		Variable		Fixed		Semifixed		Total
	Direct	Other Supplies	$4,000 5,000 $9,000	Other	$1,000 $1,000	Salaries	$10,000 $10,000	$20,000
	Indirect	Employee Benefits Housekeeping	$150 100 $250	Depreciation Administration Housekeeping	$160 500 100 $760	Maintenance Laundry	$250 100 $350	$1,360
	Totals		$9,250		$1,760		$10,350	$21,360

Figure 13–7 Laboratory Cost Behavior Organization

There is a tendency in developing management control programs, especially in the health care industry, to use one of three approaches in designating controllable costs. First, controllable costs may be defined as the total costs charged to the department; the department manager would view all costs in the previous six cells of Figure 13-7. In our example, all $21,360 of cost would be viewed as controllable by the laboratory manager. In most normal situations, however, this grossly overstates the amount of cost actually controllable by a given department manager. The result of this overstatement has been negative in many situations. Department managers have rightfully viewed this basis of control as highly inequitable.

Second, controllable costs may be limited to those costs classified as direct. This system is also not without fault: specifically, there may be fixed costs attributed directly to the department that should not be considered controllable. Rent for pieces of equipment, for example, may not be under the department manager's control. There also may be indirect costs, especially costs that are variable that the department manager can control. For example, employee benefits may legitimately be the department manager's responsibility.

Third, in some situations, controllable costs may be defined as only those costs that are direct and variable ($9,000 from Figure 13-7). This limits costs that are controllable by the department manager to their lowest level. However, it excludes what could be a relatively large amount of cost influenced by the department manager. Failure to include the latter cost in the manager's control sphere may weaken management control.

LEARNING OBJECTIVE 5

Discuss the four types of costs that might be relevant when considering alternative projects.

FUTURE COSTS

Decision making involves selection among alternatives; it is a forward-looking process. Actual historical cost may be useful as a basis for projecting future costs, but it should not be used without adjustment unless it can be assumed that future conditions will be identical to past conditions.

A variety of concepts and definitions have been used in current discussion of costs for decision-making purposes. The following four types of costs are critical to most decisions that are choosing between two or more alternatives:

1. Avoidable costs
2. Sunk costs
3. Incremental costs
4. Opportunity costs

Avoidable Costs

Avoidable costs will be affected by the decision under consideration. Specifically, they are costs that can be eliminated or saved if an activity is discontinued; they will remain only if the activity continues. For example, if a hospital was considering curtailing its volume by 50 percent in response to cost-containment pressures, what would it save? The answer is those costs that are avoidable. In most situations, multiplication of current average cost per unit of output (patient days or admissions) by the projected change in output would overstate avoidable costs because much of the cost might not be able to be reduced, at least in the short run. For example, depreciation and interest expenses might not change. Variable costs are almost always a subset of avoidable costs, but avoidable costs might include some fixed costs. For example, administrative staffing might be drastically reduced in a nursing home if 50 percent of the beds were taken out of service. Most likely, administrative staffing costs would have been classified as fixed, given earlier expectations regarding volume. Most variable costs are avoidable, but some fixed costs also may be avoidable when large changes in volume are under consideration.

Sunk Costs

Sunk costs are unaffected by the decision under consideration. In the previous example, large portions of cost—depreciation, administrative salaries, insurance, and others—are sunk or not avoidable in the proposed 50 percent reduction in volume in the nursing home.

The distinction between fixed and variable costs, on the one hand, and sunk and avoidable costs, on the other, is not perfect. Many costs classified as fixed also may be thought of as sunk, but some are not. For example, malpractice insurance premiums generally may be considered fixed cost, given an expected normal level of activity. However, if the institution is considering a drastic reduction in volume, malpractice premiums may not be entirely fixed. In summary, sunk costs are almost always a subset of fixed costs, but not all fixed costs need be sunk. In the evaluation of a decision to close a hospital, most of the hospital's costs (both fixed and variable) probably would be eliminated and therefore would be categorized as avoidable and not sunk regarding the closure decision.

Incremental Costs

Incremental costs represent the change in cost that results from a specific management action. For example, someone might want to know the incremental cost of signing a managed care contract that would generate 200 new admissions a year. There is a strong relationship between incremental and avoidable costs. They can be thought of as different sides of the same coin. We use the term incremental costs to reference the change in costs that results from a management action that increases volume. The term avoidable costs defines the change in cost that results from a management action that reduces volume. For decisions involving only modest changes in output, incremental costs and variable costs may be used interchangeably. In most situations, however, incremental costs are more comprehensive. A decision to construct a surgicenter adjacent to a hospital would involve fixed and variable costs. Depreciation of the facility would be a fixed cost, but it would be incremental to the decision if a new surgicenter were constructed.

Opportunity Costs

Opportunity costs are values foregone by using a resource in a particular way instead of in its next best alternative way. Assume that a nursing home is considering expanding its facility and would use land acquired twenty years ago. If the land had a historical cost of $1 million but a present market value of $10 million, what is the opportunity cost of the land? Practically everyone would agree that if sale of the land constituted the next best alternative, the opportunity cost would be $10 million, not $1 million. Alternatively, a hospital might consider converting part of its acute care facility into a skilled nursing facility because of a reduction in demand or obsoles-

cence in the facility. The question arises, what is the value, or what would be the cost of the facility to the skilled nursing facility operation? If there is no way that the facility can be renovated or if the facility is not needed for the provision of acute care, its opportunity cost may be zero. This could contrast sharply to the recorded historical cost of the facility.

COST MEASUREMENT

In this section, we examine the methods of cost measurement for two cost categories: (1) direct and indirect cost and (2) variable and fixed cost. Both of these cost categories are useful in financial decisions, but the cost accounting system does not directly provide estimates for them.

LEARNING OBJECTIVE 6

Explain the role of direct and indirect costs in the costing process.

DIRECT AND INDIRECT COST

In most cost accounting systems, costs are classified by department or responsibility center and by type of expenditure. Costs are charged to the departments to which they are traceable. Costs are also classified by object of expenditure; they may be identified as supplies, salaries, rent, insurance, or some other category.

Departments in a health care facility can be classified generally as direct or indirect departments, depending on whether they provide services directly to the patient. Sometimes the terms revenue and nonrevenue are substituted for direct and indirect. In the hospital industry, the following breakdown is used in general-purpose financial statements:

Operating Expense Area	Type of Department
Nursing services area	Direct/revenue
Other professional services	Direct/revenue
General services	Indirect/nonrevenue
Fiscal services	Indirect/nonrevenue
Administrative services	Indirect/nonrevenue

Whatever the nomenclature used to describe the classification of departments, cost allocation is usually required. Cost allocation is the process of assigning pooled indirect costs to specific cost objects using an allocation base that represents a major function of a business. An allocation base (also called a cost driver) is an item that is used to allocate costs, based on its assumed relationship as to why the costs occurred. The better the cause and effect relationship between why the cost occurred and the allocation basis, the more accurate the cost allocation. Some common allocation bases include square footage, the number of full-time equivalent employees (FTEs), and direct-labor hours. For example, square footage is commonly used to allocate utility expenses, on the assumption that actual utility costs are proportional to the size of the space a service occupies.

The costs of the indirect, nonrevenue departments need to be allocated to the direct revenue departments for many decision-making purposes. For example, some payers reimburse on the basis of the full costs of direct departments and are interested in the costs of indirect departments only insofar as they affect the calculation of the departments' full costs (both direct and indirect). Pricing decisions need to be based on full costs, not just direct costs, if the costs of the indirect departments are to be covered equitably. It is also critical to include indirect costs when evaluating the financial return of specific programs or product lines. For example, some indirect costs would need to be assigned to an ambulatory surgery program to properly evaluate whether the program was financially viable.

Equity is a key concept in allocating indirect department costs to direct departments. Ideally, the allocation should reflect, as nearly as possible, the actual cost incurred by the indirect department to provide services for a direct department. Department managers who receive cost reports showing indirect allocations are vitally interested in this equity principle, and for good reason. Even if indirect costs are not regarded as controllable by the department manager, the allocation of

costs to a given direct department can have an important effect on a variety of management decisions. Pricing, expansion, or contraction of a department; the purchase of new equipment; and the salaries of department managers are all affected by the allocation of indirect costs. An outpatient surgery program that has unreasonable amounts of hospital overhead allocated to it may find itself noncompetitive.

Costs of indirect departments are in most cases not directly traceable to direct departments. If they were, they could be reassigned. In such cases, they must be allocated to the direct departments in some systematic and rational manner. In general, the following two allocation decisions must be made: (1) selection of the allocation basis and (2) selection of the method of cost apportionment.

Table 13–3 provides sample data for a cost allocation. In this example, there are four departments: two are indirect (laundry/linen and housekeeping), and two are direct (radiology and nursing). How much the laundry weighs is the only allocation basis under consideration for the laundry and linen department. The housekeeping department can use one of two allocation bases, either square feet of area served or hours of service actually worked.

LEARNING OBJECTIVE 7

Describe the three methods of cost allocation.

In general, there are only three acceptable methods of cost allocation:

1. Step-down method
2. Double-distribution method
3. Simultaneous-equations method

Table 13–3 Cost Allocation Example

Department	Direct Cost	Pounds of Laundry Used	Hours of Housekeeping	Square Feet
Laundry/linen	$15,000	—	150	50,000
Housekeeping	30,000	5,000	—	—
Radiology	135,000	5,000	900	10,000
Nursing	270,000	90,000	1950	140,000
Total	$450,000	100,000	3000	200,000

Most health care facilities still use the step-down method of cost allocation. In this method, the indirect department that receives the least amount of service from other indirect departments and provides the most service to other departments allocates its cost first. A similar analysis follows to determine the order of cost allocation for each of the remaining indirect departments. This determination can be subjective to allow some flexibility, as we shall observe shortly.

In the step-down allocation process illustrated in Table 13–4, the laundry and linen department allocates its cost first. Then, housekeeping allocates its direct cost, plus the allocated cost of laundry and linen, to the direct departments of radiology and nursing, based on the ratio of services provided to those departments. The numbers in parentheses represent the proportion of cost charged to that department.

The order of departmental allocation can be an important variable in a step-down method of cost allocation. Table 13–5 depicts an alternative step-down cost allocation in which housekeeping allocates its cost first, preceding the laundry and linen department.

The double-distribution method of cost allocation is just a refinement of the step-down method. Instead of closing the individual department after allocating its costs, it is kept open and receives the costs of other indirect departments. After one complete allocation sequence, the former departments are then closed, using the normal step-down method.

The simultaneous-equations method of cost allocation is used in an attempt to calculate the exact cost allocation amounts. A system of equations is established, and mathematically correct allocations are computed. In the previous example, if simultaneous equations had been used, the cost of radiology would be $145,075 and the cost of nursing would be $304,925, using the following system of equations:

Laundry cost (LC) = $15,000 + .05 HC
Housekeeping cost (HC) = $30,000 + .05 LC
Radiology cost (RC) = $135,000 + .05LC + .30HC
Nursing cost (NC) = $270,000 + .90LC + .65 HC

Finally, it should be noted that using a different allocation base can create differences in cost allocation. For example, the use of square footage for housekeeping, instead of hours served, produces the pattern of cost allocation shown in Table 13–6 when housekeeping allocates its cost first, using the step-down method.

The important point in this discussion is that full cost is not as objective and as exact a figure as one might normally think. Indirect costs can be allocated in a variety of ways that can create significant differences in full costs for given departments. This flexibility should be remembered when examining and interpreting full-cost data.

LEARNING OBJECTIVE 8

Establish the importance of the semi-variable cost function

VARIABLE AND FIXED COST

An important and widely-used cost concept is variability regarding output. It is involved in determining a number of other costs such as avoidable, sunk, incremental, and controllable costs. However, accounting records do not directly yield this type of cost information. Instead, the costs are classified by department and by object of expenditure. Thus, to develop estimates of

Table 13–4 Step–Down Allocation Method—Alternative 1

	Direct Cost	Laundry/Linen		Housekeeping (Hours)		Total
Laundry/linen	$15,000	$15,000				
Housekeeping	30,000	750	(0.05)	$30,750		
Radiology	135,000	750	(0.05)	9,711	(0.3158)	$145,461
Nursing	270,000	13,500	(0.90)	21,039	(0.6842)	304,539
Total	$450,000	$15,000		$30,750		$450,000

Table 13–5 Step-Down Allocation Method—Alternative 2

	Direct Cost	Housekeeping (Hours)		Laundry/Linen		Total
Housekeeping	$30,000	$30,000				
Laundry/linen	15,000	1,500	(0.05)	$16,500		
Radiology	135,000	9,000	(0.30)	868	(0.0526)	$144,868
Nursing	270,000	19,500	(0.65)	15,632	(0.9474)	305,132
Total	$450,000	$30,000		$16,500		$450,000

variable and fixed costs, the relevant data must be analyzed in some way.

Our discussion of cost concepts classified by variability regarding output indicated that a semivariable cost pattern might be a good representation of many types of costs. A semivariable cost function has both a fixed and variable element. A semivariable cost function often results when various types of costs are aggregated together.

LEARNING OBJECTIVE 9

Calculate estimated fixed and variable costs using one of the described methods.

ESTIMATION METHODS

Estimation of a semivariable cost function requires separation of the cost into variable and fixed components. A variety of methods, varying in complexity and accuracy, may be used. Four of the simplest methods are (1) visual-fit, (2) high-low, (3) semi-averages, and (4) regression.

To illustrate each of these methods, assume that we are trying to determine the labor cost function for the

radiology department and we have the six biweekly payroll data points presented in Table 13–7.

In the visual-fit method of cost estimation, the previous individual data points are plotted on graph paper. A straight line is then drawn through the points to provide the best fit. Visual fitting of data is a good first step in any method of cost estimation. Figure 13–8 shows a visual fitting of the previous radiology data.

The high-low method is a simple technique that can be used to estimate the variable and fixed-cost coefficients of a semivariable cost function. The variable cost parameter is solved first. It equals the change in cost from the highest to the lowest data point, divided by the change in output. In the previous radiology example, the variable hours worked would be calculated as follows:

$$\text{Variable labor hours/film} = \frac{320 - 110}{600 - 180} = \frac{210}{420} = .50$$

The fixed-cost parameter then may be solved by subtracting the estimated variable cost (determined by multiplying the variable cost parameter estimate by output at the high level) from total cost. In our radiology example, fixed labor hours would equal the following:

$$\text{Fixed labor hours per pay period} =$$
$$320 - (.50 \times 600) = 320 - 300 = 20$$

Table 13–6 Step-Down Allocation Method—Alternative 3

	Direct Cost	Housekeeping (Square Feet)		Laundry/Linen		Total
Housekeeping	$30,000	$30,000				
Laundry/linen	15,000	7,500	(0.25)	$22,500		
Radiology	135,000	1,500	(0.05)	1,184	(0.0526)	$137,684
Nursing	270,000	21,000	(0.70)	21,316	(0.9474)	312,316
Total	$450,000	$30,000		$22,500		$450,000

Table 13-7 Radiology Payroll Data

Pay Period	Number of Films (x)	Hours Worked (y)	
1	300	180	(low)
2	240	140	(low)
3	400	230	(high)
4	340	190	(high)
5	180	110	(lowest)
6	600	320	(highest)
Total	2,060	1,170	

Alternatively, it is possible to plot the high and low points and then draw a straight line through them.

The semi-averages method is similar to the high-low method regarding its mathematical solution. To derive the estimate of variable cost, the difference between the mean of the high-cost points and the mean of the low-cost points is divided by the change in output from the mean of the high-cost points to the mean of the low-cost points. In the radiology example, variable cost would be calculated as follows:

Variable labor hours/film =

$$\frac{\dfrac{320 + 230 + 190}{3} - \dfrac{180 + 140 + 110}{3}}{\dfrac{600 + 400 + 340}{3} - \dfrac{300 + 240 + 180}{3}} = \frac{246.67 - 143.33}{446.67 - 240.00} = .50$$

Fixed cost is solved in a manner identical to that used in the high-low method. In the radiology example, fixed labor hours would equal the following:

Fixed labor hours per pay period =
246.67 − (.50 × 446.67) = 23.34

The simple linear regression method (also called least-squares regression) will produce estimates of variable cost (V) and fixed cost (F) that will minimize the variance between predicted and actual observations. In essence, linear regression is a more precise version of the visual-fit method. Rather than fitting a regression line through the scatter plot data by visual inspection, linear regression uses mathematical formulas to fit the regression line. Also, unlike the high-low and semi-averages methods, the least-squares regression method takes all of the data into account when estimating the cost formula.

A general regression would be:

Total Costs = Intercept + (Coefficient × Volume)

Thus, the intercept estimates fixed costs and the regression coefficient estimates variable cost per member. Standard errors from the regression estimates are used to consider whether differences are statistically significant.

Since cost is usually plotted on the vertical axis, the vertical difference between the line and an actual data point is referred to as the estimation error. The regression line that is fitted to the data points is the one that

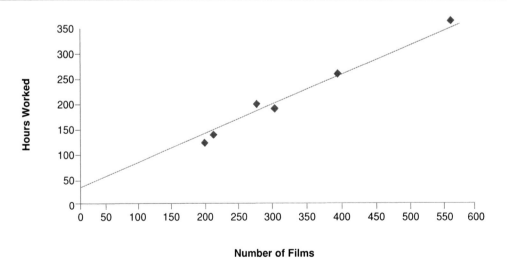

Figure 13-8 Visual Fitting of Radiology Data

minimizes the sum of the squared deviations between the estimated line and actual costs. Although the formulas that accomplish this are fairly complex (shown below), computers and many software programs, such as Excel, easily carry out these calculations. Each data point consists of the observed values of the activity level (or volume) as the X portion of the data point (the independent variable), and the cost associated with that volume level is the Y portion of each data point (the dependent variable). You simply enter the data points into the computer, and with an appropriate command, the computer and software do the rest.

In addition to estimates of the intercept (fixed cost) and slope (variable cost per unit), least-squares regression software ordinarily provides a number of other very useful statistics. One of these statistics is the adjusted R^2, called the coefficient of determination, which is a measure of the "goodness of fit." The adjusted R^2 tells us the percentage of the variation in the dependent variable (cost) that is explained by variation in the independent variable (activity). The adjusted R^2 varies from 0 percent to 100 percent, and the higher the percentage, the better (in terms of a change in the activity level explaining the change in cost).

The formulas for estimation are presented below, where Q refers to output, C refers to cost, and N refers to the number of observations:

1. $V = \dfrac{\sum QC - N\bar{Q}\bar{C}}{\sum Q^2 - N\bar{Q}^2}$

2. $F = \bar{C} - V\bar{Q}$

Applying the previous formulas to the radiology data produces the following estimates:

1. $V = \dfrac{456{,}000 - 401{,}696}{815{,}600 - 707{,}253} = .5012$

2. $F = 195 - (.5012 \times 343.33) = 22.92$

USING EXCEL FOR SIMPLE LINEAR REGRESSION

Microsoft Excel, a popular spreadsheet program, provides several built-in tools that will perform simple linear regression. Illustrated here is just one of those tools. The best way to start is to enter the data points into Excel and graph the data as a scatter plot. In addition to visually depicting the trend in the data with a

regression line, you can also calculate the equation of the regression line. This equation can either be seen in a dialogue box and/or shown on your graph. (Excel can also calculate and display the R^2.) Regression lines can be used as a way of visually depicting the relationship between the independent (x) and dependent (y) variables in the graph. A straight line depicts a linear trend in the data (i.e., the equation describing the line is of first order). (For example, y = 3x + 4.) There are no squared or cubed variables in this equation. A curved line represents a trend described by a higher order equation (e.g., $y = 2x^2 + 5x - 8$). (It is important that you are able to defend your use of either a straight or curved regression line based on the expected cost behavior.)

Figure 13–9 shows the data from the radiology payroll data as entered into Excel (see Table 13–7).[1]

Next, select the data to be graphed (in this case, the range of cells from B6 to C11). Then click on the icon to start Excel's Chart Wizard. Choose the desired chart type. In Figure 13–10, the chart type used in this example is a simple scatter plot. Continue following the prompts of the Chart Wizard until the scatter plot is produced.

Figure 13–11 shows the resulting scatter plot. With the chart selected, one of the menus within Excel is "Chart," which has the "Add Trendline" command. This command is also shown in Figure 13–11. Figure 13–12 shows the pop-up window that appears after selecting the "Add Trendline" command. Under the "Options" tab, the user can choose to have R^2 and the regression equation displayed on the chart (shown in Figure 13–12).

The four methods of estimating variable and fixed costs discussed thus far are relatively simplistic. They are useful in only limited ways to provide a basis for further discussion and analysis of what the true cost behavioral pattern might be. However, in most situations, a limited attempt, based on simplistic methods, is better than no attempt.

A slightly more sophisticated approach is multiple regression, which is an extension of the simple linear regression method. So far, we have assumed that a sin-

---

[1]The Excel examples and screen shots are from Microsoft Excel XP (version 2002) running in Windows 2000 operating system. All of the functions illustrated are available in most recent prior versions of Excel, though the exact way to access the functions might differ.

	A	B	C
1	Radiology Payroll Data		
2			
3	Pay	No. of	Hours
4	Period	Films (x)	Worked (y)
5	1	300	180
6	2	240	140
7	3	400	230
8	4	340	190
9	5	180	110
10	6	600	320
11	Total	2,060	1,170

Figure 13–9 Radiology Payroll Data Entered in Excel Spreadsheet

gle factor such as patient days drives the variable cost component of a mixed cost. This assumption is acceptable for many mixed costs, but in some situations there may be more than one causal factor driving the variable cost element. For example, shipping costs may depend on both the number of units shipped and the weight of the units. In a situation such as this, multiple regression is necessary. Multiple regression is an ana-

lytical method that is used when the dependent variable (e.g., cost) is caused by more than one factor. Although adding more factors, or variables, makes the computations more complex, the principles involved are the same as in the simple least-squares regressions discussed above. Because of the complexity of the calculations, multiple regression is nearly always done with a computer, and is easily done in Excel.

DATA CHECKS

When any of the previous methods are used, several data checks should be performed. First, the cost data being used to estimate the cost behavior pattern should be stated in a common dollar. If the wages paid for employees have changed dramatically from one year to the next, the use of unadjusted wage and salary data from the two years can create measurement problems. In our radiology example, we used a physical quantity measure of cost, namely, hours worked. A physical measure of cost should be used whenever possible.

Second, cost and output data should be matched; the figures for reported cost should relate to the activity of the period. In most situations, accounting records provide this type of relationship based on the accrual princi-

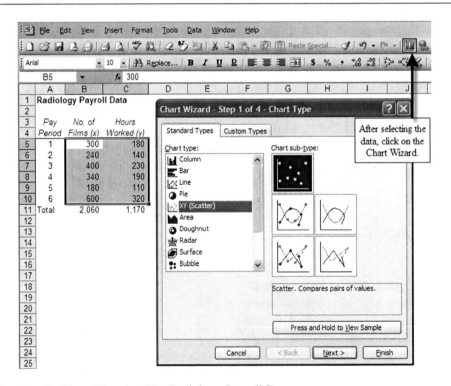

Figure 13–10 Using Excel's Chart Wizard to Plot Radiology Payroll Data

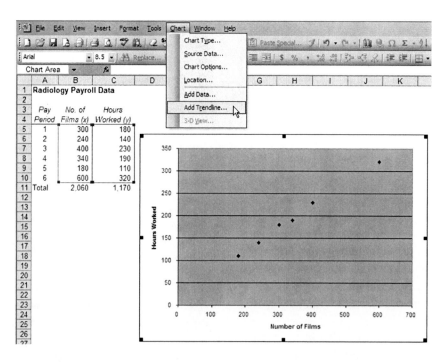

Figure 13–11 Using the "Add Trendline" Command wth Plotted Data in Excel

ple of accounting. However, in some situations, this may not happen; supply costs may be charged to a department when the items are purchased, not when they are used.

Third, the period during which a cost function is being estimated should include stable technology and a case mix. If the technology under consideration has changed dramatically during that period, there will be measurement problems. Estimating a cost function based upon two different production technologies will produce a cost function that reflects neither.

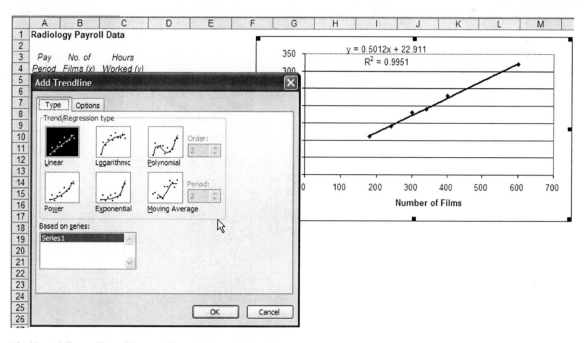

Figure 13–12 Adding a Trendline to Plotted Data in Excel

Calculate break-even volume and the volume necessary to achieve a desired net income.

BREAK-EVEN ANALYSIS

Certain techniques can be applied when analyzing the relationships among cost, volume, and profit. These techniques rely on categorizing costs as fixed and variable. They can serve as powerful management decision aids and may be valuable in a wide range of decisions. An understanding of these techniques is crucial for decision makers whose choices affect the financial results of health care facilities.

Profit in a health care facility is influenced by various factors, including the following:

* Rates or prices
* Volume
* Variable cost
* Fixed cost
* Payer mix
* Bad debts

The primary value of break-even analysis, or, as it is sometimes called, cost-volume-profit (CVP) analysis,

is its ability to quantify the relationships among the previous factors and profit.

Traditional Applications

Break-even analysis has been used in industry for decades with a high degree of satisfaction. Its name comes from the solution to an equation that sets profit equal to zero and revenue equal to costs. To illustrate, assume that a hospital has the following financial information:

Variable cost per case	$1,000
Fixed cost per period	$100,000
Price per case	$2,400

The break-even volume can be solved by dividing fixed costs by the contribution margin, which is the difference between price and variable cost.

$$\text{Break-even volume in units} = \frac{\text{Fixed Cost}}{\text{Price} - \text{Variable cost}}$$

Thus, in our hospital example, break-even volume would be the following:

$$\text{Break-even volume in units} = \frac{\$100,000}{\$2,400 - \$1,000} = 71.4 \text{ cases}$$

If volume exceeds 72 cases, the hospital will make a profit; but if volume goes below 71 cases it will incur a loss. Sometimes, a revenue and cost relationship is

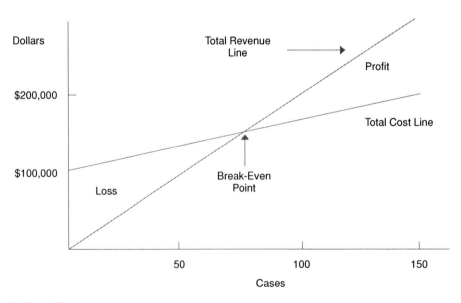

Figure 13–13 Break-Even Chart

put into graphic form to illustrate profit at various levels. Such a presentation is referred to as a break-even chart. For our hospital example, a break-even chart is shown in Figure 13–13.

In many cases, some targeted level of net income or profit is desired. The break-even model is easily adapted to this purpose; the new break-even point would become the following:

$$\text{Break-even volume in units} = \frac{\text{Fixed cost} + \text{Targeted net income}}{\text{Price} - \text{Variable cost}}$$

In our example, assuming that a profit of $6,000 was required, the new break-even point would be the following:

$$\text{Break-even volume in units} = \frac{\$100,000 + \$6,000}{\$2,400 - \$1,000} = 75.7 \text{ cases}$$

Multiple-Payer Model

Although break-even analysis is a powerful management tool, it cannot be used in the health care industry without adaptation. The major revision required relates to the revenue function. The preceding discussion of break-even analysis assumed that there was only one payer or purchaser of services. That payer was assumed to pay a fixed price per unit of product. However, this situation does not exist in the health care industry, where there may be three or more major categories of payers. For our purposes, we will assume that there are three categories of payers:

1. Cost payers (paying average cost of services provided)
2. Fixed-price payers [paying an established fee per unit of service, for example, a fixed price per diagnosis-related group (DRG)]
3. Charge payers (paying on the basis of internally set prices, but maybe discounted)

The break-even formula in these three payer situations can be generalized as follows:

$$\text{Break-even volume in units} = \frac{(1 - CO)F + NI}{(CH \times P_I) \, 1 \, (FP \times P_E) - (1 - CO)V}$$

This formula may look complex at first glance, but it is actually similar to the previous one-payer break-even formula. In fact, the previous equation can be used in the one-payer situation and provides an identical result. To aid in our understanding of the formula, we should first define the individual variables:

V = Variable cost per unit of output
F = Fixed cost per period
NI = Targeted net income
P_I = Internally set price that is paid by charge payers
P_E = Externally set price paid by fixed-price payers
CO = Proportion of cost payers
CH = Proportion of charge payers
FP = Proportion of fixed-price payers

Let us now examine each term in the equation:

- $(1 - CO)F$—This term represents the proportion of fixed costs (F) that is not paid by cost payers. Cost payers are assumed to pay their proportionate share of fixed costs. This leaves the residual portion $(1 - CO)$ unpaid; it is included in the numerator as a financial requirement that must be covered before break even occurs. If there were no cost payers, $(1 - CO)$ would be 1, and all of the fixed costs would be included. This is the case in traditional break-even analysis. For example, a hospital designated as critical access by Medicare would be paid on a cost basis and the term CO could be a large percentage of total business.
- NI—This term, targeted net income, is included as a financial requirement as in the traditional break-even formula. NI is not reduced by the cost payer portion because it is assumed that cost payers are not contributing toward meeting the net income requirement. Cost payers pay cost—nothing less and nothing more.
- $CH \times P_I$—This term represents the weighted price paid by charge payers. When added to the next term $(FP \times P_E)$, we have a measure of the price paid by the two price-paying categories of customers—charge payers and fixed-price payers. It should be emphasized that P_I represents the price received, not the charge made. For example, if ten percent of the patients paid established charges of $2,400 per case and 20 percent paid 90 percent of established charges of $2,400 per case, the following values would result:

$$CH = .10 + .20 = .30$$
$$P_I = (1.0 \times \$2,400) \times 1/3 + (.90 \times \$2,400) \times 2/3 = \$2,240$$

- $FP \times P_E$—This term represents the weighted price paid by fixed-price payers. The addition of this term to $CH \times P_I$ yields a measure of the price received for price-paying patients. The summation of the two terms can be compared with the price term used in the traditional break-even formula. Again, there may be circumstances when sub-weighting may be necessary. For example, assume that Medicare pays $2,000 per case and that 40 percent of the cases are Medicare. Also assume that ten percent of the cases are from a health maintenance organization (HMO) that pays $2,200 per case. The following values would result:

$$FP = .40 + .10 = .50$$
$$P_E = [(.40/.50) \times \$2,000] + [(.10/.50) \times \$2,200] = \$2,040$$

* $(1 - CO)V$—This term represents the net variable cost that remains after reflecting the proportion paid by cost payers. Cost payers pay their share of both fixed and variable costs. If there were no cost payers, the entire value of the variable cost per unit would be subtracted to yield the contribution margin per unit.

To determine that the traditional break-even formula is actually derived from our more general three-payer model, let us compute the break-even point using the data from the case example developed in our discussion of traditional break-even analysis:

Break-even volume in units =

$$\frac{(1 - 0) \times \$100,000 + \$6,000}{(1.0 \times \$2,4000) + (0 \times \$0) - (1 - 0)\$1,000}$$

$$= 75.7 \text{ cases}$$

Now, having tested the accuracy of the three-payer break-even formula in a one-payer situation, let us expand our initial case example to a more realistic multiple-payer situation. The data in Table 13–8 are assumed.

Also assume that the variable cost is $1,000 per case and fixed costs are $100,000 per period. In addition, the firm needs a profit of $6,000 to meet other financial requirements. The use of these data in our break-even model would produce the following result:

Break-even volume in cases =

$$\frac{(.8 \times \$100,000) + \$6,000}{(.3 \times \$2,240) + (.5 \times \$2,040) - (.8 \times \$1,000)}$$

$$= \frac{\$86,000}{\$892} = 96.413$$

Table 13–8 Multiple-Payer Case Example

Payer Proportion	Payment Method
0.20	Pay average cost
0.40	Pay $2,000 per case (fixed-price payer)
0.10	Pay $2,200 per case (fixed-price payer)
0.10	Pay 100 percent of charges, $2,400 per case
0.20	Pay 90 percent of charges, $2,160 per case

To demonstrate the accuracy of the break-even formula, we can derive the following income statement for our case example, assuming 96.4 cases as the break-even volume:

Patient revenue	
.20 × 96.4 × $2,037.34*	$39,279.92
.40 × 96.4 × $2,000.00	77,120.00
.10 × 96.4 × $2,200.00	21,208.00
.10 × 96.4 × $2,400.00	23,136.00
.20 × 96.4 × $2,160.00	41,644.80
Net patient revenue	$202,388.72
Less fixed cost	100,000.00
Less variable cost (96.4 × $1,000)	96,400.00
Net income	$ 5,988.72

*Average cost = ($100,000 + 96,400)/96.4
= $2,037.34

This income statement demonstrates that, at a volume of 96.4 patients, the firm's net income would be $5,988.72. This value does not exactly match the targeted net income level of $6,000 because of a small rounding error; the actual break-even volume was 96.413, not 96.4.

Before concluding this discussion of break-even analysis, it is useful to mention output determination. For the break-even model to be applicable, there must be one measure of output. It makes no difference whether the measure of activity is macro, such as a case, a patient day, or a covered life, or whether the measure of activity is micro, such as a procedure or a laboratory test. The following two conditions, however, are necessary:

1. It must be possible to define an average price paid for that unit for both fixed-price payers and charge payers. For example, both Medicare and

Medicaid may pay a fixed rate per case, but all charge payers may pay some percentage of the billed charges. This would require someone to aggregate average charge-payer amounts for individual billed services to an expected price per case. This might also require an assignment of a per-case amount paid by Medicare to an estimated amount for a specific service, such as a physical therapy treatment, if the focus of analysis was at the treatment level. In a situation of capitation, some transfer price must be established on a per case, per diem, or per procedure basis to apply break-even analysis if an output unit other than members or covered lives is used.

2. A variable cost per unit of the defined output measure also must be established. This may mean aggregating across departments to create a variable cost value for an aggregated output measure such as a case or a patient day. Disaggregation is not nearly as great a problem in variable cost measurement because costing systems usually provide reasonably good detail at the departmental level.

Special Applications

The break-even formula has many applications other than that of computing break-even points. Two specific applications are (1) the computation of marginal profit of volume changes and (2) rate-setting analysis.

Computation of Marginal Profit of Volume Changes

In most business situations, executives are concerned about the impact of volume changes on operating profitability. At the beginning of a budget period, management may not be sure what its actual volumes will be, but it still needs to know how sensitive profit will be to possible swings in volume. If the payer mix is expected to remain constant, the following simple formula can be used to calculate the marginal changes in profit associated with volume swings:

$$\text{Change in profit} = \text{Change in units} \times \text{Profitability index}$$
$$\text{where:}$$
$$\text{Profitability index} = CH(P_I - V) + FP(P_E - V)$$

The profitability index remains constant and is simply multiplied by projected volume change to determine the profit change. Using our earlier case example, the profitability index would be:

$$\text{Profitability index} = .3(\$2,240 - \$1,000) +$$
$$.5(\$2,040 - \$1000) = \$892$$

The value for the profitability index is actually the weighted contribution margin per unit of output. This fact is easily observed by comparing the value calculated previously with that from our three-payer break-even example. The values are the same, $892 in each case. This means that for every one unit change in output the profit will increase on average by $892. An increase of one unit will increase profit by $892, and a decrease of one unit will decrease profit by $892. A useful question to ask at this point is, how large a reduction in volume can the firm experience before its profit decreases to $2,000? Using the preceding formula, the answer would be the following:

$$\text{Change in profit} = \text{Volume change} \times \text{Profitability index}$$
$$(\$6,000 - \$2,000) = \text{Volume change} \times \$892$$
$$\text{Volume change} = 4.48 \text{ cases}$$

If volume decreases by 4.48 cases, the firm's profit will decrease to $2,000. Further analysis could be used to portray other scenarios or to answer other "what-if" type questions. In each case, the resulting data could be displayed in a table or graph.

Rate-Setting Analysis

Rate setting is an extremely important activity for most health care organizations. Rate setting or pricing was briefly covered in Chapter 5 and we will now expand our discussion to incorporate the model parameters just referenced. Usually, the objective of pricing is not usually profit maximization, but rather covering financial requirements. In general, pricing services can be stated in the following conceptual terms:

$$\text{Price} = \text{Average cost} + \text{Profit requirement} +$$
$$\text{Loss on fixed-price patients}$$

If Q represents total budgeted volume in units, we can use our earlier break-even model to develop the following pricing formula:

$$P_I = AC + \frac{NI}{CH \times Q} + \frac{(AC - P_E) \times (FP \times Q)}{CH \times Q}$$
$$\text{where:}$$
$$AC = \text{Average cost per unit} = \frac{F}{Q} + V$$

Again, it is useful to examine the individual terms to understand their conceptual relationship.

* AC—This term represents the average cost per unit. Average cost is the basis on which the firm marks up to establish a price that can meet its financial requirements.
* NI/(CH × Q)—This term divides the target net income (NI) by the number of charge-paying units (CH × Q). This payment source generates the firm's profit. Internally-set prices will not affect the amount of payment received from cost payers or fixed-price payers.
* (AC – P_E) × (FP × Q)/(CH × Q)—This term is complex but has a simple interpretation. The difference between average cost (AC) and the fixed price (P_E) represents an additional requirement that must be covered by the firm's charge-paying units. This difference per unit is then multiplied by total fixed-price payer units (FP × Q) to generate the total loss resulting from selling services to fixed-price payers. Dividing by the number of charge payers (CH × Q) translates this loss into an additional pricing increment that must be recovered from the charge payers on a per unit basis. It is important to note that if the fixed price paid by fixed-price payers (P_E) exceeds average cost (AC), this term will be negative. Prices to the charge payers then could be reduced because the fixed-price payers would be making a positive contribution to the firm's profit requirement.

To test the validity of the pricing formula, let us apply it to the data in our earlier three-payer break-even example. Assume that the volume is 96.4 cases.

$$P_I = \$2,037.34 + \frac{\$6,000}{.3 \times 96.4} + \frac{(\$2,037.34 - \$2,040) \times (.5 \times 96.4)}{.3 \times 96.4}$$

$$= \$2,037.34 + \$207.47 - 4.43 = \$2,240.38$$

The required price as determined previously, $2,240.38, is approximately equal to the price established for charge payers, $2,240. Again, a small discrepancy exists because of rounding errors.

It should be noted that $2,240 is not the actual charge or price set per case. The actual posted charge

is $2,400. PI represents the net amount actually received. Because the firm had one category of charge payers who paid 90 percent of charges, the effective price realized was only $2,240. When using this pricing formula to define hospital charges, the defined price must be increased to reflect write-off due to discounts, bad debts, or charity care. The following general formula represents the mark-up requirement:

$$Price = P_I \div (1 - Write\text{-}off\ proportion)$$

The write-off proportion is not based on total revenue; it is based only on the revenue from charge payers. For example, in our case example, the charge payers represented 30 percent of total cases. Of that 30 percent, 10 percent paid 100 percent of charges and 20 percent paid 90 percent of charges. The write-off percentage is thus the following:

$$(1/3) \times 0 + (2/3) \times .10 = .0667$$

Using this value to mark up the required net price of $2,240 would yield $2,400.

$$\$2,400 = \frac{\$2,240}{1 - .0667}$$

An important issue for many health care organizations concerns the maximization of profit per dollar of rate increase. In a number of states and regions, rate regulations impose restraints on a firm's ability to increase its rates. In addition, boards may wish to minimize rate increases in any given budgetary cycle.

The percentage of any price increase that will be realized as profit can be expressed as follows:

Percent price increase realized as profit =
(Percent charge payers) × (1 − Write-off proportion)
− Physician fee percent

Let us assume that a nursing home is interested in learning what effect a $5 increase in its per diem would have on its profitability. Its present payer mix and write-off proportions are presented in Table 13–9.

Table 13–9 Nursing Home Pricing Data

Payer Percentage	Payer Mode	Write-Off Proportion
10 percent	Medicare—pays fixed charge per diem	N/A
50 percent	Private payer—pays charges	0.1
40 percent	Medicaid—pays fixed charge per diem	N/A

Thus, a $5 per diem increase would generate $2.25 per day in additional profit.

$$50 \text{ percent} \times (1 - .10) = 45 \text{ percent}$$

Evaluating Incremental Profit of New Business

One of the most common examples of the use of marginal analysis methods is evaluating the profitability of new business. Many health care providers are being approached on an almost daily basis with a proposal for a new block of patients. For example, a preferred provider organization (PPO) may present a hospital with the opportunity to be in the PPO's network if the hospital is willing to accept a discount from its present price structure. It is easy to define a conceptual model to organize the financial evaluation of this proposal or a similar one.

Change in profit =
Change in volume × (Price per unit −
Incremental cost per unit) −
(Change in existing price × Volume affected)

The terms are defined as follows:

- Change in volume—In many cases, there will be a reasonably good measure of what the new volume will be. For example, the PPO may be able to deliver 20 new cases per year. It is important to structure a contract that has a volume trigger related to the range of discounts. If high volumes are realized, then the full discount will be granted. However, if volumes are significantly lower than expected, the discount will get smaller. This provides an incentive for the contractor to send as much volume as possible to the provider firm.
- Price per unit—This variable is almost always known with some degree of precision. In many instances, it actually may be a given figure. Prices for services are established in the contract itself.
- Incremental cost per unit—This variable is often difficult to calculate, but not impossible. If the ex-

pected change in volume is relatively small, variable cost per unit would be a good approximation.
- Change in existing price—Once a contract is signed and new business is serviced, there may be a negative effect on existing prices. If the organization has granted a discount to attract the client, it may find that its existing clients will demand similar discounts. In many areas of the country, Blue Cross Blue Shield has a most-favored nation clause that guarantees it the lowest price charged by a hospital. Any hospital that lowers prices to another payer below the Blue Cross payment rate may find itself facing an immediate reduction in price to Blue Cross and a possible lawsuit. The presence of cost payers also will create an automatic reduction in price. As more volume is delivered, the cost per unit will decrease as fixed costs are spread over more units. This means that cost payers will automatically benefit from increases in volume.

SUMMARY

Cost accounting systems can be designed to provide different measures of cost for different decision-making purposes. This is a desirable characteristic, not an exercise in playing with numbers. To understand what measure of cost is needed for a specific purpose, the decision maker must have some knowledge of the variety of alternative concepts of cost. The terms covered in this chapter should be useful in helping decision makers define their needs more precisely.

Break-even analysis presents management with a set of simple analytical tools to provide information about the effects of costs, volume, and prices on profitability. In this chapter, we examined the application of several break-even models for health care providers with three categories of payers. These models should help analysts understand the conceptual framework for improving profitability in their health care organization.

ASSIGNMENTS

1. What are the two major categories of decisions that use cost information?

2. What does it mean to state that a cost is direct?

3. Define the terms variable costs and fixed costs. Give some examples of each.

4. Is it true that indirect costs should never be included in the determination of controllable costs?

5. A hospital is considering using a vacant wing to set up a skilled nursing facility. How might you determine what the cost of the vacant space was if it was used for the skilled nursing facility.

6. A free-standing ambulatory care center averages $60 in charges per patient. Variable costs are approximately $10 per patient, and fixed costs are about $1.2 million per year. Using these data, how many patients must be seen each day, assuming a 365-day operation, to reach the break-even point?

7. You are attempting to develop a break-even for a capitation contract with a major HMO. Your hospital has agreed to provide all inpatient hospital services for 10,000 covered lives. You will receive $38 per member per month (PMPM) to cover all inpatient services. It is anticipated that 93 admissions per 1000 covered lives will be provided with an average length of stay equal to 5.0, or 465 days per 1000.

   You anticipate that your hospital will incur fixed costs, or readiness to serve costs, of $1,860,000 for these 10,000 covered lives. Variable costs per patient day are expected to be $600.

   Calculate the break-even point in patient days under this contract.

8. Your hospital's board of trustees has just determined that the maximum revenue increase it will permit next year is five percent. It also has specified maximum and minimum rate increases by department. Data for the hospital's five departments are depicted in Table 13–10.

Table 13–10 Rate Optimization Data

| | Current Charges | Budgeted Cost | Payer Composition Percentage | | | | Physician Fee | Rate Change Percentage | |
			Cost	Fixed Price	Charge	Bad Debt		Minimum	Maximum
Nursing	$2,000	$2,200	30	30	40	10	0	5	20
Emergency room	200	190	70	10	20	10	0	0	10
Operating room	300	330	35	40	25	20	0	10	25
Laboratory	1,000	750	50	30	20	15	10	−10	20
Anesthesiology	360	300	40	30	30	10	30	0	10
	$3,860	$3,770							

Given the previous information, develop a rate change plan that will maximize the hospital's net income yet still adhere to the board's guidelines.

9. Develop an estimate of fixed and variable costs for labor expenses based on the data presented in Table 13–11. Develop your estimates by using the high-low and semi-averages methods, and simple regression.

Table 13–11 Data for Variable/Fixed Cost Example

Period	Output in Units	Hours Worked
1	16,156	3525
2	19,160	4151
3	17,846	3829
4	20,238	4454
5	21,198	4657
6	14,640	3406

10. An interdepartmental service structure and its direct costs are depicted in Table 13–12. Compute the total costs, direct and allocated, for each of the three revenue centers using the direct and step-down methods of cost apportionment.

Table 13–12 Data for Cost Allocation Example

Department	Direct Costs	Percentage of Service Consumed By					
		S1	S2	S3	R1	R2	R3
Service center 1	$10,000	—	10	10	40	20	20
Service center 2	12,000	10	—	10	20	40	20
Service center 3	10,000	10	10	—	20	20	40
Revenue center 1	30,000						
Revenue center 2	25,000						
Revenue center 3	50,000						

11. Your hospital was denied a contract with an HMO last year. Legal counsel believes that there was a breach of contract and wishes to bring suit against the HMO for damages. The chief executive officer has asked you to work with the controller to develop a defensible measure of the damages experienced during the last year. Explain how you would organize your work to estimate the amount of damages.

SOLUTIONS AND ANSWERS

1. The two major categories of decisions that use cost data are planning and control. Planning decisions usually require costs that are accumulated by program or product line, whereas control decisions usually require costs that are accumulated by responsibility centers or departments.

2. A direct cost can be traced or associated with a specific cost object, usually related to a department or responsibility center.

3. A variable cost changes proportionately with volume. Common examples are materials and supplies. A fixed cost does not change with volume, but remains constant. Common examples are rent, depreciation, and interest. Fixed costs are usually constant only for some "relevant range" of volume. For example, depreciation probably will increase if a facility experiences volume increases that exceed existing capacity.

4. It is not invariably true that indirect costs should never be included in the determination of controllable costs. There are some costs that may be classified as indirect, but could be controlled by a manager. For example, housekeeping costs may be classified as an indirect cost to the physical therapy department. However, the actual amount of housekeeping services required by the physical therapy department may be affected by the actions of the physical therapy department manager.

5. The opportunity cost of the space—that is, its value in the next best alternative use—should be measured. Possible alternative uses might be as physician offices or as sleeping accommodations for patient families.

6. The number of patients that must be seen is 65.75 per day, based on the following calculation:

$$\text{Annual break-even volume} = \frac{1,200,00}{\$50} = 24,000 \text{ patients per year}$$

$$\text{Daily break-even volume} = \frac{24,000}{365} = 65.75$$

7. Fixed annual revenue = 10,000 × $38 × 12   = $4,560,000
   Fixed costs   = $1,860,000
   Variable cost per patient day   = $600

$$\text{Break-even point} = \frac{\$4,560,000 - \$1,860,000}{\$600} = 4500 \text{ patient days}$$

   If utilization is above 4500 patient days, the hospital will lose money. See Figure 13–14 to illustrate this concept.

8. The rate change plan could be developed in the manner depicted in Table 13–13.

   Results of loading as much of the rate increase as possible into nursing are depicted in Table 13–14.

9. Table 13–15 depicts estimates of fixed and variable costs for labor expenses that could be developed.

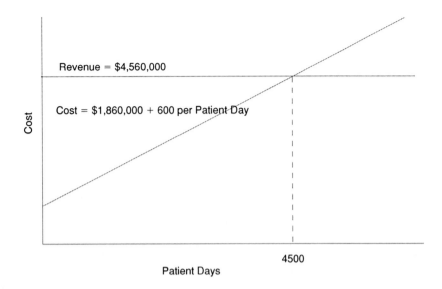

Figure 13-14 Break-Even Point.

Table 13-13 Departmental Price Change
Coefficients

Department	Percentage of Price Realized As Profit
Nursing	40.0% × .9 = 36.0%
Emergency room	20.0% × .9 = 18.0%
Operating room	25.0% × .8 = 20.0%
Laboratory	(20.0% × .85) − 10.0% = 7.0%
Anesthesiology	(30.0% × .9) − 30.0% = −3.0%

Table 13-14 Optimal Departmental Charges

Department	Current Charges	Required Minimum	Additional Charges	Final Charges
Nursing	$2,000	$100	$163	$2,263
Emergency room	200	—	—	200
Operating room	300	30	—	330
Laboratory	1,000	(100)	—	900
Anesthesiology	360	—	—	360
	$3,860	$30	$163	$4,053

Table 13-15 Variable and Fixed Cost Estimates

	Variable Hours/Unit	Fixed Hours
High-low method	0.1908	613
Semi-averages method	0.2093	193
Simple regression	0.1990	375

10. The total costs for the three revenue centers would be as depicted in Table 13–16.

Table 13–16 Solution for Cost Allocation Example

Department	Direct Apportionment Method Direct Costs	S1	S2	S3	Total
Service center 1	$10,000	$10,000	$12,000	$10,000	
Service center 2	12,000				
Service center 3	10,000				
Revenue center 1	30,000	5,000	3,000	2,500	40,500
Revenue center 2	25,000	2,500	6,000	2,500	36,000
Revenue center 3	50,000	2,500	3,000	5,000	60,500
Total	$137,000				$137,000

Department	Step-Down Method Direct Costs	S1	S2	S3	Total
Service center 1	$10,000	$10,000			
Service center 2	12,000	1,000	$13,000		
Service center 3	10,000	1,000	1,444	$12,444	
Revenue center 1	30,000	4,000	2,889	3,111	$40,000
Revenue center 2	25,000	2,000	5,778	6,222	39,000
Revenue center 3	50,000	2,000	2,889	3,111	58,000
Total	$137,000				$137,000

11. A reasonable framework for the estimation of damages would be the equation introduced earlier in this chapter:

$$\text{Change in profit} =$$
$$\text{Change in volume} \times (\text{Price per unit} - \text{Incremental cost per unit}) -$$
$$(\text{Change in existing price} \times \text{Volume affected})$$

The change in volume would be an estimate of the lost volume resulting from the breach of contract. Price per unit could be obtained from a price schedule used by the HMO to pay the hospital or other similar hospitals. Incremental cost per unit could be approximated by variable cost. Finally, if the hospital has cost payers, some recognition must be given to the higher levels of payment made by cost payers because of the lower volumes, which would have raised average cost per unit as a result of the presence of fixed costs. In short, the hospital would have experienced an increase in its existing price from its cost payers.

Chapter 14

Product Costing

LEARNING OBJECTIVES

After studying this chapter, you should be able to do the following:

1. Explain how activity-based costing differs from traditional costing.
2. Describe the relationship between planning, budgeting, and control.
3. Explain the five basic steps of budgeting.
4. Explain the concepts of standard cost profiles, service units, and standard treatment protocols.
5. Explain variance analysis, including why and how it is used by management.
6. Describe the concept of relative value units.

REAL-WORLD SCENARIO*

During the early 1990s, Blue Cross and Blue Shield of Florida, Inc. (BCBSF) faced an increasingly competitive and complex marketplace for its health care products and services, and its management structure and processes did not respond adequately to the market's different needs. To solve this problem, BCBSF identified specific objectives and strategies that divided the state into regions and market segments and sought to improve its management information tools and processes.

BCBSF has a variety of products, customers, and delivery options that demand special services. Because the company has large work units and shared processes, managers need to be able to accurately identify the processes and administrative costs associated with the various products and customers. They do this through the cost for pricing (CFP) cost assignment process.

Each activity in the company is undertaken for one of three general purposes: (1) to build or maintain a product, (2) to serve or sell to a customer, or (3) to perform general corporate duties. Furthermore, all costs incurred by the company must be recovered through the amounts that are charged to customers. Therefore, one policy decision made during the CFP design phase was to allocate all costs to products and customers.

Source: Reprinted with permission from K. L. Thurston, D. M. Deleman, and J. B. MacArthur, "Cost for Pricing at Blue Cross and Blue Shield of Florida." *Management Accounting Quarterly.* Spring 2000: 4–13.

Some of the company's activity costs relate directly to specific products and customers, which makes them easy to allocate if the correct basis (that is, cost driver) data are provided. Other activities are conducted in support of broad categories of customers or products or even other cost centers. The allocations of these activity costs are more difficult to relate to specific products or customers and require that cost center managers identify who is supported and to what extent they consume the cost center resources. Finally, some activities are performed for the company as a whole or for the benefit of all customers and cannot be related to specific products or customers at all. These activity costs are allocated across all customers based on the total corporate activity.

A major advantage of cost for pricing is that it tracks and reports the costs associated with performing activities as they relate to particular products and customers in a timely, customized, and inexpensive manner. For example, the cost of providing customer service activities to a small group customer with a health maintenance organization (HMO) may be different from the cost of providing customer service activities to a larger, multistate customer that has a preferred provider organization (PPO) product. This type of cost information is useful for pricing and profitability analysis. Also, management uses CFP information to identify and analyze cost variances and to benchmark and develop improvement programs. The model allows the company to manage and lower administrative expenses by providing more specific information about where these costs are incurred and their purpose.

For example, the identification and costing of nonvalue-added administrative activities (processing unnecessary forms or performing redundant activities) can prompt management efforts to lower costs through the reduction and eventual elimination of such activities. The resources released could be used to improve the performance of value-added activities. Also, benchmarking may reveal high-cost activities that subsequent investigations show are the result of quality problems. For instance, low-quality explanations by associates to clients about their health insurance or the sale of inappropriate health insurance products to clients may lead to excessive written, telephone, and walk-in inquiries from subscribers. In addition to creating dissatisfied customers, these practices are likely to lead to higher salary costs from the increased staffing needed to address the extra customer service inquiries.

Practically every health care provider expresses a strong and urgent interest in developing better cost accounting systems. The basis for this interest is easy to understand and relates to the nature of payment systems for health care providers. Before 1983, hospitals and many other health care providers were paid on the basis of actual cost. Hospitals, for example, were paid on a cost basis by Medicare, many Blue Cross Blue Shield plans, and most Medicaid programs. In this type of payment environment, costing was important, but allocation of costs to heavily cost-reimbursed areas was emphasized, rather than accurate costing. Reimbursement maximization, not accurate costing, was the primary objective. With the advent of prospective payment systems in the early 1980s and the growing importance of managed care in the late 1980s, hospitals and other health care providers became concerned with the actual cost of service delivery. Providers wanted to know what the actual costs of producing a medical or surgical procedure were so they could compare these costs with the revenue received and make more intelligent decisions about products and product lines.

Interest in costing is not confined to the health care industry. Industry in general has expressed a renewed interest in accurate costing that is related to heightened global competition. Perhaps the most often-used buzz word for improved costing systems in the '90s has been activity-based costing or ABC. ABC is a relatively new term that describes a system of costing that assigns costs to products or customers based on the resources they consume. This is not a new objective. All costing systems try to relate resource consumption to cost objects. The new feature of ABC relates to the identification of activities that are essential to the production of a product or service. It is these activities that are costed and then related to the completed product.

Explain how activity-based costing differs from traditional costing.

ACTIVITY-BASED COSTING

Activity-based costing (ABC) is a costing method designed to provide managers with cost information for strategic and other decisions that potentially affect capacity and therefore "fixed" costs. The managerial accounting field has been migrating away from traditional, department-based costing to activity-based costing (ABC). Most experts agree that ABC should be used as a supplement to, rather than as a replacement for, the company's formal cost accounting system. ABC is now in place in a large number of organizations, including many health systems.

The essence of ABC is that it is not an accounting system, but an economic model. That is to say, ABC does not replace financial accounting or any systems that count the purchase, sale, or use of resources. The same statement can be made for traditional, department- or product-based costing. But unlike traditional methods that "roll-together" information from financial accounting systems, ABC explicitly integrates multiple concepts of resources simultaneously in order to attribute costs to their causes. The following figures depict how ABC fits into the accounting structure of an organization:

1. Activity analysis occurs in the first stage of an ABC model (see Figure 14–1).
2. ABC unbundles the traditional cost view by responsibility center and restates costs according to

how resources are used (see Figure 14–2). ABC traces, and does not allocate, costs.
3. Activity analysis occurs at subsequent stages of an ABC model by further dividing activities into their attributes. The level of analysis varies based upon the use of the information (see Figure 14–3).
4. The "ABC Cross" demonstrates how the information generated under ABC models is used for costing (objects) and management (performance). See Figure 14–4.

Following is a summary set of steps for implementing activity-based costing.

1. Identify and define activities and activity pools.
2. Wherever possible, directly trace costs to activities and cost objects.
3. Assign costs to activity-cost pools.
4. Calculate activity rates.
5. Assign costs to cost objects using the activity rates and activity measures.
6. Prepare management reports.

Traditional cost accounting methods suffer from several defects that can result in distorted costs for decision-making purposes. All costs—even those that are not caused by any specific service/product—are allocated to services. And sometimes indirect costs that are caused by certain services are not assigned to those services. Traditional methods also allocate the costs of idle capacity to products. In effect, products are charged for resources that they do not use. And finally, traditional methods tend to place too much reliance on unit-level allocation bases, such as direct labor and number of procedures. This results in overcosting high-volume products/services and undercosting low-volume products/services and can lead to mistakes when making decisions.

Activity-based costing estimates the costs of the resources consumed by cost objects, such as products and

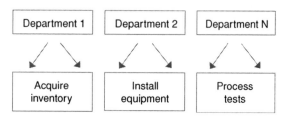

Figure 14–1 First Stage of Activity-Based Costing—Activity Analysis

Chart of Accounts View	
Salaries	600,000
Equipment	210,000
Supplies	40,000
Use and Occupancy	30,000
Total	880,000

Activity-Based View	
Create protocols	21,500
Maintain protocols	37,500
Train employees	21,000
Admit patients	46,000
Provide services	736,000
Transfer patients	18,000
Total	880,000

Figure 14–2 Activity-Based Costing Grouping of Costs Compared with Traditional Methods

customers. The approach taken in activity-based costing assumes that cost objects generate activities that in turn consume costly resources. Activities form the link between costs and cost objects. Activity-based costing is concerned with overhead—both manufacturing overhead and selling, general, and administrative overhead. The accounting for direct labor and direct material is usually unaffected.

A related concept to activity-based costing that increasingly is being adopted by some organizations is activity-based management (ABM). Whereas ABC attempts to measure a single product's true cost, ABM uses cost information to evaluate an entire operation. For both ABC and ABM, retooling the company's information systems to provide the data in such a way as to allow ABC/ABM analysis can be a massive undertaking. An organization must have clear reasons and must expect clear benefits from implementing these systems.

The approach to costing in this chapter builds on the principles of ABC as just described, but we shall refer to activity-based costing concepts more generally as product costing. The critical objective is to determine the cost of resources for either a product or a customer.

LEARNING OBJECTIVE 2

Describe the relationship between planning, budgeting, and control.

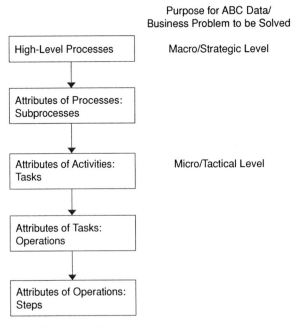

Figure 14–3 Level of Activity Analysis Related to Use

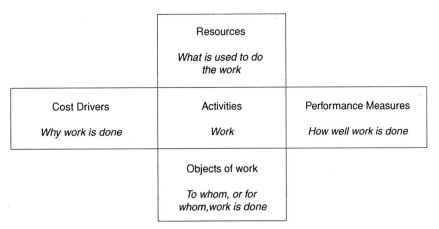

Figure 14–4 ABC Cross—How Activity-Based Costing Information is Used

RELATIONSHIP TO PLANNING, BUDGETING, AND CONTROL

Cost information is of value only as it aids in the management decision-making process. Figure 14–5 presents a schematic that summarizes the planning-budgeting-control process in a business. Of special interest is the decision output of the planning process. The planning process should detail the products or product lines that the business will produce during the planning horizon, typically a period of three to five years.

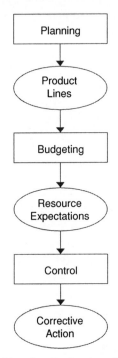

Figure 14–5 The Planning-Budgeting-Control Process

Product and Product Line

The terms "product" and "product line" seem simple and easy to understand regarding most businesses. For example, a finished car is the product of an automobile company; individual types of cars then may be grouped to form product lines, such as the Chevrolet product line of General Motors.

Can this definition of a product be transposed to the health care sector? Many people think that products cannot be defined so easily in health care firms. The major dilemma seems to arise in the area of patients versus products. In short, is the product the patient or is it the individual services provided, such as laboratory tests, nursing care, and meals? In most situations, we believe that the patient is the basic product of a health care firm. This means that the wide range of services provided to patients—such as nursing, prescriptions, and tests—are to be viewed as intermediate products, not final products. There is, in fact, little difference between this interpretation and that applied in most manufacturing settings. For example, automobile fenders are, on one hand, a final product; on the other, they are only an intermediate product in preparation of the final product, the completed automobile. Ultimately, it is the automobile that is sold to the public, not the fenders. In the same vein, it is the treated patient who generates revenue, not the individual service provided in isolation. Indeed, a hospital that provided only laboratory tests would not be a hospital, but rather a laboratory. In short, patients must exist for an individual or an entity to be a health care provider.

Product lines represent an amalgamation of patients in a way that makes business sense. Sometimes people use the term "strategic business units" to refer to areas of activity that may stand alone. For our purpose, a product line is a unit of business activity that requires a go or no-go decision. For example, eliminating one diagnosis related group (DRG) is probably not possible because that DRG may be linked to other DRGs within a clinical specialty area; it may be impossible to stop producing DRG 36 (retinal procedures) without also eliminating other DRGs, such as DRG 39 (lens procedure). Thus, in many cases, it is the clinical specialty, for example, ophthalmology, that defines the product line.

Budgeting and Resource Expectations

The budgeting phase of operations involves a translation of the product-line decisions made earlier into a set of resource expectations. The primary purpose of this is twofold. First, management must assure itself that there will be a sufficient funds flow to maintain financial solvency. Just as you and I must live within our financial means, so must any health care business entity. Second, the resulting budget serves as a basis for management control. If budget expectations are not realized, management must discover why not and take corrective actions. A budget or set of resource expectations can be thought of as a standard costing system. The budget represents management's expectations of how costs should behave, given a certain set of volume assumptions. It is important to remember that it is the forecasted or budgeted costs of a product that are of the greatest interest to management. Historical costs are useful, but only insofar as those costs indicate future costs.

LEARNING OBJECTIVE 3

Explain the five basic steps of budgeting.

The key aspect of budgeting is the translation of product-line decisions into precise and specific sets of resource expectations. This involves five basic steps:

1. Define the volumes of patients by case type to be treated in the budget period.
2. Define the standard treatment protocol by case type.

3. Define the required departmental or activity center volumes.
4. Define the standard cost profiles for departmental or activity center outputs.
5. Define the prices to be paid for resources.

The primary output of the budgeting process is a series of departmental or activity center budgets that explicates what costs should be during the coming budget period. Two separate sets of standards are involved in the development of these budgets (these standards are described later in the chapter).

We will now use a simple, hypothetical nursing home example to illustrate how these five steps would be integrated into the budgeting process. We will assume that our nursing home is a 100-bed facility with a simple organizational structure. It only has three departments: a dietary department, a nursing department, and an administration department.

Define Volumes of Patients (Step 1)

The first step in any budgetary process is to estimate the critical volume statistics. These statistics, when defined, will enable managers to determine levels of activity in each of the departments. In our nursing home example, we will assume that the facility will average 95 percent occupancy, or 34,675 patients, during the next year. For most nursing homes, patient days would be the critical measure of patient volume. In a hospital, it might be discharges, patient days, and outpatient visits. Ideally, these macro measures then would be broken down further into more specific case types. For example, in a nursing home we might categorize patients by their acuity or Resource Utilization Groups (RUGs), whereas a hospital might use DRG categories, and a medical group might use procedure codes.

Define Standard Treatment Protocol (Step 2)

The second step in the budgetary process is to define the relationship between patient volumes and departmental volumes. If 34,675 patients are seen in our nursing home next year, what does that mean in terms of individual departmental activity for the dietary, nursing, and administration departments?

The major connection here is the determination of a "standard treatment protocol." What departmental service is required to provide a patient day of care? In our nursing-home example, we will assume that there are only two real products required to treat a nursing home patient: (1) three patient meals per patient day and (2) two hours of nursing time.

Define Required Departmental Volumes (Step 3)

Given the standard treatment protocol defined in Step 2, it is relatively easy to determine departmental volumes. To treat 34,675 patients, our nursing home will need to provide the following service:

3 Meals × 34,675 = 104,025 Meals in dietary
2 Nursing hours × 34,675 = 69,350 Nursing hours

LEARNING OBJECTIVE 4

Explain the concepts of standard cost profiles, service units, and standard treatment protocols.

Define Standard Cost Profiles (Step 4)

Given the level of activity required in the departments, it is now time to define the "standard cost profiles." This set of standards simply relates departmental volume to expected resource levels. In short, what resources are required to provide a patient day of care? We will assume that the departmental managers have developed the following standard cost profiles. Dietary will be purchasing individual food packages from an outside vendor for every meal.

Dietary
  1 purchased food package
  10 minutes of dietary labor

Nursing
  1 hour of RN labor
  1 hour of aide labor

Administration
  5 full-time equivalents (FTEs) to provide 34,675 patient days of care

You will notice that the administration department has a requirement for resources, but it did not specify any service required in Step 2, the standard treatment protocol specification. There will be a number of areas, such as administration, in which there is no clear connection between service and patient volume. It is possible only on a macro basis to determine staffing or resource profiles for a specified range of activity, for example, 34,675 patient days.

One of the major advantages of ABC cited by proponents is better costing of overhead areas like administration. This better costing results from detailed analysis of the activities performed in the overhead areas. For example, administration may be broken into several patient-related activities, such as billing and purchasing. The costs for these activities then may be traced or assigned directly to the product—a patient day in our nursing home example. At some point, however, most overhead areas cannot be further divided into activity centers with product-traceable outputs, and the remaining costs must be assigned to the products in some reasonable manner.

Define Resource Prices (Step 5)

The last step in completing the budget is to determine the expected resource prices to be in effect during the budget period. Those prices are determined below:

Purchased food package	$4/meal
Dietary labor	$12/hour
RN labor	$30/hour
Aide labor	$16/hour
Administrative labor	$48,000/FTE

Table 14–1 summarizes the completed budget for the nursing home example, assuming that 34,675 patient days of care are provided next year.

Control and Corrective Action

The control phase of business operations monitors actual cost experience and compares it with budgetary

Table 14–1 Nursing Home Budget

Department	Costs
Dietary	
Purchased food packages ($4.00 × 3 × 34,675)	$416,100
Dietary labor ($12 × (1/6) × 3 × 34,675)	208,050
Total dietary	$624,150
Nursing	
RN labor ($30 × 34,675)	$1,040,250
Aide labor ($16 × 34,675)	554,800
Total nursing	$1,595,050
Administration	
Salaries (5 × $48,000)	$240,000
Total cost	$2,459,200

expectations. If there are deviations from expectations, management analyzes the causes of the deviation. If the deviation is favorable, management may seek to make whatever created the variance a permanent part of operations. If the variance is unfavorable, action will be taken in an attempt to prevent a recurrence. Much of the control phase centers around the topic of variance analysis, which is explored in depth in Chapter 16.

THE COSTING PROCESS

Most firms, whether they are hospitals, nursing homes, or steel manufacturers, have similar costing systems. In fact, in most cases, the similarities outweigh the differences. Figure 14–6 presents a schematic of the cost-measurement process that exists in most businesses.

Valuation

Valuation always has been a thorny issue for accountants—one that has not been satisfactorily resolved even today. We need only to consider the current controversy over replacement costs versus historical costs to realize the full problem. For discussion purposes, we have chosen to split the valuation process into two areas: (1) basis and (2) assignment over time. These two areas are not mutually exclusive; to some degree, they overlap. However, both areas determine the total value of a resource that is used to cost a final product.

The valuation basis is the process by which a value is assigned to each and every resource transaction occurring between the entity being accounted for and an-

other entity. In most situations, this value is historical cost.

Having established a basis value for the resource transaction, there are two major types of situations when that value will have to be assigned over time: First, the value may be expended before the actual reporting of expense; the best example of this is depreciation. Second, the expense may be recognized before an actual expenditure. Normal accruals such as wages and salaries are examples of this situation. As the period being costed increases, the problems caused by assignment over time become less severe. For example, if the period being costed is one year, normal accruals for wages and salaries represent a very small percentage of total wage and salary costs. It may be perfectly acceptable to simply use the actual dollar amount paid for wages and salaries. But, if the period being costed is one week, estimates of costs or accruals must be made because no actual wages may have been paid during the one-week period.

Allocation

The end result of the cost-allocation process is the assignment of all costs or values determined during the valuation phase of costing to direct departments. A direct department provides a service or product directly traceable to a patient. Two phases of activity are involved in this assignment: First, all resource values to be recorded as expenses during a given period are assigned or allocated to the direct and indirect departments as direct expenses. Second, once the initial cost assignment to individual departments has been made, a further allocation is required. In this phase, the ex-

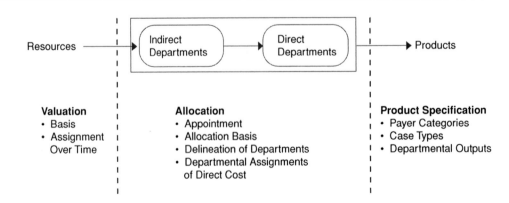

Figure 14–6 The Cost Measurement Process

penses of the indirect departments are assigned to the direct departments.

By using this framework for analysis, costing issues may be subcategorized. In the initial cost-assignment phase, the following two major decisions appear to be involved in the costing process: (1) assigning the cost to departments and (2) defining the indirect and direct departments.

In the first category, a situation may arise in which the departmental structure currently specified is not questioned, but some of the initial value assignments are. For example, premiums paid for malpractice insurance might be charged to administration, or they may be charged directly to the nursing and professional departments that are involved. In the second category, a situation may arise in which the existing departmental structure has to be revised. For example, the administration department may be divided into several new departments, such as nonpatient telephone, data processing, purchasing, admitting, business office, and other. Splitting an existing department into a number of activity centers may greatly improve the costing process and is a significant part of so-called ABC systems. The analysis focuses on the discovery of activities that are related to the products being produced. For example, admitting activities may be a significant activity within the administration department that is clearly traceable to an individual patient. Dividing administration into admitting and other activity centers may greatly improve the accuracy of individual costing and permit management to better measure the actual costs of producing a product. There are numerous examples of overhead departments that could be split into component activities that then may be traced to the patient or procedure being produced.

During the second phase of cost allocation—the reassignment from indirect departments to direct departments—the following two primary decisions are involved: (1) selection of the cost-apportionment method and (2) selection of the appropriate allocation basis. Regarding the first category, cost-apportionment methods—such as step-down, double distribution, and simultaneous equations methods—are simply mathematical algorithms that redistribute cost from existing indirect departments to direct departments, given defined allocation bases. An example of the second type of decision is the selection of square feet or hours worked for housekeeping as an appropriate allocation basis for an indirect department. Sometimes the term "cost driver" is used to describe the selection of an appropriate allocation base. Ideally, the allocation basis selected should be the variable that has the most direct or causal relationship to cost. For example, square feet would not appear to be as accurate an allocation basis or cost driver for housekeeping as hours worked.

Product Specification

In most health care firms, there are two phases in the production (or treatment) process. The schematic in Figure 14–7 illustrates this process and also introduces a few new terms.

In Stage 1 of the production process, resources are acquired and consumed within departments or activity centers to produce a product, defined as a service unit (SU). Here, two points need to be emphasized. First, all departments have SUs, but not all departments have the same number of SUs. For example, the nursing department may provide the following four levels of care: acuity levels 1, 2, 3, and 4. A laboratory, in contrast, may have 100 or more separate SUs that relate to the provision of specific tests. Second, not all SUs can be directly associated with the delivery of patient care; some of the SUs may be only indirectly associated with patient treatment. For example, housekeeping cleans laboratory areas, but there is no direct association between this function and patient treatment. However, the cleaning of a patient's room could be regarded as a service that is directly associated with a patient.

Stage 2 of the production process relates to the actual consumption of specific SUs during the treatment of a patient. Much of the production process is managed by the physician. This is true regardless of the setting (hospital, nursing home, home health care firm, or clinic). The physician prescribes the specific SUs that will be required to treat a given patient effectively.

The lack of management authority in this area complicates management's efforts to budget and control its costs. This is not meant to be a negative criticism of current health care delivery systems; all of us would prefer to have a qualified physician rather than a lay health care executive direct our care. Yet, this is perhaps the area of greatest difference between health care firms and other business entities. Management at General Motors can decide which automobiles will have factory-installed air conditioning and tinted glass, and which will not. In contrast, a health care executive will have great difficulty in attempting to direct a physician to

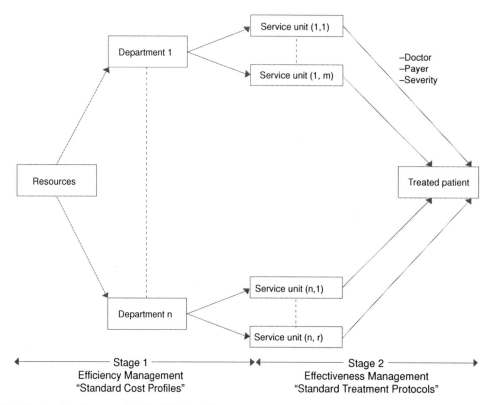

Figure 14-7 The Production Process for Health Care Firms

either prescribe or not prescribe a given procedure in the treatment of a patient.

Health care products to be costed may vary depending on the specific decision being considered. At one level, management may be interested in the cost of a specific SU or departmental output. Prices for some SUs (for example, radiograph procedures) may have to be established, and to do that management must know their costs. In other situations, knowing the cost for one treated patient or for a group of treated patients may be desired. For example, management may wish to bid on a contract to provide home health services to a health maintenance organization (HMO). In this case, it is important for management to understand what the costs of treating HMO patients are likely to be. If the contract is signed, management then needs to determine the actual costs of treating the patients from the HMO to measure the overall profitability from that segment of the business. Alternatively, it may be necessary to group patients by specialty. A hospital may wish to know whether it is losing money from treating a particular DRG entity or some grouping of DRGs, such as obstetrics. This kind of cost information is especially critical to man-

agement decision making related to the expansion or contraction of specific clinical service areas and the recruitment of new medical staff.

STANDARD DEVELOPMENT

The key to successful product costing is management's ability to develop and maintain the following two systems: (1) a system of standard cost profiles and (2) a system of standard treatment protocols. The relationship between these two systems is shown in Figure 14-7. The "linchpin" between them is the SU concept. Specifically, management must know what it costs to produce an SU, and it must know what particular SUs are needed to treat a given patient.

Standard Cost Profiles

The standard cost profile (SCP) is not a new concept; it has been used in manufacturing cost accounting systems for many years. For our purposes, there are two key elements in an SCP: (1) the definition of the SU being costed and (2) the profile of resources required to produce the SU.

As noted earlier, the number of SUs in a given department may vary; some departments may have one, whereas others may have 100 or more. If the number of SUs is very large, however, there may be an unacceptable level of costing detail involved to make the system feasible. In these situations, it may be useful to aggregate some of the SUs. For example, the laboratory may perform 1000 or more tests. In this situation, it may make sense to develop cost profiles for only the most commonly performed tests and to use some arbitrary assignment method for the remaining noncommon tests.

The SU does not have to be a product or service that is directly provided or performed for a patient. Many indirect departments do not provide services or products to the patient; instead, their products or services are consumed by other departments, both direct and indirect. However, many indirect departments have SUs that are provided directly to the patient. For example, the dietary department, often regarded as an indirect department, may not have revenue billed for its product to the patient. However, a meal that the dietary department furnishes to a patient is an SU that is just as direct as a laboratory test or a chest radiograph. In a similar vein, housekeeping may provide cleaning for a patient's room that is, in effect, a direct service consumed by the patient.

Thus, SUs may be categorized as either direct or indirect. A direct SU is associated with a given patient. An indirect SU is provided to another department of the hospital, as opposed to a patient. The differentiation between direct and indirect SUs is important, not only in the development of standard cost profiles, but also in the development of standard treatment protocols. Direct SUs must be identified when standard treatment protocols are defined, whereas indirect SUs need not be specifically identified, although some estimate of allocated cost is often required.

In the development of an SCP for a given SU, the following resource expense categories are listed: (1) direct expenses (labor, materials, and departmental overhead) and (2) allocated overhead. Ideally, the expense also should be categorized as variable or fixed. This distinction is particularly important in certain areas of management decision making, as noted in Chapter 13. Specifically, the differentiation between variable and fixed cost is critical to many incremental pricing and volume decisions. It is also important in flexible budgeting systems and management control. These topics are explored in greater depth in Chapters 15 and 16.

Table 14–2 presents an SCP for a regular patient meal in a dietary department. The total cost of providing one regular patient meal, or SU 181, is $5.40. The variable cost per meal is $2.80, and the average fixed cost per meal is $2.60.

In most situations, direct labor is the largest single expense category. In our dietary meal example, this is not true because the direct material cost, mostly raw food, is larger. It is possible, and in many cases desirable, to define direct labor costs by labor category. Thus, in our dietary meal example, we might provide separate listings for cooks, dietary aides, and dishwashers.

An important point here is the division of cost into fixed and variable quantities. Table 14–2 indicates that

---

Table 14–2 Standard Cost Profile for a Dietary/Regular Patient Meal, Service Unit 181

Cost Category	Quantity Variable	Required Fixed	Unit Cost	Variable Cost	Average Fixed Cost	Average Total Cost
Direct labor	0.05	0.05	$16.00	$0.80	$0.80	$1.60
Direct materials	1.00	0.00	2.00	2.00	0.00	2.00
Department overhead	0.00	1.00	1.00	0.00	1.00	1.00
Allocated costs						
Housekeeping	0.00	0.10	2.00	0.00	0.20	0.20
Plant operation	0.00	1.00	0.20	0.00	0.20	0.20
Administration	0.00	0.02	20.00	0.00	0.40	0.40
Total				$2.80	$2.60	$5.40

.05 units of variable labor time is required per meal, and .05 units of fixed labor is required per meal. (In Chapter 13 we discussed several methods for splitting costs into fixed and variable elements.) The fixed-cost assignment is an average based on some expected level of volume. This is an important point to remember when developing SCPs; a decline in volume below expected levels will increase the average cost of production because the fixed cost is spread over fewer units of output.

The third column of Table 14–2 presents unit cost. This represents management's best guess as to the cost or price of the resources to be used in the production process. Our dietary meal SCP indicates a price of $16 per unit of direct labor. This value reflects the expected wage per hour to be paid for direct labor in the dietary department. Again, it might be possible and desirable to divide direct labor further into specific job classifications. This usually permits better costing, but it also requires more effort.

Any fringe benefit cost associated with labor should be included in the unit cost. For example, the average direct hourly wage in our dietary meal example might be $12.80 per hour, but fringe benefits may average 25 percent of salaries or $3.20 per hour (.25 × $12.80). In this case, the effective wage would be $16 per hour, which is the reported cost per hour in Table 14–2.

Departmental overhead consists of expenses that are charged directly to a department and do not represent either labor or materials. Common examples are equipment costs, travel allowances, expenses for outside-purchased services, and cost of publications. Usually, these items do not vary with level of activity or volume, but remain fixed for the budgetary period. If this is the case, assignment to an SCP can be based on a simple average. For example, assume that our dietary department expects to provide 200,000 regular patient meals next year. Assume further that the department has been authorized to spend $200,000 in discretionary areas that constitute departmental overhead. The average cost per meal for these discretionary costs would be $1.00 and would be fixed.

Allocated costs are probably the most difficult to assign in most situations. In our dietary example, we include only three allocated cost areas. This is probably a low figure; a number of other departments most likely would provide service to the dietary department and should be properly included in the SCP.

There are two major alternatives to using estimates of allocated costs in an SCP. First, individual costing studies could be performed, and services from one department to another could be recorded. This process may be expensive, however, and not worth the effort. For example, if separate meters were installed, utility costs could be associated with each user department. However, the installation of such meters is probably not an effective expenditure of funds; costing accuracy would not be improved enough to justify the extra expenditure.

The second alternative would be a simple averaging method. All overhead costs might be aggregated and apportioned to other departments on the basis of direct expenses, FTEs, or some other criterion. This method is relatively simple, but its accuracy would be suspect if significant variation in departmental utilization exists.

We believe that the best approach to costing is to identify all possible direct SUs. These SUs, which can be directly associated with a patient, are much more numerous than one would expect. For example, a meal provided to a patient is a direct SU, but is currently treated as an indirect product in most costing systems. Laundry and linen departments have certain SUs that are directly associated with a patient, such as clean sheets and gowns. Housekeeping provides direct services to patients when its personnel clean rooms. The administration and medical records departments also provide specific direct services to patients in the form of processed paper work and insurance forms. If such costs, currently regarded as indirect, were reclassified as direct, there would be a substantially lower level of indirect costs that would require allocation. This would improve the costing of patients—the health care product—and make the allocation of indirect costs less critical. Currently, indirect costs in many health care settings are in excess of 50 percent of total cost. With better identification of services or SUs, we believe that level could be reduced to 25 percent or lower. This identification of services or activities is the "heart" of ABC costing systems.

Standard Treatment Protocols

There is an analogy between a standard treatment protocol (STP) and a job-order cost sheet used in industrial cost accounting. In a job-order cost system, a separate cost sheet is completed for each specific job. This is necessary because each job is different from jobs performed in the past and jobs to be performed in the future. Automobile repairs are an excellent example of a job-order cost system. A separate cost sheet is prepared for each job. That cost sheet then serves as the bill or invoice to the customer.

Health care firms also operate in a job-cost setting. Patient treatment may vary significantly across patients. The patient's bill may be thought of as a job-order cost sheet in that it reflects the actual services provided during the course of the patient's treatment. Of course, not all of the services provided are shown in the patient's bill. For example, meals provided are rarely charged for as a separate item.

In a typical job-order cost setting, standards may not always be applied. When you leave your car at the dealership for servicing, the dealer does not prepare a standard job-order cost sheet. Dealers have no incentive to do this because they expect that customers will pay the actual costs of the service when they pick up their cars. If they do not, the dealer may take possession of the car as collateral.

In the past, a similar situation existed among health care firms; the client or patient would pay for the actual cost of services provided. Today, this is no longer true for the majority of health care products. Today, most health care firms are paid a fixed fee or price regardless of the range of services provided. Medicare's DRG payment system is an example of this type of payment philosophy. Health care providers who have accepted capitation have an additional dilemma because cost is now a function of both utilization and cost per episode. The provider must estimate the number of episodes of care, as well as the cost per episode. It is similar to an automobile manufacturer providing a warranty. The manufacturer must determine both the frequency of claims and the average cost per claim.

Little revenue realized by a health care provider is derived from cost payers in today's marketplace; and the majority of revenue is fixed price on either a case, per diem, procedure, or capitated basis. Because the revenue is fixed, understanding the cost of a treatment protocol is essential to effective management. Table 14–3 shows a hypothetical STP for DRG 208 (disorder of biliary tract). (This STP is for illustrative purposes only; it should not be regarded as a realistic STP for DRG 208.) In this STP, costs are split into fixed and variable components. Thus, the STP requires 25 patient meals at a variable cost of $2.80 per meal and a fixed cost of $2.60 per meal. The basis for these data is the SCP (see Table 14–2). As noted earlier, this division between fixed and variable costs is extremely valuable for management when it makes its planning and control decisions. For example, if Medicare paid the hospital $2,800 for every DRG 208 patient treated, we would conclude that, at least in the short run, the hospital would be financially

better off if it continued to treat DRG 208 cases, because the payment of $2,800 exceeds the variable cost of $2,034 and the hospital is therefore making a contribution to fixed costs.

Table 14–3 depicts two areas in which no actual quantity is specified: pharmacy prescriptions and other laboratory tests. In these instances, the total cost of the services is instead divided between fixed and variable costs. Because of the large number of products provided in each of these two areas, it would be impossible to develop an SCP for each product item. However, some of the heavier volume laboratory tests or pharmacy prescriptions may be separately identified and costed; for example, laboratory complete blood count is listed as a separate SU.

Some of the items shown in Table 14–3 may not be reflected in a patient's bill. For example, patient meals, linen changes, room preparation, and admission processing, usually would not be listed in the bill. Also, separation of nursing care by acuity level may not be identified in the bill; many hospitals do not distinguish between levels of nursing care in their pricing structures.

A final point to emphasize is that not all SUs will show up in an STP. Only those SUs that are classified as direct are listed. A direct SU can be directly traced or associated with patient care. The costs associated with the provision of indirect SUs are allocated to the direct SUs. At the same time, the objective should be to create as many direct SUs as possible. The creation of traceable SUs is one of the objectives of ABC systems.

LEARNING OBJECTIVE 5

Explain variance analysis, including why and how it is used by management.

VARIANCE ANALYSIS

In general, given the systems of standards discussed previously (SCPs and STPs), the following four types of variances may be identified in the variance analysis phase of control:

1. Price (rate)
2. Efficiency
3. Volume
4. Intensity

Table 14-3 Standard Treatment for DRG 208/Disorder of Biliary Tract

Service Unit No.	Service Unit Name	Quantity	Variable Cost/ Unit	Fixed Cost/ Unit	Total Cost/ Unit	Total Variable Cost	Total Fixed Cost	Total Cost
1	Admission process	1	$96.00	$104.00	$100.00	$96.00	$104.00	$200.00
7	Nursing care level 1	1	160.00	80.00	240.00	160.00	80.00	240.00
8	Nursing care level 2	7	170.00	90.00	260.00	1,190.00	630.00	1,820.00
9	Nursing care level 3	1	220.00	90.00	310.00	220.00	90.00	310.00
29	Pharmacy prescriptions		76.00	38.00	114.00	76.00	38.00	114.00
38	Chest radiograph	1	24.00	16.00	40.00	24.00	16.00	40.00
46	Laboratory complete blood count	1	8.00	7.00	15.00	8.00	7.00	15.00
49	Other laboratory tests		170.00	110.00	280.00	170.00	110.00	280.00
57	Patient meals	25	2.80	2.60	5.40	70.00	65.00	135.00
65	Linen changes	5	1.20	1.00	2.20	6.00	5.00	11.00
93	Room preparation	1	14.00	6.00	20.00	14.00	6.00	20.00
Totals						$2,034.00	$1,151.00	$3,185.00

The first three types of variances are a direct result of the development of the SCPs; they are the product of departmental activity. A rate or price variance is the difference between the price actually paid and the standard price multiplied by the actual quantity used. The equation is as follows:

Price variance = (Actual price − Standard price) × Actual quantity

For example, assume that our dietary department of Table 14–2 produced 1500 patient meals for the period in question when budgeted volume was 1600 meals. To produce these meals, it used 180 hours of labor and paid $16.50 per hour. In this case, the price or rate variance would be the following:

($16.50 − $16.00) × 180 hours = $90.00

This variance would be unfavorable because the department paid $16.50 per hour when the expected rate was $16.00.

An efficiency variance reflects productivity in the production process. It is derived by multiplying the difference between actual quantity used and standard quantity by the standard price:

Efficiency variance = (Actual quantity − Standard quantity) × Standard price

In our dietary example, the efficiency variance would be

(180 hours − 155 hours) × $16 = $400

Standard labor is derived by multiplying the variable labor requirement of .05 by the number of meals produced, or 1500. This means that expected or standard variable hours required would be 75 hours (.05 × 1500). The budgeted fixed-labor requirement of 80 hours is added to the variable labor requirement to produce a total labor requirement of 155 hours (80 + 75). In our example, the department used 25 more hours of labor than had been expected. As a result, it incurred an unfavorable efficiency variance of $400.

The volume variance reflects differences between expected output and actual output. It is a factor to be considered in situations involving fixed costs. If no fixed costs existed, the resources required per unit would be constant. This would mean that the cost per unit of production should be constant. For most situations, this is not a reasonable expectation; normally, fixed costs are present.

The volume variance is derived by multiplying the expected average fixed cost per unit by the difference between budgeted volume and actual volume. The equation is as follows:

Volume variance = (Budgeted volume − Actual volume) × Average fixed cost per unit

In the case of direct labor in our dietary example, the volume variance would be an unfavorable $80 assuming budgeted volume was 1500 patient days:

(1,600 − 1,500) × $.80 = $80

Notice that in our example, the total of these variances equals the difference between actual costs incurred for direct labor and the standard cost of direct labor assigned to the SU, a patient meal:

Actual direct labor	
($16.50 × 180 hours)	$2,970
Less standard cost	
($1.60 × 1500 meals)	2,400
Total variance	$570
Price variance	$90.00
Efficiency variance	400.00
Volume variance	80.00
Total variance	$570.00

The intensity variance is the difference between the quantity of SUs actually required when treating a patient and the quantity necessary in the STP. For example, if 20 meals were provided to a patient categorized in DRG 208, there would be a favorable variance of five meals, given the STP data of Table 14–3 which forecast 25 meals per each case of DRG 208.

Intensity variances are generically defined as follows:

Intensity variance = (Actual SUs − Standard SUs) ×
Standard cost per SU

Thus, in our example, the intensity variance for the DRG 208 patient regarding meals would be a favorable $27.00 ([20 meals − 25 meals] × $5.40).

It may be useful to divide intensity variances into fixed and variable elements. In our example, it is probably not fair to state that $27.00 was saved because five fewer meals were delivered. Five times $2.80, the variable cost, may be a better reflection of short-term realized savings.

One final statement about variance analysis: It is important to specify the party responsible for variances. This is, after all, part of the rationale for standard costing—to be able to take corrective action through individuals to correct unfavorable variances. In our example, three variances—price, efficiency, and volume—are distinguished in the departmental accounts. However, the department manager may not be responsible for all of this variation, especially in the volume area. Usually, department managers have little control over volume; they merely react to the volume of services requested from their departments.

The intensity variance can be largely associated with a given physician. Most of the SUs are of a medical nature, resulting from physician decisions regard-

ing testing or length of stay (LOS). It may be helpful, therefore, to accumulate intensity variances by physicians. Periodic discussions regarding these variations can be most useful to both the health care executive and the physician. Ideally, physicians should participate actively in the development of STPs.

LEARNING OBJECTIVE 6

Describe the concept of relative value units.

RELATIVE VALUE UNIT COSTING

In a number of settings, the costing of individual products is difficult to accomplish and may not be worth the time and effort required. For example, medical groups often produce a large number of different medical procedures. Ancillary providers, such as laboratories or imaging centers, may produce hundreds of different procedures. Costing of any specific procedure is virtually impossible. Imagine for a moment the effort involved in costing a routine visit to a physician's office. Once you identified the individual activities involved in the delivery of service and the indirect support costs associated with service delivery, it would be an accounting "nightmare" to assign those costs to 100 or more procedures routinely performed in the doctor's office.

One solution that is used in many settings is relative value unit (RVU) costing. In RVU costing, some relative weights are assigned for each of the commonly-produced outputs. For medical groups, the most commonly-accepted classification of outputs is current procedural terminology (CPT) codes. Medicare uses CPT codes in its resource-based relative value system discussed in Chapter 2. These assigned weights can be used to cost individual procedures. For example, consider an ophthalmology practice that performs only two procedures (Table 14–4).

If we assume that the total expenses of the practice are presented as in Table 14–5, we then could develop a cost per procedure using the RVU concept.

The cost for each of the two procedures would then be calculated as shown in Table 14–6.

Various types of budgets then can be produced based on RVU weights. RVU-weighted office visits or procedures are ones that have been adjusted for the

Table 14–4 Relative Value Weights

CPT #	Number of Procedures	Physician Work Weight	Total Work Units	Practice Weight	Total Practice Units	Malpractice Weight	Total Malpractice Units
67800	1,000	1.5	1,500	1.0	1,000	0.05	50
66985	500	8.5	4,250	14.0	7,000	0.75	375
Total	1,500		5,750		8,000		425

Table 14–5 Cost per Weighted Procedure

	Total Expenses	Total Weighted Units	Cost Per Weighted Unit
Physician compensation	$200,000	5,750	$34.78
Practice expenses	450,000	8,000	56.25
Malpractice expense	7,500	425	17.65

amount of resources they consume. It is necessary to make these adjustments because various types of visits and procedures require different resources. Each organization must develop its own appropriate categorization scheme that applies to its services.

Table 14–6 Cost per Procedure

	CPT 67800	CPT 66985
Physician work units	1.50	8.50
× cost per unit	$34.78	$34.78
Physician cost per procedure	$52.17	$295.63
Practice work units	1.00	14.00
× cost per unit	$56.25	$56.25
Malpractice cost per procedure	$56.25	$787.50
Malpractice work units	0.05	0.75
× cost per unit	$17.65	$17.65
Malpractice cost per procedure	$0.88	$13.24
Total cost per procedure	$109.30	$1,096.37

SUMMARY

Product costing has become much more critical to health care executives today than it was before 1983. The emphasis on prospective prices and competitive discounting creates a real need to define costs. For health care purposes, the product is a treated patient. Various aggregations of patients also may be useful. For example, we may want to develop cost data by DRG, by clinical specialty, or by payer category.

To develop a standard cost system in a health care firm, two sets of standards must be defined. First, a series of SCPs must be developed for all SUs (intermediate departmental products) produced by the firm. This part of standard costing is analogous to that of most manufacturing systems. Second, a set of STPs must be defined for major patient-treatment categories. These STPs must identify all the service units to be provided in the patient treatment. Physician involvement is critical in this area.

The purpose of standard costing is to make planning decisions, such as those involved in pricing and product mix, more precise and meaningful. Standard costing is also useful when making control decisions. Variance analysis is based on the existence of standard cost and the periodic accumulation of actual cost data. Timely analysis of variances can help management achieve desired results.

ASSIGNMENTS

1. An HMO has asked your hospital to provide all of its obstetric services. It has offered to pay your hospital $2,000 for a normal vaginal delivery, without complications (DRG 373). You have looked at the STP for this DRG and discovered that your hospital's cost is $2,400. What should you do?

2. Dr. Jones is scheduled to meet with you this afternoon. She has been an active admitter, but you would like to see her practice increase. After reviewing Dr. Jones' financial report, shown in Table 14–7, what recommendations would you make?

3. Using the data presented in Table 14–8, explain why some DRGs have negative values for deductions.

4. In Table 14–8, DRG 14 has the largest revenue of all the case types listed, yet it lost money. Why?

5. The data in Table 14–9 represent a cost accountant's effort to define the variable cost for DRG 104 (cardiac valve procedures with cardiac catheter). Evaluate this method.

Table 14–7 Dr. Jones' Financial Report

DRG Number	Type Description	No. of Discharges	ALOS*	Comp. LOS*	LOS Var	Total Charges	Deductions	Net Revenue	Variable Cost	Gross Margin	Fixed Cost	Net Income
0316	Renal failure	7	11.7	6.7	5.0	$19,371	$4,484	$14,887	$7,372	$7,515	$6,926	$589
0315	Other kidney & urinary tract O.R. procedures	5	42.4	12.7	29.7	28,945	6,270	22,675	12,375	10,300	8,866	1,434
0468	Extensive O.R. procedure unrelated to principal diagnosis	5	32.2	11.3	20.9	87,309	12,739	74,570	33,421	41,149	30,955	10,194
0130	Peripheral vascular disorders w CC	3	6.0	8.8	-2.8	8,166	1,834	6,332	3,055	3,277	3,297	(20)
0138	Cardiac arrhythmia & conduction disorders w CC	3	4.3	7.4	-3.1	3,524	1,027	2,497	1,351	1,146	985	161
0182	Esophagitis, gastroent & misc digest disorders age >17 w CC	3	7.3	6.7	0.6	14,171	3,427	10,744	5,308	5,436	5,503	(67)
0331	Other kidney & urinary tract diagnoses age >17 w CC	3	8.7	7.6	1.1	10,983	2,539	8,444	3,900	4,544	4,390	154
0024	Seizure & headache age >17 w CC	2	16.0	6.8	9.2	4,625	1,156	3,469	1,651	1,818	1,459	359
0127	Heart failure & shock	2	4.0	10.4	-6.4	1,827	592	1,235	606	629	348	281
0140	Angina pectoris	2	7.0	6.6	0.4	5,290	1,179	4,111	2,079	2,032	1,765	267
0188	Other digestive system diagnoses age >17 w CC	2	9.5	6.5	3.0	4,733	1,148	3,585	1,551	2,034	1,926	108
0296	Nutritional & misc metabolic disorders age >17 w CC	2	8.0	8.9	-0.9	2,840	625	2,215	1,103	1,112	995	117
0321	Kidney & urinary tract infections age >17 w/o CC	2	23.0	4.6	18.4	12,377	248	12,129	4,103	8,026	4,505	3,521
0442	Other O.R. procedures for injuries w CC	2	6.5	11.6	-5.1	11,415	2,629	8,786	4,533	4,253	4,082	171
0443	Other O.R. procedures for injuries w/o CC	2	8.5	5.6	2.9	8,974	2,227	6,747	3,392	3,355	3,225	130
0452	Complications of treatment w CC	2	44.5	6.0	38.5	1,827	482	1,345	562	783	693	90
0467	Other factors influencing health status	2	1.5	3.1	-1.6	1,461	396	1,065	452	613	518	95
0010	Nervous system neoplasms w CC	1	35.0	13.5	21.5	267	99	168	62	106	35	71
0016	Nonspecific cerebrovascular disorders w CC	1	8.0	11.0	-3.0	4,984	1,093	3,891	2,064	1,827	2,034	(207)
0066	Epistaxis	1	7.0	4.6	2.4	302	112	190	86	104	68	36
0085	Pleural effusion w CC	1	19.0	12.1	6.9	675	251	424	393	31	220	(189)
0088	Chronic obstructive pulmonary disease	1	3.0	9.1	-6.1	2,634	694	1,940	1,087	853	946	(93)
0112	Percutaneous cardiovascular procedures	1	9.0	26.2	-17.2	6,357	1,380	4,977	2,445	2,532	2,482	50
0120	Other circulatory system O.R. procedure	1	71.0	16.4	54.6	10,448	3,461	6,987	2,862	4,125	2,178	1,947
0143	Chest pain	1	6.0	4.2	1.8	5,659	1,179	4,480	2,333	2,147	2,070	77
0144	Other circulatory system diagnoses w CC	1	2.0	9.3	-7.3	2,085	439	1,646	858	788	713	75
0152	Minor small & large bowel procedures w CC	1	93.0	13.7	79.3	1,084	403	681	241	440	149	291
0171	Other digestive system O.R. procedures w CC	1	35.0	6.9	28.1	2,136	793	1,343	555	788	358	430
0175	G.I. hemorrhage w/o CC	1	6.0	5.8	0.2	3,734	883	2,851	1,676	1,175	1,027	148
0224	Shoulder, elbow, or forearm proc, exc major joint proc, w/o CC	1	23.0	4.3	18.7	10,977	5,544	5,433	3,672	1,761	4,165	(2,404)
OP 30	Case types	62	17.9	8.6	9.3	$279,180	$59,333	$219,847	$105,148	$114,699	$96,883	$17,816

*ALOS = average length of stay. LOS = length of stay.
  See Appendix 2-B for key to abbreviations.

Table 14–8 Financial Statement by DRG Category

DRG Number	Description	Total Charges	Total Deductions	Net Revenue	Variable Cost	Total Gross Margin	Margin Percent	Fixed Cost	Net Income	Income Percentage
0001	Craniotomy age >17 except for trauma	$14,115	$3,317	$10,798	$4,709	$6,089	43.1	$4,192	$1,897	13.4
0002	Craniotomy for trauma age >17	1,170	435	735	302	433	37.0	220	213	18.2
0004	Spinal procedures	5,553	(251)	5,804	2,278	3,526	63.5	1,596	1,930	34.8
0005	Extracranial vascular procedures	14,814	2,310	12,504	5,641	6,863	46.3	4,898	1,965	13.3
0006	Carpal tunnel release	12,488	1,991	10,497	4,441	6,056	48.5	4,649	1,407	11.3
0007	Periph & cranial nerve & other nerv syst proc w CC	2,586	(1,900)	4,486	586	3,900	150.8	424	3,476	134.4
0008	Periph & cranial nerve & other nerv syst proc w/o CC	6,742	605	6,137	2,577	3,560	52.8	2,806	754	11.2
0010	Nervous system neoplasms w CC	36,194	5,602	30,592	13,594	16,998	47.0	13,625	3,373	9.3
0011	Nervous system neoplasms w/o CC	9,075	2,869	6,206	3,058	3,148	34.7	2,885	263	2.9
0012	Degenerative nervous system disorders	49,084	11,628	37,456	18,392	19,064	38.8	18,500	564	1.1
0013	Multiple sclerosis & cerebellar ataxia	4,249	532	3,717	1,448	2,269	53.4	1,417	852	20.1
0014	Specific cerebrovascular disorders except tia	129,884	37,434	92,450	48,146	44,304	34.1	45,014	(710)	-0.5
0015	Transient ischemic attack & precerebral occlusions	39,989	10,813	29,176	13,768	15,408	38.5	14,098	1,310	3.3
0016	Nonspecific cerebrovascular disorders w CC	7,272	1,713	5,559	2,855	2,704	37.2	2,496	208	2.9
0017	Nonspecific cerebrovascular disorders w/o CC	544	11	533	147	386	71.0	223	163	30.0
0018	Cranial & peripheral nerve disorders w CC	12,807	895	11,912	4,305	7,607	59.4	4,680	2,927	22.9
0019	Cranial & peripheral nerve disorders w/o CC	4,083	(160)	4,243	1,311	2,932	71.8	1,535	1,397	34.2
0020	Nervous system infection except viral meningitis	8,246	619	7,627	2,405	5,222	63.3	2,519	2,703	32.8
0021	Viral meningitis	3,443	1,334	2,109	1,180	929	27.0	971	(42)	-1.2
0022	Hypertensive encephalopathy	589	147	442	194	248	42.1	135	113	19.2

Table 14–9 Format for Defining Variable Cost for DRG 104 (Cardiac Valve Procedures with Cardiac Catheter)

Department	Average Charges	Ratio of Direct Costs to Charges	Estimated Costs	Estimated Variable Costs (As Percent of Total Estimated Costs)	Estimated Variable Costs
General nursing	$1,240	0.71	$880	70	$616
Special care unit	1,810	0.68	1,231	70	862
Central supply	180	0.28	50	75	38
Laboratory	270	0.47	127	10	13
EKG	50	0.37	19	20	4
EEG	60	0.38	23	20	5
Nuclear medicine	190	0.37	70	30	21
Diagnostic radiology	95	0.38	36	25	9
Operating room	650	0.47	306	65	199
Emergency department	105	0.49	51	40	21
Transfusion	405	0.63	255	70	179
Pharmacy	320	0.28	90	75	67
Anesthesiology	180	0.44	79	30	24
Respiratory therapy	295	0.35	103	25	26
Physical therapy	85	0.61	52	25	13
Clinic	110	0.53	58	30	17
Totals	$6,045		$3,430		$2,114

SOLUTIONS AND ANSWERS

1. Hopefully, the STP for DRG 373 separates the costs into variable and fixed elements. If the variable cost is less than $2,000, your hospital may earn some marginal profit from the additional business. However, it would be useful to get some idea of current experience for the HMO's current population. There may be some patient-management differences, especially regarding length of stay that could result in more or less cost.

2. Most of the income generated by Dr. Jones is in areas where the LOS is significantly above the normal level. For example, DRGs 468, 321, and 120 accounted for 85 percent of the total income that she generated for the hospital. In each of these three DRG categories, her lengths of stay were well above normal. Because these cases were profitable, they must not have been billed to Medicare. If it is likely that some of your major payers may shift to a prospective case payment basis, you may not want to encourage Dr. Jones to increase her practice. The data in her financial report indicate a relatively high LOS in almost all areas.

3. DRG 7 has a minus $1,900 deduction. This means that payment received for treating this DRG category exceeded charges by $1,900. This probably reflects payment by Medicare in excess of charges. This situation may change if other hospitals have a similar experience because Medicare may change its payment. Presently, however, DRG 7 is a profitable product for the hospital (134.4 percent).

4. The deductible provision provides one reason why DRG 14 lost money. Approximately 29 percent of the DRG charges were written off. You may want to pay special attention to the firm's STP for this case type. Perhaps the firm's LOS or ancillary services are excessive.

5. The first potential weakness in the cost accountant's method is the use of a cost-to-charge ratio. There is no guarantee that charges for departmental services always will be related to costs. Use of a cost to charge method assumes that all procedures within a department are priced at a constant markup from cost. Often, this is not true because some procedures may have higher markups. A hospital may raise prices more on procedures with a higher percentage of patients who pay on a billed charges basis. The cost-to-charge method may also miss a large block of indirect departmental costs that may be variable. Finally, the method simply does not relate well to the two-stage definition of standard costs involving SCPs and STPs, as discussed in this chapter. In fairness, it must be noted that the cost accountant's method would cost significantly less than other methods, and it is not clear whether the improved accuracy that might result from some other, more sophisticated, system would be worth the extra cost.

Chapter 15

The Management Control Process

LEARNING OBJECTIVES

After studying this chapter, you should be able to do the following:

1. Define a budget and describe how management uses it.
2. Explain the concept of management control and how budgeting is used as part of it.
3. List sources of differences between budgeted and actual amounts.
4. Explain the budgeting process.
5. List the major types of budgets and describe how they are used.
6. Describe the concept of zero-base budgeting.
7. Explain how benchmarking is performed at the department level.

REAL-WORLD SCENARIO

James Olin has been recently named supervisor of the endoscopy lab. He has compared recent cost reports with his departmental budget; he is especially interested in his labor costs over the last three biweekly cost periods, which have shown increasingly unfavorable variances. A summary of the data James is reviewing is shown below:

	Period 1	Period 2	Period 3
Procedures	330	315	300
Actual Hours Worked	4310	4251	4193
Budgeted Hours	4290	4095	3900
Difference	20 Unfavorable	156 Unfavorable	293 Unfavorable
Budgeted Hours per Procedure	13.0	13.0	13.0
Hours Worked per Procedure	13.1	13.5	14.0

The budgeted value for worked hours per procedure is 13.1 and James can see that his labor hours utilization variance is increasing and becoming more unfavorable. The CFO has also noticed the unfavorable variation in James's area and has asked for an explanation and a plan to bring his actual costs in line with budgeted values. While James is new to his role as supervisor, he has been involved in the department for five years as a nurse and is very familiar with the operation. It is his opinion that there is no excess labor and that his employees are stretched to their limits already. A reduction in staff of 293 hours during the last biweekly pay period to meet budget would have removed 3.66 FTEs and put a tremendous strain on the department's ability to provide quality care on a timely basis. James is further confused because he already cut his work force by 117 hours, or nearly 1.5 FTEs since the first payroll period, to balance with a decrease in the number of procedures being performed.

The more that James thinks about this issue, the more he becomes convinced that the problem must be related to the decrease in volume. He reasons that some of his staff must be available irrespective of the actual volume of procedures performed. A review of current staff positions leads him to believe that approximately 38 FTE staff members must be in place to adequately provide services, given the current delivery structure of his department. With 38 required staff members, James figures that 3040 hours (38 x 80 hours per payroll period) of staff time are required, irrespective of actual volume. Most of his staffing budget is therefore fixed and would not decline with volume reductions.

James recently read about a concept of budgeting referred to as "flexible budgeting," a method that is appropriate when costs in a department are comprised of both fixed and variable elements. James is preparing to develop a flexible budget for his department and present this information to the CFO.

Thirty years ago, the word "budgeting" could not have been found in the vocabularies of many health care executives. Today, this is no longer true. Most hospitals and other health care firms now develop and use budgets as an integral part of their overall management control process.

To a large extent, the attention health care providers pay to budgeting is attributable to changes in the environment. Over the last twenty years, the health care industry has experienced a dramatic shift in its revenue function from cost-related to fixed prices on either a procedure, case, or covered-life basis. Firms that sell products or services in markets where prices are fixed must control their costs. Budgeting is, of course, a logical way for any business organization to control its costs.

External market forces thus certainly have stimulated the development of budgets in the health care industry; but most likely, such budgets would have been developed in any case. Hospitals and health care firms have grown larger and more complex, in both organization and finances; and budgeting is imperative in organizations in which management authority is delegated to many individuals.

LEARNING OBJECTIVE 1

Define a budget and describe how management uses it.

ESSENTIAL ELEMENTS

For our purposes, a budget is defined as a quantitative expression of a plan of action. It is an integral part of the overall management control process of an organization.

Young and Anthony (1999) discuss management control in great detail. They define it as a process by which managers ensure that resources are obtained and used effectively and efficiently while accomplishing an organization's objectives.

Efficiency and Effectiveness

In the previous definition, special emphasis is placed on attaining efficiency and effectiveness. In short, they determine the success or failure of management control.

These two terms have precise meanings. Often, people talk about the relative efficiency and effectiveness of their operations as if efficiency and effectiveness were identical, or at least highly correlated. They are neither identical, nor are they necessarily correlated. An operation may be effective without being efficient, or vice versa. A well-managed operation ideally should be both effective and efficient. Efficiency is easier to measure and its meaning is fairly well understood; efficiency is simply a relationship between outputs and inputs. For example, a cost per patient day of $1,100 is a measure of efficiency—it tells how many resources, or inputs, were used to provide one day of care, the measure of output.

Managers and other persons wishing to assess performance in the health care industry are increasing their use of efficiency measures. In most situations, efficiency is measured by comparison with some standard. Several basic considerations should be understood if efficiency measures are to be used intelligently. First, output measures may not always be comparable. For example, comparing the costs per patient day of care in a 50-bed rural hospital with those in a 1000-bed teaching hospital is not likely to be meaningful. A day of care in a teaching hospital typically entails more service. Second, cost measures may not be comparable or useful for the specific decision being considered. For example, two operations may be identical, but one may be in a newer facility and thus have a higher depreciation charge; or the two operations may account for costs differently. One hospital may use an accelerated depreciation method, such as the sum of the year's digits, whereas the other may use straight-line depreciation. Third, the cost concepts used may not be relevant to the decision being considered. For example, a certificate-of-need review to decide which of two hospitals should be permitted to develop a cardiac catheterization lab obviously will consider cost. However, comparing the full costs of a procedure in each institution and selecting the least expensive one could produce bad results. For this specific decision, the full-cost concept is wrong. Incremental or variable cost is the relevant cost concept in this case. Chapter 13 discusses these cost concepts. The focus of interest is on what the future additional cost would be, not what the historical average cost was.

Effectiveness is concerned with the relationship between an organization's outputs and its objectives or goals. A health care firm's typical goals might include solvency, high quality of care, low cost of patient care, institutional harmony, and growth. Measuring effectiveness is more difficult than measuring efficiency for at least two reasons. First, defining the relationship between outputs and some goals may be difficult because many firms' goals or objectives are not likely to be quantified. For example, exactly how does an alcoholism program contribute to quality of care? Still, objectives and goals usually can be stated more precisely in quantitative terms. In fact, they should be quantified to the greatest extent possible. In the alcoholism program example, quality scales, such as frequency of repeat visits or new patients treated, might be developed.

Second, the output usually must be related to more than one organization goal or objective. For example, both solvency and reasonable cost are legitimate objectives for a hospital. Yet, continuing a home health operation might affect solvency negatively and simultaneously reduce patient treatment costs. How should decision makers weigh these two criteria to determine an overall measure of effectiveness?

Control Unit

In most health care facilities, management controls various responsibility centers. These centers are generally referred to as departments. Figure 15–1 presents an organizational chart of a hospital and its departments.

Usually, the departments perform special functions that contribute to overall organization goals, either directly or indirectly. They receive resources or inputs and produce services or outputs. Figure 15–2 illustrates this relationship.

Responsibility centers are the focus of management control efforts. Emphasis is placed on the effectiveness of their operations. Measurement problems occur when the responsibility structure is not identical to the program structure. Decision makers are frequently interested in a program's total cost. Yet, in the case of a burn-care program, for example, it is unlikely that all the resources used in the program will be assigned to it directly; the costs of medical support services (such as physical therapy, laboratory, and radiology services, as well as other general and administrative services) will not likely be contained in the burn-care unit. Program lines typically run across responsibility center or departmental lines. This necessitates cost allocations for decisions that require program cost information. It should be remembered that when cost allocations are involved, the accuracy of the information, as well as its comparability, may be suspect. For example, one may be interested in the specific costs of a burn-care program, but then find that those costs must be allocated from various departments or responsibility centers, such as laboratory, radiology, and housekeeping departments.

Responsibility centers vary greatly, depending on the controlling organization. For a regulatory agency, the responsibility center might be an entire health care firm; for a health care firm manager, it may be an individual department; for a department manager, it may be a unit within the department. The only requirement is that a designated person be in charge of the identified responsibility center.

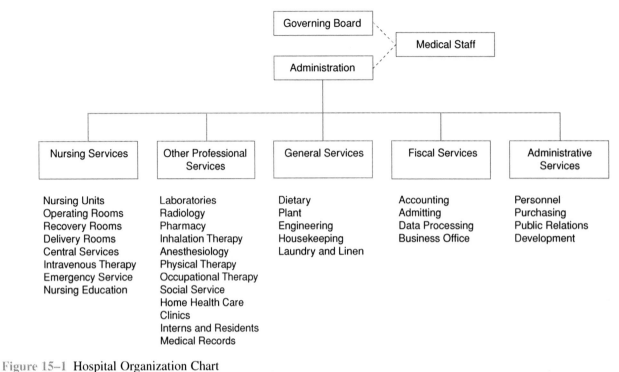

Figure 15–1 Hospital Organization Chart

LEARNING OBJECTIVE 2

Explain the concept of management control and how budgeting is used as part of it.

PHASES OF MANAGEMENT CONTROL

Figure 15–3 illustrates the relationship of various phases of the management control process with itself and with the planning process. Management control relies on the existence of goals and objectives; without them, the structure and evaluation of the management control process is incomplete. Poor or no planning usually limits the value of management control. Effectiveness becomes impossible to assess without stated goals and objectives; in such cases, one can focus only on measuring and attaining efficiency. The

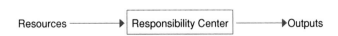

Figure 15–2 Responsibility Center Production Relationship

organization can assess only whether it has produced outputs efficiently; it cannot evaluate the desirability of those outputs.

For the purposes of this discussion, we shall be concerned with the four phases of management control as defined by Anthony and Young. They are as follows:

1. Programming
2. Budgeting
3. Accounting
4. Analysis and reporting

Programming

Programming is the phase of management control that determines the nature and size of programs that an organization will provide to accomplish its stated goals and objectives. It is the first phase of the management control process and interrelates with planning. In some cases, the boundary dividing the two activities may in fact be difficult to establish. Programming usually lasts three to five years—longer than budgeting, but shorter than planning.

Programming decisions deal with new and existing programs. The methodology for programming is

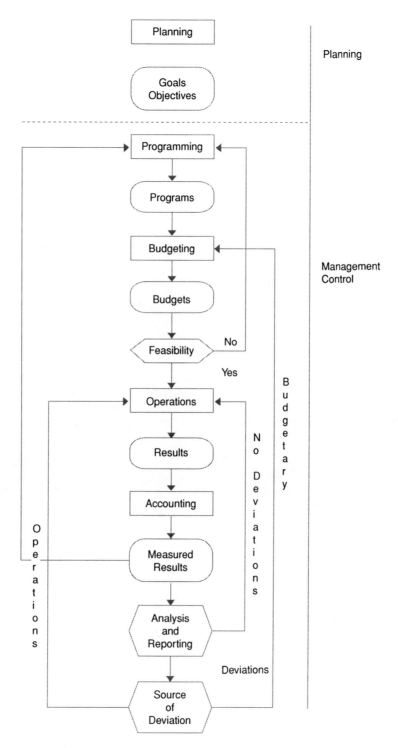

Figure 15–3 The Management Control Process

different in these two areas. Programming decisions for new programs involve capital investment or capital budget decision making (this process is examined more extensively in Chapter 18). The method

for making programming decisions for existing programs is often referred to as zero-base review, or zero-base budgeting, which will be discussed later in this chapter.

To illustrate the programming process, assume that a stated objective of a hospital organization is to develop and implement an ambulatory care program in the community. The decision makers in the programming phase of management control would take this stated objective and evaluate alternative programs to accomplish it, such as a surgicenter, an outpatient clinic, or a mobile health-screening unit. After this analysis, a decision might be made to construct a ten-room surgicenter on a lot adjacent to the hospital. This would be a program decision.

Budgeting

Budgeting is the management control phase of primary interest. It was defined earlier as a quantitative expression of a plan of action. Budgets are usually stated in monetary terms and cover a period of one year.

The budgetary phase of management control follows the determination of programs in the programming phase. In many cases, no real review of existing programs is undertaken; the budgeting phase then may be based on a prior year's budget or on the actual results of existing programs. Proponents of zero-base budgeting have identified this practice as a major shortcoming.

The budgeting phase primarily translates program decisions into terms that are meaningful for responsibility centers. The decision to construct a ten-room surgicenter will affect the revenues and costs of other responsibility centers, such as the laboratory, radiology, the anesthesiology departments, and the business office. The effects of program decisions thus must be carefully and accurately reflected in the budgets of each of the relevant responsibility centers.

Budgeting also may change programs. A more careful and accurate estimation of revenues and costs may prompt one to reevaluate prior programming decisions and deem them financially unfeasible. For example, the proposed ten-room surgicenter may be shown, through budget analysis, to produce a significant operating loss. If the hospital cannot or will not subsidize this loss from other sources, the programming decision must be changed. The size of the surgicenter may be reduced from ten rooms to five to make the operation "break even."

Accounting

Accounting is the third phase of the management control process. Once the decision about which programs to implement has been made and budgets have

been developed for them along responsibility center lines, the operations phase begins. The accounting department accumulates and records information on both outputs and inputs during the operating phase.

It is important to note that cost information is provided along both program and responsibility center lines. Responsibility center cost information is used in the reporting and analysis phase to determine the degree of compliance with budget projections. Programmatic cost information is used to assess the desirability of continuing a given program at its present size and scope in the programming phase of management control.

Analysis and Reporting

The last phase of management control is analysis and reporting. In this phase, differences between actual costs and budgeted costs are analyzed to determine the probable cause of the deviations; they are then reported to the individuals who can take corrective action. The method used in this phase is often referred to as variance analysis, which is discussed in greater detail in Chapter 16. Those doing the analysis and reporting rely heavily on the information provided from the accounting phase to break down the reported deviations into categories that suggest causes.

LEARNING OBJECTIVE 3

List sources of differences between budgeted and actual amounts.

In general, there are three primary causes for differences between budgeted and actual costs:

1. Prices paid for inputs were different from budgeted prices.
2. Output level was higher or lower than budgeted.
3. Actual quantities of inputs used were different from budgeted levels.

Within each of these causal areas, differences may arise from either budgeting or operations. A budgetary problem is usually not controllable; no operating action can be taken to correct the situation. For example, the surgicenter may have budgeted for ten registered nurses (RNs) at $4,000 each per month. However, if there was no way to employ ten RNs at an average wage less than $4,200 per month, the budget would have to be adjusted to reflect the change in expectations. Alternatively, the problem may arise from operations and be controllable. Perhaps the nurses of the surgicenter are more experienced and better trained than expected. If this is true, and the mix of RNs originally budgeted is still regarded as appropriate, some action should be taken to change the actual mix over time.

LEARNING OBJECTIVE 4

Explain the budgeting process.

THE BUDGETING PROCESS

Elements and Participants

Budgeting is regarded by many as the primary tool that health care managers can use to control costs in their organizations. The objectives of budgetary programs, as defined by the American Hospital Association, are five:

1. Define in statistical and monetary terms the operating plans of the hospital.
2. Describe the allocation of available resources for most effectively attaining the objectives in the operating plan.
3. Provide a basis for evaluating the financial performance of the plans.
4. Provide a useful tool for the control of costs.
5. Present a tool for communicating short range plans and financial requirements both within the organization and to the hospital's community.

The budgetary process encompasses a number of interrelated, but separate budgets. Figure 15–4 provides a schematic representation of the budgetary process and the relationships between specific types of budgets.

The individuals and roles involved in the budgetary process may vary. In general, the following individuals or parties may be involved:

* Governing board
* Chief executive officer (CEO)
* Controller
* Responsibility center managers
* Budgetary committee

The governing board's involvement in the budgetary process is usually indirect. The board provides the goals, objectives, and approved programs that are used as the basis for budgetary development. In many cases, it formally approves the finalized budget, especially the cash budget and budgeted financial statements; these are critical when assessing financial condition, which is a primary responsibility of the board.

The chief executive officer (CEO) or administrator of the health care facility has overall responsibility for budgetary development. The budget is the administrator's tool in the overall program of management by exception, which enables the CEO to focus only on those areas where problems exist.

Controllers often serve as budget directors. Their primary function is facilitation: they are responsible for providing relevant data on costs and outputs and for providing budgetary forms that may be used in budget development. They are not responsible for either making or enforcing the budget.

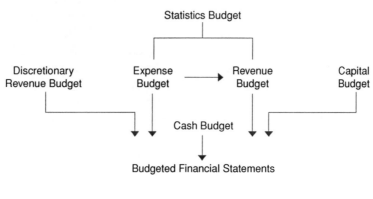

Figure 15–4 Integration of the Budgetary Process

Responsibility centers are the focal points of control. Managers of departments should be actively involved in developing budgets for their assigned areas and are responsible for meeting those budgets.

Many large health care firms use a special budgetary committee to aid in budget development and approval. Typically, this committee is composed of several department managers and headed by the controller. A committee structure such as this can help legitimize budgetary decisions that might appear arbitrary and capricious if made unilaterally by management.

LEARNING OBJECTIVE 5

List the major types of budgets and describe how they are used.

STATISTICS BUDGET

Development of the statistics budget is the first step in budgeting. It provides the basis for subsequent development of the revenue and expense budgets. Together, these three budgets are sometimes referred to as the operating budget.

The objective of the statistics budget is to provide measures of workload or activity in each department or responsibility center for the next budget period. The following three issues are involved in this task:

1. Output expectations
2. Responsibility for estimation
3. Estimation methodology

Output Expectation

Sales forecasts in many businesses reflect management's output expectations—how much of the business' product can be sold, given certain promotional efforts. There is some question about the extent to which health care firms can determine their volume of service, at least within the usual budgetary period. Although volume may change in the long run through the development or discontinuation of certain programs, most health care firms implicitly assume while developing their statistics budget that they cannot affect their overall volume during the next budgetary period. Instead, they assume that they will provide services to meet their actual demand. This leads to a reliance on past period service levels to forecast demand. Assuming that demand patterns in the budget period will be similar to prior periods can, however, be a costly mistake. First, foreseeable but uncontrollable forces may dramatically alter service patterns. For example, retirement of key medical staff with no replacement could drastically reduce admissions. Second, the health care facility may in fact control service levels in the short run and do so in a way that reduces costs. For example, a hospital may decide to develop clinical pathways in conjunction with its physicians, thus reducing total volume and total cost.

Responsibility for Estimation

The second issue regarding the statistics budget is the assignment of responsibility for developing projected output or workload indicators. Should department managers provide this information themselves, or should top management provide it to them? In some situations, department managers may tend to overstate demand. Overstatement of demand implies a greater need for resources within their own area and creates potential budgetary slack if anticipated volumes are not realized. Information coming from top management may be the converse: understatement of demand resulting in a lower total cost budget that might not provide adequate resources to meet actual output levels. Thus, negotiation often becomes necessary when determining demand for budgetary purposes.

Estimation Methodology

The last area of statistics budget development concerns problems of estimation. In most health care facilities, department activity depends on a limited number of key indicators, such as patient days, outpatient visits, or covered lives.

Prior values for these indicators can be related to departmental volume through statistical analysis. The major problem becomes one of accurately forecasting values for the indicators.

The use of seasonal, weekly, and daily variations in volume poses an important estimation problem. Too often, yearly volume is assumed to be divided equally between the monthly periods throughout the year, even when that is clearly not the case. Recognition of seasonal, weekly, and daily patterns of variation in volume can in fact create significant opportunities for cost reduction, especially in labor staffing.

Finally, types of output at the departmental level are often varied in nature. In fact, a department normally produces more than one type of output; for example, a laboratory may provide literally thousands of different tests. In such situations, a weighted unit of service is needed, such as the relative value units (RVUs) used in areas such as laboratory and radiology. Using weighted unit measures in the statistics budget is especially important when the mix of services is expected to change. Assume that a hospital is rapidly increasing its volume in outpatient clinics. This expansion in volume will increase activity in many other departments, including the pharmacy department. If, in such a situation, the filling of an outpatient prescription requires significantly more effort than the filling of an inpatient prescription, the use of an unweighted activity measure for prescriptions could provide misleading information for budgetary control purposes. Much less labor might be budgeted than is actually needed.

EXPENSE BUDGET

With estimates of activity for individual departments developed in the statistics budget, department managers can proceed to develop expense budgets for their areas of responsibility. Expense budgeting is the area of budgeting "where the rubber meets the road." Management cost control efforts are finally reflected in hard numbers that the departments must live with—in most cases, for the budget period. Major categories of expense budgets at the departmental level include payroll, supplies, and other. In some situations, a budget for allocated costs from indirect departments also may be included, although departmental managers usually do not do this.

In our discussion of expense budgeting, we shall focus on the following four issues of budgeting that are of general interest:

1. Length of the budget period
2. Flexible or forecast budgets
3. Standards for price and quantity
4. Allocation of indirect costs

Length of the Budget Period

Generally speaking, there are two alternative budget periods that may be used—fixed and rolling. Of the two, a fixed budget period is much more frequently used in the health care industry. A fixed budget covers some defined time from a given budget date, usually one year. This contrasts with a rolling budget, in which the budget is periodically extended on a frequent basis, usually each month or every three-month quarter. For example, in a rolling budget period with a monthly update, the entity always would have a budget that projected at least eleven more months. The same is not true in a fixed budget, in which case at fiscal year end, there may be only one week or one month remaining.

A rolling budget has many advantages, but it requires more time and effort and therefore more cost. Among its major advantages are the following:

- More realistic forecasts, which should improve management planning and control
- Equalization of the workload of budget development during the entire year
- Improved familiarity and understanding of budgets by department managers

Flexible or Forecast Budgets?

The use of a flexible budget versus a forecast budget has been discussed heavily in the health care finance field. Presently, few health care firms use a formal system of flexible budgeting. However, flexible budgeting is a more sophisticated method of budgeting than typical forecast budgeting and is being adopted by more and more health care firms as they become experienced in the budgetary process.

A flexible budget adjusts targeted levels of costs for changes in volume. For example, the budget for a nursing unit operating at 95 percent occupancy would be different from the budget for that same unit operating at 80 percent occupancy. A forecast budget, in contrast, would make no formal differentiation in the allowed budget between these two levels.

The difference between a forecast and a flexible budget is illustrated by the historical data and projected use levels for the laboratory presented in Table 15–1. The forecast levels of volume in RVUs for 2007 are identical to the actual volumes of 2006, except that a ten percent growth factor is assumed. The department manager using this statistics budget must develop a budget for hours worked in 2007. A common approach to this task is to assume that past work experience indicates future requirements. In this case,

Table 15–1 Laboratory Productivity Data

	2006 Actual Hours Worked	RVUs	2007 Expected RVUs
January	2,825	5,700	6,270
February	2,700	5,200	5,720
March	2,900	6,000	6,600
April	2,875	5,900	6,490
May	2,825	5,700	6,270
June	2,700	5,200	5,720
July	2,750	5,400	5,940
August	2,625	4,900	5,390
September	2,725	5,300	5,830
October	2,750	5,400	5,940
November	2,750	5,400	5,940
December	2,775	5,500	6,050
Total	33,200	65,600	72,160

Note: 2006 average hours/RVU = 33,200/65,600 = .5061.

Table 15–2 Alternative Hours-Worked Budget for Laboratory

	Forecast Budget*	Flexible Budget
January	3,043	2,967**
February	3,043	2,830
March	3,043	3,050
April	3,043	3,022
May	3,043	2,967
June	3,043	2,830
July	3,043	2,885
August	3,043	2,747
September	3,043	2,857
October	3,043	2,885
November	3,043	2,885
December	3,043	2,912
Total	36,516	34,837

*(.5061 × 72,160)/12 = 3,043.35.
**January value = 1,400 + (.25 × 6,270).

the average value for hours of work required per RVU in 2006 was 0.5061. A common method for developing a forecast budget is to multiply this value of 0.5061 by the estimated total workload for the budget period, which is expected to be 72,160, and spread the total product equally over each of the twelve months. This is the forecast budget depicted in Table 15–2.

A major difference between a flexible budget and a forecast budget is that a flexible budget must recognize and incorporate underlying cost behavioral patterns. In this laboratory example, hours worked might be written as a function of RVUs as follows:

Hours worked = (1,400 hours per month) + (.25 × RVUs)

Application of this formula to the budgeted RVUs expected in 2007 yields the flexible budget presented in Table 15–2.

Two points should be made before concluding our discussion of flexible budgeting versus forecast budgeting. First, a flexible budget may be represented as a forecast budget for planning purposes. For example, in the laboratory scenario of Table 15–2, the flexible budget would provide an estimated hours-worked requirement of 34,837 hours for 2007. However, in an actual control period evaluation, the flexible budget formula would be used. To illustrate, assume that the actual RVUs provided

in January 2007 amounted to 6,500 instead of the forecasted 6,270. Budgeted hours in the flexible budget then would not total 2,967 but 3,025:

1,400 + (.25 × 6,500) = 3,025

This value would be compared with the actual hours worked, not the initially forecasted 2,967.

Second, dramatic differences in approved costs can result from the two methods. Recognizing that the underlying cost behavioral patterns can change the estimated resource requirements approved in the budgetary process. In the laboratory example in Table 15–2, the forecast budget calls for 36,516 hours versus the flexible budget hours requirement of 34,837. The difference results from the method used to estimate hours worked. In a forecast budget method, the prior average hours per RVU relationship is used. In most situations, average hours or average cost should be greater than variable hours or variable cost. In departments with expanding volume, the estimated requirements for resources could be overstated. This is the situation in our laboratory example where volume increased ten percent from the prior year. Because some of the labor cost was fixed (1400 hours per month), the increase in total labor costs was not proportional. The converse may be true in departments with declining volume. In many cases, the use of forecast budgeting methods is based on the incorporation of prior average cost relationships. This error is not made with flexible budgeting methods because their use depends on explicit incorporation of cost behavioral patterns that distinctly recognize variable and fixed costs.

A flexible budget makes sense when there are expenses that could vary with small changes in volume. Expense categories such as supplies are usually variable in nature. Labor costs may or may not be variable. The use of part-time labor, overtime, and outside pools all tend to make labor costs variable. In general, greater variability or uncertainty in volume forecasts should lead management to adopt more flexible staffing policies.

Standards for Price and Quantity

Earlier, three factors were identified that can create differences between budgeted and actual costs: volume, prices, and usage or efficiency. The use of flexible budgeting is an attempt to improve the recognition of deviations caused by changes in volume. The use of standards for prices and wage rates, coupled with standards for physical quantities, is an attempt to improve the recognition of deviations from budgets that result from prices and usage.

For example, assume that the flexible budget-hours requirement for the laboratory example is still hours worked = $1,400 + (.25 \times \text{RVUs})$. Assume further that the budgeted wage rate is $20 per hour and the actual RVUs for January 2007 amounted to 6500. Total payroll cost for hours worked (excluding vacations and sick pay) is assumed to be $68,200 with 3100 hours actually worked (average wage rate of $22 per hour). The variance analysis report presented in Table 15–3 would be applicable to the laboratory department.

The total unfavorable variance of $7,700 results from a $6,200 unfavorable price variance and a $1,500 unfavorable efficiency variance. Splitting the variance in this manner helps management quickly identify possible causes. For example, the $6,200 price variance may be due to a negotiated wage increase of $2 per hour. If this is the case, the department manager is clearly not responsible for the variance. If, however, the difference is due to an excessive use of overtime personnel or a more costly mix of labor, then the manager may be held responsible for the difference and should attempt to prevent the problem from occurring again. The unfavorable efficiency variance of $1,500 reflects excessive use of labor during the month in the amount of 75 hours. An explanation for this difference should be sought and steps taken to prevent its recurrence.

Standard costing techniques have been used in industry for many years as an integral part of management control. Although it is true that input and output relationships may not be as objective in the health care industry as they are in general industry, this does not imply that standard costing cannot be used. In fact, there are many areas of activity within a health care facility that have fairly precise input-output relationships—housekeeping, laundry and linen, laboratory, radiology, and many others. Standard costing can prove to be a valuable tool for cost control in the health care industry, if properly applied (this topic is explored in greater detail in Chapter 16).

Table 15–3 Standard Cost Variance Analysis for Labor Costs, Laboratory, January 2007

1. Price variance = (Actual hours worked) $\times$ (Actual wage rate)
      − (Actual hours worked) $\times$ (Budgeted wage rate)
      = $(3,100 \times \$22.00) - (3,100 \times \$20.00)$
      = $6,200 [Unfavorable]

2. Efficiency variance = (Actual hours worked) $\times$ (Budgeted wage rate)
         − (Budgeted hours worked) $\times$ (Budgeted wage rate)
         = $(3,100 \times \$20.00) - (3,025 \times \$20.00)$
         = $1,500 [Unfavorable]

3. Total variance = $6,200 + $1,500 = $7,700 [Unfavorable]

Note: Actual wage rate = $68,200/3,100 = $22.00. Budgeted wage rate = $20.00. Actual hours worked = 3,100. Budgeted hours worked = $(1,400) + (.25 \times 6,500) = 3,025$.

Allocation of Indirect Costs

There probably has been more internal strife in organizations over the allocation of indirect costs than over any other single budgetary issue. A comment often heard is, "Why was I charged $10,000 for housekeeping services last month when my department didn't use anywhere near that level of service?"

A strong case can in fact be made for not allocating indirect costs in budget variance reports. In most normal situations, the receiving department has little or no control over the costs of the servicing department. Allocation may thus raise questions that should not be raised. Although it is true that indirect costs need to be allocated for some decision-making purposes, such as pricing, they are generally not needed for evaluating individual responsibility center management.

However, an equally strong argument can be made for including indirect costs in the budgets of benefiting departments. They are legitimate costs of the total operation and department managers should be aware of them. If department managers' decisions can influence costs in indirect areas, these managers should be held accountable for those costs. For example, maintenance, housekeeping, and other indirect costs can be influenced by the decisions of benefiting departments. Ideally, a charge for these indirect services should be established and levied against the using departments, based on their use. Labeling the cost of indirect areas as totally uncontrollable can stimulate excessive and unnecessary use of indirect services, and thus have a negative impact on the total cost control program in an organization.

REVENUE BUDGET

The revenue budget can be set effectively only after the expense budget and the statistics budget have been developed. Revenues must be set at levels that cover all associated expenses, plus provide a return on invested capital. This is a fundamental rule of finance and is equally valid for both voluntary, not-for-profit firms and investor-owned firms. Moreover, some of the total revenue actually realized by a health care facility is directly determined by expenses because of the presence of cost reimbursement formulas.

Rate Setting

In this discussion of the revenue budget, we shall focus on only one aspect of revenue budget development—pricing or rate setting. Specifically, we shall illustrate the rate-setting model discussed in Chapters 5 and 13 through an additional example.

Figure 15–5 illustrates the rate-setting model. Sources of information to define the variables of the model are identified. However, the following three parameters have no identified source:

1. Desired profit
2. Proportion of charge-paying patients
3. Proportion of charge-paying patient revenue not collected

In most situations, separate figures for the percentage of write-offs on charge-paying patients and the percentage of charge-paying patients are not available on a departmental basis. Sometimes the best information

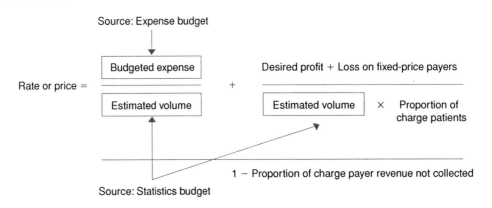

Figure 15–5 Rate Setting in the Revenue Budget

available may be the percentage of bad-debt write-offs on total revenue for the institution as a whole. Using the example data for Department 1 in Table 15–4, a one percent write-off on 20 percent of the patients who paid charges in the department implies that five percent of the charge-paying patient revenue in that department is written off (one percent divided by 20 percent is five percent). The corresponding figure for Department 2 is 50 percent (30 percent divided by 60 percent). Using these data, and substituting the total or aggregate values for the percentage write-offs on charge-paying patients and the percentage of charge-paying patients, the following rates would be established:

$$\text{Department 1 price} = \frac{\dfrac{\$10,000}{100} + \dfrac{\$500}{100 \times .4}}{1 - .3875} = \$183.67$$

$$\text{Department 2 price} = \frac{\dfrac{\$10,000}{100} + \dfrac{\$500}{100 \times .4}}{1 - .3875} = \$183.67$$

Proper reflection of the departmental values, however, would produce the following rates:

$$\text{Department 1 price} = \frac{\dfrac{\$10,000}{100} + \dfrac{\$500}{100 \times .2}}{1 - .05} = \$131.58$$

$$\text{Department 2 price} = \frac{\dfrac{\$10,000}{100} + \dfrac{\$500}{100 \times .6}}{1 - .50} = \$216.67$$

In the former case, the use of aggregate or average values produces an inequitable pricing structure. The price for Department 1 was initially overstated, whereas the price for Department 2 was initially understated. If equity in rate setting is an objective, reliance on average values can prevent the development of an equitable rate structure along departmental lines. In many cases, the errors may be significant.

Desired Profit Levels

Determining a desired level of profit is not easy. In many cases, it is a subjective process, made to appear objective through the application of a quantitative profit requirement. For example, desired profit may be arbitrarily set at some percentage of budgeted expenses, such as ten percent above expenses, or as a certain percentage of total investment. However, desired levels of profit can, in general, be stated as the difference between financial requirements and expenses as follows:

Desired profit = Budgeted financial requirements − Budgeted expenses

Budgeted financial requirements are cash requirements that an entity must meet during the budget period. Four elements usually constitute total budgeted financial requirements:

1. Budgeted expenses, excluding depreciation
2. Requirements for debt principal payment
3. Requirements for increases in working capital
4. Requirements for capital expenditures not financed with debt

Budgeted expenses at the departmental level should include both direct and indirect (or allocated) expenses. Depreciation charges are excluded because depreciation is a noncash requirement expense.

Debt principal payments include only the principal portion of debt service due. In some cases, additional reserve requirements may be established, which may

Table 15–4 Rate-Setting Example Data

	Department 1	Department 2	Total
Loss on fixed price payers	—	—	—
Desired profit	$500	$500	$1,000
Budgeted expense	$10,000	$10,000	$20,000
Estimated volume	100	100	—
Percentage bad debt	1.00	30.00	15.50
Percentage charge-paying patients	20.00	60.00	40.00
Percentage bad debt on charge-paying patients	5.00	50.00	38.75

require additional funding. Interest expense is already included in budgeted expenses and should not be included in debt principal payments.

Working capital requirements also represent a financial requirement that must be built into the pricing structure because working capital is not included as an element of expense. The maintenance of necessary levels of inventory, accounts receivable, and precautionary cash balances requires an investment. Changes in the total level of this investment must be funded from cash, additional indebtedness, or a combination of the two. Planned financing of increases in working capital is a legitimate financial requirement.

Capital expenditure requirements may be of two types. First, actual capital expenditures may be made for approved projects. Those projects not financed with indebtedness require a cash investment. Second, prudent fiscal management requires that funds be set aside and invested to meet reasonable requirements for future capital expenditures. This amount should be related to the replacement cost depreciation of existing fixed assets.

Any loss incurred on fixed-price payers, such as Medicare, must be added to the desired profit target. The amount of the loss would represent the projected difference between allocated costs or expenses and net revenue received from fixed-price payers. If revenues from fixed-price payers exceed costs, the difference would be subtracted from the profit target. For example, if a firm received $5,000,000 in revenue from Medicare and incurred $4,800,000 in costs to provide care to Medicare patients, the difference of $200,000 would be subtracted from the desired profit target. The effect would be lower required rates or prices. (Chapters 5 and 13 provide more detail on price setting.)

A logical question is, "How is the desired profit requirement allocated to individual departments?" Usually, it is just assigned on the basis of some percentage of budgeted expenses. If a nursing home budgets $5 million in expenses and determines that $500,000 profit is required, each department might set its rates to recover ten percent above its expenses. However, the importance of cost reimbursement and bad debts at the departmental level also should be considered.

Discretionary Revenue Budget and Capital Budget

Discretionary revenue may be important, especially for institutions with large investment portfolios. A good management control system will have a budget for expected return on investments. Variations from the expected level then would be investigated. In some cases, changes in investment management may be necessary.

Capital budgeting can give many health care managers a major control tool. It can significantly affect the level of cost. This is especially true not only when the initial capital costs associated with given capital expenditures are considered, but also when considering the associated operating costs for salaries and supplies. (The capital budgeting process is examined in detail in Chapter 18.)

THE CASH BUDGET AND BUDGETED FINANCIAL STATEMENTS

The cash budget is management's best indicator of the organization's expected short-run solvency. It translates all of the previous budgets into a statement of cash inflows and outflows. The cash budget is usually broken down by periods, such as months or quarters, within the total budget period. An example of a cash budget is shown in Table 15–5.

Departmental expense budgets, departmental revenue budgets, a discretionary revenue budget, and a capital budget that do not provide a sufficient cash flow can necessitate major revisions. If the organization cannot or will not finance the deficits, the budgets must be changed to maintain the solvency of the organization. A poor cash budget could cause an increase in rates, a reduction in expenses, a reduction in capital expenditures, or many other changes. These changes and revisions must be made until the cash budget reflects a position of short-run solvency.

The two major financial statements that are developed on a budgetary basis are the balance sheet and the statement of revenue and expense. These two statements are indicators of both short- and long-run solvency; however, they are more important in assessing long-run solvency. Changing projections in either statement might cause changes in any of the other budgets.

In short, the budgeted financial statements and the cash budget test the adequacy of the entire budgetary process. Budgets that result in an unfavorable financial position, as reflected by the budgeted financial statements and the cash budget, must be adjusted. Solvency is a goal that most organizations cannot sacrifice. Cash budgeting is explored in greater detail in Chapter 22.

Table 15–5 Cash Budget, Budget Year 2007

| | 1st Quarter | | | | | |
	January	February	March	2nd Quarter	3rd Quarter	4th Quarter
Receipts from operations	$300,000	$310,000	$320,000	$1,000,000	$1,100,000	$1,100,000
Disbursements from operations	280,000	280,000	300,000	940,000	1,000,000	1,000,000
Cash available from operations	$20,000	$30,000	$20,000	$60,000	$100,000	$100,000
Other receipts						
Increase in mortgage payable				500,000		
Sale of fixed assets		20,000				
Unrestricted income—endowment			40,000	40,000	40,000	40,000
Total other receipts	$ —	$20,000	$40,000	$540,000	$40,000	$40,000
Other disbursements						
Mortgage payments			150,000		150,000	
Fixed-asset purchase				480,000		
Funded depreciation			30,000	130,000	30,000	30,000
Total other disbursements	$ —	$ —	$180,000	$610,000	$180,000	$30,000
Net cash gain (loss)	20,000	50,000	(120,000)	(10,000)	(40,000)	110,000
Beginning cash balance	100,000	120,000	170,000	50,000	40,000	—
Cumulative cash	$120,000	$170,000	$50,000	$40,000	$ —	$110,000
Desired level of cash	100,000	100,000	100,000	100,000	100,000	100,000
Cash above minimum needs (financing needs)	$20,000	$70,000	$(50,000)	$(60,000)	$(100,000)	$10,000

ZERO-BASE BUDGETING

Zero-base budgeting is a term that has gained much publicity. It has been touted as management's most effective cost containment tool. It also has been described as the biggest hoax of the century. The truth lies somewhere in the middle.

Zero-base budgeting, or zero-base review, as some prefer to call it, is a way of looking at existing programs. It is part of programming, but it focuses on existing programs instead of new programs. Zero-base budgeting assumes that no existing program is entitled to automatic approval. Many individuals have identified automatic approval with existing budgetary systems that are based on prior-year expenditure levels.

Zero-base budgeting is a process of periodically reevaluating all programs and their associated levels of expenditures. The process involves looking at the entire budget and determining the efficacy of the entire expenditure. It thus requires a tremendous effort and investment of time. It cannot be done well on an annual basis. Management decides the frequency of this reevaluation and may vary it from every year to every five years. This is why many refer to it as zero-base review instead of zero-base budgeting. Some have suggested that a zero-base review of a given activity would be appropriate every five years.

Although most decision makers agree with the concept of zero-base budgeting, in practice it poses the following two significant questions:

1. What evaluation methodology should be used in zero-base budgeting?
2. Who should be involved in the actual decision-making process?

In each case, the answers are important to the success or failure of the zero-base budget program. Yet, there still is not complete agreement among experts regarding the answers.

Nearly everyone would agree that cost-benefit analysis should be the evaluation methodology of zero-base budgeting. There are two important questions related to the application of cost-benefit analysis to zero-base budgeting programs: (1) Are the services that are presently provided being delivered in an efficient manner? (2) Are these services being delivered in an effective manner in terms of the organization's goals and objectives? A procedure for quantitatively answering these two questions involves the following seven sequential steps:

1. Define the outputs or services provided by the program or departmental area.
2. Determine the costs of these services or outputs.
3. Identify options for reducing the cost through changes in outputs or services.
4. Identify options for producing the services and outputs more efficiently.
5. Determine the cost savings associated with options identified in Steps 3 and 4.
6. Assess the risks, both qualitative and quantitative, associated with the identified options of Steps 3 and 4.
7. Select and implement those options with an acceptable cost/risk relationship.

LEARNING OBJECTIVE 7

Explain how benchmarking is performed at the departmental level.

BENCHMARKING AT THE DEPARTMENTAL LEVEL

One of the critical aspects of management control at the departmental or responsibility center level is access to relevant productivity standards. How much labor should be used to produce a certain level of output? In general, there are three sources of productivity standards:

* Internally-developed historical standards
* Engineered standards
* Comparative group standards

Internally-developed standards based upon historical performance are the easiest and least costly method of productivity standard development. It is also the most commonly used method. For example, a hospital laundry and linen department may have a historical average of 20 hours of labor per 1000 pounds of laundry. That historical average could be used to budget labor hours for the coming year. The biggest disadvantage of using this method is that historical averages don't provide information about relative efficiency. Is 20 hours of labor per 1000 pounds of laundry an efficient level of productivity or not?

Engineered standards can be developed with internal staff, or they can be developed with the help of outside consultants. The key aspect to this method is an exhaustive study of the work setting and the definition of normative standards of productivity. For example, a consultant might determine that only 14 hours of labor is required per 1000 pounds of laundry. Significant opportunities for cost reduction may result because of this engineered standard. The management problem of achieving this standard still remains, however, and there is no guarantee that the projected savings can be realized soon, if ever. Management must act on the information that it was given if it is to realize savings. The primary disadvantage of engineered standards is cost. The use of specialized internal staff or outside consultants can be expensive.

Comparative group productivity standards are available in most health care industry sectors. Sometimes associations that represent health care firms collect data and distribute them to members, or private firms also may provide comparative group standards from survey data they have collected. Table 15–6 provides some hospital departmental standards from Cleverley & Associates in Worthington, Ohio. The data indicate that the average direct cost in 150- to 250-bed hospitals laundry departments was $527.00 per 1000 pounds.

Comparative group data are usually less expensive to obtain than engineered standards, but there are several drawbacks. First, is the productivity standard com-

Table 15–6 Productivity and Cost Standards for Selected Hospital Departments

Department	Output Unit	Direct Cost per Output Unit
Nursing		
Intensive care unit	Patient days	$636.76
General routine care	Patient days	270.82
Nursery	Patient days	225.18
Professional Services		
Operating room	Weighted procedure	$17.80
Radiology-diagnostic	Weighted procedure	27.52
Laboratory	Weighted procedure	31.60
Physical therapy	Weighted procedure	40.25
General Services		
Laundry and linen	1000 pounds	$527.00
Housekeeping	100 square feet	589.00
Food services	Meals	6.80

Source: Cleverley & Associates, Departmental Benchmarking Report, 2006, U.S. Average for Hospital between 150 to 250 beds.

parable across all departments in the group? To be comparable, both the measure of cost and output must be defined in the same manner by all reporting members. For example, is the number of pounds of laundry measured wet or dry? Does the measure of labor hours include vacation and sick time? Second, knowing there is a difference between a group average and your department's performance doesn't tell you why the difference exists. Our laundry may require 20 hours per 1000 pounds and the national average may be 12 hours, but how can we achieve that standard? Perhaps the equipment used is old and requires more labor costs. The difference does imply that something is wrong and that change is needed, but communication with other group members may be necessary to realize savings. Many of the comparative group reporting services provide mechanisms for inter-firm communication to learn and adopt best practices. Ultimately, the objective is to achieve superior performance, as Figure 15–6 illustrates.

SUMMARY

This chapter has focused on the process of management control that is used in organizations. Most management control processes involve the following four

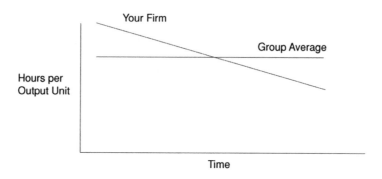

Figure 15–6 Closing the Performance Gap

phases of activity: programming, budgeting, accounting, and analysis and reporting. Budgeting is an activity that many department managers view as the primary focus of management control because of its direct focus on resource allocation and emphasis on efficiency. Efficiency standards are primary inputs in the budgeting process and are often provided through comparative benchmarking data.

REFERENCES

R. N. Anthony and D. W. Young, *Management Control in Non-Profit Organizations*, 6th Edition, Burr Ridge, IL: Irwin/McGraw-Hill, 1999.

Truman H. Esmond, Jr., *Budgeting for Effective Hospital Resource Management*, Chicago: American Hospital Association, 1990, page 26.

ASSIGNMENTS

1. Under what conditions is a flexible budget likely to be more effective than a forecast budget?

2. Can an organization be efficient but not effective? Discuss the circumstances in which this could be true.

3. The first step in the budgeting process is to develop the statistics budget. Why is this true?

4. Ann Walker, CPA, is the controller for your hospital. For a long time, Ms. Walker has been concerned about management control in the hospital and she finally has developed a new departmental labor control system. It is based on the data in Table 15–7 for the obstetrics nursing unit.

Table 15–7 Budget Data for Obstetrics Example

Period	Patient Days	Hours Worked	Rate	Total Cost
1	350	1,550	$27.00	$41,850
2	400	1,700	27.60	46,920
3	300	1,400	26.40	36,960
4	375	1,625	27.60	44,850
5	450	1,850	27.60	51,060
Total	1875	8,125		$221,640

Note: Average rate = $27.28 = $221,640/8,125. Average hours/patient day = 4.33 = 8,125/1,875.

Using these data, Ms. Walker developed a two-factor variance model for labor costs in the obstetrics department. In Period 1, the variances in this model would be as follows:

Labor rate variance = ($27.00 − $27.28) × 1,550 = −$434.00 (Favorable)

Labor usage variance = [1,550 − (4.33 × 350)] × $27.28 = $941.16 (Unfavorable)

A similar model for labor control has been adopted in all other departments. As the chief executive officer of the hospital, are you satisfied with this labor control system? What suggestions for revisions would you make?

5. Floyd Farley is the maintenance department head. His department is participating in a wage-incentive program in which he and his staff receive 20 percent of the department's income as supplemental income. Net income is defined as $25 multiplied by maintenance staff hours charged, less direct departmental expense. Do you see any problems with this system? If so, how might they be solved?

6. You have been asked to prepare a flexible budget for a 40-bed nursing unit. A schedule of staffing requirements by occupancy is presented in Table 15–8.

Table 15–8 Staffing Budget for Nursing Unit

	Below 60% Occupancy	60 to 80% Occupancy	80 to 100% Occupancy
First shift			
Head nurse	1	1	1
Registered nurse	1	1	2
Licensed practical nurse	1	1	1
Aide	1	2	2
Second shift			
Registered nurse	2	2	2
Licensed practical nurse	1	1	1
Aide	2	3	3
Third shift			
Registered nurse	1	1	1
Licensed practical nurse	1	1	1
Aide	0	1	2

Daily personnel costs by job title and shift	**Daily Cost**
Head nurse	$175
Registered nurse—first shift	135
Second and third shifts	155
Licensed practical nurse—first shift	85
Second and third shifts	100
Aides—first shift	70
Second and third shifts	75

Prepare a budget for management that shows expected personnel costs for this nursing unit by occupancy level.

7. You must establish a pricing schedule for laboratory procedures. From a total hospital perspective, management has decided that the hospital must earn 5 percent above costs. The hospital has established that it loses 10 percent on each fixed-price payer (Medicare). That is, for every $100 of cost incurred to treat a fixed-price payer, the hospital receives only $90 in payment. You must build both the required profit and the expected loss on fixed-price payers into your rate structure. Payer mix for the laboratory is expected to be as presented in Table 15–9.

Table 15–9 Laboratory Pricing Data

	Budgeted RVUs Inpatient	Outpatient	Total
Medicare	200,000	50,000	250,000
Medicaid	40,000	10,000	50,000
Blue Cross	80,000	20,000	100,000
Commercial insurance and HMOs	60,000	10,000	70,000
Bad debt and charity	15,000	15,000	30,000
Total RVUs	395,000	105,000	500,000

Medicare pays on a fixed price per diagnosis-related group for all inpatients. There is thus no separate payment for laboratory tests. Medicaid pays average costs for both inpatient and outpatient tests. Medicare also pays on a fee schedule for outpatient tests. On average Medicare receives 80 percent of cost for outpatient lab tests. Blue Cross pays 95 percent of charges for both inpatient and outpatient procedures. All other commercial insurance and health maintenance organization (HMO) patients pay 100 percent of charges. If budgeted expenses are $1,000,000 ($2.00 per RVU), what price must be set to meet management's profit expectations?

8. How would you calculate the amount of revenue to be realized as cash from patient sources in a fiscal period?

9. What is the major conceptual difference between zero-base budgeting and conventional budgeting?

10. In a hospital operation, what key variables are important when projecting volume at departmental levels?

SOLUTIONS AND ANSWERS

1. Two conditions are necessary for a flexible budget to be more useful than a forecast budget. First, there must be some indication that costs are variable, at least in part. Second, there must be some variability in activity levels, that is, volume is not expected to be constant in each period.

2. Efficiency relates to the costs per unit of output produced. Effectiveness relates to the attainment of organizational objectives given its outputs. It is possible for a firm to be efficient, but not effective. For example, a hospital might provide inpatient care at an extremely low cost. However, this might not be effective if the provision of the inpatient care is accomplished at rates that threaten the hospital's goal of financial solvency.

3. Figure 15–4 indicates that the statistics budget provides input for the development of the expense budget and the revenue budget. Projection of both expenses and revenues is a function of expected volume and variability of volume over the budget period. In cases when volume is expected to vary significantly, management may try to make more of their costs variable to maximize their ability to control costs, given volume changes. For example, more variable staffing may be used through the use of part-time employees, nursing pools, or overtime.

4. The primary weakness of Ms. Walker's model is its failure to incorporate fixed labor requirements. A flexible budgeting system should be put into effect instead. Using a high-low method, the following budget parameters for hours required can be estimated:

$$\text{Variable hours} = \frac{1{,}850 - 1{,}400}{45 - 300} = 3.0 \text{ hours per patient day}$$

$$\text{Fixed hours per period} = 1{,}850 - (3.0 \times 450) = 500 \text{ hours per period}$$

The deviation in hours worked per period is removed when the fixed labor requirement is recognized (Table 15–10).

Table 15–10 Flexible Budget Comparison of Actual versus Budgeted Hours

Period	Actual Hours	Budgeted Hours (500 + 3.0 × PD)	Difference
1	1,550	1,550	0
2	1,700	1,700	0
3	1,400	1,400	0
4	1,625	1,625	0
5	1,850	1,850	0

5. Mr. Farley has an incentive to engage his staff in what might be needless maintenance. This could be controlled by setting limits on the absolute level of incentive payment that could be earned, for example, by basing the incentive payments on the difference between actual and budgeted costs or by establishing control systems for authorizing maintenance work.

6. The budget in Table 15–11 could be developed to show daily standard personnel costs by occupancy level for the nursing unit.

Table 15–11 Nursing Unit Budget

	Occupancy		
	Below 60%	60% to 80%	80% to 100%
First shift			
Head nurse	$175	$175	$175
Registered nurse	135	135	270
Licensed practical nurse	85	85	85
Aide	70	140	140
Second shift			
Registered nurse	310	310	310
Licensed practical nurse	100	100	100
Aide	150	225	225
Third shift			
Registered nurse	155	155	155
Licensed practical nurse	100	100	100
Aide	0	75	150
Total standard personnel costs	$1,280	$1,500	$1,710

7. Using the formula in Figure 15–5, the following rate structure can be established to meet management's profit expectations:

$$\text{Price} = \frac{\dfrac{\$1,000,000}{500,000} + \dfrac{(\$50,000 + \$60,000)}{500,000 \times .40}}{1 - .175} = \$3.0909$$

$$\text{Desired profit} = .05 \times \$1,000,000 = \$50,000$$

$$\text{Loss on Medicare Inpatient} = .4 \times \$1,000,000 \times .10 = \$40,000$$

$$\text{Loss on Medicare Outpatient} = .10 \times \$1,000,000 \times .20 = \$20,000$$

$$\text{Total charge volume in RVUs} = \text{BC } (100,000) + \text{Bad Debt } (30,000) + \text{Commercial } (70,000) = 200,000$$

$$\text{Proportion of charge payers} = (100,000 + 70,000 + 30,000)/500,000 = .40$$

$$\text{Total charge volume not paid in RVUs} = \text{BC } (5,000) + \text{BD } (30,000) + \text{Comm } (0) = 35,000$$

$$\text{Proportion of charge payer revenue not collected} = 35,000/200,000 = .175$$

Budgeted Income

Medicare inpatient (.4 × $1,000,000 × .9)	$360,000
Medicare outpatient (.1 × $1,000,000 × .8)	80,000
Medicaid (.1 × $1,000,000)	100,000
Blue Cross (100,000 × $3.0909 × .95)	293,636
Commercial insurance and HMO (70,000 × $3.0909)	216,364
Bad debt and charity	0
Total revenue	$1,050,000
Less expenses	1,000,000
Budget profit	$ 50,000

8. Cash realized from patient sources could be expressed as follows:

   Cash flow = Net patient revenue + Beginning patient accounts receivable −
   Ending patient accounts receivable

9. Zero-base budgeting starts from a zero base. That is, all expenditures must be justified in the budgeting review. Conventional budgeting looks primarily at expenditures that are above prior levels.

10. The volume of actual cases treated (discharges or admissions) and outpatient activity are the key variables that affect departmental volumes. For example, laboratory tests are usually related to discharges and outpatient visits. Patient days are derived from discharges by assuming an average length of stay. Refinements in forecasting can be achieved by projecting case mix. Finally, more or fewer ancillary services per discharge may be required, depending on the type of case.

Chapter 16

Cost Variance Analysis

After studying this chapter, you should be able to do the following:

1. Describe alternative cost control approaches.
2. Describe the two major theories used for the detection of out-of-control costs.
3. Define variance analysis and how it is used by management.
4. Calculate the various types of cost variances.
5. Explain and calculate price, efficiency, and volume variances.

Linda Wills, CEO at Buckeye Valley Community Hospital, is preparing for the monthly board meeting. She was contacted earlier in the day by one of the board members, Doug Marshall, who was very upset by the plunge in hospital profit. Preliminary projections show the hospital closing the year with a loss of $7.5 million. As a banker, Doug is concerned about the pressure that puts on the hospital and questions whether the hospital will be in compliance with its debt service coverage covenants. Doug has always questioned the management ability of Linda's staff, and especially their ability to control costs. The data clearly show that the hospital's primary problem is related to cost. Revenues have been increasing slowly because of restricted government payments and deeply discounted managed care contracts, while costs have been escalating.

Data presented at the last board meeting showed hospital costs-per-adjusted discharge increasing by eight percent last year. This fact just irritated Doug and sent him off on a 30-minute tirade about how his business wouldn't survive if he let his costs increase at that magnitude. Linda and her CFO tried to explain the issues involved in dealing with health care costs in general, and hospital costs in particular. All these arguments fell on Doug's deaf ears. He closed the meeting with a challenge to Linda and her staff. He asked them to explain why costs increased eight percent with specific details, not generalities. Linda has tried to do this and thought of a couple of specific procedures that might help drive some of these points home.

She chose Single Vessel PTCA, which experienced an increase in costs of 21.7 percent, from $7,605 to $9,254. The increase in cost had puzzled most of Linda's management staff because length of stay actually dropped from 4.9 days to 4.3 days. Nursing costs fell, but ancillary costs skyrocketed. Upon examination, all of the increase was tracked to medical supplies. Most of the cardiologists performing this procedure had decided to use a new closure device that improves the quality of care, but is very costly. Many other examples in different product segment areas could also be explained when the costs of the procedure were compared at the revenue code level between years. Linda has directed the financial staff to document changes in costs for major procedures during the last year using variance analysis at the revenue code level. She is hopeful that this type of information will help answer Doug's questions as well as focus her staff on areas where costs can be controlled.

Cost variance analysis is of great potential importance to the health care industry. Successful use of cost variance analysis requires a sound system of standard setting, or budgeting, and a related system of cost accounting. Perhaps the major factor impeding the widespread adoption of more effective cost variance analysis in the health care industry has been the lack of interaction between it and existing systems of cost accounting.

Cost accounting systems usually serve two basic informational needs. First, they supply data essential for product or service costing. Second, they provide information for managerial cost control activity. This second role is the major topic of this chapter.

LEARNING OBJECTIVE 1

Describe alternative cost control approaches.

COST CONTROL

The following conceptual model is used to discuss the major alternatives to cost control in organizations:

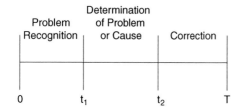

In general, there are three distinct time phases in an out-of-control situation:

1. Recognition of problem (0 to t_1)
2. Determination of problem or cause (t_1 to t_2)
3. Correction of problem (t_2 to T)

The unit of time used in the previous representation may be minutes, hours, days, weeks, or even months.

The important point is that the longer the problem remains uncorrected (0 to T), the greater the cost to the organization.

The term "efficiency cost" is sometimes used to describe the total cost incurred by an organization as a result of an out-of-control situation. Efficiency cost may be represented as follows:

Efficiency cost = T × R × P
where:
T = total time units that the problem remains uncorrected
R = loss or cost per time unit
P = probability that the problem occurrence is correctable

The objective of management should be to minimize the efficiency cost in any given situation. While accomplishing this objective, two major alternatives are available to management: (1) the preventive approach and (2) the detection-correction (DC) approach.

In the preventive approach, management attempts to minimize the efficiency cost by minimizing the probability that a problem will occur (P). One of the major methods for reducing the value of P centers on staffing. Management attempts not only to hire the most competent individuals available, but also to provide them with relevant training programs and materials to ensure consistently high levels of performance. The nature of the reward structure, both monetary and nonmonetary, also enters into this management strategy. The preventive approach is obviously used by most organizations, but the emphasis on it is usually greater in small organizations. In these organizations, the number of people supervised by one manager is usually smaller and the evaluation of individual performance is more direct.

The DC approach seeks to minimize efficiency cost by minimizing the time that a problem remains uncorrected (T). This method is directly related to the effectiveness of variance analysis. Effective variance analysis should result in a reduction of both the recognition of problem phase (0 to t_1) and the determination of cause phase (t_1 to t_2). The actual correction phase (t_2 to T) relies primarily on the effective motivation of management.

The development of cost variance analysis systems to reduce the recognition and determination phases usually involves the expenditure of funds. Prudent management dictates that the marginal expenditures of funds for system improvements be evaluated by their expected reductions in efficiency cost. For example, the frequency of reporting could be altered to reduce the problem recognition phase, or the number of cost areas reported could be increased to improve both recognition and determination times. However, these improvements are likely to result in increased cost and may not be justified. Areas of relatively small dollar expenditure or largely uncontrolled costs thus are not prime candidates for major system improvements.

INVESTIGATION OF VARIANCES

In the DC approach to cost control, cost variances are the clues that both signal that a potential problem exists and suggest a possible cause. These variances are usually an integral part of any management-by-exception plan of operations. A decision to investigate a given variance is not an automatic occurrence. It involves some financial commitment by the organization, and thus should be weighed carefully against the expected benefits. Unfortunately, management rarely knows whether any given variance is due to a random or noncontrollable cause or to an underlying problem that is correctable or controllable.

Many organizations have developed rules to determine what variances will be investigated. Common examples of such rules are to investigate the following:

* All variances that exceed an absolute dollar size (for example, $500)
* All variances that exceed budgeted or standard values by some fixed percentage (for example, ten percent)
* All variances that have been unfavorable for a defined number of periods (for example, three periods)
* Some combination of the previous rules

Actual specification of criteria values in the previous rules is highly dependent on management judgment and experience. A variance of $1,000 may be considered normal in some circumstances and abnormal in others.

LEARNING OBJECTIVE 2

Describe the two major theories used for the detection of out-of-control costs.

At some point, management may wish to determine whether the historical criteria values should be changed. In that case, some method of testing whether the historical values are acceptable or not acceptable must be developed. In general, there are two possible theories that may be used to develop this information: (1) classical statistical theory and (2) decision theory.

CLASSICAL STATISTICAL THEORY

One of the most commonly used means to determine which cost variances to investigate is the control chart. The control chart is often used to monitor a physical process by comparing output observations with predetermined tolerance limits. If actual observations fall between predetermined upper and lower control limits on the chart, the process is assumed to be in control.

Control charts can be established for determining when a cost variance should be investigated. The major assumption underlying the traditional development of control charts is that observed cost variances are distributed in accordance with a normal probability distribution. In a normal distribution, it can be anticipated that approximately 68.3 percent of the observations will fall within one standard deviation (s) of the mean ($\bar{x}$), 95.5 percent will fall within two standard deviations ($\bar{x} \pm 2\sigma$), and 99.7 percent will fall within three standard deviations ($\bar{x} \pm 3\sigma$).

The control limits for any given variance will then be set at the following:

$$\bar{x} \pm K\sigma$$

If the costs of investigation are high relative to the benefits in a given situation, then K may be set to a high value (for example, 3.0). This will ensure that few investigations will be made and that some out-of-control situations may continue. Conversely, if benefits are high relative to the costs of investigation, then lower values of K may be selected that will ensure that more investigations will be performed and that some situations that are not out of control will be investigated.

To develop the control chart, the underlying distribution must be specified. An assumption that the distribution is normal means that the analyst must define both the mean ($\bar{x}$) and the standard deviation (σ). In most situations, this specification will result from an analysis of prior observations. The ratio of the mean to the standard deviation is defined as the "coefficient of variation." Operations that have large coefficients of variation often represent greater control problems. To illustrate this process, assume that the pattern of labor variances in Table 16–1 occurred during the 13 bi-weekly pay periods:

The mean ($\bar{x}$) of these observations is calculated as follows:

$$\bar{x} = \frac{\sum x_i}{n} = \frac{0}{13} = 0$$

An estimate of the standard deviation (σ) is calculated as follows:

$$\sigma = \sqrt{\frac{\sum (x_i - \bar{x})^2}{n - 1}} = 437.80$$

If the labor cost variances in this example are expected to follow a normal distribution in the future with ($\bar{x}$) = 0 and σ = \$437.80, control limits for investigation at the 95-percent level could be defined by multiplying the estimated standard deviation by two. The following control chart would result:

$$\bar{x} + 2\sigma = 875.60$$
$$\bar{x} = 0$$
$$\bar{x} - 2\sigma = -875.60$$

Any observation falling within the control limits would not be investigated, whereas variances falling outside the established limits would be investigated.

The major deficiency in the classical statistical approach is that it does not relate the expected costs of investigation and benefits with the probability that the variance signals are out of control. The control chart can signal when a situation is likely to be out of control, but it cannot directly evaluate whether an investigation is warranted.

Table 16–1 Labor Variances by Pay Period

Pay Period	Variances (x^i)
1	800
2	400
3	−500
4	−100
5	200
6	−700
7	500
8	−300
9	−200
10	300
11	200
12	−200
13	−400
	0

DECISION THEORY

Decision theory provides a framework for directly integrating the probability of the system being out of control and the costs and benefits of investigation into a definite decision rule. Central to this approach is the payoff table, which specifically considers costs and benefits. Table 16–2 provides an example of a payoff table, where:

I = cost of investigation
C = cost of correcting an out-of-control situation
L = cost of letting an out-of-control situation continue (expected loss)

The payoff table is a conceptualization of the actual decision evaluation process. It can be applied to any cost variance situation. The objective is to minimize the actual cost for a given situation. To accomplish this, estimates of the probabilities for the two states, in control and out of control, are required.

Assume that P denotes the probability that the system is in control and that (1 − P) represents the probability

Table 16–2 Variance Investigation Payoff Table

	State	
Action	In Control	Out of Control
Investigate	I	I + C
Do not investigate	O	L

that the system is out of control. The expected cost of the two courses of action can be defined as follows:

Expected cost of investigating =
$$(P \times I) + (1 - P)(I + C) = I + (1 - P)C$$

Expected cost of not investigating =
$$(P \times O) + (1 - P)L = (1 - P)L$$

By setting the two expected costs equal to each other, we can determine the value of P to which the decision-maker is indifferent. This break-even probability would be calculated as follows:

$$P^* = 1 - \frac{I}{L - C}$$

Evaluation of this formula provides a nice summarization of earlier comments concerning the costs and benefits of investigating variances. In situations of high investigation costs (I) and low net benefits (L − C), the critical value of P (P*) becomes low. This, of course, means that to justify an investigation, the probability that the system is actually in control (P) must be very low, or, alternatively, the probability that the system is actually out of control (1 − P) must be large.

To use the decision theory model just described, the analyst must have estimates of I, C, L, and P. In most situations, there is a reasonable expectation that I and C will be relatively constant. These costs are usually directly related to the labor involved in the analysis. L, however, usually varies, depending on the size of the cost variance. In short, the loss depends on the proportion of the variance to be saved in future periods and the number of periods over which the loss is expected to occur if the situation is not corrected.

The value of P is, in many respects, the most difficult of the parameter values to specify. Either objective or subjective approaches may be used. An objective method may be used to develop an estimated probability distribution for the system. If the underlying distribution is assumed to be normal, estimating the mean and standard deviation from prior observations will enable the analyst to specify the distribution from this estimated distribution. The probability that any given system is under control (P) then can be defined.

Subjective estimates of P are possible on both a prior basis and an ex post facto basis. A subjective normalized distribution of variances can be built in advance as a basis for the estimate. The analyst might ask department managers between which two values

they would expect 50 percent of actual observations to fall. In a normal distribution, 50 percent of the observations will fall within plus or minus two-thirds of one standard deviation. If the budget cost for labor in a department is $4,000 per pay period, the department manager might specify that he or she expects actual observations to fall between $3,700 and $4,300 50 percent of the time. Using this information, a normalized distribution could be defined as presented in Figure 16–1.

Subjective estimates of P also may be made after an actual variance occurred and then related directly to the actual size of the cost variance. This assessment then can be related to a table of critical values of P necessary for an investigation decision of a given variance. This permits analysts to directly use sensitivity analysis in their decisions. For example, assume that I is $100 and that C is $200. Assume further that L is equal to two times the absolute size of the variance. Table 16–3 defines the critical values of P based upon the previous information. For example, if the variance was $200, the critical value of P would be 0.50 (1 − (100/(400 − 200))).

This table is relatively straightforward. As the dollar size of the variance increases, the probability that the system is under control must increase to justify a "do not investigate" decision. For example, if a variance of $600 occurred, the analyst must believe that there is at least a 90-percent probability that the system is under control.

LEARNING OBJECTIVE 3

Define variance analysis and how it is used by management.

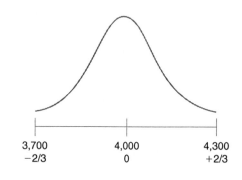

Figure 16–1 Normal Distribution of Labor Cost Utilization

Table 16–3 Relationship of P* to Variance Size

Critical Value of P (P*)	Size of Variance
0.50	$200
0.75	300
0.83	400
0.88	500
0.90	600

VARIANCE ANALYSIS CALCULATIONS

Variance analysis is simply an examination of the deviation of an actual observation from a standard. For the purposes of this chapter, the following two types of standards for comparative purposes are used: (1) prior-period values and (2) budgeted values. In each case, the objective of cost variance analysis is to explain why actual costs are different, either from budgeted values or from prior-period actual values. This objective is an important element in the cost-control process of the organization.

Prior-Period Comparisons

Relevant Factors

An evaluation of the difference between current levels of cost and prior costs should suggest to management which factors have contributed to the change. In general, the following three major factors influence costs: (1) input prices, (2) productivity of inputs, and (3) output levels.

Input prices usually are expected to increase over time. It is important, however, from management's perspective, to evaluate what portion, if any, of that increase was controllable or avoidable. Rapidly increasing prices for some commodities may signal opportunities for resource substitutions, for example, by switching to a less expensive mix of labor or substituting one supply item for another. In fact, measuring productivity has become increasingly important in the health care industry as a result of the emphasis on cost containment. One of the major difficulties in evaluating productivity, however, has been the changing nature of health care services. Comparison of productivity within a hospital for two periods requires that the services in each period be identical. For example, a comparison of full-time equivalents (FTEs) per patient day in 2007 with FTEs per patient day of care in 2004 is meaningless unless a patient day of care in 2007 is identical to a patient day of care in 2004. Finally, changes in output levels also influence the level of costs. This influence may occur in two ways. First, the absolute level of output provided may affect the quantity of resources necessary to produce the output level. Second, service intensity may affect resource requirements. Any increase in the number of services required per unit of output will directly affect costs. For example, a change in the number of laboratory procedures performed per patient day of care probably will affect the total cost per patient day of care.

This discussion can be summarized in the following cost function:

$$\text{Total cost} = P \times \frac{I}{X} \times \frac{X}{Q} \times Q$$

where:

P = input prices
I = physical quantities of inputs
X = services required per unit of output
Q = output level

In the previous cost equation, P represents the effect of input prices, I/X represents the effect of productivity, X/Q represents the effect of service intensity, and Q represents the influence of output. Changes in cost can result from changes in any one of these four terms.

LEARNING OBJECTIVE 4

Calculate the various types of cost variances.

MACROANALYSIS

There are many occasions when it is important to discover and communicate the causes for cost increases at the organizational level, whether that organization is a hospital, nursing home, or surgicenter. For example, your board may want to know why your total costs have increased 60 percent in the last three years. A useful framework can be developed to provide answers to questions such as this, provided that some critical pieces of information can be defined.

- There must be one measure of activity or output for the entire organization. This might be an adjusted discharge, patient day, visit, or other measure.

• It must be possible to define a measure of activity for each department within the organization and to define a cost per unit for that measure. It may not be necessary to define an output unit for indirect departments—those departments that do not directly provide a product or service to the patient—provided that the costs of the indirect departments have been allocated to the direct departments.

We will now develop a model and example for a hospital to illustrate the use of this macroanalysis. First, we will assume that our measure of activity is an adjusted discharge. The term "adjusted" simply reflects that outpatient activity has been recognized. This recognition may have occurred through a simple ratio of inpatient revenue to total patient revenue at the organizational level or at the individual departmental level.

The general cost per adjusted discharge (CPD) can be defined in the following equation:

$$CPD = C \times Q$$

where:

C = cost (direct and indirect) per unit of output in each department
Q = units of output in each department required per adjusted discharge

The following example is now presented to help clarify the previous concepts. The data in Table 16–4 represent cost and volume information for the year 2007. These data are compared with cost and volume data for 2005.

In this example, the CPD increased 31.6 percent from 2005 to 2007. Causes for the increase could be partitioned into the following two possible areas:

1. Intensity of service—More units of intermediate services are required per discharge, such as laboratory tests and days in intensive care unit.
2. Cost—Cost increases could have resulted from higher prices paid for inputs such as wage and salary, changes in the nature of the service provided (such as a change in the proportion of routine chest radiographs to computed tomography scans), or a change in efficiency of production.

The following two indices, HCI (Hospital Cost Index) and HII (Hospital Intensity Index) capture the impact of each of these two areas.

$$\frac{CPD^t}{CPD^0} = \frac{C^t Q^t}{C^0 Q^0} = HCI \times HII$$

The HCI is defined as the following:

$$HCI = \frac{C^t Q^0}{C^0 Q^0}$$

The HCI measures the change in cost attributed to both price increases and productivity changes. The other index, HII, is defined as the following:

$$HII = \frac{C^0 Q^t}{C^0 Q^0}$$

The HII measures the change in cost due to changes in service intensity.

Using this framework in our example data would yield the following values:

$$HCI = \frac{\begin{array}{l}(\$714.29 \times .4000) + \\ (\$308.12 \times 6.6000) + \\ (\$500.00 \times 1.5000) + \\ (\$85.71 \times 5.0000) + \\ \underline{(\$285.71 \times 2.0000)}\end{array}}{\begin{array}{l}(\$562.50 \times .4000) + \\ (\$252.52 \times 6.6000) + \\ (\$472.22 \times 1.5000) + \\ (\$75.00 \times 5.000) + \\ (\$150.00 \times 2.0000)\end{array}}$$

$$\frac{\$4,069}{\$3,275} = 1.242$$

$$HII = \frac{\begin{array}{l}(\$562.50 \times .4828) + \\ (\$252.52 \times 6.1552) + \\ (\$472.22 \times 1.7241) + \\ (\$75.00 \times 6.0345) + \\ \underline{(\$150.00 \times 2.4138)}\end{array}}{\begin{array}{l}(\$562.50 \times .4000) + \\ (\$252.52 \times 6.6000) + \\ (\$472.22 \times 1.5000) + \\ (\$75.00 \times 5.0000) + \\ (\$150.00 \times 2.0000)\end{array}}$$

$$\frac{\$3,455}{\$3,275} = 1.055$$

The previous calculations show that the increase in CPD from 2005 to 2007 could be broken down as follows:

Percentage increase due to cost increases	24.2%
Percentage increase due to intensity	5.5
Joint cost and intensity	1.9
Total increase	31.6%

Table 16–4 Summary of Cost per Discharge (2007 and 2005)

2007 Cost Summary
(11,600 Discharges)

Department	Volume	Cost (000s)	Cost/ Unit (C^t)	Units/ Discharge (Q^t)
Intensive care unit	5,600	$4,000	$714.29	0.4828
Routine nursing	71,400	22,000	308.12	6.1552
Operating room	20,000	10,000	500.00	1.7241
Laboratory	70,000	6,000	85.71	6.0345
Radiology	28,000	8,000	285.71	2.4138
		$50,000		

Note: 2007 CPD = $50,000,000/11,600 = $4,310.34.

2005 Cost Summary
(12,000 Discharges)

Department	Volume	Cost (000s)	Cost/ Unit (C^t)	Units/ Discharge (Q^t)
Intensive care unit	4,800	$2,700	$562.50	0.40000
Routine nursing	79,200	20,000	252.52	6.60000
Operating room	18,000	8,500	472.22	1.50000
Laboratory	60,000	4,500	75.00	5.00000
Radiology	24,000	3,600	150.00	2.00000
		$39,300		

Note: 2005 CPD = $39,300,000/12,000 = $3,275.00.

For those who wish to further break down the causes for the increase in CPD during the two-year period, some individual departmental analysis could be done. For example, in 2007, the average laboratory CPD was $517.22 ($85.71 × 6.0345), compared with $375.00 ($75.00 × 5.000) in 2005. This represents a 37.9 percent increase and could be broken down into cost and intensity factors also. The next section applies variance analysis using prior period values to individual departments or cost centers within a health care firm.

DEPARTMENTAL ANALYSIS OF VARIANCE

The preceding indices are useful for analyzing cost changes at the total facility level. In such situations, a measure of output for the facility as a whole—such as patient days, admissions, discharges, visits, or enrollees—would be used. Although this type of analysis may be useful, it is also often desirable to analyze the reasons

for cost changes at the departmental level. In general, the primary reason for a cost change at the departmental level between two periods can be stated as a function of the following three factors:

1. Changes in input prices
2. Changes in input productivity (efficiency)
3. Changes in departmental volume

LEARNING OBJECTIVE 5

Explain and calculate price, efficiency, and volume variances.

The following three variances can be calculated to compute the effects of cost changes at the departmental level:

Price variance = (present price − old price) × present quantity

Efficiency variance = (present quantity − expected quantity at old productivity) × old price

Volume variance = (present volume − old volume) × old cost per unit

These formulas may be applied to the laundry example found in Table 16–5. It is assumed that the laundry has only two inputs: soap and labor.

With these calculations, Table 16–6 summarizes the factors that created cost changes in the laundry department and indicates that increased volume was the largest source of the total change in cost. It is often useful to factor this volume variance into two areas:

Intensity = (change in volume due to intensity difference) × old cost per unit

Pure volume variance = (change in volume due to change in overall service) × old cost per unit

Here, the intensity variance represents the change in volume due to increased intensity of service. For example, in 2007, 2.25 pounds of laundry were provided per patient day (180,000/80,000). The corresponding value for 2005 was 2.00 pounds per patient day (140,000/ 70,000). The two volume variances would be the following:

Intensity variance = ([2.25 − 2.00] × 80,000) × $1.870 = $37,400

Pure volume variance = 2.00 × (80,000 − 70,000) × $1.870 = $37,400

The system of cost variance analysis described previously should be a useful framework in which to discuss factors causing changes in departmental costs. Aggregation of some resource categories probably will be both necessary and desirable. There would be little point in calculating price and efficiency variances for each of 100 or more supply items. Only major supply categories should be examined. The supply items that

---

Table 16–5 Cost Data for Linen/Linen Department

	2005	2007
Pounds of laundry	140,000	180,000
Units of soap	1,400	1,800
Soap units per pound of laundry	0.01	0.01
Price per soap unit	$40.00	$50.00
Productive hours worked	19,600	27,000
Productive hours per pound of laundry	0.14	0.15
Wage rate per productive hour	10.50	12.00
Total cost	$261,800	$414,000
Cost per pound	$1.870	$2.300
Patient days	70,000	80,000
Pound of laundry per patient day	2.00	2.25

Price variances
  Soap = ($50.00 − $40.00) × 1,800 = $18,000 [Unfavorable]
  Labor = ($12.00 − $10.50) × 27,000 = $40,500 [Unfavorable]
Efficiency variances
  Soap = (1,800 − [.01 × 180,000]) × $40.00 = $0
  Labor = (27,000 − [.14 × 180,000]) × $10.50 = $18,900 [Unfavorable]
Volume variances
  Volume variance = (180,000 − 140,000) × $1.870 = 74,800 [Unfavorable]

Table 16–6 Variance Analysis Summary

Causes of Laundry Department Cost Change, 2002 to 2004

	Dollars	% Change
Increase in wages	$40,500	26.6
Increase in soap price	18,000	11.8
Decline in labor efficiency	18,900	12.4
Increase in volume	74,800	49.1
Total change in cost	$152,200	100.0

are aggregated together could not be broken down in terms of individual price and efficiency variances because there would be no common input quantity measure. For example, the addition of pencils, sheets of paper, and boxes of paper clips would not produce a comparable unit of measure. For these smaller areas of supply or material costs, a simple change in cost per unit of departmental output may be just as informative as detailed price and efficiency variances.

VARIANCE ANALYSIS IN BUDGETARY SETTINGS

A final area in which variance analysis can be applied is the operation of a formalized budgeting system. The presentation that follows assumes a budgeting system that is based on a flexible model. This means that the management must have identified those elements of cost that are presumed to be fixed and those that are presumed to be variable in the budgetary process. Although relatively few health care organizations use flexible budgeting models at the present time, a trend toward their adoption is emerging. In this context, the variance analysis models examined here may be applied to any budgetary situation, fixed or flexible.

The cost equation for any given department may be represented as follows:

$$Cost = F + (V \times Q)$$

where:

F = fixed costs
V = variable costs per unit of output
Q = output in units

The fixed and variable cost coefficients are the sum of many individual resource quantity and unit price products. These terms can be represented as follows:

$$F = I_f \times P_f$$
$$V = I_v \times P_v$$

where:

I_f = physical units of fixed resources
P_f = price per unit of fixed resources
I_v = physical units of variable resources per unit of output
P_v = price per unit of variable resources

In most budgeting situations, there are three levels of output or volume that are critical in cost variance analysis. The first is the actual level of volume produced in the budget-reporting period. This level of activity is critical because if management has established a set of expectations concerning how costs should behave (given changes in volume from budgeted levels), an adjustment to budgeted cost can be made for a change in volume.

The second critical level is that of budgeted or expected volume. It is on this expected volume level that management establishes its commitments for resources, and therefore incurs cost. An unjustified faith in volume forecasts can lock management into a sizable fixed-cost position, especially regarding labor costs.

The third critical level is that of standard volume. Standard volume is equal to actual volume, unless there is some indication that not all of the output was necessary. For example, a utilization review committee may determine that a certain number of patient days were medically unnecessary or that some surgical procedures were not warranted. Alternatively, in some indirect departments, such as maintenance, it may be important to identify the difference between actual and standard, or necessary, output. The cost effect of these output decisions needs to be isolated, and control should be directed to the individual(s) responsible.

The expected level of costs incurred at each of the three levels of volume (actual, budgeted, and standard) may be expressed as follows:

$$FB^a = F + (V \times Q_a)$$
$$FB^b = F + (V \times Q_b)$$
$$FB^s = F + (V \times Q_s)$$

where:

FB^a = flexible budget at actual output level
FB^b = flexible budget at budgeted output level
FB^s = flexible budget at standard output level
Q^a = actual output
Q^b = budgeted output
Q^s = standard output

The major categories of variances now can be defined to explain the difference between actual cost (AC) and applied cost ($Q^s \times FB^b/Q^b$). See Table 16–7.

For control purposes, it is important to further break down the spending variance into individual resource categories, and also to isolate the change due to price and efficiency factors. This will not only better isolate control for budget deviations, but also improve the problem definition and determination phase times discussed earlier in the detection-correction approach to cost control. The spending variances are broken down as follows:

Efficiency = $(I^a - I^b)P^b$
Price = $(P^a - P^b)I^a$

where:

I^a = actual physical units of resource
I^b = budgeted physical units of resource
P^a = actual price per unit of resource
P^b = budgeted price per unit of resource

With this background, we must now relate the structure we developed for standard costing in Chapter 14 to our analyses of budgetary variances. The following two sets of standards are involved: (1) standard cost profiles (SCPs) and (2) standard treatment protocols (STPs). SCPs are developed at the departmental level. They reflect the quantity of resources that should be used and the prices that should be paid for those resources to produce a specific departmental output unit, which can be defined as a service unit (SU). Table 16–8 provides an SCP for a nursing unit, with the SU defined as a patient day.

Using Table 16–8, a standard variance analysis could be performed for any period. For example, the data in Table 16–9 reflect actual experience in the most recent month.

Table 16–7 Categories of Budgetary Variances

Variance Name	Definition	Cause
Spending	$(AC - FB^a)$	Price and efficiency
Utilization	$(Q^a - Q^s) \times (FB^b/Q^b)$	Excessive services
Volume	$(Q^b - Q^a) \times (F/Q^b)$	Difference from budgeted volume

In this example, the nursing unit would have incurred actual expenditures of $99,300 during the month. It would have charged its standard cost times the number of patient days to treated patients:

Cost charged to patients = $97,080 = $161.80 × 600

The total variance to be accounted for would be the difference ($99,300 – $97,080), or $2,220, which is an unfavorable variance. The individual variances that constitute this total are shown in the following calculations:

1. Spending variances
   • Efficiency variances $([I^a - I^b]P^b)$
     a. Head nurse = (180 − 189) × $30.00 = $270.00 (Favorable)
     b. RN = (1,800 − 1,830) × $24.00 = $720.00 (Favorable)
     c. LPN = (1,200 − 1,200) × $16.00 = 0
     d. Aides = (2,400 − 2,430) × $10.00 = $300.00 (Favorable)
     e. Supplies = (1,300 − 1,200) × $4.40 = $440.00 (Unfavorable)
   • Price variances $([P^a - P^b]I^a)$
     a. Head nurse = ($31.00 − $30.00) × 180 = $180.00 (Unfavorable)
     b. RN = ($25.00 − $24.00) × 1,800 = $1,800.00 (Unfavorable)
     c. LPN = ($16.20 − $16.00) × 1,200 = $240.00 (Unfavorable)
     d. Aides = ($9.60 − $10.00) × 2,400 = $960.00 (Favorable)
     e. Supplies = ($4.80 − $4.40) × 1,300 = $520.00 (Unfavorable)
2. Volume variance $([Q^b - Q^a] [F/Q^b])$
   • Volume variance = (630 − 600) × $43.00 = $1,290.00 (Unfavorable)

Efficiency—Head nurse	$270.00	(Favorable)
Efficiency—RN	720.00	(Favorable)
Efficiency—LPN	0.00	
Efficiency—Aides	300.00	(Favorable)
Efficiency—Supplies	440.00	(Unfavorable)
Price—Head nurse	$ 180.00	(Unfavorable)
Price—RN	1,800.00	(Unfavorable)
Price—LPN	240.00	(Unfavorable)
Price—Aides	960.00	(Favorable)
Price—Supplies	520.00	(Unfavorable)
Volume	1,290.00	(Unfavorable)
Total	$2,220.00	(Unfavorable)

A few additional statements about the calculation of the efficiency variances may be necessary. The formula states that the difference between actual quantity (I^a)

Table 16–8 Standard Cost Profile for Nursing Unit

Standard Cost Profile
Nursing Unit Number 6
Patient Day = Service Unit
Expected Patient Days = 630

Resource	Quantity Variable	Quantity Fixed	Unit Cost	Variable Cost	Average Fixed Cost	Average Total Cost
Head nurse	0.00	0.30	$30.00	$0.00	$9.00	$9.00
Registered Nurse (RN)	2.00	1.00	24.00	48.00	24.00	72.00
Licensed Practical Nurse (LPN)	2.00	0.00	16.00	32.00	0.00	32.00
Aides	3.00	1.00	10.00	30.00	10.00	40.00
Supplies	2.00	0.00	4.40	8.80	0.00	8.80
Total				$118.80	$43.00	$161.80

and budgeted quantity (I^b) is multiplied by budgeted price (P^b). The most difficult calculation is that for budgeted quantity. It represents the quantity of resources that should have been used at the actual level of output, or the sum of the budgeted fixed requirement plus the variable requirement at actual output (600 patient days). Table 16–10 shows the calculation of fixed and variable requirements for the individual resource categories.

The calculation for volume variance also may require some further explanation. This variance is simply the product of the difference between budgeted and actual volume ($Q^a - Q^b$) and the average fixed cost budgeted (F/Q^b). The average fixed cost, as calculated in the SCP amounted to $43.00. You will notice that in our example volume variance is unfavorable because actual volume of patient days (600) was less than budgeted patient days (630). Because actual volume was

less than that budgeted, the average fixed cost per unit will increase. The reverse situation would have existed if actual volume had exceeded budgeted volume. In that situation, the volume variance would have been favorable.

The third type of variance, utilization variance, results from a difference between actual volume and standard volume, or the quantity of volume actually needed. The measure of standard volume is generated from the STPs, which define how much output or how many SUs are required per treated patient type.

Let us generate a hypothetical set of data to apply to our nursing unit example. Assume that the patients treated in Nursing Unit Number 6 are all in diagnosis related group (DRG) 209 (major joint procedures) and are all associated with one physician, Dr. Mallard. Our STP for DRG 209 calls for a 5-day length of stay. A review of Dr. Mallard's patient records reveals that only

Table 16–9 Actual Cost for Nursing Unit

Actual Month's Cost
Nursing Unit Number 6
Actual Patient Days = 600

Resource	Quantity Used	Unit Cost	Total Cost
Head nurse	180	$31.00	$5,580
Registered Nurse (RN)	1,800	25.00	45,000
Licensed Practical Nurse (LPN)	1,200	16.20	19,440
Aides	2,400	9.60	23,040
Supplies	1,300	4.80	6,240
Total			$99,300

Table 16–10 Calculation of Budgeted Resource Requirements

1 Resource Category	2 Average Fixed Requirement/ Unit	3 Budgeted Fixed Requirement (Col. 2 × 630)	4 Average Variable Requirement/ Unit	5 Budgeted Variable Requirement (Col. 4 × 600)	6 Total Requirement (Col. 3 + Col. 5)
Head nurse	0.30	189	0.00	0	189
Registered Nurse (RN)	1.00	630	2.00	1,200	1,830
Licensed Practical Nurse (LPN)	0.00	0	2.00	1,200	1,200
Aides	1.00	630	3.00	1,800	2,430
Supplies	0.00	0	2.00	1,200	1,200

560 patient days of care should have been used (112 cases at 5 days per case). Dr. Mallard had forty patients with lengths of stay greater than 5 days. These forty patients accounted for an excess of 80 patient days. Dr. Mallard also had 20 patients with shorter lengths of stay. These patients offset 40 days of the 80-day surplus. Thus, although 600 patient days of care were provided, only 560 should have been used. This creates an unfavorable utilization variance, calculated as the product of budgeted cost per unit and the difference between actual and standard volume. In our example of Nursing Unit Number 6, the utilization variance would be as follows:

$$\text{Utilization variance} = (600 - 560) \times \$161.80 = \$6,472.00 \text{ (Unfavorable)}$$

This variance is not charged to the nursing department. It is charged to the manager of patient treatment, which in this case is Dr. Mallard.

Figure 16–2 depicts the flow of costs and the variances associated with each account. This delineation of variances serves as a powerful tool for analyzing actual cost variances from budgeted cost levels. The existence of a flexible budget model is not a prerequisite to its use. The only real prerequisite is that major resource cost categories be separated into price and utilization components. Because effective cost control appears to be predicated on a separate analysis of price and utilization decisions, this does not seem too difficult a task, considering the potential payoff. Finally, it should be noted that there is no requirement to formally include these variances in the budget-reporting

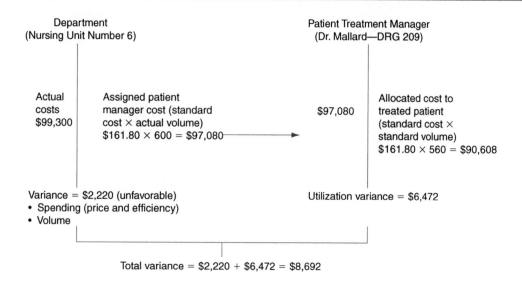

Figure 16–2 Variance Analysis Summary

models. They can be calculated on an ad hoc basis to investigate and explain large cost variances.

VARIANCE ANALYSIS IN MANAGED CARE SETTINGS

Variance analysis is an important analytical tool that has become useful to managed care firms that are seeking to monitor and control their costs. Because most managed care firms operate with relatively small margins, and because most of their costs are variable, changes in budgetary assumptions can have a sizable influence on costs and, therefore, profitability.

The following relationships will help us to formulate a variance analysis model that will separate cost variations into factors that are suggestive of cause and should lead to corrective actions more quickly.

Total cost = Inpatient cost (IPC) + Outpatient cost (OPC)

Inpatient Cost (IPC)
IPC = Admissions × Cost per admission
Admissions = Enrollees (E) × Admissions per member (APM)
Cost per admission = Cost per admission at case mix of 1.0 (CPA) × Admission case-mix index (ACMI)
IPC = E × APM × CPA × ACMI

Outpatient Cost (OPC)
OPC = Visits × Cost per visit
Visits = Enrollees (E) × Visits per member (VPM)
Cost per visit = Cost per visit at case mix of 1.0 (CPV) × Visit case-mix index (VCMI)
OPC = E × VPM × CPV × VCMI

The previous formulas define the following primary cost drivers:

1. Enrollment (E)
2. Utilization (APM or VPM)
3. Efficiency (CPA or CPV)
4. Patient mix (ACMI or VCMI)

Costs in a managed care setting can increase because of changes in any one of these four factors. An increase in enrollment most likely will lead to an increase in costs, but this increase may be offset by an increase in revenues, and profits may actually improve. Utilization increases most likely will lead to an

increase in costs because more units of service, either more admissions or more visits, are being provided per member. Increases in cost per unit (CPA or CPV) would signal a decline in efficiency and lead to an increase in costs. If the managed care organization is not fully integrated and is not affected by increased production costs, this may not be a concern. If, however, the managed care firm owns the providers of care, then increases in their costs will adversely affect profitability of the consolidated firm. Finally, changes in patient mix, ACMI or VCMI, can adversely affect costs. Utilization of more costly procedures can have a negative effect on profits.

To illustrate the use of this framework, a case example is presented in Table 16–11.

The total variance to account for in the case presented in Table 16–11 is shown in Table 16-12.

The numbers indicate that costs were much higher than expected, but they do not relay the cause of the variance. The definition of individual variances can help explain causes for the total variance and suggest possible solutions. We know from the case in Table 16–11 that there were 880 actual inpatient admissions and that the actual cost per case was $5,304, which generated actual inpatient costs of $4,667,520. There were 750 budgeted inpatient admissions, and budgeted costs per case were $5,000, which generated an expected or budgeted cost of $3,750,000. Costs were higher than budgeted because we admitted more patients and the cost to treat them was higher than expected. Let's use the framework described previously to partition the total variance into areas that might suggest possible causes and solutions.

Volume-Related Variances

We know that we admitted 130 more patients than expected (880 − 750) and experienced 10,000 more outpatient visits than expected (55,000 − 45,000). This deviation in volume can result from two possible causes:

- Changes in enrollees
- Changes in utilization rates

Enrollment Variances

Enrollment variances are simply the product of budgeted cost per unit times the change in enrollment

Table 16–11 Managed Care Budget to Actual Comparison

	Budgeted	Actual
Enrollees (E)	10,000	11,000
Admissions per member (APM)	0.075	0.080
Admissions (E × APM)	750	880
Visits per member (VPM)	4.5	5.0
Visits (E × VPM)	45,000	55,000
Cost per admission (CPA)	$5,000	$5,200
Admission case-mix index (ACMI)	1.0	1.02
Actual cost per admission (CPA × ACMI)	$5,000	$5,304
Cost per visit (CPV)	$75	$80
Visit case-mix index (VCMI)	1.10	1.15
Actual cost per visit (CPV × VCMI)	$82.50	$92.00
Inpatient costs	$3,750,000	$4,667,520
Outpatient costs	$3,712,500	$5,060,000
Total costs	$7,462,500	$9,727,520

times budgeted utilization. The formulas for these variances are presented in Table 16–13.

Utilization Variances

Utilization variances are simply the product of the change in volume due to the change in usage rates calculated at the actual number of enrollees times budgeted cost per unit (Table 16–14).

Note that the change in inpatient volume attributed to enrollment variance is 75 (1,000 × .075) and that the change in inpatient volume attributed to utilization variance is 55 (.005 × 11,000). Added together, the two variances total 130, which was the difference between budgeted and actual inpatient cases. In a similar manner, the outpatient volume difference of 10,000 can be factored into 4,500 attributed to enrollment variance and 5,500 attributed to utilization variance. Multiplying these variations in volume by the budgeted costs of $5,000 per case and $82.50 per visit yield the variances calculated previously.

Cost-Related Variances

The actual cost of treating an inpatient case was $5,304 compared to a budgeted cost per case of $5,000, a difference of $304 per case. The outpatient difference between actual and budgeted cost per visit was $9.50 ($92.00 − $82.50). These differences in costs contributed to the overall unfavorable variance, but as before, there are two possible causes for this deviation in cost per unit:

- Changes in the efficiency of production
- Changes in the case mix of patients seen

Efficiency Variance

Efficiency variances are a reflection of a change in the underlying cost of production, keeping case mix constant. The efficiency variance is the product of the difference between actual and budgeted costs for a constant case mix equal to one times the actual case mix of

Table 16–12 Summary of Cost Variance

	Inpatient Costs	Outpatient Costs	Total Costs
Actual costs	$4,667,520	$5,060,000	$9,727,520
Less budgeted costs	3,750,000	3,712,500	7,462,500
Variance	$917,520	$1,347,500	$2,265,020

Table 16–13 Variance Definitions—Enrollment

Variance Formula	Calculation	Variance
Inpatient = $(E^a - E^b) \times APM^b \times CPA^b \times ACMI^b$	$(11,000 - 10,000) \times .075 \times \$5,000 \times 1.0$	\$375,000
Outpatient = $(E^a - E^b) \times VPM^b \times CPV^b \times VCMI^b$	$(11,000 - 10,000) \times 4.5 \times \$75 \times 1.1$	\$371,250
Total enrollment variance		\$746,250

patients seen times actual volume of patients (Table 16–15). Differences could result from increases in actual costs for an integrated delivery system, which owned one or more of the delivery providers. Differences could also result in a non-integrated delivery system because more enrollees sought care at higher priced providers.

Case-Mix Variances

Case-mix variances reflect the change in cost per unit that has resulted not from a change in efficiency, but from a change in case mix of patients seen. This variance may not be controllable by the providers and may be a reflection of the nature of the insured population. Case-mix variances are the product of the change in case mix times the expected cost per unit at a case-mix standard value of one times the actual volume (Table 16–16).

The variation in cost per case was \$304, of which \$204 is attributed to efficiency variation and \$100 is attributed to case-mix variation. The difference in cost per outpatient visit was \$9.50, of which \$5.75 is attributed to efficiency variation and \$3.75 is attributed to case-mix variation. Multiplying these differences by the actual volumes of patients seen (880 cases and 55,000 visits) produces the variances reported previously.

It is now possible to summarize the variance analysis performed to date in a structure that may help management direct their attention to areas needing correction. This is done in Table 16–17.

Table 16–17 shows that the majority of the total variance can be attributed to enrollment variance and utilization variance. Of the two, enrollment variances accounted for approximately 32.9 percent of the total variation and is not likely to be a problem because increased enrollment most likely was offset by increased

Table 16–14 Variance Definitions—Utilization

Variance Formula	Calculation	Variance
Inpatient = $(APM^a - APM^b) \times E^a \times CPA^b \times ACMI^b$	$(.080 - .075) \times 11,000 \times \$5,000 \times 1.0$	\$275,000
Outpatient = $(VPM^a - VPM^b) \times E^a \times CPV^b \times VCMI^b$	$(5.0 - 4.5) \times 11,000 \times \$75 \times 1.10$	\$453,750
Total utilization variance		\$728,750

Table 16–15 Variance Definitions—Efficiency

Variance Formula	Calculation	Variance
Inpatient = $(CPA^a - CPA^b) \times ACMI^a \times E^a \times APM^a$	$(\$5,200 - \$5,000) \times 1.02 \times 11,000 \times .080$	\$179,520
Outpatient = $(CPV^a - CPV^b) \times VCMI^a \times E^a \times VPM^a$	$(\$80 - \$75) \times 1.15 \times 11,000 \times 5.0$	\$316,250
Total efficiency variance		\$495,770

Table 16-16 Variance Definitions—Case Mix

Variance Formula	Calculation	Variance
Inpatient = (ACMI[a] − ACMI[b]) × CPA[b] × E[a] × APM[a]	(1.02 − 1.0) × $5,000 × 11,000 × .080	$88,000
Outpatient = (VCMI[a] − VCMI[b]) × CPV[b] × E[a] × VPM[a]	(1.15 − 1.10) × $75 × 11,000 × 5.0	$206,250
Total case-mix variance		$294,250

revenues. The utilization variances accounted for 32.2 percent of the total variation and could represent a serious problem that should be examined. Continuation of this trend could destroy the firm's profitability.

SUMMARY

In general, within the framework for cost control, the following two approaches are possible: (1) preventive and (2) detection-correction (DC). The DC approach is usually based on some system of variance analysis. From a decision-theory perspective, the investigation of a variance is based on the cost of investigation, the probability that a correctable problem exists, the potential loss if the problem is not corrected, and the costs of problem correction. It may not always be possible to develop truly objective measures for these values, but sensitivity analysis may offer a useful aid in such situations.

Table 16-17 Individual Variance Analysis Summary

Variance Cause	Inpatient Amount	Inpatient %	Outpatient Amount	Outpatient %	Amount	Total %
Enrollment	$375,000	40.8	$371,250	27.6	$746,250	32.9
Utilization	275,000	30.0	453,750	33.7	728,750	32.2
Efficiency	179,520	19.6	316,250	23.5	495,770	21.9
Case Mix	88,000	9.6	206,250	15.3	294,250	13.0
Total	$917,520	100.0	$1,347,500	100.0	$2,265,020	100.0

ASSIGNMENTS

1. Two general types of approaches to internal control are preventive and detection-correction approaches. Preventive approaches stress the elimination of problems, whereas detection-correction approaches stress the early recognition and correction of problems. What sorts of things could you do if you used a preventive approach to reduce costs?

2. What is a coefficient of variation, and how can that information be used in budgeting?

3. Which would you investigate first—a budget variance that is 1.0 standard deviation away from the expected value or one that is 1.5 standard deviations away from the value? Why?

4. When is the use of a flexible budget likely to be most effective?

5. Standard cost accounting systems often separate variance into price and efficiency components. Why?

6. Why might the use of a multivariable flexible budget reduce the time involved in investigating variances?

7. Ned Zechman is the dietary manager of a large convalescent center. He is disturbed by highly unfavorable variances in his food budget over the past three months. Ned has been reducing both the quantity and quality of delivered meals, but to date, there has been no reflection of this in his monthly budget variance report. A recent organizational change brought in Pat Schumaker, who is now responsible for all purchasing activity, including dietary. All purchased food costs are charged to dietary at the time of purchase. What do you think might explain Ned's problem, and how would you determine the cause?

8. Assume that the budgeted cost for a department is $10,000 per week and the standard deviation is $500. The decision to investigate a variance requires a comparison of expected benefits with expected costs. Suppose an unfavorable variance of $1,000 is observed. The normal distribution indicates the probability of observing this variance is .0228 if the system is in control. Furthermore, assume that the benefits would be 50 percent of the variance and that investigation costs are $200. Should this variance be investigated? Assume that the variance is still $1,000, but it is favorable. Should it still be investigated?

9. Departmental costs may be out of control if either the variance is outside specified limits or the number of successive observations, above or below expected costs, is excessive. The binomial distribution can be used as a basis for determining what is or is not excessive. If we assume that the probability of being either above or below budgeted costs is .50, then the probability of n successive observations of actual costs being greater than budgeted costs is $.50^n$. What is the probability of observing six successive periods in which actual costs are greater than budgeted costs?

10. You are evaluating the performance of the radiology department manager. The SU, or output, for this department is the number of procedures. A static budget was prepared at the beginning of the year. You are now examining that budget in relation to actual experience. The relevant data are included in Table 16–18.

Table 16–18 Radiology Department Data

	Actual	Original Budget	Variance
Procedures	100,000	120,000	20,000 (Unfavorable)
Variable costs	$1,200,000	$1,320,000	$120,000 (Favorable)
Fixed costs	600,000	600,000	—
Total costs	$1,800,000	$1,920,000	$120,000 (Favorable)

The department manager is pleased because he has a favorable $120,000 cost variance. Evaluate the effectiveness claims of the manager using the budgetary variance model described in this chapter.

11. The data in Table 16–19 were assembled for a laundry department during the period from 2005 to 2007.

Table 16–19 Laundry Department Data

	2005	2007
Weighted patient days	24,140	24,539
Pounds of laundry	333,225	328,624
Pounds per day	13.80385	13.39191
Hours worked	6,665	6,901
Hours per pound	0.020	0.021
Average salary per hour	$10.50	$11.00
Total salary cost	$69,977	$75,912
Salary cost per pound	$0.210	$0.231
Supply units	3,332	3,286
Supply units per pound	0.01	0.01
Cost per supply unit	$2.69	$3.18
Total supply cost	$8,979	$10,466
Total cost	$78,956	$86,378
Cost per pound	$0.2369	$0.2628

Break down the total change in cost ($7,422) into the variance categories described in this chapter, that is, price, efficiency, intensity volume, and pure volume variances.

12. John Jones, CEO at Valley Hospital, is concerned by the rapid increase in cost per case during the last five years at his hospital. Five years ago, his average cost per case was $9,295; it is now $14,355. Using the data in Table 16–20, help John understand what factors have fueled the increase in costs during the last five years.

Table 16–20 Valley Hospital DRG Costs

	Total Cost	Volume	Average Cost
Present			
DRG 106	$150,000	10	$15,000
DRG 107	200,000	20	10,000
DRG 103	95,000	1	95,000
	$445,000	31	$14,355
Five Years Ago			
DRG 106	$114,750	9	$12,750
DRG 107	192,000	24	8,000
DRG 103	0	0	0
	$306,750	33	$9,295

13. You have just taken a position as a financial analyst with the American Health Plan, a partially integrated delivery system, contracting with major employers for health care services. The financial and utilization data in Table 16–21 were presented to you regarding the previous completed year.

Table 16–21 American Health Plan Budget

	Budgeted	Actual
Enrollees	10,000	11,000
Patient days per 1,000 enrollees	600	550
Patient days	6,000	6,050
Visits per member	5.0	5.5
Visits	50,000	60,500
Cost per patient day	$1,000	$1,100
Cost per visit	$65	$62
Inpatient costs	$6,000,000	$6,655,000
Outpatient costs	$3,250,000	$3,751,000
Total costs	$9,250,000	$10,406,000
Per member per year costs	$925	$946

You have been asked to make some sense of this data and factor the total variance of $1,156,000 ($10,406,000 − $9,250,000) into some subaccounts that suggest possible causes. Please review these data and calculate the following variances for both inpatient and outpatient categories:

- Enrollment variance
- Utilization variance
- Efficiency variance (note that there is no case-mix intensity standard)

SOLUTIONS AND ANSWERS

1. The following are some of the things you could do, using a preventive approach: improve employee training, increase inspection of material, improve equipment maintenance, and increase supervision.

2. The coefficient of variation is the ratio of the standard deviation to the mean. A large value implies great variability in the results. In a budgeting context, operations with large prior coefficients of variation typically require a more sophisticated budget model, such as a flexible budget, to account for deviations from average performance.

3. The budget variance that is 1.5 standard deviations from expected performance is more likely to be controllable and should be investigated first. However, adjustments for the relative differences in investigation costs and variance size should be considered.

4. A flexible budget is likely to be most effective when costs in a department are not fixed and are expected to vary with changes in output or other variables.

5. In many situations, separating variances into price and efficiency components is helpful because one person does not have decision responsibility for both purchases and usage. Even in situations when one person does have responsibility for both components, the separation is useful because it provides information for focused management correction.

6. A multivariable flexible budget model defines more than one factor that influences costs. For example, a nursing unit may have its staffing costs affected by both volume of patients and the acuity of patients. To the extent that a multivariable budget model reflects cost behavior more accurately, it may provide a better indication of when actual costs are out of control. This may reduce unnecessary investigations or justification efforts.

7. Prices paid for food may have increased significantly either because of recent changes in food prices or because of ineptness or fraud on the part of Mr. Schumaker. An audit of purchasing costs should be initiated, especially if other departments in the center have similar problems.

8. The following calculations should be made as a basis for deciding whether an investigation should be conducted:

   Expected benefits = .5 × $1,000 × (1 − .0228)* = $488.60
   Expected costs = $200
   *(1 − .0228) = Probability that the variance is not a random occurrence

   Yes, the variance should be investigated, because the expected benefits are greater than the expected costs. Even if the variance is favorable, it should be investigated, because it may indicate that the budget is not accurate. A reduction of the budget may promote a future reduction in costs.

9. The probability of observing six successive periods in which actual costs are greater than budgeted costs is $.50^6 = .0156$.

10. In your evaluation, you can calculate spending and volume variances for the radiology department. The total variance would be calculated as:

Actual cost less assigned cost (Actual costs less actual volume times budgeted cost per unit), or

$1,800,000 − [100,000 × ($1,920,000 / 120,000)] = $200,000 (Unfavorable)

The radiology department has an unfavorable variance of $200,000, as opposed to a favorable variance of $120,000. This $200,000 unfavorable variance can be broken into spending and volume variances:

Spending variance = Actual costs − Budgeted fixed costs − Budgeted variable cost
= $1,800,000 − $600,000 − ($11 × 100,000) = $100,000 (Unfavorable)

Volume variance = (Budgeted volume − Actual volume) × Budgeted average fixed cost
= (120,000 − 100,000) × ($600,000/120,000) = $100,000 (Unfavorable)

The department manager may not be responsible for the volume variance, but the unfavorable spending variance of $100,000 should be analyzed to see what caused it. More detail would permit further breakdowns by price and efficiency variances.

11. The causes of the change in cost and the resulting variances for the laundry department are presented in Table 16–22.

Table 16–22 Variances for Laundry Department

Variance Category	Amount of Variance	Variance Sign	Percentage (%)
Labor price	$3,451	(Unfavorable)	46.5
Supply price	$1,610	(Unfavorable)	21.7
Labor efficiency	$3,451	(Unfavorable)	46.5
Supply efficiency	0		0.0
Pure volume	$1,305	(Unfavorable)	17.6
Intensity volume	($2,395)	(Favorable)	(32.3)
Total	$7,422		100.0

Labor price = ($11.00 − $10.50) × 6,901 = $3,451 (Unfavorable)
Supply price = ($3.18 − $2.69) × 3,286 = $1,610 (Unfavorable)
Labor efficiency = (.021 − .020) × 328,624 × $10.50 = $3,451 (Unfavorable)
Supply efficiency = (.01 − .01) × 328,624 × $2.69 = 0
Pure volume = (13.80385 × [24,539 − 24,140]) × $.2369 = $1,305 (Unfavorable)
Intensity volume = ([13.80385 − 13.39191] × 24,539) × $.2369 = $2369 (Favorable)

12. The primary cause for the increase in cost has been the initiation of a new DRG category (103) that is expensive to produce. This case illustrates the importance of case mix and severity-adjusting cost data. Table 16–23 breaks the variances into price and cost and volume variances.

Table 16–23 Valley Hospital Variance Analysis

Variance Analysis by DRG

	Cost	Volume	New	Total
DRG 106	$22,500	$12,750	$—	$35,250
DRG 107	40,000	(32,000)	—	8,000
DRG 103	—	—	95,000	95,000
	$62,500	($19,250)	$95,000	$138,250

13. Table 16–24 provides the variances in the required categories.

Table 16–24 American Health Plan Variances

	Inpatient	Outpatient	Total
Enrollment	$600,000	$325,000	$925,000
Utilization	(550,000)	357,500	(192,500)
Efficiency	605,000	(181,500)	423,500
Total	$655,000	$501,000	$1,156,000

The calculations for the variances are the following:

Enrollment:

Inpatient = 1,000 × .600 × $1,000 = $600,000 (Unfavorable)
Outpatient = 1,000 × 5.0 × $65 = $325,000 (Unfavorable)

Utilization:

Inpatient = (.550 − .600) × 11,000 × $1,000 = −$550,000 (Favorable)
Outpatient = (5.5 − 5.0) × 11,000 × $65 = $357,500 (Unfavorable)

Efficiency:

Inpatient = ($1,100 − $1,000) × 6,050 = $605,000 (Unfavorable)
Outpatient = ($62 − $65) × 60,500 = −$181,500 (Favorable)

The data suggest that the vast majority of the variance was created by an increase in enrollment. Of the total $1,156,000 variance, $925,000 was the result of an increase in enrollment. This should not be a concern. There was, however, an increase in the price paid for inpatient care from $1,000 per day to $1,100 per day. It is not clear whether this is a result in the intensity of patients seen, or the use of more expensive hospitals. Inpatient utilization decreased significantly and created a favorable variance of $550,000. On the outpatient side, the situation was reversed. Outpatient utilization increased, resulting in an unfavorable variance of $357,500, whereas outpatient efficiency or prices paid actually declined, resulting in a favorable variance of − $181,500.

Chapter 17

Financial Mathematics

LEARNING OBJECTIVES

After studying this chapter, you should be able to do the following:

1. Explain why a dollar today is worth more than a dollar in the future.
2. Define the terms future value and present value.
3. Explain the difference between an ordinary annuity and an annuity due.
4. Calculate the future value of an annuity.

REAL-WORLD SCENARIO

The critical aspect of understanding the value of any stock relates in part to the time value of money. The price of a stock is the sum of its anticipated future earnings or cash flow, adjusted by the time value of money and the uncertainty or risk of these future earnings. The "cost of capital" could be thought of as the investment hurdle or opportunity cost for similar risk investments. In other words, it is the minimum return an investor will accept to invest in a stock of similar risk.

Typically, this rate is greater than a return on U.S. Treasury securities. In March of 2006, ten-year Treasury note rates, which are guaranteed by the federal government, were around 4.7%. If an investor did not expect to achieve a return of at least 4.7% on a stock investment, then there would be no reason to take on the risk. However, over the past 70 years, most investors have received a premium of 6 to 7% above the bond rate to compensate for this risk. In other words, stocks have outpaced government bonds by 6 to 7%. Thus, the value of stock hinges upon two factors: the cost of capital, and the expected future earnings or cash flow streams, which is dependent upon the time value of money.

In this chapter, we examine the concepts and methods of discounting sums of money received at various points in time through the use of compound interest formulas and tables. This material is of special importance in the context of the next three chapters on capital project analysis, Chapter 18), consolidations and mergers (Chapter 19), and capital formation (Chapter 20). The present abbreviated discussion of financial mathematics is intended as a review for those who have had prior exposure; if this material is new to the reader, some background reading may be necessary.

LEARNING OBJECTIVE 1

Explain why a dollar today is worth more than a dollar in the future.

The two major questions in the financial decision-making process of any business are the following: (1) Where shall we invest our funds? (2) How shall we finance our investment needs? Investment decisions involve expending funds today while expecting to realize returns in the future. Financing decisions involve the receipt of funds today in return for a promise to make payments in the future. The evaluation of the relative attractiveness of alternative investment and financing opportunities is a major task of management. Differences in the timing of either receipts or payments can have a significant impact on the ultimate decision to invest or finance in a certain way. A payment that is made or received in the first year has a greater value than an identical payment made or received in the tenth year. The concept underlying this point is often referred to as the time value of money. A time value for money is simply the assignment of a cost or interest rate for money.

Money or funds can be thought of as a commodity, like any other commodity that can be bought or sold. The price for the commodity called money is often stated as an interest rate, for example, ten percent per year. An interest rate of ten percent per year implies exchange rates between money at different periods. When the interest rate is ten percent, a dollar received one year from today is worth only .9091 of a dollar received today, and a dollar received ten years from today is worth only .3855 of a dollar today. Compound interest rate tables are merely values that provide relative weighting for money received or paid during different periods at specified prices or interest rates. With these relative weightings, money received or paid in different time periods can be added or subtracted to produce some logical meaningful result. The major purpose of compound interest tables is to permit addition and subtraction of money paid or received during different periods. The resulting sums are usually expressed in dollars at one of the two following time points: (1) present value and (2) future value.

LEARNING OBJECTIVE 2

Define the terms future value and present value.

The compound interest tables provided in this chapter are categorized as either present value or future value tables. The present value tables provide the relative weights that should be used to restate money of future periods back to the present. Future value tables provide the relative weighting for restating money of one period to some designated future period.

SINGLE-SUM PROBLEMS

Future Value—Single Sum

There are many situations in which a business would be interested in the future value of a single sum. For example, a nursing home may want to invest $100,000 today in a fund to be used in two years for replacing items. It would like to know what sum of money would be available two years from now.

This type of problem is easily solved, using the values presented in Table 17–1. The first step in solving the problem is to set up a time graph. This involves the following four variables that make up any simple compound interest problem:

1. Number of periods during which the compounding occurs (n)
2. Present value of future sum (p)
3. Future value of present sum (f)
4. Interest rate per period (i)

If you know the values of any three of these variables, you can solve for the fourth. The time graph is a simple device that helps you to conceptualize the problem and identify the known values to permit the problem to be solved. In the previous nursing home investment example, a ten percent interest rate per period would be reflected in Figure 17–1.

The value 0 on this time graph represents the present time, whereas the values 1 and 2 represent Year 1 and Year 2. In the nursing home example, we know three of the four variables and can, therefore, solve the problem through substitution in the following formula:

$$f = p \times f(i,n)$$

Table 17–1 Future Value of $1 Received in n Periods

Period	2%	4%	6%	8%	10%	12%	14%
1	1.0200	1.0400	1.0600	1.0800	1.1000	1.1200	1.1400
2	1.0404	1.0816	1.1236	1.1664	1.2100	1.2544	1.2996
3	1.0612	1.1249	1.1910	1.2597	1.3310	1.4049	1.4815
4	1.0824	1.1699	1.2625	1.3605	1.4614	1.5735	1.6890
5	1.1041	1.2167	1.3382	1.4693	1.6105	1.7623	1.9254
6	1.1262	1.2653	1.1485	1.5869	1.7716	1.9738	2.1950
7	1.1487	1.3159	1.5036	1.7138	1.9487	2.2107	2.5023
8	1.1717	1.3686	1.5938	1.8509	2.1436	2.4760	2.8526
9	1.1951	1.4233	1.6895	1.9990	2.3579	2.7731	3.2519
10	1.2190	1.4802	1.7908	2.1589	2.5937	3.1058	3.7072
11	1.2434	1.5395	1.8983	2.3316	2.8531	3.4785	4.2262
12	1.2682	1.6010	2.0122	2.5182	3.1384	3.8960	4.8179
13	1.2936	1.6651	2.1329	2.7196	3.4523	4.3635	5.4924
14	1.3195	1.7317	2.2609	2.9372	3.7975	4.8871	6.2613
15	1.3459	1.8009	2.3966	3.1722	4.1772	5.4736	7.1379
16	1.3728	1.8730	2.5404	3.4259	4.5950	6.1304	8.1372
17	1.4002	1.9479	2.6928	3.7000	5.0545	6.8660	9.2765
18	1.4282	2.0258	2.8543	3.9960	5.5599	7.6900	10.5752
19	1.4568	2.1068	3.0256	4.3157	6.1159	8.6128	12.0557
20	1.4859	2.1911	3.2071	4.6610	6.7275	9.6463	13.7435
30	1.8114	3.2434	5.7435	10.0627	17.4494	29.9599	50.9502
40	2.2080	4.8010	10.2857	21.7245	45.2593	93.0510	188.8835

The factor f(i,n) is the future value of $1 invested today for n periods at i rate of interest per period. These values can be found in Table 17–1, using the previous generic formula. The following calculation then can be made to solve the problem:

$$f = \$100,00 \times f(10\%,2) \text{ or}$$
$$f = \$100,000 \times 1.210 \text{ or}$$
$$f = \$121,000$$

In some situations, it may be the interest rate that we wish to determine. Assume that we can invest $8,576 today in a discounted note that will pay us $10,000 two years from today. Figure 17–2 summarizes the problem.

The following calculation then can be made to solve the problem:

$$\$10,000 = \$8,576 \times f(i,2) \text{ or}$$
$$f(i,2) = 1.166$$

A check of the values in Table 17–1 indicates that the interest rate would be 8 percent (f[8%,2] = 1.166). If the previous value had not exactly matched a figure in the table, some interpolation would have been required.

A microcomputer or a calculator with a financial mathematics function also could be used to solve the previous types of problems. It is still useful, however, to set up a time graph to conceptualize the problem

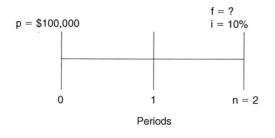

Figure 17–1 Future Value of Present Sum

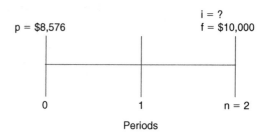

Figure 17–2 Solving for the Interest Rate

before entering numbers into the calculator or computer.

Present Value—Single Sum

In some situations, it is the present value of a future sum that is of interest. This type of problem is similar to those we examined regarding the future value of a single sum. In fact, the same table of values could be used, except that now we would use division rather than multiplication.

The general equation used to solve present-value, single-sum problems is the following:

$$p = f \times p(i,n)$$

The factor $p(i,n)$ represents the present value of $1 received in n periods at an interest rate of i. Values for $p(i,n)$ can be found in Table 17–2.

Assume that your health maintenance organization (HMO) has a $100,000 debt service obligation due in two years. You are interested in learning how much money must be set aside today to meet the obligation if the expected yield on the investment is 12

percent. The relevant time graph is depicted in Figure 17–3.

The calculation to solve the problem would be the following:

$$p = f \times p(i,n) \text{ or}$$
$$p = \$100,000 \times p(12\%,2) \text{ or}$$
$$p = \$100,000 \times .7972 \text{ or}$$
$$p = \$79,720$$

It is important to note that the values of Table 17–1 and Table 17–2 are reciprocals of each other. That is:

$$f(i,n) = 1/p(i,n)$$

In effect, this means that only one of the two tables is necessary to solve either a present-value or future-value problem involving a single sum.

ANNUITY PROBLEMS

Future Value

In many business situations, there is more than one payment or receipt. In the case of multiple payments or

Table 17–2 Present Value of $1 Due in n Periods

Period	2%	4%	6%	8%	10%	12%	14%
1	0.9804	0.9615	0.9434	0.9259	0.9091	0.8929	0.8772
2	0.9612	0.9246	0.8900	0.8573	0.8264	0.7972	0.7695
3	0.9423	0.8890	0.8396	0.7938	0.7513	0.7118	0.6750
4	0.9238	0.8548	0.7921	0.7350	0.6830	0.6355	0.5921
5	0.9057	0.8219	0.7473	0.6806	0.6209	0.5674	0.5194
6	0.8880	0.7903	0.7050	0.6302	0.5645	0.5066	0.4556
7	0.8706	0.7599	0.6651	0.5835	0.5132	0.4523	0.3996
8	0.8535	0.7307	0.6274	0.5403	0.4665	0.4039	0.3506
9	0.8368	0.7026	0.5919	0.5002	0.4241	0.3606	0.3075
10	0.8203	0.6756	0.5584	0.4632	0.3855	0.3220	0.2697
11	0.8043	0.6496	0.5268	0.4289	0.3505	0.2875	0.2366
12	0.7885	0.6246	0.4970	0.3971	0.3186	0.2567	0.2076
13	0.7730	0.6006	0.4688	0.3677	0.2897	0.2292	0.1821
14	0.7579	0.5775	0.4423	0.3405	0.2633	0.2046	0.1597
15	0.7430	0.5553	0.4173	0.3152	0.2394	0.1827	0.1401
16	0.7284	0.5339	0.3936	0.2919	0.2176	0.1631	0.1229
17	0.7142	0.5134	0.3714	0.2703	0.1978	0.1456	0.1078
18	0.7002	0.4936	0.3503	0.2502	0.1799	0.1300	0.0946
19	0.6864	0.4746	0.3305	0.2317	0.1635	0.1161	0.0829
20	0.6730	0.4564	0.3118	0.2145	0.1486	0.1037	0.0728
30	0.5521	0.3083	0.1741	0.0994	0.0573	0.0334	0.0196
40	0.4529	0.2083	0.0972	0.0460	0.0221	0.0107	0.0053

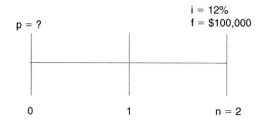

Figure 17–3 Present Value of a Future Sum

receipts, when each payment or receipt is constant per time period, we have an annuity situation. Figure 17–4 depicts a time graph for an annuity.

LEARNING OBJECTIVE 3

Explain the difference between an ordinary annuity and an annuity due.

In the graph in Figure 17–4, F represents the future value of the invested annuity deposits at the end of period n. (Note that F is used to denote future value for annuities, while f is used for single sums.) The values for R represent the periodic deposits that are constant for each period. It should be emphasized that the deposits are made at the end of each period. Such a system of deposits is often described as an ordinary annuity. The values presented in Tables 17–3 and 17–4 assume an ordinary annuity situation in which deposits or receipts occur at the end of the period.

LEARNING OBJECTIVE 4

Calculate the future value of an annuity.

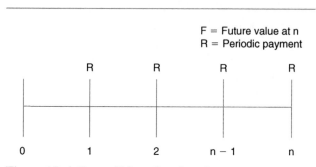

Figure 17–4 Future Value of an Annuity

The basic equation for a future value annuity is:

$$F = R \times F(i,n)$$

The factor F(i,n) represents the future value of $1 invested each period for n periods at i rate of interest. Values for F(i,n) can be found in Table 17–3. Again, if three of the four variables (F, R, i, and n) in the previous equation are known, the equation can be solved to determine the fourth. Thus, if we know F, i, and n, we can solve for R.

Assume that a hospital wants to know what the value of $50,000 worth of annual deposits in a trust fund for professional malpractice insurance will be in three years if the fund earns 8 percent per year. The time graph for this problem is depicted in Figure 17–5.

The calculation to solve the problem would be as follows:

$$
\begin{array}{c}
F = R \times F(i,n) \text{ or} \\
F = \$50,000 \times F(8\%,3) \text{ or} \\
F = \$50,000 \times 3.2464 \text{ or} \\
F = \$162,320
\end{array}
$$

The values in Table 17–3 also could be determined through simple addition of the values for a single sum in Table 17–1. This can be seen easily by further examining our hospital example. Table 17–5 summarizes the relevant data.

Notice that the future value total in Table 17–5 is identical to that in the earlier annuity formula. Also note that the summation of the individual future value factors yields the value of the annuity factor (3.2464). In general, a future value annuity factor can be expressed as follows:

$$F(i,n) = f(i,1) + f(i,2) + \ldots + f(i,n + 1) + 1.0$$

In many situations, a financial mathematics problem may be part annuity and part single sum. In such cases, the use of a time graph will help you spot this duality and solve the problem correctly. Assume that a hospital has a sinking fund payment requirement for the last ten years of a bond's life. At the end of that period, there must be $45 million available to retire the debt. The hospital has created a $5 million fund today, twenty years before debt retirement, to offset part of the future sinking fund requirement. If the investment yield is expected to be ten percent per year, what annual deposit must be made to the sinking fund? Figure 17–6 summarizes the problem.

Table 17–3 Future Value of $1 Received Each Period for n Periods

Period	2%	4%	6%	8%	10%	12%	14%
1	1.0000	1.0000	1.0000	1.0000	1.0000	1.0000	1.0000
2	2.0200	2.0400	2.0600	2.0800	2.1000	2.1200	2.1400
3	3.0604	3.1216	3.1836	3.2464	3.3100	3.3744	3.4396
4	4.1216	4.2465	4.3746	4.5061	4.6410	4.7793	4.9211
5	5.2040	5.4163	5.6371	5.8666	6.1051	6.3528	6.6101
6	6.3081	6.6330	6.9753	7.3359	7.7156	8.1152	8.5355
7	7.4343	7.8983	8.3938	8.9228	9.4872	10.0890	10.7305
8	8.5830	9.2142	9.8975	10.6366	11.4359	12.2997	13.2328
9	9.7546	10.5828	11.4913	12.4876	13.5795	14.7757	16.0853
10	10.9497	12.0061	13.1808	14.4866	15.9374	17.5487	19.3373
11	12.1687	13.4864	14.9716	16.6455	18.5312	20.6546	23.0445
12	13.4121	15.0258	16.8699	18.9771	21.3843	24.1331	27.2707
13	14.6803	16.6268	18.8821	21.4953	24.5227	28.0291	32.0887
14	15.9739	18.2919	21.0151	24.2149	27.9750	32.3926	37.5811
15	17.2934	20.0236	23.2760	27.1521	31.7725	37.2797	43.8424
16	18.6393	21.8245	25.6725	30.3243	35.9497	42.7533	50.9804
17	20.0121	23.6975	28.2129	33.7502	40.5447	48.8837	59.1176
18	21.4123	25.6454	30.9057	37.4502	45.5992	55.7497	68.3941
19	22.8406	27.6712	33.7600	41.4463	51.1591	63.4397	78.6992
20	24.2974	29.7781	36.7856	45.7620	57.2750	72.0524	91.0249
30	40.5681	56.0849	79.0582	113.2832	164.4940	241.3327	356.7868
40	60.4020	95.0255	154.7620	259.0565	442.5926	767.0914	1,342.0251

The first step is to determine the future value of the $5 million deposit, which is

$$f = \$5,000,000 \times f(10\%,20) \text{ or}$$
$$f = \$5,000,000 \times 6.7275 \text{ or}$$
$$f = \$33,637,500$$

This means that the amount of money that must be generated by the ten sinking fund deposits must equal $11,362,500 ($45,000,000 − $33,637,500). The following calculation provides the solution:

$$F - f = R \times F(i,n) \text{ or}$$
$$\$11,362,500 = R \times F(10\%,10) \text{ or}$$
$$\$11,362,500 = R \times 15.9374 \text{ or}$$
$$R = \$712,946$$

Present Value

While determining the present value of an annuity, the procedure is analogous to that used to determine the future value of an annuity, except that our attention is now on present value rather than future value. Figure 17–7 represents the typical present value annuity problem.

As noted earlier, this is an ordinary annuity situation because the payments are at the end of the period. The basic equation used to solve a present-value annuity problem is the following:

$$P = R \times P(i,n)$$

The factor P(i,n) represents the present value of $1 received at the end of each period for n periods when i is the rate of interest. Values for P(i,n) are found in Table 17–4. (Note that P is used to denote an annuity problem, while p is used to denote a single sum problem.)

Assume that a hospital is considering buying an older hospital and consolidating its operations in another nearby facility. An actuary has estimated that pension payments of $100,000 per year for the next four years will be required to satisfy the obligation to vested employees. The hospital wants to know what the present value of this obligation is so that it can be subtracted from the negotiated purchase price. The obligation's discount rate is assumed to be 12 percent. The time graph for this problem is depicted in Figure 17–8.

The calculation to solve the problem is as follows:

$$P = \$100,000 \times P(12\%,4) \text{ or}$$
$$P = \$100,000 \times 3.0373$$
$$P = \$303,730$$

Table 17–4 Present Value of $1 Received Each Period for n Periods

Period	2%	4%	6%	8%	10%	12%	14%
1	0.9804	0.9615	0.9434	0.9259	0.9091	0.8929	0.8772
2	1.9416	1.8861	1.8334	1.7833	1.7355	1.6901	1.6467
3	2.8839	2.7751	2.6730	2.5771	2.4869	2.4018	2.3216
4	3.8077	3.6299	3.4651	3.3121	3.1699	3.0373	2.9137
5	4.7135	4.4518	4.2124	3.9927	3.7908	3.6048	3.4331
6	5.6014	5.2421	4.9173	4.6229	4.3553	4.1114	3.8887
7	6.4720	6.0021	5.5824	5.2064	4.8684	4.5638	4.2883
8	7.3255	6.7327	6.8017	5.7466	5.3349	4.9676	4.6389
9	8.1622	7.4353	7.3601	6.2469	5.7590	5.3282	4.9464
10	8.9826	8.1109	7.8869	6.7101	6.1446	5.6502	5.2161
11	9.7868	8.7605	8.3838	7.1390	6.4951	5.9377	5.4527
12	10.5753	9.3851	8.8527	7.5361	6.8137	6.1944	5.6603
13	11.3484	9.9856	9.2950	7.9038	7.1034	6.4235	5.8424
14	12.1062	10.5631	9.7122	8.2442	7.3667	6.6282	6.0021
15	12.8493	11.1184	9.7122	8.5595	7.6061	6.8109	6.1422
16	13.5777	11.6523	10.1059	8.8514	7.8237	6.9740	6.2651
17	14.2919	12.1657	10.4773	9.1216	8.0216	7.1196	6.3729
18	14.9920	12.6593	10.8276	9.3719	8.2014	7.2497	6.4674
19	15.6785	13.1339	11.1581	9.6036	8.3649	7.3658	6.5504
20	16.3514	13.5903	11.4699	9.8181	8.5136	7.4694	6.6231
30	22.3965	17.2920	13.7648	11.2578	9.4269	8.0552	7.0027
40	27.3555	19.7928	15.0463	11.9246	9.7791	8.2438	7.1050

Present-value annuity problems can be thought of as a series of individual single-sum problems. The present-value annuity factor P(i,n) is the sum of the individual single-sum values of Table 17–2. The data in Table 17–6 summarize this calculation in our hospital example.

The small differences between the annuity values and the single-sum values in Table 17–6 are due to rounding errors.

The present-value annuity factor [P(i,n)] can be expressed as follows:

$$P(i,n) = p(i,1) + p(i,2) + ... + p(i,n)$$

In most business situations, ordinary annuity problems do not arise. The classic exception to the ordinary annuity situation is a lease with front-end payments. Assume that a clinic wants to lease a computer for the next five years with quarterly payments of $1,000 due at the beginning of each quarter. If the clinic's discount rate is 16 percent per annum, what is the present value of the lease liability? The relevant time graph is presented in Figure 17–9.

The graph in Figure 17–9 indicates that the clinic has a nineteen-period ordinary annuity, with each period lasting three months. The effective interest rate for each quarter is four percent. The present value of the first payment is $1,000 because it occurs at the beginning of the first quarter. The following calculation provides the solution to the problem:

P = $1,000 + $1,000 × P(4%,19) or
P = $1,000 + $1,000 × 13.1339 or
P = $14,134

SUMMARY

In the area of financial mathematics, compound interest rate tables provide us with values with which we

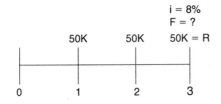

i = 8%
F = ?

50K   50K   50K = R

0   1   2   3

Figure 17–5 Determining the Future Value of an Annuity

Table 17–5 Using Sum of Simple Future Value Factors to Calculate Annuity Value

| Year | Future Value Factor (8%) | Future Value | Year Invested | | |
			1	2	3
1	1.1664	$58,320	$50,000		
2	1.0800	54,000		$50,000	
3	1.0000	50,000			$50,000
Total	3.2464	$162,320			

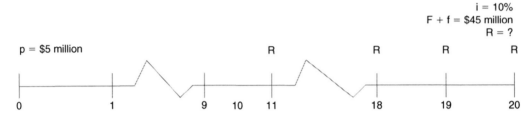

Figure 17–6 Determining the Annual Sinking Fund Deposit

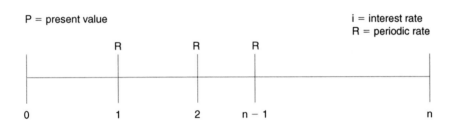

Figure 17–7 Typical Present Value Annuity

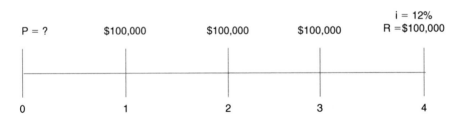

Figure 17–8 Present Value of the Pension Obligation

Table 17–6 Using Sum of Simple Present Value Factors to Calculate Annuity Value

| Year | Present Value Factor (12%) | Present Value | Year of Payment | | | |
			1	2	3	4
1	0.8929	$89,290	$100,000			
2	0.7972	79,720		$100,000		
3	0.7118	71,180			$100,000	
4	0.6355	63,550				$100,000
Total	3.0374	$303,740				

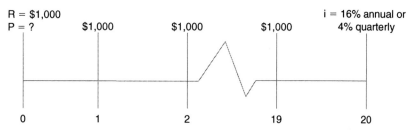

Figure 17–9 Present Value of a Lease Liability

can weight money flows that are received or paid during different periods. The relative weighting assigned to each period's money flow is a function of the price of money, or the interest rate. The relative weightings permit us to add or subtract money flows from different periods and produce a meaningful measure. The value of money is usually expressed in terms of present value or value at some future specified date.

ASSIGNMENTS

1. Steven Hudson has agreed to settle a debt of $100,000 by paying $14,903 per year for ten years. What effective rate of interest is Steven paying under this agreement?

2. Findling Hospital is planning a major expansion project. The construction cost of the project is to be paid from the proceeds of serial notes. The notes are of equal amounts and include a provision for interest at an annual rate of eight percent payable semiannually over the next ten years. It is expected that receipts from the hospital will provide for the repayment of principal and interest on the notes. Allan Klein, controller of the hospital, has estimated that the cash flow available for repayment of principal and interest will be $450,000 per year. The construction project is expected to cost $3,420,000. Can the hospital meet the peak debt service with existing cash flows?

3. Jerry Scott has just accepted a position with a state agency that has a retirement pension plan calling for joint contributions by the employee and the employer. Jerry is now ten years from retirement age of 65 and expects to contribute $400 per year to the plan, which would make him eligible for payments of $1,000 per year for the remainder of his life, starting in ten years. Because this retirement plan is optional, Jerry is considering the alternative of investing annually an amount equal to his $400 per year contribution. If Jerry assumes that his investments would earn eight percent annually, and that his life expectancy is eighty years, should he invest in his own plan or should he make contributions to his employer's fund?

4. Meany Hospital wishes to provide for the retirement of an obligation of $10,000,000 that becomes due July 1, 2015. The hospital plans to deposit $500,000 in a special fund each July 1 for eight years, starting July 1, 2007. On that same initial date, the hospital wishes to deposit an amount that, with accumulated interest at ten percent compounded annually, will bring the total value of the fund to the required $10,000,000 at July 1, 2015. What dollar amount should the hospital deposit?

5. Jim Hubert, an investment banker with The Ohio Company, is arranging a financing package with Bill Andrews, president of Liebish Hospital. The financing package calls for $20 million in bonds to be repaid in 20 years. A decision must be made regarding the amount that must be deposited on an annual basis in a sinking fund. It is estimated that the sinking fund will earn interest at the rate of eight percent compounded annually. What dollar amount must be set aside annually in the sinking fund to meet the $20 million payment in the twentieth year?

6. General Hospital is evaluating a zero-interest capital financing alternative. General would borrow $100,000,000 and receive $62,100,000 in cash. The $100,000,000 note would carry no interest payment, but would be due at the end of the fifth year. The lender would require an annual sinking fund payment over the next five years to meet the maturity value of $100,000,000. If the fund is scheduled to earn interest at the rate of six percent annually, what amount must be deposited annually?

7. ABC Hospital is embarking on a major renovation program. The total cost of construction will be $50,000,000. Payments will be $10,000,000 at the end of Year 1, $30,000,000 at the end of Year 2, and $10,000,000 at the end of Year 3. ABC wants to set aside sufficient funds today to meet the expected construction draws. If the fund can be expected to earn eight percent per annum, what amount should be set aside?

8. If you issue $100,000 of ten-percent bonds with interest payable semiannually over the next 5 years, what is the market value of the bonds if the required market rate of interest is 12 percent annually? Assume that no payment of principal is made until maturity.

9. You have agreed to buy an adjacent medical office building with quarterly payments of $100,000 for the next six years. Payments are due at the beginning of each quarter. If the cost of money to you is 16 percent per annum, would you pay $1,200,000 in cash today to the present owners?

10. You plan to invest $1 million per year for the next three years to meet future professional liability payments. If the fund earns interest at a rate of ten percent per annum, how large will the balance be in five years? Assume that no payments for claims are made until then.

1. The graph in Figure 17–10 and the following calculations show the effective rate of interest Steven is paying.

$$P = R \times P(i,n)$$
$$\$100,000 = \$14,903 \times P(i,10)$$
$$P(i,10) = 6.710$$
$$i = 8\%$$

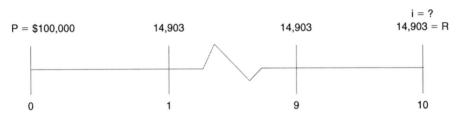

P = \$100,000   14,903   14,903 $i = ?$ \
                                                       14,903 = R

0   1   9   10

Figure 17–10 Steve Hudson's Rate of Interest

2. In this hospital expansion project, it is necessary to recognize that debt service will be at the maximum or peak in the first year. This is the pattern that results with a serial note. Thus:

$$\text{Debt principal payment} = \$3,420,000/20 = \$171,000 \text{ every six months}$$
$$\text{Interest in first six months} = .04 \times \$3,420,000 = \$136,800$$
$$\text{Interest in second six months} = .04 \times (\$3,420,000 - \$171,000) = \$129,960$$
$$\text{Total first-year debt service} = \$171,000 + \$136,800 + \$171,000 + \$129,960 = \$608,760$$

Thus, Findling Hospital's project cannot be financed with the existing cash flow of \$450,000.

3. The graph in Figure 17–11 and the following calculations are relevant to Jerry's retirement fund decision.

Calculation of the value of the state agency's payments at Year 10 is as follows:

$$P = \$1,000 \times P(8\%,15)$$
$$P = \$1,000 \times 8.559$$
$$P = \$8.559$$

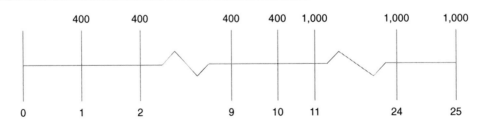

400   400   400   400 1,000   1,000   1,000

0   1   2   9   10   11   24   25

Figure 17–11 Jerry Scott's Annual Investments

Calculation of the value of Jerry's deposits at Year 10 is as follows:

$$F = \$400 \times F(8\%,10)$$
$$F = \$400 \times 14.4866$$
$$F = \$5,795$$

Thus, Jerry is better off with the state agency's retirement plan. His deposits of $400 would not provide a fund large enough to give him $1,000 a year for 15 years.

4. The relevant calculations for Meany Hospital are as follows and depicted in Figure 17–12.

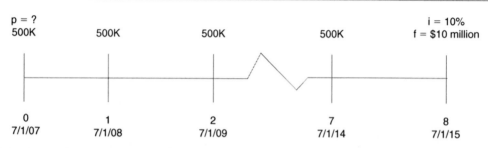

p = ?
500K   500K   500K   500K   i = 10%
                                      f = $10 million

0	1	2	7	8
7/1/07	7/1/08	7/1/09	7/1/14	7/1/15

Figure 17–12 Meany Hospital Required Fund Deposit

Calculation of the value of annual deposits at July 1, 2015 is as follows:
Future Value of Deposits = $500,000 × f(10%,8) + [$500,000 × F(10%,7)]f(10%,1)

$$F = \$500,000 \times 2.1436 + (\$500,000 \times 9.4872) \times 1.10$$
$$F = \$1,071,800 \times \$5,217,960 = \$6,289,760$$

Calculation of the required deposit at July 1, 2007 is as follows:

Required amount at July 1, 2015 must equal $10,000,000 − $6,289,760, or $3,710,240.

$$p = \$3,710,240 \times p(10\%,8) = \text{required deposit at July 1, 2007}$$

$$p = \$3,710,240 \times .467$$

$$p = \$1,732,682 = \text{deposit required at July 1, 2007}$$

5. Figure 17–13 and the following calculations show the dollar amount that must be set aside annually in the sinking fund to meet the $20 million repayment in the 20th year.

$$F = R \times F(i,n)$$
$$\$20,000,000 = R \times F(8\%,20)$$
$$\$20,000,000 = R \times 45.7620$$
$$R = \$437,044$$

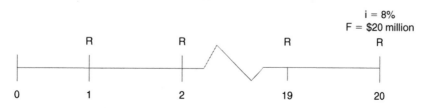

i = 8%
F = $20 million
R   R   R   R

0	1	2	19	20

Figure 17–13 Liebish Hospital Sinking Fund

6. Figure 17–14 and the following calculations show the amount that General Hospital will have to deposit in the sinking fund each year.

$$F = R \times F(i,n)$$
$$\$100,000,000 = R \times F(6\%,5)$$
$$\$100,000,000 = R \times 5.6371$$
$$R = \$17,739,618$$

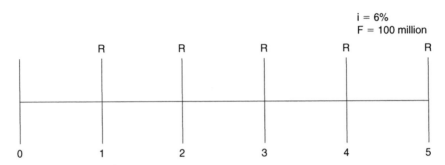

Figure 17–14 General Hospital Annual Sinking Fund

7. Figure 17–15 and the following calculations show the amount that ABC Hospital must set aside to meet expected construction draws.

$$p = \$10,000,000 \times p(8\%,1) + \$30,000,000 \times p(8\%,2) + \$10,000,000 \times p(8\%,3)$$
$$p = \$10,000,000 \times .926 + \$30,000,000 \times .857 + \$10,000,000 \times .794$$
$$p = \$42,910,000$$

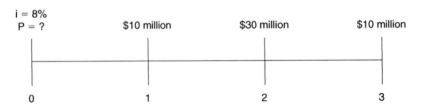

Figure 17–15 ABC Hospital Fund Requirement

8. The market value of the bonds may be calculated as follows (Figure 17–16):

$$\text{Market Value} = \$5,000 \times P(6\%,10) + \$100,000 \times p(6\%,10)$$
$$\text{Market Value} = \$5,000 \times 7.360 + \$100,000 \times .558$$
$$\text{Market Value} = \$92,600$$

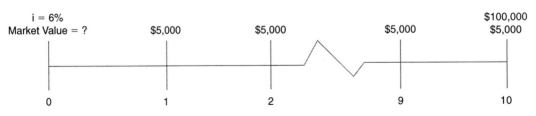

Figure 17–16 Market Value of Bonds

9. To determine whether you should pay $1,200,00 in cash today to the present owners, Figure 17–17 and the following calculations are relevant.

$$P = \$100,000 + \$100,000 \times P(4\%,23)$$
$$P = \$100,000 + (\$100,000 \times 14.857)$$
$$P = \$1,585,700$$

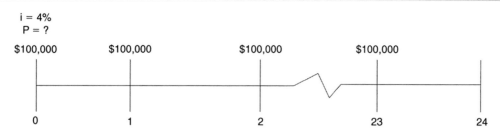

Figure 17–17 Present Value of the Installment Sale

Yes, you should make the $1,200,000 cash payment to the present owners. The present value of an outright purchase price of $1,200,000 is less than the present value of the installment sale arrangement.

10. Figure 17–18 and the following calculations show the amount of the fund balance in five years.

$$\text{Fund value} = \$1,000,000 \times F(10\%,3) \times f(10\%,2)$$
$$\text{Fund vaue} = \$1,000,000 \times 3.310 \times 1.210$$
$$\text{Fund value} = \$4,005,100$$

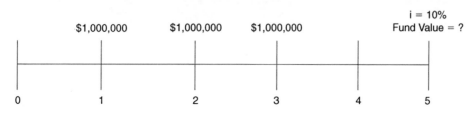

Figure 17–18 Required Fund Balance in Five Years

Chapter 18

Capital Project Analysis

LEARNING OBJECTIVES

After studying this chapter, you should be able to do the following:

1. Explain who is involved in the capital investment decision process.
2. Describe the kinds of decisions that are made in capital investment decision analysis.
3. Explain the four stages of the capital decision-making process.
4. List some of the kinds of information that are needed to evaluate a capital investment project.
5. Calculate a project's net present value, profitability index, and equivalent annual cost.
6. Explain the concept of a discount rate and what the weighted average cost of capital is.

REAL-WORLD SCENARIO

The phone rang in the office of Jack Smith, an executive at Specialized Medical Devices, Inc. (SMD), a firm that manufactures specialized digital mammography devices. On the line was Dr. Sipparo, Chief of Radiology at Academic Medical Center (AMC). Dr. Sipparo explained that she needed Jack's help in understanding an analysis prepared by the staff of Robert Alexander, Academic Medical Center's Chief Executive Officer, of the pending purchase of new imaging equipment for the evaluation of patients presenting for breast cancer screening. AMC is evaluating two types of imaging equipment—standard screen-film mammography equipment and a machine offered by SMD that allows for full-field digital mammography (FFDM) with tomosynthesis. Dr. Sipparo explained the situation as follows:

Based on his staff's cost analysis, Robert Alexander believes the hospital should purchase the conventional mammography equipment rather than the digital mammography machine. The physicians in the radiology department are very upset by this. They want the hospital to purchase the tomosynthesis scanner because it incorporates the latest imaging technology. In addition, Dr. Sipparo is not convinced by the CEO's staff's analysis that the conventional equipment is really the better choice, even from a purely financial perspective.

The capital budget committee meets next week, and Dr. Sipparo needs help. She has asked Jack to evaluate the analysis prepared by Dr. Alexander's staff and to recommend changes to the analysis if he feels that they are warranted.

Digital mammography, which eliminates the film and lab costs associated with conventional mammography, provides the ability to combine multiple images taken from slightly different angles into three-dimensional (3D) images. Tomosynthesis is a relatively new technology that has been developed for use with digital mammography and it allows for multiple high-resolution cross-sectional images of the breast to be obtained at the same dose as conventional screen-film mammography.

Tomosynthesis proponents argue that this 3D image may allow for both improved detection of breast cancer and for fewer false positive screening mammograms. In current practice, 7 to 15 percent of women undergoing mammography screening may be recalled for additional mammography or ultrasound images. Approximately 50 percent of these women may have a suspicious-looking area on the mammogram; this area results from normal breast tissues from several areas of the breast becoming superimposed to look like a lesion or other abnormality. Tomosynthesis, which allows cross-sectional viewing of the breast, may allow the radiologist to differentiate between superimposed tissue and actual lesions, thereby allowing for a reduction in the recall rate. Reducing the recall rate is an important goal because of the patient's anxiety associated with being asked to return for additional views. It is also possible that tomosynthesis may increase the positive biopsy rate. Tomosynthesis might also allow the complete patient workup in one visit for many women, a significant accomplishment given the noncompliance with recommended follow-up appointments after abnormal screening studies.

Robert Alexander remains skeptical, however. He is concerned that full-field digital mammography with tomosynthesis will increase the hospital's initial fixed costs of screening, while many of the reduced costs will accrue to the patient and to the payer, for which the hospital is not remunerated or tangibly rewarded. He also is concerned about the increased time it will take for radiologists to learn how to use this new technology.

Robert's staff had analyzed the two alternatives using an equivalent annual cost (EAC) method. Because the alternatives have different useful lives, EAC appeared to be the best way to determine which type of equipment would be more cost effective for the hospital. Essentially, EAC is the amount of an annuity that has the same life and present value as the investment option being considered. Thus, Dr. Alexander based the cost comparison on the initial outlay costs of both types of imaging equipment and on the annual maintenance, personnel-related and other costs associated with the two equipment types. Dr. Alexander wants to purchase the conventional mammography equipment because it results in lower costs for AMC.

Dr. Sipparo, however, remains convinced that FFDM with tomosynthesis is the right decision. She believes the technology is superior, offers better care, and ultimately, will reduce many of the long-term costs associated with breast cancer screening and diagnosis. Without a strong financial background, she is unsure how to convince Dr. Alexander of this, which is why she contacted Mr. Smith. She wanted his help to prepare an alternative analysis using the latest financial decision-making tools.

Capital project analysis occurs during the programming phase of the management control process. Whereas zero-base budgeting or zero-base review can be considered as the programming phase of management control concerned with old or existing programs, capital project analysis is the phase primarily concerned with new programs. Here, it is broadly defined to include the selection process of investment projects.

Capital project analysis is an ongoing activity, but it is not usually summarized annually in the budget. The capital budget is the yearly estimate of resources that will be expended for new programs during the coming year.

Capital budgeting may be considered as less comprehensive and shorter term than capital project analysis.

Explain who is involved in the capital investment decision process.

PARTICIPANTS IN THE ANALYTICAL PROCESS

The capital decision-making process in the health care industry is complex for several reasons. First, a health care firm, whether nonprofit or investor-owned, is likely to have more complex and less quantifiable objectives than firms in other industries. Provision of care to the indigent and community access to services, as well as attention to quality standards are often critical objectives for health care firms in addition to profits. Second, the number of individuals involved in the process, either directly or indirectly, is likely to be greater in the health care industry than in most other industries. Figure 18–1 illustrates the relationships of various parties involved in the capital decision-making process of a health care facility.

External Participants

Financing Sources

The option of obtaining funds externally for many new programs is an important variable in the capital decision-making process. A variety of individual organizations are involved in the credit determination process, including investment bankers, bond rating agencies, bankers, and feasibility consultants. Many of these entities and their roles are discussed in Chapter 20. At this juncture, it is important to recognize that, collectively, these entities may influence the amount of money that can be borrowed and the terms of the borrowing, and this can affect the nature and size of capital projects undertaken by a given health care facility.

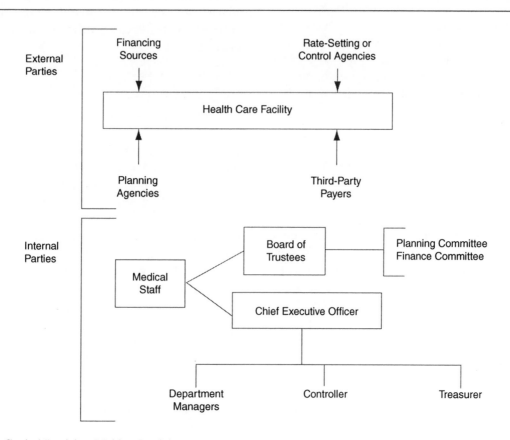

Figure 18–1 Capital Decision-Making Participants

Rate-Setting and Rate-Control Agencies

Some states control or limit the rates that hospitals and other health care firms can charge for services. The influence exerted by rate-setting or rate-control organizations on capital decision making is indirect, but still extremely important. Control of rates can limit both short-term and long-term profitability. This control can reduce a health care firm's ability to repay indebtedness, and thus limit its access to the capital markets. More directly, rate-setting organizations can limit the amount of money available for financing capital projects by reducing the amount of profits that may be retained. One of the major effects of rate control is to significantly reduce the level of capital expenditures by health care firms.

Third-Party Payers

Like rate-setting and rate-control agencies, third-party payers can indirectly influence the capital decision-making process. Through their reimbursement provisions, third-party payers can affect both capital expenditure levels and sources of financing. For example, many people believe that third-party cost reimbursement provides a strong incentive for increased capital spending; in most situations, such cost reimbursement provides for the reimbursement of depreciation and interest expense, which then may be used to repay financial requirements associated with any indebtedness. As a result, the risk associated with hospital indebtedness is reduced. In the past, third-party cost reimbursement favorably affected the availability of credit. Conversely, recent departures from cost reimbursement have had an adverse impact on credit availability.

Planning Agencies

In many states, state approval of capital expenditures is still required. Planning agencies review certificate-of-need applications and their recommendations are then passed on to the state authority responsible for final approval or disapproval. An unfavorable decision by the state may be appealed in court.

Internal Participants

Board of Trustees

Ultimately, the board of trustees is responsible for the capital expenditure and capital financing program of the health care firm. However, in most situations, the board delegates this authority to management and special board committees. The board's major function should be to clearly establish defined goals and objectives. The statement of goals and objectives is a prerequisite to the programming phase of management control, which includes capital expenditure analysis. Without a clear statement of goals and objectives, capital expenditure programs cannot be adequately defined and analyzed.

Another role of this governing board should be to approve a preliminary five-year capital expenditure program. This capital expenditure program should link back to the strategic financial plan discussed in Chapter 12. The list of capital expenditures should be generated by management and should reflect not just a "wish list" of capital expenditures that would be desirable to make, but should represent management's best guess concerning what future capital expenditures will be essential to meet and maintain the organization's mission.

Planning Committee

Many health care facility boards of trustees have established planning committees whose primary function is to define, analyze, and propose programs to help the organization attain its goals and objectives. These committees are specialized groups within the board of trustees that are directly involved in capital expenditure analysis.

Finance Committee

Some boards of trustees also have established finance committees that have authority in several key financial functional areas, including budgeting and capital financing. In these two particular areas, a finance committee may be involved with translating programs (perhaps identified by the planning committee) into financing requirements. These requirements may be operational or capital. The finance committee's major responsibility is to ensure adequate financing to meet program requirements. Many of the finance committee's budgetary functions are delegated to the controller; many of its capital financing functions are delegated to the treasurer.

Chief Executive Officer

The chief executive officer (CEO) is responsible on a day-to-day basis for implementing approved capital expenditure programs and developing related financing plans. The CEO must develop an organizational system that responds to the requests of department managers and medical staff for capital expenditures. Much of the authority vested in the chief executive officer's position is delegated by the board of trustees.

The administration also may seek board approval for its own programs.

Department Managers

Department managers make most of the internal requests for capital expenditure approval. In many health care facilities, formal systems for approving capital expenditures have been developed to receive, process, and answer departmental requests. The allocation of a limited capital budget to competing departmental areas is a difficult task for management. Careful definition of the criteria for capital decision making can help make this problem less political and more objective.

Medical Staff

Medical staff demands for capital expenditures are a problem unique to the health care industry. Medical staff members, in most situations, are not employees of the health care firm but rather use it to treat their private patients. Because of their ability to change a firm's utilization dramatically and thus affect financial solvency, administrators listen to, and frequently honor, medical staff members' wishes. Health care firms thus encounter strong pressure from individuals who have little financial interest in the organization and whose financial interest may, in fact, be contrary to that of the health care firm.

Controller

The controller facilitates approval of capital expenditures. The controller is usually responsible for developing capital expenditure request forms and for assisting department managers with preparing their capital expenditure proposals. The controller usually serves as an analyst, assisting the administrator with allocating the budget to competing departmental areas. In many small health care firms, the controller's function may be merged with that of the treasurer.

Treasurer

The treasurer is responsible for obtaining funds for both short- and long-term programs. The treasurer may work with the finance committee to negotiate for funds necessary to implement approved programs.

LEARNING OBJECTIVE 2

Describe the kinds of decisions that are made in capital investment decision analysis.

CLASSIFICATION OF CAPITAL EXPENDITURES

A capital expenditure is a commitment of resources that is expected to provide benefits during a reasonably long period, at least two or more years. Any system of management control must take into account the various types of capital expenditures. Different types of capital expenditures create different problems; they may require specific individuals to evaluate them or special methods of evaluation.

The more important classifications of capital expenditures are:

* the period during which the investment occurs.
* the types of resources invested.
* the dollar amounts of capital expenditures.
* the types of benefits received.

Period of Investment

Determining the amount of resources committed to a capital project depends heavily on the definition of the period. For example, how would you determine the capital expenditures needed by a project that had a low initial investment cost, but will have a significant investment cost in future years? Should just the initial capital expenditure be considered, or should total expenditures over the life of the project be considered? If the latter is the answer, is it appropriate just to add the total expenditures together, or should expenditures made in later years be weighted to reflect their lower present value? If so, at what discount rate? These are not simple questions to answer, but they are important when evaluating capital projects.

A classic example of this type of problem in the health care industry is the initiation of programs that have been funded by grants. In many such situations, there appears to be little or no investment of capital, because the amounts are funded almost totally through the grant. The programs thus appear to be highly desirable. However, if there is a formal or informal commitment to continue the programs for a longer period, capital expenditures and additional operating funds for later periods may be required. In such cases, it is imperative that the grant-funded projects be classified separately and their long-run capital cost requirements be identified. The health care facility may very well not have a sufficient capital base to finance a program's continuation. Thus, granting agencies should assess the health care facility's financial capability to continue funded programs after the grant period expires.

Types of Resources Invested

When discussing capital expenditures, many people are apt to limit their attention just to the expenditure or resources invested in capital assets, that is, tangible fixed assets. This narrow focus has several shortcomings, however, and may result in ineffective capital expenditure decisions.

First, focusing on tangible fixed assets implies ownership; yet, many health care facilities lease a significant percentage of their fixed assets, especially in the major movable equipment area. If a lease is not construed to be a capital expenditure, it may escape the normal review and approval system. Lease payments should be considered capital expenditures. Furthermore, the contractual provisions of the lease should be considered when determining the total expenditure amount. Weight should be given to future payments or to the alternative purchase price of the asset.

Second, the capital costs of a capital expenditure are only one part of total cost; indeed, in the labor-intensive health care industry, capital costs may be just the "tip of the iceberg." All of the operating costs associated with beginning and continuing a capital project should be considered. Programs with low capital investment costs may not be considered as favorable when their operating costs are taken into account.

Lifecycle costing is a method for estimating the cost of a capital project that reflects total costs, both operating and capital, over the project's estimated useful life. The lifecycle cost of all contemplated programs should be considered; failure to do this can cause errors in the capital decision-making process, especially in the selection of alternative programs. Consider, for example, two alternative renal dialysis projects; both may have the same capacity, but one may have a significantly greater investment cost because it uses equipment requiring less monitoring and lower operating costs. Failure to consider the operating cost differences between these two projects may bias the decision in favor of the project with lower capital expenditures and result in higher expenses in the long run.

Amounts of Expenditures

Different systems of control and evaluation are required for different-sized projects. It would not be eco-

nomical to spend $500 in administrative time evaluating the purchase of a $100 calculator. Nor would it be wise to spend only $500 to evaluate a $25 million building program. Obviously, control over capital expenditures should be conditioned by the total amount involved; and, if appropriate, the amount should be based on the total lifecycle cost.

Control of capital expenditures in most organizations, including health care firms, typically follows one of three patterns:

1. Approval required for all capital expenditures
2. Approval required for all capital expenditures above a pre-established limit
3. No approval required for individual capital expenditure projects below a total budgeted amount

Retaining final approval of all capital expenditures allows management to exert maximum control over the resource-spending area. However, the cost of management time to develop and review expenditure proposals is high. In most organizations of any size, management review of all capital expenditure requests is not productive. However, some review is needed, so a limit must be established. For example, a given responsibility center or department need not submit any justification for individual capital expenditure projects requiring less than $500 in investment costs. In such cases, there is usually some formal or informal limitation on the total dollar size of the capital budget that will be available for small-dollar capital expenditures. This prevents responsibility center managers from making excessive investments in capital expenditures that have no formalized reviewing system.

Another form of management control over capital expenditures is an absolute dollar limit; that is, any responsibility center manager may spend up to an authorized capital budget on any items in question. The real negotiation involves determining the size of the capital budget that will be available for individual departments. However, this system, although least costly in terms of review time, does not ensure that the capital expenditures actually made are necessarily in the best interests of the organization.

Types of Benefits

Depending on the types of benefits envisioned for a capital expenditure, different systems of management control and evaluation may be necessary. For example, investment in a medical office building results in different benefits than investment in an alcoholic rehabilitation unit. Such differences make it inappropriate to rely exclusively on any one method of evaluating projects. It is important to note that traditional methods of evaluating capital budgeting may not be appropriate in the health care industry. Traditional methods evaluate only the financial aspects of a capital expenditure. However, projects in the health care industry may produce benefits that are much more important than a reduction in cost or an increase in profit.

The following are major categories of investment in which benefits may be differentially evaluated:

* Operational continuance
* Financial
* Other

The first category of investment produces benefits that permit continued operations of the facility along present lines. Here, the governing board or management must usually answer the following two questions: (1) Are continued operations in the present form desirable? (In most cases, the answer is yes.) (2) Which alternative investment project can achieve continued operations in the most desirable way (for example, with lowest cost, patient safety, and so on)? A classic example of this type of investment is based on a licensure requirement for installation of a sprinkler system in a nursing home. Failure to make the investment may result in discontinuance of operations.

The second category of investment provides benefits that are largely financial, in terms of either reduced costs or increased profits to the organization. Many people may believe that these two are identical, that is, that reduced costs imply increased profits. However, as we will determine, this may not be true if cost reimbursement for either operating or capital costs is present. The important point to remember is that if the major benefits are financial, traditional capital budgeting methods may be more appropriate.

The third category of investments is a catch-all category. Investments here would range from projects that activate major new medical areas (such as outpatient or mental health services) to projects that improve employee working conditions (such as employee gymnasiums). In this category, benefits may be more difficult to quantify and evaluate. Traditional capital-budgeting methods thus may be appropriate only in the selection of less costly ways to provide designated services.

THE CAPITAL PROJECT DECISION-MAKING PROCESS

Making decisions that will be the basis on which capital projects will be undertaken is not an easy task. In many respects, this may represent the most difficult and important management decision area. The allocation of limited resources to specific project areas will directly affect the efficiency and effectiveness and, ultimately, the continued viability of the organization.

LEARNING OBJECTIVE 3

Explain the four stages of the capital decision-making process.

For our purposes, we can divide the capital decision-making process into four interrelated activities or stages:

1. Generation of project information
2. Evaluation of projects
3. Decisions about which projects to fund
4. Project implementation and reporting

LEARNING OBJECTIVE 4

List some of the kinds of information that are needed to evaluate a capital investment project.

Generation of Project Information

In this stage of the decision-making process, information is gathered that can be analyzed and evaluated later. This is an extremely important stage because inadequate or inaccurate information can lead to poor decision making. Specifically, there are six major categories of information that should be included in most capital expenditure proposals:

1. Alternatives available
2. Resources available
3. Cost data
4. Benefit data
5. Prior performance
6. Risk projection

Alternatives Available

A major deficiency related to many capital expenditure decisions is the failure to consider possible alternatives. Often, capital expenditures are presented on a "take it or leave it" basis, yet there usually are alternatives. For example, different manufacturers might be selected, different methods of financing could be used, or different boundaries in the scope of the project could be defined.

Resources Available

Capital expenditure decisions are not made in a vacuum. In most situations, there are constraints on the amount of available funding. This is the whole rationale behind capital expenditure decision making: scarce resources must be allocated among a virtually unlimited number of investment opportunities. There is little question that top-level management needs information concerning the availability of funding.

However, there is some question about its importance at the departmental level. On one hand, a budgetary constraint may temper requests for capital expenditures. On the other hand, it may encourage a department manager to submit only those projects that are in the department's best interests. These may, in fact, conflict with the broader goals and objectives of the organization as a whole.

Cost Data

It goes without saying that cost information is an important variable in the decision-making process. In all cases, the lifecycle costs of a project should be presented. Limiting cost information to capital costs can be counterproductive.

Benefit Data

We can divide benefit data into the following two categories: quantitative and nonquantitative. Some believe that many of the benefit data in the health care industry are nonquantitative. To a large extent, quantitative data are viewed as being synonymous with financial data. And because financial criteria are sometimes viewed as less important in the nonprofit health care industry, the assumption is that quantitative data are also less important. This is not true. Quantitative data can and should be used. Effective management control is predicated on the use of numbers that relate to the organization's stated goals and objectives.

It may not be easy to develop quantitative estimates of benefits, but it is not impossible. For example, assume that a hospital in an urban area opens a clinic in a medically underserved area. One of the stated goals for the clinic is the reduction of unnecessary use of the hospital's emergency room for nonurgent care. A realistic and quantifiable benefit of this project should be a numerical reduction in the use of the hospital's emergency room for nonurgent care by individuals from the clinic area. However, no quantitative assessments are either projected or reported; the only quantitative statistics used are those of a financial nature. The management control process in this situation is less valuable than it should have been.

Prior Performance

Information on prior operating results of projects proposed by responsibility center managers can be useful. A comparison of prior actual results with forecast results can give a decision maker some idea of the manager's reliability in forecasting. In too many cases, project planners are likely to overstate a project's benefits if the project interests them. Review of prior performance can help a manager evaluate the accuracy of the projections.

It is generally acknowledged that most people requesting capital expenditure approval for their projects will overstate benefits (revenues) and understate costs. This type of behavior is not necessarily intentional, but may reflect sincere faith and interest in the project. Individuals reviewing proposals must recognize this inherent bias and also recognize that not all people make the same magnitude of errors in forecasts.

Risk Projection

Nothing is certain in this world except death and taxes, especially when evaluating capital expenditure projects. It is important to ask "what-if" questions. For example, how would costs and benefits change if volume changed? Volume of service is a key variable in most capital expenditure forecasts, and its effects should be understood. In some situations, requiring projections for the highest, the lowest, and the most likely projections of volume can help answer the questions. The same types of calculations can be made for other key factors, such as prices of key inputs and technologic changes. This is an important area to understand because some capital expenditure projects are inherently more risky than others. Specifically, programs with extremely high proportions of fixed or sunk costs are much more sensitive to changes in volume than those with low percentages of fixed or sunk costs.

Evaluation of Projects

Although financial criteria are clearly not the only factors that should be evaluated while making capital expenditure decisions, there are few, if any, capital expenditure decisions that can omit financial considerations. Our focus is on the following two prime financial criteria: solvency and cost.

Solvency

A project that cannot show a positive rate of return in the long run should be questioned. If implemented, such a program will need to be subsidized by some other existing program area. For example, should a hospital subsidize an outpatient clinic? If so, to what extent? This is the kind of policy and financial question the governing board of the organization needs to determine. The fairness of some patients subsidizing other patients is one of the basic qualitative issues in capital project analysis. Operation of an insolvent program eventually can threaten the solvency of the entire organization. Thus, organizations that plan to subsidize insolvent programs must be in good financial condition, and assessment of financial condition can be done only after the organization's financial statements are examined.

Cost

Cost is the second important financial concern. An organization needs to select the projects that contribute most to the attainment of its objectives, given resource constraints. This type of analysis is often called cost-benefit analysis. Benefits differ from project to project. While evaluating alternative programs, decision makers must weight those benefits according to their own preferences and then compare them with cost.

There is a second dimension to the cost criterion. All projects that are eventually selected should cost the least to provide the service. This type of evaluation is sometimes called cost effectiveness analysis. Least cost should be defined as the present value of both operating and capital costs (methods for determining this are discussed later in the chapter).

Decisions about Which Projects to Fund

At this juncture of the capital expenditure decision-making process, it is time to make the decisions. The decision makers possess lists of possible projects that may be funded. Each project should represent the lowest cost of providing the desired service or output. In addition, various benefit data on each project should be described. These data should be consistent with the criteria that the decision makers used in their capital expenditure decision making.

To illustrate this process, assume that the members of the governing board are deciding on how many, if any, of three proposed programs they will fund in the coming year. The three programs are a burn care unit, a hemodialysis unit, and a commercial laboratory. Assume further that the members have decided that there are only four criteria of importance to them:

1. Solvency
2. Incremental management time required
3. Public image
4. Medical staff approval

Because none of the three projects clearly dominates, it is not clear which, if any, should be funded. Thus, the decision makers must weight the criteria according to their own preferences and determine the overall ranking of the three projects. For example, one manager might weight solvency and management time highly, relative to public image and the medical staff, and thus select the commercial laboratory project. Another manager might weight medical staff and public image more heavily, and thus select the hemodialysis or burn care unit project.

In this example, the three projects can be ranked in terms of their relative standing on each of the four criteria in Table 18–1.

Project Implementation and Reporting

Most capital expenditure control systems are concerned primarily, if not exclusively, with analysis and evaluation prior to selection. However, a real concern should be focused on whether the projected benefits are actually being realized as forecast. Without this feedback on the actual results of prior investments, the capital expenditure control system's feedback loop is not complete.

The following are some of the specific advantages of establishing a capital expenditure review program:

Table 18–1 Capital Project Ranking

	Project		
Criterion	Hemodialysis Unit	Burn-Care Unit	Commercial Laboratory
Solvency	2	3	1
Management time	2	3	1
Public image	2	1	3
Medical staff	1	2	3

• Capital expenditure review could highlight differences between planned versus actual performance that may permit corrective action. If actual performance is never evaluated, corrective action may not be taken. This could mean that the projected benefits might never be realized.

• Use of a review process may result in more accurate estimates. If people realize that they will be held responsible for their estimates, they may tend to be more careful with their projections. This will ensure greater accuracy in forecast results.

• Forecasts by individuals with a continuous record of biased forecasts can be adjusted to reflect that bias. This should result in a better forecast of actual results.

JUSTIFICATION OF CAPITAL EXPENDITURES

In most health care organizations, there is a formalized process for approval of a capital expenditure. Usually, this approval process is initiated by a department or responsibility center manager through the completion of a capital expenditure approval form. An example of a completed capital expenditure approval form is shown in Exhibit 18–1. Both the approval form and the approval process may vary across health care organizations, depending on the nature of the management control process in each case.

The approval form in Exhibit 18–1 is, in fact, more comprehensive than that used in most health care organizations. Thus, it provides a detailed summary of the following key aspects involved in capital expenditure approval:

• Amount and type of expenditure
• Attainment of key decision criteria
• Detailed financial analysis

In most firms, small capital expenditures are usually not subjected to detailed analysis and do not require justification. For example, capital expenditures less than $2,000 are not reviewed according to the instructions in Exhibit 18–1. This does not mean that a department has an unlimited capital expenditures budget if it spends less than $2,000 per item; the department is most likely subject to some overall level for small capital expenditures. For example, a department such as physical therapy might have an $8,000 limit on small capital expenditure items. No justification for capital expenditure items less than $2,000 would be required if the aggregate limit of $8,000 is not violated.

Replacement items also are specially recognized. In the example in Exhibit 18–1, a replacement expenditure less than $20,000 is not subject to review. The rationale for this higher limit relates to the operational continuance of capital expenditures. Replacement expenditures are often viewed as essential to the continuation of existing operations. They are, therefore, not as closely evaluated as are expenditures for new pieces of equipment.

In any decision-making process, it is important to carefully define the criteria that will be used in the selection process. The example in Exhibit 18–1 has three categories of criteria:

1. Need (management goals, hospital goals)
2. Economic feasibility
3. Acceptability (physicians, employees, community)

Most capital expenditure forms probably would request that data regarding economic or financial feasibility be included. Exhibit 18–1 provides data in other areas as well and also includes a means for scoring the project. For the specific project being appraised, a raw score of 16 and a priority score of 5 resulted. Different values could be obtained by changing the form's measures and their relative weightings.

Exhibit 18–1 Completed Capital-Expenditure Approval Form

Appraisal Sheet for Capital-Expenditure Proposals

Department and number _____ Surgery #818 _____

Date of request for purchase _____ 1/7/07 _____

Summary description of item or package of items (attach original request for purchase)

IABP (intra-aortic balloon pump) Model 10 with cardiac output computer and recorder
_____

_____

Total capital expenditure, including training, renovation, and purchase of equipment (attach list)	$19,500
Undepreciated value of equipment being replaced	0
Total cost of implementation	$19,500

Appraisal Instructions

Level I — Complete a Level I assessment for any one of the following:
1. A new item having a total capital expenditure exceeding $2,000
2. A replacement item having a total capital expenditure exceeding $20,000
3. A proposed capital expenditure requiring an evaluation before a purchase (or lease) decision may be made

Level II —Complete both a Level I and a Level II assessment for any proposed capital expenditure that meets any of the following criteria:

1. It exceeds $100,000.
2. It initiates or modifies the scope of type of health services rendered in the community and may require a certificate of need.
3. It requires a more extensive evaluation than offered by a Level I review.

Appraisal Outcome	By (initials)	Date	Priority Status
Request denied	_____	_____	_____
Request accepted and pending	_____	_____	_____
Request approved	_____	_____	_____

Level I Review—Complete the following assessment for any proposed capital expenditure requiring either a Level I or Level II review.

A. Need
1. Indicate whether the proposed capital expenditure contributes directly to the achievement of any of the following management goals (check those that apply):
   _____ Revenue
   _____ Hospital improvement study
   _____ Productivity
   ___X___ Quality assurance
   _____ Employee development
   _____ Management services consultant package
   _____ Other goal (specify)

2. Indicate whether the proposed capital expenditure contributes directly to the achievement of any of the following hospital goals (check one or more goals):
   ___X___ Patient care
   _____ Medical and allied health education
   ___X___ Community service

continues

Exhibit 18–1   continued

_____ Cost containment
_____ The leadership role
_____ Clinical research

3. Provide the following information on historical and projected utilization of items for the provision of patient care services. (See the finance department for assistance in completing this section.)

   a. For replacement items only:

      1) Identify units of service, if any, provided through the utilization of existing equipment; the actual volume of services provided during the most recent year for which statistics are available; the current patient charge, if any, for these services; and the annual revenue realized.

	Unit of Service	Historical Annual Volume	Patient Charge	Annual Revenue
1.	_____	_____	_____	_____
2.	_____	_____	_____	_____
3.	_____	_____	_____	_____
4.	_____	_____	_____	_____
Total			$	

      2) Serial number of item _____

      3) Fixed asset tag number _____

   b. For both new and replacement items:

      1) Identify the units of service, if any, to be offered through acquisition of the proposed item and the estimated volume of services to be provided annually. If known, provide the proposed patient charge per unit of service.

	Unit of Service	Estimated Annual Volume	Proposed Patient Charge
1.	Ped open heart	161	$459.16 (average)
2.	_____	_____	_____
3.	_____	_____	_____

      2) Identify any other services of which volume of utilization will be affected through acquisition of the proposed item: _____

      3) Percentage of charge patients for department (from cost report):   93.1
      4) Estimated useful life of equipment: 10   years

4. Document the reasons justifying the acquisition of the proposed capital expenditure, particularly as they relate to the achievement of hospital, departmental, and management goals and objectives.
   We presently borrow General Hospital's balloon pumps three or four times per month. This is a life-saving device. Without it, some patients cannot survive open-heart surgery.

continues

Exhibit 18–1 continued

B. Economic feasibility
 1. Estimate any change in the annual operating costs associated with acquisition of this proposed capital expenditure. (See the finance department for assistance in completing this section.)

Change in Annual Operating Cost

Personnel	_____
Employee benefits @ 23%	_____
Physician cost	_____
Materials and supplies	_____
Maintenance contracts	_____
Insurance	_____
Other depreciation	$1,950
Total change in annual operating cost	$1,950

Provide documentation in support of the previous estimates.

 2. Financial analysis (to be completed by finance):

Estimated Cost to Purchase IABP Model 10 with Cardiac Output Computer

Cash Expenditure	Cost Reimbursement @ 26%	Net Cash (Disbursed) Received	Present Value @ 6%
($19,500)	$507	($18,993)	($17,918)
	507	507	451
	507	507	426
	507	507	402
	507	507	379
	507	507	357
	507	507	337
	507	507	318
	507	507	300
	507	507	283
($19,500)	$5,070	($14,430)	($14,665)

Total present value (cost)   ($14,665)

 3. Space analysis:
  a. Change in the number of square feet of space required for item: n/a
  b. Is existing department space available for the item?

  (Circle one) (Yes) No

If not, document plan for acquiring additional space.

C. Acceptability
 1. Physician impact of the capital-expenditure decision:
  a. What is the scope of any physician-attitude change? (Check one.)
   _____ 1) No change. (Skip to Section C-2.)
   ___X___ 2) One or two physicians will be affected.
   _____ 3) The majority of the physicians in a hospital service will be affected.

continues

Exhibit 18-1 continued

    b. What is the *intensity* of the effect on physician attitude? (Check two answers—one for acceptance and one for non-acceptance.)

Not accepted:

       _____ 4) The affected physicians will move their practices to other hospitals.

       __X__ 3) The affected physicians will tend to reduce their practices at the hospital.

       _____ 2) The affected physicians, at the very least, will be disgruntled and will tend to discuss in the community and with other physicians the lack of the expenditure or project.

       _____ 1) The physicians will be aware of the lack of support for the project and will be less likely to believe that the hospital is maintaining a proper level of patient care.

       _____ 0) No effect.

Accepted:

       _____ 0) No effect.

       _____ 1) The affected physicians will be aware of the expenditure or project and will be satisfied that the hospital is maintaining a high level of patient care.

       __X__ 2) The affected physicians will be very impressed and will tend to discuss the expenditure or project favorably in the community and with other physicians.

       _____ 3) The affected physicians will tend to increase their practices moderately in the hospital.

       _____ 4) The affected physicians will move their patients to the hospital.

2. Employee impact of the capital-expenditure decision:

    What is the effect on the attitude of hospital employees? (Check two answers—one for acceptance and one for non-acceptance.)

Not accepted:

       _____ 4) Major and widespread negative impact on employee morale and attitude toward the hospital.

       _____ 3) Widespread disappointment with the hospital and some general negative effect on the hospital's image among employees.

       __X__ 2) Negative reaction from a limited group of employees (in two or more departments).

       _____ 1) Negative reaction from a limited group of employees in one department.

       _____ 0) No effect.

Accepted:

       __X__ 0) No effect.

       _____ 1) Limited reaction from a few employees.

       __X__ 2) Positive reaction from a limited group of employees (one or two departments).

       _____ 3) Positive impact on nearly all employees.

       _____ 4) Major and widespread impact with long-term effect on employee attitude toward the hospital.

3. Community impact of the capital-expenditure decision:

    What is the expected community impact? (Check the answers below that best describe the expected community impact; check one for acceptance and one for non-acceptance.)

Not accepted:

       _____ 4) Intense and widespread negative reaction in the community will affect the hospital's image.

       __X__ 3) A widespread negative effect on the hospital's general image and reputation will result.

       _____ 2) Limited negative effect on the hospital's general image and reputation will result.

       _____ 1) The attitudes of relatively few people will be negatively affected.

       _____ 0) No effect.

Accepted:

       _____ 0) No effect.

       _____ 1) Relatively few people will be positively affected.

       _____ 2) Certain groups in the community will be favorably impressed.

       __X__ 3) A widespread positive effect on the hospital's image and reputation will result.

       _____ 4) Significant and widespread positive community reaction will contribute significantly to the hospital's general image and reputation.

continues

Exhibit 18–1 continued

APPRAISAL SCORE SHEET FOR
CAPITAL EXPENDITURE PROPOSALS

	Assigned Value	Raw Score	Priority Instruction	Priority Score
A. Need				
1) If proposal directly contributes to one or more management goals (I-A-1)	+1	+1		
2) If proposal directly contributes to one or more hospital goals (I-A-2)	+1	+1		
(For Level II reviews only)				
3) Performance expectations (II-A-4)				
If negative or questionable	−1			
If positive	+1			
4) If certificate-of-need approval is necessary but unlikely (II-A-5)	−3	___	Enter positive raw score as	___
Subtotal, need score		2	priority score.	2
B. Economic feasibility				
1. If annual operating costs (including depreciation) are reduced (I-B-1-a)	+1			
2. Return on investment (I-B-2-a)				
If greater than 7.5%	+2			
If positive	0			
If negative	−2	−2		
3. If significant additional space is required (I-B-3)	−1			
(For Level II reviews only)				
4. If external financing is required (II-B-1)	−1	___	Enter positive raw score as	___
Subtotal, economic score		−2	priority score.	
C. Acceptability				
1. Physician attitude			If scopes core is greater than 2, enter raw score in priority score column.	
a. Scope (enter score for response to question I-C-1-a)	1 to 3	2		

continues

Exhibit 18–1 continued

b. Intensity (add responses to question I-C-1-b)	0 to 8	5	If raw score exceeds 4, the excess is priority score.	1
2. Employee attitude (add responses to question I-C-2)	0 to 8	4	If raw score exceeds 4, the excess is priority score.	
3. Community attitude (add responses to question I-C-3)	0 to 8	6	If raw score exceeds 4, the excess is priority score.	2
Subtotal, acceptability score		16	Total priority	3
Total raw score		16	score	5

Note: A capital-expenditure proposal may be approved, disapproved, or deferred on the basis of an appraisal of the raw scores for need, economy, and acceptability, considered either independently or together. An approved capital-expenditure proposal is ranked according to its priority score for future appropriation of capital-expenditure funds.

The important point to recognize is that project selection usually involves the consideration of criteria other than financial criteria. Failure to collect data on the attainment of those additional criteria for specific projects often will lead to more subjectivity in the process. Without such relevant data, individuals may make inferences that are not legitimate.

A key aspect of the capital expenditure approval process is the financial or economic feasibility of the project. In most capital expenditure forms, there is some summary statistic that measures the project's overall financial performance. In general, such measures are usually categorized as either (1) discounted cash-flow methods (DCF) or (2) nondiscounted cash-flow methods. In the present discussion, we will not be concerned with nondiscounted cash-flow methods because they are usually regarded as less sophisticated than DCF methods.

LEARNING OBJECTIVE 5

Calculate a project's net present value, profitability index, and equivalent annual cost.

DISCOUNTED CASH FLOW METHODS

In this section, we examine three DCF methods that are relatively easy to understand and use:

1. Net present value
2. Profitability index
3. Equivalent annual cost

Before examining these three methods, a word of caution is in order. In our view, the calculation of specific DCF measures is an important, but not a critical, phase of capital expenditure review. We strongly believe that the most important phase in the capital expenditure review process is the generation of quality project information. Specifically, the set of alternatives being considered must include the best ones; it does a firm little good to select the best five projects from a list of ten inferior ones. Beyond that, the validity of the forecasted data is critical; small changes in projected volumes, rates, or costs can have profound effects on cash flow. Determination of possible changes in volumes, costs, or rates is much more important than discussions about the appropriate discount rate or cost of capital.

Each of the previous three DCF methods is based on a time-value concept of money. Each is useful in evaluating a specific type of capital expenditure or capital financing alternative. Specifically, their areas of application are:

Method of Evaluation	Area of Application
Net present value	Capital financing alternative
Profitability index	Capital expenditures with financial benefits
Equivalent annual cost	Capital expenditures with nonfinancial benefits

Net Present Value

A net present value (NPV) analysis is a useful way to analyze alternative methods of capital financing. In most situations, the objective in such a situation is clear: the commodity being dealt with is money, and it is management's goal to minimize the cost of financing operations. (We will consider shortly how this goal may conflict with solvency when the effects of cost reimbursement are considered.)

Net present value equals discounted cash inflows less discounted cash outflows. In a comparison of two alternative financing packages, the one with the highest NPV should be selected.

For example, assume that an asset can be financed with a four-year annual $1,000 lease payment or can be purchased outright for $2,800. Assume further that the discount rate is ten percent, which may reflect either the borrowing cost or the investment rate, depending on which alternative is relevant. (We will discuss the issue of an appropriate discount rate shortly.) The present value cost of the lease is $3,170. This amount is greater than the present value cost of the purchase, $2,800. With no consideration given to cost reimbursement, the purchase alternative is the lowest cost alternative method of financing.

In this era of prospective payment and capitation, the effects of cost reimbursement are declining for many providers with the exception of designated critical access hospitals under the Medicare program. For accuracy, however, the effects of cost reimbursement should be considered, if applicable. Reimbursement of costs would mean that the facility would be entitled to reimbursement for depreciation if the asset were purchased, or the facility would be entitled to the rent payment if the asset were leased. (Some third-party cost payers limit reimbursement on leases to depreciation and interest if the lease is treated as an installment purchase.) Assuming that straight-line depreciation is used and that 20 percent of capital expenses are reimbursed by third-party cost payers, the present value of the reimbursed cash inflow (using the discount factors from Table 17-4 in the previous chapter) would be as presented in Table 18–2.

If the asset were purchased, the organization would pay $2,800 immediately. For each of the next four years, it would be reimbursed for the noncash expense item of depreciation in the amount of $700 per year ($2,800 ÷ 4). However, because only 20 percent of the patients are capital cost payers, only $140 per year would be received (.20 × $700). If the asset was leased, the organization would be permitted reimbursement of the lease payment in the amount of $1,000 per year. However, because only 20 percent of the patients are capital cost payers, only $200 (.20 × $1,000) would be paid.

The NPV of the previous two financing methods for considering cost reimbursement would be as presented in Table 18–3.

In this example, it is clear that the best method of financing is outright purchase. By purchasing the asset, annual expenses will be $700 in depreciation, compared with $1,000 per year with the leasing plan. In addition, purchasing is also a plan that results in a lower NPV. Relative ratings regarding NPV could change quickly, however, given higher percentages of capital cost reimbursement. To see the impact of cost reimbursement on NPV, assume that 80 percent of capital costs will be reimbursed. When this change is reflected in the calculations in Table 18–2, leasing's NPV (−$634) is better (i.e., less negative) than purchasing's NPV (−$1,025).

Table 18–2 Present Value of Reimbursement

		Annual Reimbursement		Discount Factor		% of Cost Reimbursement		
Present value of reimbursed depreciation	=	$2,800/4	×	3.170	×	0.20	=	$444
Present value of reimbursed lease payments	=	$1,000	×	3.170	×	0.20	=	$634

Table 18–3 Net Present Value of Financing Alternatives

		Present Value of Reimbursement (Cash Inflows)		Present Value of Payments (Cash Outflows)		NPV
NPV of purchase	=	$444	=	$2,800	=	−$2,356
NPV of lease	=	$634	=	$3,170	=	−$2,536

Profitability Index

The profitability index method of capital project evaluation is of primary importance in cases when the benefits of the projects are mostly financial, for example, a capital project that saves costs or expands revenue with a primary purpose of increased profits. In these situations, there is usually a constraint on the availability of funding. Thus, those projects with the highest rate of return per dollar of capital investment are the best candidates for selection. The profitability index attempts to compare rates of return. The numerator is the NPV of the project, and the denominator is the investment cost.

$$\text{Profitability index} = \frac{\text{NPV}}{\text{Investment cost}}$$

To illustrate the use of this measure, let us assume that a hospital is considering an investment in a laundry service shared with a group of neighboring hospitals. The initial investment cost is $100,000 for the purchase of new equipment and delivery trucks. Savings in operating costs are estimated to be $20,000 per year for the entire ten-year life of the project. If the discount rate is assumed to be ten percent, the following calculations could be made, ignoring the effect of cost reimbursement and using the discount factors from Table 17–4 in the previous chapter.

Present value of operating savings =
$20,000 × 6.145 = $122,900

NPV = $122,900 − $100,000 = $22,900

$$\text{Profitability index} = \frac{\$22,900}{\$100,000} = .229$$

Values for profitability indices that are greater than zero imply that the project is earning at a rate greater than the discount rate. Given no funding constraints, all projects with profitability indices greater than zero should be funded. However, in most situations, funding constraints do exist, and only a portion of those projects with profitability indices greater than zero are actually accepted.

The previous calculations give no consideration to the effects of cost reimbursement. If we assume that 50 percent of the facility's capital expenses are reimbursed and 50 percent of its operating expenses are reimbursed, then the following additional calculations must be made:

Present value of reimbursed depreciation =

($100,000/10) × 6.145 × .50 = $30,725

Present value of lost reimbursement from operating savings = $20,000 × 6.145 × .50 = $61,450

NPV = $22,900 + $30,725 − $61,450 = −$7,825

$$\text{Profitability index} = \frac{-\$7,825}{\$1000,00} = -.07825$$

The previous calculations require some clarification. We are adjusting the initially calculated NPV of $22,900 to reflect the effects of cost reimbursement. Depreciation is the first item to be considered. Because 50 percent of the facility's patients are associated with capital cost reimbursement formulas, it can expect to receive 50 percent of the annual depreciation charge of $10,000 ($100,000/10) or $5,000 per year as a reimbursement cash flow. The present value of this stream, $30,725, is added to the initial net present value of $22,900.

The second item to be considered is the operating savings. If the investment is undertaken, the facility can anticipate a yearly savings of $20,000 for the next ten years. However, that savings will reduce its reimbursable costs by $20,000 annually, which means that 50 percent of that amount, or $10,000, will be lost annually in reimbursement. The present value of that loss for the ten years is $61,450, which is subtracted from the initial NPV. The effect of cost reimbursement thus reduces increased costs associated with new programs, but it also reduces the cost savings associated with new programs.

The preceding example illustrates an important financial concept discussed in Chapter 3. When cost reimbursement exists, as it does for critical access hospitals under Medicare, there is less incentive to invest in projects that reduce costs. In the previous example, the laundry facility's profitability index decreased from .229 to −.07825 when the effects of capital and operating cost reimbursement were considered.

Equivalent Annual Cost

Equivalent annual cost (EAC) is of primary value when selecting capital projects for which alternatives exist. Usually, these are capital expenditure projects that are classified as operational continuance or other. (The profitability index measure just discussed is used for projects in which the benefits are primarily financial in nature.)

Equivalent annual cost is the expected average cost, considering both capital and operating cost, over the life of the project. It is calculated by dividing the sum of the present value of operating costs over the life of the project and the present value of the investment cost by the discount factor for an annualized stream of equal payments (as derived from Table 17–4 in the previous chapter):

$$EAC = \frac{Present\ value\ of\ operating\ cost\ +\ Present\ value\ of\ investment\ cost}{Present\ value\ of\ annuity}$$

To illustrate use of this measure, assume that an extended care facility must invest in a sprinkler system to maintain its license. After investigation, two alternatives are identified. One sprinkler system would require a $5,000 investment and an annual maintenance cost of $500 during each year of its estimated ten-year life. An alternative sprinkler system can be purchased for $10,000 and would require only $200 in maintenance cost each year of its estimated twenty-year life. Ignoring cost reimbursement and assuming a discount factor of ten percent, the following calculations can be made:

EAC of a $5,000 sprinkler system:

Present value of operating costs =
$500 × 6.145 = $3,073

Present value of investment = $5,000
EAC ($5,000 sprinkler system) =

$$\frac{\$3,073 + \$5,000}{6.145} = \$1,314$$

EAC of a $10,000 sprinkler system:

Present value of operating costs =
$200 × 8.514 = $1,703

Present value of investment = $10,000

EAC ($10,000 sprinkler system) =

$$\frac{\$1,703 + \$10,000}{8.514} = \$1,375$$

From this analysis, it can be determined that the $5,000 sprinkler system would produce the lowest equivalent annual cost, $1,314 per year, compared with the $1,375 equivalent annual cost of the $10,000 system.

Two points should be made regarding this analysis. First, the equivalent annual cost method permits comparison of two alternative projects with different lives. In this case, a project with a ten-year life was compared with a project with a twenty-year life. It is assumed that the technology will not change and that in ten years the relevant alternatives still will be the two systems being analyzed. However, in situations of estimated rapid technologic changes, some subjective weight should be given to projects of shorter duration. In the previous example, this is no problem, because the project with the shorter life also has the lowest equivalent annual cost.

Second, equivalent annual cost is not identical to the reported or accounting cost. The annual reported accounting cost for the two alternatives would be the annual depreciation expenses plus the maintenance cost. Thus:

Accounting expense per year
($5,000 sprinkler system) =

$$\frac{\$5,000}{10} + \$500 = \$1,000$$

Accounting expense per year
($10,000 sprinkler system) =

$$\frac{\$10,000}{20} + \$200 = \$700$$

Reliance on such information that does not incorporate the time-value concept of money can produce misleading results, as it does in the previous example. The second alternative is not the lowest cost alternative when the cost of capital is included. In this case, the savings of $5,000 in investment cost between the two systems can be used either to generate additional investment income or to reduce outstanding indebtedness. It is assumed that the appropriate discount rate for each of these two alternatives would be ten percent.

Once again, the effects of cost reimbursement should be considered. In our example, we assume that 50 percent of the extended care facility's costs will be reimbursed. The following adjustments result:

EAC of a $5,000 sprinkler system:

Present value of reimbursed operating costs =
$500 × 6.145 × .50 = $1,536.25

Present value of reimbursed depreciation =

$$\frac{\$5,000}{10} \times 6.145 \times .50 = \$1,536.25$$

EAC of a $5,000 sprinkler system
(Reflecting cost reimbursement) =

$$\$1,314 - \frac{(\$1,536.25 + \$1,536.25)}{6.145} = \$814$$

EAC of $10,000 sprinkler system
(Reflecting cost reimbursement):

Present value of reimbursed operating costs =
$200 × 8.514 × .50 = $851.40

Present value of reimbursed depreciation =

$$\frac{\$10,000}{20} \times 8.514 \times .50 = \$2,128.50$$

EAC of $10,000 sprinkler system
(Reflecting cost reimbursement):

$$\$1,375 - \frac{(\$851.40 + \$2,128.50)}{8.514} = \$1,025$$

Again, some clarification of the calculations may be useful. To reflect the effect of cost reimbursement, the reimbursement of reported expenses for the two alternative sprinkler systems must be considered. The reported expense items for both sprinkler systems are depreciation and maintenance costs, which are referred to as operating costs. Depreciation for the $5,000 sprinkler system will be $500 per year ($5,000/10), and 50 percent of this amount ($250) will be paid for

reimbursement each year. The present value of the reimbursed depreciation ($250 × 6.145) is $1,536.25. Using the same procedure, the present value of reimbursed depreciation for the $10,000 sprinkler system is $2,128.50 ($250 × 8.514). In a similar fashion, payment for reimbursement of the maintenance costs for the two sprinkler systems also will be made. For the $5,000 system, the annual $500 maintenance cost will yield $250 in new reimbursement (.50 × $500) per year. The present value of this reimbursement inflow is $1,536.25. Using the same calculations for the $10,000 sprinkler system yields a present value of $851.40. The present values of both reimbursed depreciation and maintenance costs are then annualized and subtracted from the initially calculated equivalent annual cost to derive new equivalent annual costs that reflect cost reimbursement effects.

In this case, cost reimbursement did not change the decision. The lower-cost sprinkler system, after consideration of the effects of reimbursement, is still the best alternative.

LEARNING OBJECTIVE 6

Explain the concept of a discount rate and what the weighted average cost of capital is.

SELECTION OF THE DISCOUNT RATE

In the three DCF methods just discussed, to specify the discount rate we simply arbitrarily selected a number for each of our examples. In an actual case, however, the issue of how to select the appropriate discount rate requires careful attention.

Before discussing methods of determining the appropriate discount rate, it may be useful to evaluate the role of the discount rate in project selection. A natural question at this point is, would an alternative discount rate affect the list of capital projects selected? For example, if we used a discount rate of 10 percent and later learned that 12 percent should have been used, would our list of approved projects change? The answer is maybe. In some cases, alternative values for the discount rate would alter the relative ranking, and therefore the desirability of particular projects.

Again, we believe that the definition of the discount rate is an important issue, but not a critical one—

especially for health care organizations. This is true for several reasons. First, in the case of health care organizations, the financial criterion is not likely to be the only criterion. Other areas—such as need, quality of care, and teaching—also may be important. Second, a change in the relative ranking of projects is much more likely to result from an accurate forecast of cash flows than it is from an alternative discount rate. Efforts to improve forecasting would appear to be much more important than esoteric discussions about the relevancy of cost-of-capital alternatives.

In this context, we can examine three primary methods for defining a discount rate or the cost of capital for use in a DCF analysis:

1. Cost of specific financing source
2. Yield achievable on other investments
3. Weighted cost of capital

The cost of a specific financing source is sometimes used as the discount rate. Usually, the identified financing source is debt. For example, if a firm can borrow money at eight percent in the bond market, that rate would become its cost of capital or discount rate.

Another alternative is to use the yield rate possible on other investments. In many cases, this rate might be equal to the investment yield possible in the firm's security portfolio. For example, if the firm currently earned ten percent on its security investments, then ten percent would be its discount rate. This method, based on an opportunity cost concept, is relatively easy to understand.

The last alternative is to use the weighted cost of capital. This is the most widely-discussed and used method of defining the discount rate. In its simplest form, it is calculated as follows:

$$\text{Cost of capital} = (\% \text{ Debt} \times \text{Cost of debt}) + (\% \text{ Equity} \times \text{Cost of equity})$$

The advantage of this method is that it clearly represents the cost of capital to the firm. A major problem with its use, however, is the definition of the cost of equity capital. This is an especially difficult problem for nonprofit firms. How do you define the cost of equity capital? Detailed exploration of this issue and other aspects of discount rate selection are beyond the scope of the present discussion.

Readers who are interested in examining these topics in greater depth are referred to any good introductory finance textbook.

VALUATION

It is becoming an almost everyday occurrence to read about one health care entity buying or acquiring another related health care business. Hospitals buy other hospitals, nursing homes, physician practices, durable medical equipment firms, and other types of businesses. Nursing homes buy other nursing homes, home health firms, and other businesses. Although there are many tasks that need to be accomplished in any business acquisition, one of the most difficult and most important is valuation. Exactly what is the value of the business being acquired?

Valuation is really a subset of capital expenditure analysis. The business being acquired can be thought of as a capital expenditure that needs to be evaluated just as any other capital expenditure made in the organization. Nonfinancial criteria should be considered, and the contribution that the acquired business will make toward the acquiring firm's mission must be addressed.

SUMMARY

The capital decision-making process in the health care industry is complex, involving many independent decision makers. In this chapter, we examined the process and focused on methods for evaluating capital projects. Although capital expenditure decisions in the health care industry are not usually decided exclusively on the basis of financial criteria, most health care decision makers regard financial factors as important elements in the process. In that context, the three DCF methods we have examined can serve as useful tools in capital project analysis for health care facilities.

1. A health care firm's investment of $1,000 in a piece of equipment will reduce labor costs by $400 per year for the next five years. Thirty percent of all patients seen by the firm have a third-party payer arrangement that pays for capital costs on a retrospective basis. Thirty percent of all patients also reimburse for actual operating costs. What is the annual cash flow of the investment? Assume a five-year life and straight-line depreciation.

2. A hospital has just experienced a breakdown of one of its boilers. The boiler must be replaced quickly if the hospital is to continue operations. Should this investment be subjected to any analysis?

3. Few firms ever track the actual results achieved from a specific capital investment against projected results. What are the likely effects of such a management policy?

4. Santa Cruz Community Hospital is considering investing $90,000 in new laundry equipment to replace its present equipment, which is completely depreciated and outmoded. An alternative to this investment is a long-term contract with a local firm to perform the hospital's laundry service. It is expected that the hospital would save $20,000 per year in operating costs if the laundry service was performed internally. Both the expected life and the depreciable life of the projected equipment are six years. Salvage value of the present equipment is expected to be zero. Assuming that Santa Cruz Community Hospital can borrow or invest money at eight percent, calculate the payback, the NPV, and the profitability index. Ignore any reimbursement effects.

5. Frances Gebauer, president of Lucas Valley Hospital System, is investigating the purchase of 36 computer game systems for rental purposes. The sets have an expected life of two years and cost $500 apiece. The possible rental income flows are presented in Table 18–4.

Table 18–4 Rental Revenues from Computer Game Systems

Year 1		Year 2	
Rental Income	Conditional Probability	Rental Income	Conditional Probability
$12,000	0.40	$4,000	0.40
		7,000	0.60
		6,000	0.30
$15,000	0.60	8,000	0.70

If funds cost Lucas Valley ten percent, calculate the expected NPV of this project.

6. Mr. Dobbs, administrator at Innovative Hospital, is considering opening a new health screening department in the hospital. However, he is concerned about the financial consequences of this action, because the Board has indicated the current financial position of the hospital is not good; thus the project must pay for itself. As a result, Mr. Dobbs is especially interested in the establishment of a rate for the service and wishes to consult with you for your expert financial advice. He has prepared the cost and utilization data found in Table 18–5 for your review.

Table 18–5 Projected Costs of Health Screening Unit

Year	Variable Cost	Fixed Costs*	Patients Screened
1	$ 96,000	$120,000	2,400
2	144,000	135,000	3,600
3	192,000	150,000	4,800
4	192,000	150,000	4,800
5	192,000	150,000	4,800

* Includes annual depreciation of $70,000.

Mr. Dobbs is aware of the rapid pace of technologic change and anticipates that the current equipment, costing $350,000, will need to be replaced at the end of Year 5 for $500,000. He is not concerned about price inflation for his other operating costs because he believes that the increased costs can be recovered by increased charges. However, he is concerned about establishing a current charge for the new service that will generate a fund of sufficient size to meet the Year 5 replacement cost. Mr. Dobbs believes that any invested funds will earn interest at a rate of eight percent compounded annually. Assume that all payments and receipts are made at year end. What rate would you recommend charging for the new health screening service? Assume this rate to be effective for the entire five-year period.

7. Scioto Valley Convalescent Center is considering buying a $25,000 computer to improve its medical record and accounting functions. It is estimated that this investment will reduce operating costs by $7,000 per year. The computer has an estimated five-year life with an estimated $5,000 salvage value. What is this investment's profitability index if the discount rate is eight percent? Ignore reimbursement considerations.

8. In Assignment 7, assume that costs are reimbursed 30 percent. Further assume that Scioto Valley is a tax-paying entity with a marginal tax rate of 40 percent. What is the profitability index for this project now?

SOLUTIONS AND ANSWERS

1. The cash flow of the equipment investment by the health care firm will be equal to the annual reimbursed depreciation plus the reduced operating costs net of the cost reimbursement effect and may be calculated as follows:

$$\text{Cash flow} = \text{Annual depreciation} \times \text{Proportion of capital cost payers}$$
$$+ (\text{Annual operating savings} \times [1 - \text{Proportion of operating cost payers}])$$
$$= \$200 \times .30 + (\$400 \times [1 - .30])$$
$$= \$60 + \$280 = \$340$$

2. The investment in a new boiler would benefit the hospital in the area of operational continuance. Failure to make the needed investment would mean discontinued service. In this case, less analysis is needed, but care still should be exercised when identifying alternatives. The lowest-cost alternative to meet the need should be selected.

3. If it does not compare actual with projected results, management may lose some of the benefits that were originally expected to be realized with its investment. If the control loop is not closed, management will not know (and therefore cannot correct for) deviations from forecasted results. It is also possible that some department managers will overstate benefits for their favorite capital projects and that such actions will not be perceived as having any adverse consequences, because no comparison of forecast with actual results was made.

4. The calculations in Table 18–6 show the payback, the NPV, and the profitability index for the laundry service investment.

Table 18–6 Laundry Alternative Analysis

$$\text{Payback} = \text{Investment cost/Annual cash flow} =$$
$$\$90,000/\$20,000 = 4.5 \text{ years}$$

$$\text{Net present value} = \text{Present value of cash inflows} -$$
$$\text{Investment cost}$$
$$= \$20,000 \times P(8\%,6) - \$90,000$$
$$= \$20,000 \times 4.623 - \$90,000 = \$2,460$$

$$\text{Profitability index} = \text{Net present value/Investment cost} =$$
$$\$2,460/\$90,000 = .0273$$

---

5. The NPV of Lucas Valley's computer game system purchase project is shown in the data in Table 18–7.

Table 18–7 Expected NPV of TV Purchase

Item	Amount	Year	Probability	Expected Value	Present Value Factor	Expected Present Value
Rental income	$12,000	1	0.40	$4,800	0.9090	$4,363.20
Rental income	15,000	1	0.60	9,000	0.9090	8,181.00
Rental income	4,000	2	0.16	640	0.8260	528.64
Rental income	7,000	2	0.24	1,680	0.8260	1,387.68
Rental income	6,000	2	0.18	1,080	0.8260	892.08
Rental income	8,000	2	0.42	3,360	0.8260	2,775.36
TV cost	(18,000)	0	1.00	(18,000)	1.0000	(18,000.00)
Expected NPV						$127.96

6. The first step in determining the rate that Mr. Dobbs should charge for the new health screening service is to calculate the present value of the cash flow requirements that need to be covered by the charge for the service (Table 18–8).

Table 18–8 Present Value of Cash Operating Expenses

Item	Amount	Year	Present Value Factor (8%)	Present Value
Costs less depreciation	$146,000	1	0.926	$135,196
Costs less depreciation	209,000	2	0.857	179,113
Costs less depreciation	272,000	3	0.794	215,968
Costs less depreciation	272,000	4	0.735	199,920
Costs less depreciation	272,000	5	0.681	185,232
Replacement	500,000	5	0.681	340,500
				$1,255,929

The second step is to define the rate that will generate the required present value as calculated in Table 18–8. If we define r as the required rate per screening, the following calculation can be made:

$$\$1,255,929 = (2,400 \times r \times p[8\%,1]) + (3,600 \times r \times p[8\%,2])$$
$$+ (4,800 \times r \times p[8\%,3]) + (4,800 \times r \times p[8\%,4])$$
$$+ (4,800 \times r \times p[8\%,5])$$

$$\$1,255,929 = (2,400r\,[.926]) + (3,600r\,[.857]) + (4,800r\,[.794])$$
$$+ (4,800r\,[.735]) + (4,800r\,[.681])$$

$$\$1,255,929 = 15,915.6r$$

$$r = \frac{\$1,255,929}{15,915.6}$$

$$r = \$78.91$$

7. The profitability index for the computer investment by Scioto Valley Convalescent Center is calculated as follows:

Present value of cash inflows = ($7,000 × P[8%,5]) + ($5,000 × p[8%,5])
= ($7,000 × 3.993) + ($5,000 × .681)
= $31,356

$$\text{Profitability index} = \frac{\$31,356 - \$25,000}{\$25,000} = .254$$

8. The calculation of the profitability index for the computer investment in these new circumstances is now the following:

Calculation of present value of cash inflows:

Operating savings $7,000 × (1 − .30) × (1 − .40) × 3.993 =	$11,739
Reimbursed depreciation $4,000 × .30 × (1 − .40) × 3.993 =	2,875
Depreciation tax shelter effect $4,000 × .40 × 3.993 =	6,389
Salvage value $5,000 × .681 =	3,405
Total present value	$24,408

$$\text{Profitability index} = \frac{(\$24,408 - \$25,000)}{\$25,000} = -0.0237$$

Chapter 19

Consolidations and Mergers

LEARNING OBJECTIVES

After studying this chapter, you should be able to do the following:

1. Understand the terminology used in the field of consolidations, mergers, and acquisitions.
2. Explain some of the possible reasons why consolidations, mergers, and acquisitions occur.
3. Explain McKinsey & Company's five steps of planning for a merger or acquisition.
4. Understand common methods for valuation of a potential target firm.
5. Apply analytical methods and tools to value potential acquisitions.

REAL-WORLD SCENARIO

Chad Pemberton, CEO of Linworth Medical Center, has been approached by a major investor-owned hospital chain about Linworth's possible acquisition of one of their local hospitals. Chad knows that other hospitals in town have received similar overtures because the chain has made known their intent to sell this hospital within a year. The acquisition hospital, Orca Memorial, had been part of another investor-owned chain until six months ago, when it was acquired by the present system in a stock swap arrangement. Orca Memorial does not meet the present system's criteria for ownership. It is the only investor-owned hospital in town and has experienced several years of declining profitability. Chad is very interested in acquiring this hospital because his major competitors have all been engaged in merger mania during the last three years. Chad's hospital is the only remaining non-aligned hospital in town. Chad's declining market share has hurt him at the negotiating table with major health plans.

While Chad is very interested in buying Orca Memorial, he is concerned about the possible price that he may have to pay to acquire the hospital. Linworth's board is very conservative and does not want to expose the hospital to a burdensome level of debt or to erode their sizable cash reserve position. This situation has been made more complex by the current lack of profitability at Orca Memorial. Kyle Carpenter, the board chairperson at Linworth Medical Center, has told Chad on numerous occasions that he will examine the numbers very closely and will not approve any acquisition above a fair market value.

Chad's dilemma is: Just what is a 'fair market value' given the historic lack of earnings? Chad believes that his management team could turn Orca Memorial around in two years and restore it to profitability, but Mr. Carpenter is very skeptical about rose-colored projections of future profitability.

Chad is examining the following financial summary for Orca Memorial hoping to find a way to convince the board to move forward:

Hospital beds	125
Total operating revenue	$57,042,000
Total expenses	$57,629,000
Net income before tax	−$587,000
Interest expense	0
Depreciation expense	$3,100,000
Book value	$25,800,000

There is strong evidence to indicate that a $14 million bid would buy Orca Memorial. Chad believes that Orca is a 'steal' at $14 million because the assets alone are valued at $25.8 million with no outstanding long-term debt. Chad has also learned that investor-owned chains are also being valued at 1 to 1.4 times sales, which makes Orca Memorial worth $57 to $80 million. Earnings Before Interest, Taxes, Depreciation, and Amortization (EBITDA) multiples for investor-owned hospitals are averaging 6 to 7 times EBITDA , which would create a valuation of $15.1 to $17.6 million. The more Chad examines the data the more he becomes convinced that a bid of $14 million for Orca Memorial makes good economic sense. He is still concerned, however, about his ability to convince Mr. Carpenter and other board members that they should move forward with a bid.

It is becoming an almost everyday occurrence to read about one health care entity buying or acquiring another related health care business. Hospitals buy other hospitals, nursing homes, physician practices, durable medical equipment firms, and other types of businesses. Nursing homes buy other nursing homes, home health firms, and other businesses. The way that these firms combine is through acquisition, merger, or consolidation. The objective of this chapter is to define what is meant by consolidations, mergers, and acquisitions and to understand why they happen. The impact of these deals on shareholders (in the case of for-profit firms) of both the acquiring and acquired companies is investigated, and the reasons why some mergers succeed while others fail are examined. Finally, in order to determine the value of a firm, several valuation frameworks are provided.

LEARNING OBJECTIVE 1

Understand the terminology used in the field of consolidations, mergers, and acquisitions.

DEFINING THE TERMS

Mergers and acquisitions (M&A) have long played an important role in the growth of firms. Growth is generally viewed as vital to the well-being of a firm. There are three basic ways to acquire another company:

- A merger or consolidation
- An acquisition of the stock of the target company
- An acquisition of the target company's assets but not its corporate shell

In a consolidation, two or more corporations combine to form a brand new corporation. A merger is the combination of two or more companies, with one continuing as a legal entity while all others cease to exist; the former company's assets and liabilities become part of the continuing company. In both a merger and a consolidation, the surviving corporation has direct ownership of the assets and liabilities of the target company (or companies).

An acquisition of stock differs from a merger in two important respects. First, the target company remains in existence as a separate legal entity. Second, because the legal person, i.e., the target corporation, is still in existence, the acquiring company owns stock of the target, not the target corporation's individual assets such as inventory, equipment or land. In many respects, this type of transaction is very similar to purchasing publicly-traded stock in the open market, except the acquirer of the stock buys a majority of the outstanding shares.

An acquisition of assets is not exactly like either a merger or an acquisition of stock, but it is more similar to the former. Like a merger, the acquiring company ends up directly owning the target corporation's assets. However, it may or may not directly have responsibility for liabilities. That depends on the parties' bargain. Moreover, the sale of assets does not directly affect the legal entity (the target corporation). The target corporation can either continue to exist or be liquidated. Thus, if assets, but not liabilities, are acquired and if the target's corporate shell remains as the holder of the funds given for the target's assets, a merger and an acquisition of assets are similar, but also meaningfully different. On the other hand, if all the assets and all the liabilities are acquired and if the target's corporate shell is liquidated and consideration from the acquiring company is distributed to the target corporation's shareholders, a merger and acquisition of assets are functionally identical.

There are several different types of mergers. Horizontal mergers involve two firms operating in the same kind of business. Vertical mergers involve different stages of production and operations; and conglomerate mergers involve firms engaged in unrelated business activity. Acquisition means that company X buys company Y and acquires control. An example of a horizontal acquisition is Duke University Health System's 1998 purchase of Durham Regional Hospital. An example of vertical integration is when a medical center purchases a skilled nursing facility, when it previously did not offer such services.

When discussing M&As, there are a number of other terms that are often used. Leveraged buyouts (LBOs) involve the purchase of the entire public stock interest of a firm, or division of a firm, financed primarily with debt. If the transaction is by management, it is referred to as a management buyout (MBO). If the shares are owned exclusively by the acquiring party (e.g., management), rather than third-party investors, the transaction is called 'going private,' and there is no market for trading its shares. Joint ventures involve the joining together of two or more firms in a project or

even in a new company founded jointly by the two companies. In these cases, equity participation and control are decided by mutual agreement in advance of the joint venture.

Sell-offs are considered the opposite of mergers and acquisitions. The two major types of sell-offs are spin-offs and divestitures. In a spin-off, a separate new legal entity is formed with its shares distributed to existing shareholders of the parent company in the same proportions as in the parent company. In contrast, divestitures involve the sale of a portion of the firm to an outside party with cash or equivalent consideration received by the divesting firm.

MERGER AND ACQUISITION ACTIVITY

As with many industries, the health care industry long has reflected the belief that 'bigger is better.' Health care systems have existed for decades. Table 19–1 shows that this trend continued even into the early 2000s, as the number of acute-care hospitals declined, while revenue increasingly was concentrated in the larger hospitals. In many sectors of health care, however, merger activity began to slow in the early 2000s due to a variety of factors (see Table 19–2). The sector labeled 'Other' includes a variety of health care companies and services, such as dental care practices, outpatient surgery centers, institutional pharmacies, hospices, ambulance companies, and disease management companies, among others.

Some specific information regarding hospital industry merger and acquisition activity is presented in Table

Table 19–1 Number of Acute-Care Hospitals by Annual Revenue, 1997–2004

Annual Revenue	Number of Hospitals		
	1997	*2000*	*2004*
< $5 million	210	219	194
$5–$10 million	369	282	214
$10–$50 million	1,609	1,497	1,374
$50–$100 million	827	797	781
$100–$200 million	719	732	794
> $200 million	613	661	737
	4,347	4,188	4,094

Source: Cleverley and Associates' *State of the Hospital Industry, 2006 Edition.*

Table 19–2 Number of Health Care Sector Mergers and Acquisitions 2003 to 2004

| Sector | Change in Number of Transactions | | |
	No. of 2004 Deals	No. of 2003 Deals	Percentage Change
Behavioral	20	11	81.8
Home Health	29	na	na
Hospitals	59	38	55.3
Labs, MRI, and Dialysis	36	37	−2.7
Long-Term Care	85	na	na
Managed Care	37	29	27.6
Physician Medical Group	36	27	33.3
Rehabilitation	10	17	−41.2
Other	111	123	−9.8
Total	423	410	3.2

Source: Irving Levin Associates, www.levinassociates.com

19–3. The data show that the number of multiple hospital deals is increasing relative to single facility deals. The valuation multiples show some variability across the three years shown, but the price to EBITDA multiple have been fairly consistent and average around 8.0. Some examples of the largest M&A deals in 2004 are shown in Table 19–4.

Though partially offset by the Balanced Budget Relief Act (BBRA), the Balanced Budget Act of 1997 put reimbursement pressure on many health care sectors, leading to deteriorating financial condition and less financial and operating flexibility. In 1999, the stock prices of many publicly-owned companies in the industry traded at all-time lows. Some signs of financial health began to reappear during 2000 and have continued forward.

In recent years, some of the hospital mergers were severed by consent of the parties involved. The ability to recognize cost efficiencies from certain mergers has been questionable, especially in situations where medical professionals are anxious to maintain their independence to determine medical protocols and treatments.

Second, in certain markets there is now an 'undoing' of previous consolidations. Many physician practice management groups have broken up as a result of the management companies' failure to deliver on promised business efficiencies. In the managed care sector, HMOs have been accused of hampering the ability of physicians to deliver medical care, and a consumer and medical backlash against HMO business practices has been unleashed. Many hospital consolidations have failed to realize the expected efficiencies of management and operations.

A major increase in health care expenditures looms on the horizon. Many private insurance plans are anticipating double-digit price increases for the remainder of the decade ending 2010. This increase in cost comes as a result of rapidly-rising prescription drug costs and the rising cost of new treatment modalities.

Significant health plan mergers are still taking place with the primary objective of market share capture. For example, the Wellpoint-Anthem merger of 2005 and smaller targeted acquisitions by United Healthcare have created two very large nationally visible plans.

Table 19–3 Hospital Valuation Statisitics 2002 to 2004

| | Hospital Valuation Statisitics | | |
	2004	2003	2002
Median Price to Revenue Multiple	0.53	0.76	0.70
Median Price to EBITDA Multiple	8.1	6.5	8.0
Single Hospital Transactions	40	28	11
Multiple Hospital Transactions	19	10	47

Source: Irving Levin Associates, www.levinassociates.com

Table 19–4 Large 2004 Healthcare Transactions

Acquiring Firm	Acquired Firm	Dollar Value
Anthem, Inc.	Wellpoint Health Networks	$16.4 Billion
United Health Group, Inc.	Oxford Health Plans	$4.9 Billion
Anthem, Inc.	Trigon Healthcare	$4.2 Billion
United Health Group, Inc.	Mid Atlantic Medical	$2.9 Billion
Welsh, Carson, Anderson & Stowe	Select Medical Corporation	$2.3 Billion
First Health Group	Coventry Health Care	$1.9 Billion
The Blackstone Group	Vanguard Health Systems	$1.75 Billion
LifePoint Hospitals	Province Healthcare	$1.7 Billion
Texas Pacific Group	Iasis Healthcare Corp.	$1.4 Billion
Wellpoint Health Networks	Right Choice Managed Care	$1.3 Billion

Source: Irving Levin Associates, www.levinassociates.com

The two plans each had fiscal year 2005 revenues of $45 billion.

LEARNING OBJECTIVE 2

Explain some of the possible reasons why consolidations, mergers, and acquisitions occur.

OVERVIEW OF THEORIES OF MERGER & ACQUISITION ACTIVITY

Numerous theories have been proposed to explain M&A activity, and more specifically, the reasons why mergers and acquisitions occur. Some of the reasons firms give for wanting to acquire or merge with another firm are to increase market share, to expand the firm's geographic reach, to expand quickly into new products or services, to gain immediate financial results (such as tax savings or to quickly grow revenue or earnings), or to gain strategic or financial synergistic effects. These theories focus on efficiency, synergy, motivation of the managers, as well as the factors that influence them in engaging in M&A activity.

Efficiency Theories

Efficiency theories are the most optimistic views about the potential of mergers for social benefits. By merging two companies there is a possibility of lower unit costs, stronger purchasing power, or gain of management efficiencies. Economies of scale are an example of an efficiency that might be gained through a merger. The differential efficiency theory argues that there are differences in the effectiveness of management between two companies. In theory, if the management of Firm A is more efficient than the management of Firm B, after Firm A acquires Firm B, then the efficiency of Firm B is brought up to the level of efficiency of Firm A. Efficiency represents the real gain in merging businesses.

Efficiency theories also include the possibility of achieving some form of synergy. If synergy occurs, the value of the combined firm exceeds the value of the individual firms brought together by the mergers. This theory makes the assumption that economies of scale do exist in the industry and that prior to the merger, the firms were operating at a level of activity that fell short of achieving the potentials for economies of scale. One potential problem in merging firms with existing organizations is the question of how to combine and coordinate the efficient parts of the organizations and eliminate duplication and inefficiencies.

Information Theories

Information theories refer to the revaluation of the ownership shares of firms based upon new information that is generated during the merger negotiations, the tender offer process, or the joint venture planning. This is explained in two ways. The first is the kick-in-the-pants explanation where management is stimulated to implement a higher-valued operating strategy. The second is the sitting-on-a-gold-mine hypothesis where negotiations or tendering activity may involve the dissemination of new information or lead the market to judge that the bidders have superior information. The market may then revalue previously 'undervalued' shares.

Agency Problems

An agency problem arises when managers, or agents acting on behalf of the principals (all shareholders), own no shares or only a fraction of the shares of the firm. This partial ownership may cause managers to work less vigorously than otherwise and/or consume more perquisites (also known as "perks"; examples are lavish trips, expense accounts, club memberships, etc.) because the majority of the owners bear most of the cost.

There are two different theories that emerge from the agency problem. Some believe that the threat of a takeover may mitigate the agency problem by substituting for the need of individual shareholders to monitor the managers. If the managers have a stake in the business, they will do what is best for the company, thus doing what is best for all shareholders. However, others argue that mergers may be a manifestation of the agency problem since managers are motivated to increase the size of their firms further, and consequently, adopt lower investment hurdle rates.

Market Power

Another reason given for mergers is that they will increase a firm's market share. In a horizontal merger, if a company acquires one of its competitors, then it will have a greater share of the market. Greater market share should permit the firm to achieve pricing leverage in its market. This means that the firm can either negotiate higher rates with managed care firms or simply establish higher posted prices for its services. The government is very interested in merger cases where a potential for abuse of market power exists; most of the mergers where this possibility exists are carefully reviewed for antitrust issues.

Tax Considerations

Tax considerations are also a reason for a merger. One example is where a firm is sold with accumulated tax losses. In some instances, a firm with tax losses can shelter the positive earnings of another firm with which it is joined. Consequently, the acquiring firm gains value for its shareholders by having to pay fewer taxes than it would have without the acquisition.

FACTORS AFFECTING M&A ACTIVITY

In order to successfully complete an M&A transaction, a number of factors must be present. These factors include: corporate will (the company's goals and strategy), funding, relative values of the two companies, a conducive economic environment, as well as some other factors. Because these and other factors must be 'in sync,' there tend to be cycles in merger and acquisition activity.

Factors affecting M&A activity can be categorized as external and internal. External factors include: monetary policy, general economic activity, political issues, and regulatory policy (competition policy, foreign investment policy). Monetary policy affects M&A activity because, generally speaking, when interest rates are high, stocks are out of favor (valuations are low) and well-funded companies can buy others at a good price. Low valuation multiples for stocks can also hamper merger and acquisitions because the acquiring company's currency, its own stock, may be depressed. The internal factors that can influence M&A activity, such as management capabilities and type of product, vary from company to company and from industry to industry. When one combines the internal and external factors, the result is an M&A cycle. The predominant influence at any one peak or trough may differ. However, typically a peak is a time when corporations have access to funds, valuations are low, interest rates are low, and bank financing is available.

WHY DO MERGERS SUCCEED OR FAIL?

Any company contemplating an acquisition must familiarize itself with the simple facts that external growth is extremely competitive and the probability of increasing its shareholders' wealth via M&A is low. In the case of mergers, the average return (around the time of the announcement) to shareholders of the acquired company is 20 percent while the average return to the acquiring company is 0 percent. In the case where a tender offer for takeover has occurred (i.e., a company makes a public offer to the shareholders of a target company), the acquired company's shareholders receive an average return of 30 percent, while the shareholders of the acquiring company receive 4 percent.

Clearly, the acquired company's shareholders can expect significant returns whereas the acquiring company's shareholders do not see the gains they might expect. Some research tends to paint a bleak picture with respect to the success of mergers and acquisitions. In an analysis conducted by McKinsey & Company consultants of 116 acquisition programs undertaken between 1972 and 1983, 61 percent were failures, 23 percent were successes and 16 percent unknown (Copeland, Koller, & Murrin, 2000). (An acquisition was deemed successful if it earned its cost of equity capital or better on funds invested in the acquisition program. In other words, income after taxes as a percentage of equity invested in the acquisition had to exceed the acquirer's opportunity cost of equity.) If the successes and failures are probed further by looking at the rates by type of acquisition, a company acquiring another company in a related business has a greater chance of success than one acquiring a company in an unrelated business.

With those statistics suggesting high failure rates of mergers and acquisitions, the question remains: Why acquire or merge? There are a number of reasons that can be cited for the failures. Poor management and unfortunate circumstances (bad luck) are two such reasons. However, the most likely is that acquirers pay too much.

Companies overpay for a variety of reasons. One reason is that acquirers are overoptimistic in their assumptions. Assumptions, such as rapid growth continuing indefinitely, a market rebounding from a cyclical slump or a company 'turning around,' can sometimes lead acquirers to overpay. A second possible reason is an overestimation of the synergies that the merged company will experience. One of the most difficult aspects of the merger is the integration of the two firms afterwards. Suppose Company X is known for having a strong marketing department. Company Y takes over Company X and assumes in its valuation that it will be able to take advantage of this marketing strength. However, as a result of the merger, key people from Company X exit the merged company, leaving the firm with a weaker marketing department than the acquiring company had hoped. The third possible reason for overpaying is simply that the acquiring company overbids. In the heat of the deal, the acquirer may find it all too easy to bid up the price beyond the limits of reasonable valuations. A fourth possible reason is poor post-acquisition integration. Integration can be difficult and during this time, relationships with customers, employees, and suppliers can easily be disrupted, and this may cause damage to the value of the business.

LEARNING OBJECTIVE 3

Explain McKinsey & Company's five steps of planning for a merger or acquisition.

McKinsey & Company suggests a five-step program for successful mergers and acquisitions. The first step is to manage the pre-acquisition phase. It is important during the pre-acquisition phase that employees maintain the secrecy of the deal. If the secrecy is not maintained and there are rumors of a takeover attempt, the valuation of the target will increase, potentially killing the deal. It is also important that managers evaluate their own company, understand its strengths and weaknesses, and understand the industry structure. Once this is done, then managers can begin to identify the value-adding approach that will work best for their company. There are three approaches suggested by McKinsey. The first is to strengthen or leverage the company's core business; the second is to capitalize on functional economies of scale; and the third is to benefit from technology or skills transfer.

Once the approach has been identified, the next step is to screen candidates. Public companies, divisions of companies, and privately-held companies should be considered when developing a list of potential targets. In this step, McKinsey suggests that a list of 'knockout criteria' be developed. These criteria allow managers to eliminate those companies that do not 'fit' with their own company (i.e., too big, too small, availability). It is also suggested that during this part of the analysis consideration should be given to the role of lawyers, investment banks, and accountants, as they will have an impact at various stages of the process.

Once candidates have been screened and those who do not meet the initial criteria have been eliminated, the remaining candidates must be valued. The objective for the acquiring company should be to pay only one dollar more than the value to the next highest bidder, and an amount that is less than the value to the acquirer. In determining the value to the acquirer, McKinsey suggests that the value of the acquiring company be added to the value of the target company 'as is.' The value of realistic synergies must then be added, while taking into account how long it will take to capture them. The transaction costs for doing the deal are then subtracted. The result is the value of the combined post-merger company. The value gain is the combined value less the value of the acquiring company.

The fourth step is to negotiate. A key point in this part of the process is for the acquiring company to decide on a maximum reservation price and to stick to it. A negotiation strategy is established by considering the following factors: the acquisition value to the acquirer, the value of the target company to the existing owners and other potential buyers, the financial condition of the existing owners and other potential acquirers, the strategy and motivation of the existing owners and other potential acquirers, and the potential impact of antitakeover provisions.

Upon successful acquisition, the final step is to manage post-merger integration. In a study conducted by McKinsey & Company, it was noted that most acquirers destroy rather than create value after the acquisition. Prior to being acquired, 24 percent of the companies studied were performing better than the industry average and another 53 percent were performing better than 75 percent of their industry average. Post-acquisition, these percentages dropped to 10 percent and 15 percent, respectively. To improve the chances of success, McKinsey suggests that companies begin quickly and manage the process carefully. It is also important to note that this does not mean the acquiring company should impose its goals and style on the acquired company, but rather that the management team should work something out together that both companies (as a new entity) can accept and subscribe to.

LEARNING OBJECTIVE 4

Understand common methods for valuation of a potential target firm.

VALUATIONS

Although there are many tasks that need to be accomplished in any business acquisition, one of the most difficult and most important is valuation. Exactly what is the value of the business being acquired? In this section, frameworks are provided for numerous valuation methods. Figure 19–1 provides an overview of the major valuation methods. These basic valuation methods can be used in any valuation circumstance, not only with respect to M&A activity. (The final section of this chapter presents a model which highlights distinctions between the 'standard' discounted cash flow valuation model and valuation in an M&A context.)

Valuation is really a subset of capital expenditure analysis. The business being acquired can be thought of as a capital expenditure that needs to be evaluated just

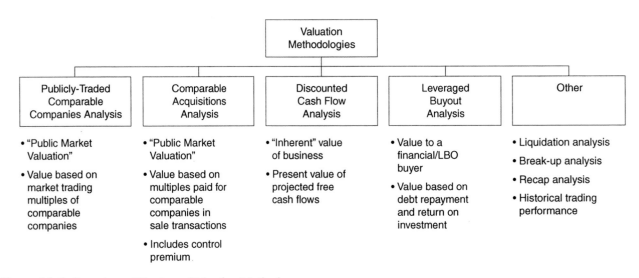

Figure 19–1 Overview of Business Valuation Methods

as any other capital expenditure made in the organization. Nonfinancial criteria should be considered, and the contribution that the acquired business will make toward the acquiring firm's mission must be addressed.

Valuation of a business is not a scientific process that results in one objective measure of value. Different measures of value result for the following three reasons:

1. Different methods of valuation are used.
2. Different expectations regarding future performance of the acquired business are assumed.
3. Different values may be assigned by different prospective buyers.

Before discussing the valuation methods in detail, descriptions of some general terms of valuation will be helpful. The equity value of a for-profit firm represents value attributable to the "owners" of the business (i.e., residual value after paying debt). The market value of a company's equity equals the product of its number of shares outstanding and its current stock price. The value of debt is typically assumed to be its market value (if observable). An organization's enterprise value (also termed firm value or total value) represents the value of all capital invested in the business, and can be expressed as follows:

Enterprise value = market value of equity + net debt,
where
Net debt = short-term debt + long-term debt
(including current portion) + minority interest +
preferred stock + capitalized leases −
(cash + cash equivalents)

Alternative Valuation Methods

In general, three major methods of valuation are often cited in practice:

1. Income/cash flow (discounted cash flow) approach
2. Asset-based approach
3. Comparable sales approach

The most common methods of valuing health care firms are usually based on some projections of income or cash flow. The three most common methods are:

1. Direct capitalization
2. Price earnings multiple
3. Discounted cash flow (DCF)

Direct Capitalization Approach

In direct capitalization, a projected value for cash flow is determined. That number is then divided by some discount rate. The discount rate ideally represents the acquiring firm's cost of capital, but it is often adjusted up or down to reflect the risk of the business being acquired. For example, if a durable medical equipment (DME) firm was thought to have cash flow of $100,000 per year for the foreseeable future and the purchasing firm's cost of capital was 12 percent, the value of the DME firm would be the following:

$$\text{Value of DME firm} = \frac{\$100,000}{.12} = \$833,333$$

To reflect greater risk in the business, the discount rate could be increased to 20 percent. This increase would effectively reduce the value to $500,000. A preferable way to reflect risk, rather than adjust the discount rate, would be to conduct a sensitivity analysis on the forecast of cash flows. It is highly desirable to have at least the following three scenarios forecast: most likely, pessimistic, and optimistic.

Price Earnings Approach

A price earnings approach is similar to direct capitalization, except that it uses earnings, rather than cash flow, to discount; and multiplication rather than division is used. The key formula in this approach is:

$$P_0 = \text{"Multiple"} \times EPS_1$$

where P_0 is the price of the share in year 0 and EPS_1 is the projected earnings per share in year 1.

In this valuation approach, the multiple is the projected Price/Earnings (P/E) Ratio. A P/E ratio for a company can be determined by looking for a similar company within the industry. A similar company is one that has similar operational characteristics (e.g., industry, product, markets, customers, etc.) and financial characteristics (size, leverage, margins, growth, etc.) as your target company. Remember the following guidelines when comparing companies: higher growth for a company results in a higher P/E ratio and higher risk results in a lower P/E ratio. When comparing companies, if one company has higher financial leverage (all else equal), it will have a lower P/E since financial leverage is related to increased risk. Similarly, a typical company in a high-growth industry will tend to have a higher P/E (all else equal) than a typical company in a low-growth industry. Table 19–5 presents

Table 19–5 Valuation Multiples (3–10–06)

	P/E Trailing 12 Months	P/E 2006	P/E 2007
Wellpoint (WLP)	19.2	16.9	14.7
HCA, Inc. (HCA)	15.4	14.6	12.9
Beverly Enterprises (BEV)	14.6	12.6	NA
Merck (MRK)	13.6	14.8	14.8
Dow/Wall Street Journal Index	17.8	15.5	13.9

price earnings multiples for selected firms in several major sectors of the health care industry. Two major points should be made with respect to the data presented there. First, P/E multiples for future earnings are usually lower than for historical earnings. This is a direct result of discounting because future earnings have lower value than current earnings and are also less certain. Second, differences in P/E multiples exist largely because of different expectations for future growth. In Table 19–5, Wellpoint (WLP) has the highest P/E multiple of any firm listed, which would suggest the market believes there is greater earnings growth for WLP than the other firms.

Assume that the previously mentioned DME firm had earnings—not cash flow—of $125,000. If the purchasing firm applied a P/E ratio of 8 to the earnings, the value would be the following:

Value of DME firm = 8.0 × $125,000 = $1,000,000

A variation of the P/E multiple is EBITDA (earnings before interest, taxes, depreciation, and amortization). The higher the EBITDA multiple, the greater the value assigned to the firm. It is important to note that using an EBITDA multiple provides an estimate of the total value of the business. To value the equity portion, only the outstanding debt must be subtracted. Table 19–6 illustrates this concept for HCA, Inc. a national, for-profit hospital company, under the assumption that its EBITDA multiple is 7.2.

Discounted Cash Flow Valuation Methods

Discounted cash flow methods are most commonly used in most health care firm valuations. The typical approach will estimate cash flows for each of the next five years. These cash flows are then discounted to reflect the present value of the firm. The last remaining requirement is to estimate what the value of the acquired firm will be at the end of year 5, or whenever annual cash flows are no longer estimated. Generically, the value of a firm would be stated as follows:

Value = Present value of estimated future cash flows
+ Present value of terminal value

Steps in the Discounted Cash Flow Approach

In the DCF approach, the value of a business is the future expected cash flow discounted at a rate that reflects the riskiness of the projected cash flows. This model is used to evaluate capital spending projects as well as entire businesses, which are effectively just collections of individual projects.

Step 1. Calculate Cost of Capital (K_d). The first step in a DCF analysis is to determine the cost of capital. The cost of capital is the minimum acceptable rate of return on new investments based on the rate investors can expect to earn by investing in alternative, identically risky securities. Using the acquiring company's target capital structure, the Weighted Average Cost of Capital

Table 19–6 HCA, Inc. Valuation (millions, except EBITDA multiple)

	Fiscal Year Ending 12/31/05
Net Income	$1,424
+ Interest	655
+ Income Taxes	725
+ Depreciation and Amortization	1,374
EBITDA	$4,178
× EBITDA multiple	7.2
Value	$30,082
− Debt	$10,475
Equity Value	$19,607
HCA Stock Value (3–10–06)	$19,453

(WACC) is calculated. The WACC is generally a weighted average of the company's cost of debt (on an after-tax basis) and cost of equity. The acquiring company uses its own cost of capital only when it can be safely assumed that the acquisition will not affect the risk profile of the acquirer. If the acquisition will affect the acquirer's risk, then the discount rate must be adjusted.

Step 2. Determine Free Cash Flows. Cash flow is usually defined more broadly than net income plus depreciation for valuation purposes. Often, the term "free" cash flows is used. Free cash flows are the ones typically used in the DCF calculation. "Free" refers to those cash flows that are available to stakeholders (e.g., equity and debt holders) after consideration for taxes, capital expenditures, and working capital needs. Cash flow should be considered as the cash flow contribution the target is expected to make to the acquiring company. The formula used to calculate free cash flows is the following:

$$EBIT \times (1 - t) + \text{Non-cash expenses} -$$
$$\text{Capital expenditures} - \text{Incremental working capital}$$

where EBIT is earnings before interest and taxes and t is the marginal tax rate of the firm. Noncash expenses include items such as depreciation and amortization. These are added back since they do not affect the company's cash position. Capital expenditures are purchases of fixed assets that are not reflected in the company's income statements, but rather are accounted for through depreciation and amortization over the life of the asset. However, capital expenditures do represent cash outlays and are subtracted from EBIT. Incremental working capital is the amount of additional cash that will be tied up in items such as accounts receivable and cash required for the operations of the merged firm. Increased working capital is often estimated as a percentage of the increase in sales. It is subtracted from EBIT as it does not represent a free cash flow to the firm.

Most analysts think of depreciation plus net income as cash flow. Interest is added back in the previous concept of free cash flow to recognize that the business may be financed in a manner different from the way it is presently financed and that financing is incorporated in the cost of capital. If a business was purchased and the existing debt of that business was assumed by the purchaser, then interest should not be subtracted because the interest expense would be a cash expense assumed by the buyer. In addition, any principal pay-

ments on debt would also be subtracted to derive free cash flow when the acquired firm's debt is being assumed. Capital expenditures are subtracted to recognize that businesses need to renovate and replace their physical assets if they are to stay in business, and in fact, this represents a reduction of available cash flow. In the same manner, expenditures for working capital also represent a drain on available funds, or free cash flow. A buildup in accounts receivable means that not all of the firm's net income is available.

The free cash flows should be determined for a particular projected time frame. This time frame should extend to a time after which it is believed the company will experience constant growth. Five to ten years is often used somewhat arbitrarily, but the exact time frame used should be tailored to the particular valuation scenario.

Step 3. Calculate Present Value of Cash Flows. Calculate the present value of the cash flows based on the determined cost of capital (K). This is a simple matter of discounting the amounts back to year 0. Generally, only one K is used throughout the entire forecast period, although it is possible that this value may change over the forecast period. Another assumption that is made in these calculations is that all cash flows occur at the end of the period.

Step 4. Add Present Value of Terminal Value. At this point, we have not accounted for the cash flows that will be generated by the entity beyond the forecast period. In order to account for this, the present value of the terminal value is added to the present value of cash flows. The terminal value is the present value of the resulting cash flow perpetuity beginning one year after the forecast period.

The most common method calculates the discounted cash flow assuming constant growth of cash flows. In order to complete this calculation, the cash flow in the year following the forecast period is calculated. Assuming the terminal value of cash flow projections is year T, the terminal value (as of year T) is:

$$\frac{CF_T \times (1 + g)}{K - g}$$

where CF_T is the cash flow in year T, g is the constant growth rate assumed for the firm beyond year T, and K is the cost of capital.

Applying the direct capitalization method to cash flows is not the only way to construct a residual value. In some cases, an estimate of the resale value of the firm might be used. Other methods might also be used in certain situations. The following point, however, is important: the residual value may be uncertain and, as a result, some alternative scenarios should be tested. One value should never be accepted. Alternative valuations under different assumptions should be sought.

Step 5. Subtract Debt and Other Obligations Assumed. When valuing equity in a firm, it must be recognized that the shareholders, as owners of the firm, have an obligation to pay any debtholders. Consequently, repayment of these obligations (the market value of the debt and any other similar obligations) must be subtracted from the present value of the cash flows of the firm.

LEARNING OBJECTIVE 5

Apply analytical methods and tools to value potential acquisitions.

VALUATION EXAMPLE

Suppose an analyst has been asked to assess the value of Meredith Dean Hospital. The analyst first determines the cost of capital for the hospital. The beta (β) for Meredith Dean Hospital is 1.38. Beta describes the sensitivity of an instrument or portfolio to broad market movements. The stock market (represented by an index such as the S&P 500 is assigned a beta of 1.0. By comparison, a portfolio (or instrument) which has a beta of 0.5 will tend to participate in broad market moves, but only half as much as the market overall. A portfolio (or instrument) with a beta of 2.0 will tend to benefit or suffer from broad market moves twice as much as the market overall.

Assume that long-term risk-free interest rates are at 5.85 percent. Using the CAPM model and assuming a market risk premium of 6 percent, the cost of equity is calculated to be:

$$K_e = R_f + \beta_{Dean}(R_M - R_f)$$
$$K_e = 5.85\% + 1.38(6\%)$$
$$K_e = 14.13\%$$

The hospital can acquire debt at a rate of 8.50 percent and has a tax rate of 45 percent. Therefore, the cost of debt is calculated to be:

$$K_d = \text{Debt} \times (1 - t)$$
$$K_d = 8.50\% (1 - 0.45)$$
$$K_d = 4.68\%$$

Assume that the hospital's balance sheet for the present year indicates a capital structure of 35 percent debt and 65 percent equity. Assuming this is also the target capital structure, the result is a WACC calculated to be:

$$K = (35\% \times 4.68) + (65\% \times 14.13)$$
$$K = (1.64\%) + (9.18\%)$$
$$K = 10.82\%$$

The next step for the analyst would be to review the financial statements provided to project expected cash flows. The EBIT can be estimated from past income statements. Over the past three years (years 0, -1 and -2), Meredith Dean Hospital has experienced an annual increase in its EBIT of over ten percent. The analyst assumes, based on industry data, that a growth level of ten percent is sustainable for the next two years, but beyond this period, the analyst believes that a growth level of two percent is more reasonable. The analyst believes that with the growth this hospital will be experiencing over the next ten years, new medical equipment will have to be installed in three years worth approximately $2 million with a depreciation rate of 30 percent. No other major capital expenditures are anticipated. However, it will be necessary for Meredith Dean Hospital to maintain its capital base. In order to do this, the analyst assumes that in all years other than year 3, the company will spend an equal amount on capital expenditures and depreciation. Working capital in the past three years has increased proportionately with increases in revenues. Therefore, see the following table for the projected free cash flows for the next five years:

Based upon the calculated cost of capital of 10.82 percent, the projected cash flows are discounted back to the present year, year 0. The result is a present value of $8,885,032. The terminal value can now be calculated. The analyst believes that annual growth of two percent is sustainable for Meredith Dean Hospital beyond year 5. Therefore, the cash flow in year 6 is calculated by increasing the cash flow in year 5 by two

Cash Flow Projections:

	Year 1	Year 2	Year 3	Year 4	Year 5
EBIT	4,675,000	5,142,500	5,245,350	5,350,257	5,457,262
EBIT (1-t)	2,571,250	2,828,275	2,884,942	2,942,641	3,001,494
+ Non-cash expenses	750,000	750,000	750,000	1,350,000	1,350,000
− Capital Expenditures	750,000	750,000	2,000,000	1,350,000	1,350,000
− Incremental working capital	300,000	330,000	336,600	343,332	350,200
Total FCF	2,271,250	2,498,275	1,298,342	2,599,309	2,651,294
Present Value (at 10.82%)	2,094,476	2,124,522	1,018,171	1,879,749	1,768,114

percent. The resulting cash flow is $2,704,320 which is the numerator in the formula below:

$$\text{Terminal Value} = \frac{CF_T \times (1 + g)}{K - g}$$

The overall result is a terminal value of $30,661,223 ($2,704,320/.0882). The present value of this terminal value is $18,344,196 ($30,661,223 discounted at 10.82 percent for five years). The sum of the present value of the year 1 through year 5 cash flows and the present value of the terminal value is $27,229,228. The company's long-term debt is then subtracted, which according to Meredith Dean Hospital's balance sheet is $7,000,000. The analyst has, therefore, come up with a value for Meredith Dean Hospital of $20,229,228. These calculations are only the beginning of the analyst's work. The next step would then be to do some sensitivity analysis to test the assumptions made. Is the 10.82 percent discount rate appropriate? Is an ongoing growth rate of two percent reasonable in the hospital industry? After completing this analysis, the analyst will be left with a range of values based on different assumptions.

The Cost of Equity in Not-for-Profit and Private Firms

When valuing not-for-profit or private companies, it is difficult to estimate the cost of equity. There is no equity information to use for calculating the firm's beta. A common solution is to take an average beta of comparable publicly-traded companies. Be careful, however, to unlever the betas of the public companies (using their respective debt-to-equity ratios) to arrive at their asset betas. Then, average the asset betas of the public companies and "re-lever" for the company being evaluated using its debt-to-equity ratio.

Asset-Based Valuation Method

Asset-based approaches to valuation rely on the availability of objective measures for the assets being acquired. Usually, three alternative asset-based valuation approaches are identified. One approach is simply to take the tangible book value of the acquired firm's assets. Although this method is objective, there is great doubt about the relevance of the resulting value. For example, consider a computed tomography (CT) scanner that was acquired two years ago at a cost of $700,000 that now has a book value of $500,000, which reflects two years of depreciation. The $500,000 value is most likely not a good measure of this asset's value to an acquiring firm.

A second asset-based method would be to use the replacement cost of the assets. For example, assume that the CT scanner in the previous example now has a current replacement cost of $1,400,000. Recognizing two years' worth of depreciation would produce an adjusted replacement cost of $1,000,000.

Current replacement cost	$1,400,000
− Allowance for depreciation	400,000
Estimated replacement cost	$1,000,000

This estimate of value would be useful for a firm that anticipated using the CT scanner in the future. Replacement cost is often associated with "a going concern" basis of operation. A "going concern" basis simply means the business is expected to continue and will not be terminated. The acquired firm will continue to operate basically as it currently does and, therefore, the existing capital assets will be needed.

The third asset-based approach assumes that the assets are not really needed and will be sold. For example, the CT scanner referenced previously will be sold in a secondhand market for $600,000. This value is often associated with liquidation.

Comparable Sales Approaches

Comparable sales methods are widely used in real estate valuation. Real estate appraisers will look at properties similar to the one being valued that have sold in that location during a recent time interval. This method of valuation is not often used for health care businesses because there are not enough comparable sales to make the valuation meaningful. Common rules of thumb based on sales around the country are sometimes used. For example, nursing homes may sell in a range of $15,000 to $45,000 per bed depending on the payer mix and the present age of the facility. Other health care examples would include physician practice acquisition and health maintenance organizations (HMOs). Most physician practices are acquired for $100,000 to $200,000 per physician, whereas HMOs typically sell for $200 to $600 per member. Although these comparable sales values are useful, they usually are only a benchmark against which a calculated value is determined from an appraisal based on income or cash flow.

Breakup Value

Another way to value a company is by assessing its breakup value. In this method, the book value of the assets of the target company is added to the value of any hidden assets such as real estate, brand names, and copyrights. The market value is then assessed for each piece if it were to be sold separately. There are a number of reasons why the pieces sold separately might be worth more than the whole. These include hidden assets, improved earnings through cost savings, unused debt capacity or tax implications, or the breakup has not been carefully researched or followed. This approach attempts to determine what others would pay to gain control of each piece.

Goodwill

It is also important to understand the term "goodwill." Goodwill is defined as the price or value paid for a business less the fair market value of the tangible assets acquired. For example, assume that a hospital paid $4,000,000 for a 100-bed nursing home. All of the tangible assets of the nursing home would be appraised at fair market value. A piece of land may have a recorded cost of $100,000 on the nursing home's books, but its

current market value might be $800,000. The fair market value of the land would be $800,000. Alternatively, some equipment items might be reduced below their historical cost because they are no longer of value.

Goodwill is an intangible asset that, until recently, was amortized over future years. The next section describes a recent change in the accounting for goodwill. For example, assume that the fair market value of the acquired assets in the nursing home was $3,000,000. The amount of goodwill would be $1,000,000 ($4,000,000 − $3,000,000) and would have been written off as a cost of operation in the future. Goodwill plus fair market value will equal the price paid for the business.

ACCOUNTING FOR BUSINESS COMBINATIONS

Until 2001, there had been two methods used to account for mergers: purchase accounting and pooling of interests. Under purchase accounting, target assets are reported at fair market value. Anything paid above this amount is considered goodwill. In July 2001, however, the Financial Accounting Standards Board (FASB) issued Statement 141—Business Combinations, and Statement 142—Goodwill and Other Intangible Assets.

Statement 141 required that the purchase method of accounting be used for all business combinations initiated after June 30, 2001, effectively prohibiting the use of the pooling-of-interests method. Pooling of interests allowed companies to ignore goodwill, instead combining all assets without recording the premium paid above fair market value of tangible assets. Management of acquiring companies often favored this method because of its simplicity and because of the avoidance of recording goodwill. Many accountants criticized the method, however, arguing that it allowed corporations to make overpriced acquisitions without having to suffer the consequences in their earnings.

Statement 142 changed the accounting for goodwill from an amortization method to an impairment-only approach, meaning that the amortization of goodwill, including goodwill recorded from past business combinations, ceased upon adoption of that statement, which for companies operating with calendar year-ends, was January 1, 2002. Until this statement was issued, accounting rules required companies to amortize goodwill assets over periods up to 40 years.

ANTITRUST CONSIDERATIONS

Much of the legal environment for health care was discussed in Chapter 4. Here, we will highlight the main areas of health care law that relate to mergers and acquisitions. State and federal agencies can challenge mergers and acquisitions on antitrust grounds. Merger decisions of the Federal Trade Commission (FTC) and the Department of Justice (DOJ) are based on careful definition of the relevant hospital market, examination of that market's concentration, consideration of other independent hospitals in the market, and an assessment of whether efficiencies gained from the merger might offset anticompetitive effects.

The DOJ and the FTC created an antitrust safety zone for small acute-care hospital mergers. Reasoning that mergers of such small hospitals will likely have more benefit by keeping them open, the agencies will not challenge mergers and acquisitions where at least one of the hospitals has fewer than 100 beds and an average daily census of fewer than 40 patients during the last three years.

Aside from the safety zone, the government uses five steps to analyze firm mergers. As explained by Dean Harris in *Healthcare Law and Ethics* (1999), these five steps are:

1. **Definition, measurement, and concentration of the relevant market**—This is done using the Herfindahl-Hirschman Index (HHI), which is calculated by squaring the market shares (where the market share percentage is first multiplied by 100) of each firm in its relevant market. A post-merger HHI below 1000 suggests an unconcentrated market and is unlikely to be challenged. On the other hand, an HHI above 1800 might suggest an overly concentrated market and might draw more scrutiny. For example, consider a market with ten providers each currently having ten percent market share. The present HHI in this market would be 1000. If two of the firms merged, the new HHI would be 1200. The critical argument in many situations is the definition of the market. Expanding the market boundaries will produce lower HHI values.
2. **Potential adverse effects on competition from the merger**—The concern here is that third-party payers have enough bargaining power to negotiate with providers on quality and price.

3. **Determine if new firms entering the market would be likely to prevent those anticompetitive effects**—This relates to barriers to entry (e.g., certificate of need, political barriers, and cost) for competitive firms. If the barriers to entry are low, the threat of new entrants might be enough to stop the post-merger firm from exercising all of its market power. If barriers to entry are high, however, the merged firm might have undue liberty to aggressively wield its power.
4. **Determine if there are any significant net efficiencies as a result of the merger**—Federal regulators will be looking for tangible economies of scale, not just speculative claims by the potential merger parties.
5. **Determine if either party to the merger is a "failing firm"**—If the acquired firm would likely go bankrupt absent the merger, then federal regulators will be less likely to block the merger, reasoning that the merger does not really remove a viable competitor from the marketplace.

The federal government has permitted states to enact special legislation that permits them to exempt health care facilities from federal antitrust review through the issuance of a "Certificate of Public Advantage (COPA)." In most cases, issuance of a COPA requires the merging parties to estimate potential cost savings resulting from a merger and to reflect those reductions in future rates. Control is then exercised over the merged facilities through rate review and controls on net patient revenue.

SUMMARY

The health care business environment is characterized by change, including the level of technology, reimbursement methods, and labor availability. The general trend in health care has been toward consolidation. Most health care managers today will be involved in some capacity with a type of consolidation, merger, or acquisition of another entity. Thus, they should understand why and how these acquisitions occur. Although purely financial considerations might not dominate the decision criteria, the financial implications of any possible deal must be considered. In that context, the valuation methods we have examined can serve as useful tools in capital project analysis for health care facilities. Just as importantly, understanding how value will be added through the deal is critical to the success of the new, combined entity. Finally, re-member that every type of consolidation involves change for the employees, customers, and patients of all the effected firms. Thus, just as financial planning is important, so too is planning for the effects on the people involved. Managers must therefore be prepared to deal with numerous post-deal issues that invariably will arise.

REFERENCES

T. Copeland, T. Koller, and J. Murrin, *Measuring and Managing the Value of Companies* (Indianapolis: John Wiley & Sons, 2000).

D. Harris, *Healthcare Law and Ethics: Issues for the Age of Managed Care* (Washington DC: AUPHA Press, 1999).

1. Two hospitals are considering merging their laundry departments and constructing a new facility to take care of their future laundry requirements. Some relevant cost data are presented in Table 19–7.

Table 19–7 Laundry Merger Data

	Hospital A	Hospital B	Merged C
Variable cost/pound	0.030	0.032	0.024
Pounds of laundry	300,000	700,000	1,000,000
Fixed costs/year			
Depreciation (lease)	$1,000	$5,000	$8,000
Maintenance	1,400	2,500	3,000
Administrative salaries	8,000	16,000	20,000
Transportation	0	0	3,000
Total fixed cost	$10,400	$23,500	$34,000

The new laundry facility will cost approximately $40,000 to construct and will be located between the two hospitals in a leased building. Average life of the equipment is assumed to be eight years, which generates a $5,000 yearly depreciation charge. Lease payment is fixed at $3,000 per year for the next eight years. Financing for the project will be generated from available funds in each institution: $12,000 from Hospital A and $28,000 from Hospital B. Expenses will be shared using the same ratios (30 and 70 percent). Both hospitals use a discount factor of ten percent on their cost-reduction investment projects. Given this information, do you think the merger would be beneficial to both hospitals? What other information would you like to have to help you evaluate this investment project?

2. In the preceding laundry merger problem, assume that Hospital B would expect to replace its present equipment with new equipment in two years at a cost of $64,000. The equipment would have an eight-year life. Ignoring cost-reimbursement considerations, does the merger make economic sense for Hospital B under these conditions?

3. You have been asked to provide an estimate of the value for a nursing home that your client is interested in buying. Financial data and projections are presented in Table 19–8.

Table 19–8 Projected Nursing Home Cash Flows

	Year 1	Year 2	Year 3	Year 4	Year 5
Net Income	$2,000	$2,200	$2,400	$2,700	$3,000
+Depreciation	1,400	1,500	1,700	2,000	2,200
– Working capital	500	600	700	800	1,000
– Capital expenditures	4,000	4,000	5,000	300	300
Free cash flow	($1,100)	($900)	($1,600)	$3,600	$3,900

Use an assumed discount rate of ten percent to value the firm, and assume that the fifth-year cash flow will carry into the future. After you have completed your valuation, what additional information or steps would you suggest to the client?

4. Assume that as of January 2, 2002, Trigon Healthcare sold at $48.75 per share with 175,215,000 outstanding shares. This creates a market value of Trigon Healthcare shares of $8,541,731,250 ($48.75 × 175,215,000).

Calculate the multiple of EBITDA that Trigon Healthcare is trading, assuming the values in Table 19–9.

Table 19–9 Trigon Healthcare Valuation Data

Net income	$285,964,000
Interest	771,000
Income taxes	170,205,000
Depreciation and amortization	94,458,000
EBITDA	$551,398,000
Debt	$38,970,000

SOLUTIONS AND ANSWERS

1. The relevant data and calculations in the laundry service merger between Hospital A and Hospital B are presented in Table 19–10.

Table 19–10 Discounted Cash Flow Analysis of Laundry Merger

	Hospital A	Hospital B
Cash outflow—unmerged		
Variable costs	$9,000	$22,400
Maintenance	1,400	2,500
Salaries	8,000	16,000
Total	$18,400	$40,900
Cash outflow—merged		
Variable costs	$7,200	$16,800
Lease	900	2,100
Maintenance	900	2,100
Salaries	6,000	14,000
Transportation	900	2,100
	$15,900	$37,100
Net savings	$2,500	$3,800

Hospital A:
Present value of savings = $2,500 × P(10%,8) = $2,500 × 5.335 = $13,337.50
Profitability index = $1,337.50/$12,000.00 = .111

Hospital B:
Present value of savings = $3,800 × P(10%,8) = $3,800 × 5.335 = $20,273
Profitability index = −$7,727/28,000 = −.276

Thus, given present data, the merger would be beneficial to Hospital A, but not to Hospital B. A key piece of additional data that is needed is the replacement cost of the existing equipment. If Hospital B would need to acquire new equipment in the near future, the merger also might be favorable to it. The effects of cost reimbursement also should be considered.

2. The laundry merger project in these new circumstances would require use of the equivalent annual cost method. The alternative of a merger (Figure 19–2) would have an eight-year life, whereas the alternative not including a merger (Figure 19–3) would have a ten-year cycle.

Hospital B Merged Equivalent Annual Cost

$$\text{Equivalent annual cost} = \frac{[\$37,100 \times P(10\%,8)] + \$28,000}{P(10\%,8)}$$

$$\text{Equivalent annual cost} = \frac{[\$37,100 \times 5.335] + \$28,000}{5.335}$$

$$= \$42,348$$

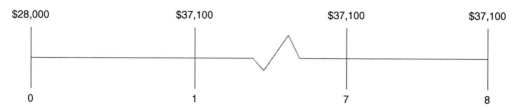

Figure 19–2 Cost of Merger—Hospital B

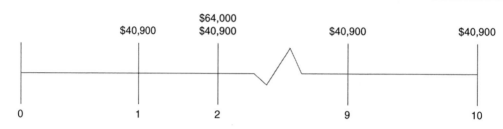

Figure 19–3 Costs Unmerged—Hospital B

Hospital B Unmerged Equivalent Annual Cost

$$\text{Equivalent annual cost} = \frac{[\$40{,}900 \times P(10\%,10)] + [\$64{,}000 \times p(10\%,2)]}{P(10\%,10)}$$

$$\text{Equivalent annual cost} = \frac{[\$40{,}900 \times 6.145] + [\$64{,}000 \times .826]}{6.145}$$

$$= \$49{,}503$$

The alternative of a merger is now more desirable for Hospital B because it has a lower equivalent annual cost compared with the alternative that does not include a merger.

Table 19–11 Nursing Home Valuation

Present Value of Cash Flows	Amount	Present Value Factor	Present Value
Year 1	($1,100)	0.909	($1,000)
Year 2	(900)	0.826	743
Year 3	(1,600)	0.751	(1,202)
Year 4	3,600	0.683	2,459
Year 5	3,900	0.621	2,422
Present value of residual value cash flows after year 5	$39,000	0.621	$24,220
Total value			$26,156

3. Using the data in Table 19–8, along with the present value factors from Table 17–2, the estimate of value in Table 19–11 would result. The largest driver of the current valuation is the residual value. Validity of this forecast is therefore critical.

4. (EBITDA $\times$ Multiple) $-$ Debt $=$ Market Value

($551,398,000 $\times$ Multiple) $-$ $38,970,000 $=$ $8,541,731,000

$$\text{EBITDA Multiple} = \frac{\$8,580,701,000}{\$551,398,000} = 15.56$$

Chapter 20

Capital Formation

After studying this chapter, you should be able to do the following:

1. Identify the sources of equity financing.
2. Explain the factors that influence the desirability of alternative sources of financing.
3. Explain what an investment banker does.
4. List the major bond-rating agencies and explain their role in the debt market.
5. List some of the pros and cons of retiring debt early.

REAL-WORLD SCENARIO

James Keeler, CFO at Bennett Medical Center, is reviewing the Center's most recent audited financial statements that were delivered that morning by the auditors. For the past year, Bennett Medical Center has been in violation of its debt service coverage ratio in the trust indenture related to its 2006 revenue bond financing. The required debt service coverage ratio in the trust indenture is 1.05, and Bennett Medical Center's last fiscal year debt service coverage ratio was 1.01.

Mr. Keeler has known of the debt service coverage violation for some time, and in fact alerted the bond trustee to this issue six months ago. The bond trustee presented two options. First, they could have called the entire $80 million issue immediately, which would have forced Bennett Medical Center into bankruptcy. Second, they could appoint an outside consultant to work with the hospital to correct the current debt service coverage deficiency. Fortunately, the trustee chose to appoint an outside consulting firm three months ago to work with Mr. Keeler and others on the hospital staff to correct the current cash flow deficiency.

Mr. Keeler's concern was how the auditor would treat the current noncompliance with its debt service coverage provision. The auditor could have qualified its opinion and reclassified the entire $80 million of long-term bonded debt to a current liability. Alternatively, the auditor could have chosen a footnote disclosure to the financial statements. Mr. Keeler was relieved to find that the auditor had chosen the latter alternative. The footnote in the most recent audited financial statement states that Bennett Medical Center is in violation of their debt service coverage covenant and that an outside consulting firm has been selected. The auditor then stated, "Accordingly, the 2006 Revenue Bonds have been classified as noncurrent liabilities in the accompanying balance sheet."

Mr. Keeler realizes that significant changes must be made to return the hospital to solvency, but is confident that major strides can be made in the upcoming year to push their debt service coverage ratio above the required value of 1.05 and remove the operating constraints imposed by the bond trustee.

In this chapter, we will examine the concepts and principles of capital formation in the health care industry. Few areas are more important to the financial well-being of a health care firm. A firm that cannot obtain the amounts of capital specified in its strategic financial plan will not be able to achieve its long-term objectives. Indeed, if the firm finds it difficult to acquire any amount of capital at a reasonable cost, its future survival may be questionable. Successful firms have the capability to provide capital financing when needed and at a cost that is reasonable.

Two key questions are relevant to our discussion of capital formation in the health care industry. First, how much capital is needed? Ideally, the firm should have defined its capital needs in its strategic financial plan. Capital needs should include working capital requirements and replacement reserves, as well as the funding needs for buildings and equipment.

Second, what sources of capital financing are available? At the time of this writing, the future availability of tax-exempt financing is unclear. Tax-exempt financing has been the largest source of capital for the hospital industry for the last 20 years. If it were eliminated, financing patterns would experience a major shift. The exact direction of this shift is unclear at this time, although it would seem that taxable sources of debt would have to be substituted for tax-exempt sources.

Table 20–1 presents a summary of investment and financing patterns in the hospital industry for the years 2001 and 2003.

In general, we can classify the sources of financing into the following two categories: (1) equity and (2) debt. In the hospital industry, approximately 50 percent of total assets are financed with equity and 50 percent are financed with debt. However, financing patterns may vary somewhat in different sectors of the health care industry. For example, many long-term care facilities have much higher proportions of debt. Debt financing in such facilities may run as high as 90 percent.

Table 20–1 Acute Care Hospitals' Consolidated Balance Sheets, 2001 and 2003

	2001 (000)	2003 (000)	% Change
Cash	$8,077	$9,955	23.3
Accounts Receivable	18,307	19,792	8.1
Inventory	1,451	1,688	16.3
Other Current Assets	5,163	6,544	26.7
Total Current Assets	$32,998	$37,979	15.1
Net Property, Plant, & Equipment	$46,468	$51,155	10.1
Investments	15,559	17,501	12.5
Other Assets	14,529	17,936	23.4
Total Assets	$109,554	$124,571	13.7
Current Liabilities	$18,061	$20,078	11.2
Long Term Liabilities	33,576	37,630	12.1
Equity	57,917	66,863	15.4
Total Liabilities & Equity	$109,554	$124,571	13.7

Source: Cleverley & Associates, *State of the Hospital Industry, 2005 Edition.*

LEARNING OBJECTIVE 1

Identify the sources of equity financing.

EQUITY FINANCING

In general, the following are the only ways in which a firm can generate new equity capital: (1) profit retention, (2) contributions, and (3) sale of equity interests. We already have stressed in past chapters the importance of earning adequate levels of profit. Hence, our discussion at this point is focused primarily on contributions and sales of new equity. A contribution may be given to a firm for a variety of reasons. Normally, in tax-exempt health care firms, a contribution is given with no expectation of a future return. The donor may derive some immediate or deferred tax benefit, but there is no expectation of a financial return to be paid by the health care entity. In contrast, contributions are given to a taxable health care entity with the expectation of a future financial return. The contribution may be in the form of a stock purchase or a limited partnership unit. It is important to note that this form of contribution also may be available to tax-exempt entities through a corporate restructuring arrangement. We will discuss this point in more detail shortly.

Philanthropy is definitely not dead in our nation. In 2004, approximately 2.1 percent of our nation's gross domestic product, or $248.5 billion, was in the form of philanthropic gifts. Tables 20–2 and 20–3 provide data showing the sources and the distribution of giving for the years 1995, 2000, and 2004. These data present an encouraging picture. Total giving increased during the 19-year period of 1995 to 2004 on an inflation-adjusted basis by 62 percent. Individuals were clearly the largest source of giving, representing about 76 percent of total giving.

To be successful, a major philanthropic program should have the following key elements:

- A "case statement." This document should carefully and persuasively define why you need money.
- A designated development officer. This individual may not be a full-time employee, but duties and expectations should be precisely defined. Incentives for development officers should be related to expectations for giving.
- Trustee and medical staff involvement. People give to people, not to organizations.
- Prospect lists. You should know who in the community are prime prospects for giving.
- Programs for giving. This is critical. You should have a variety of methods and means to encourage giving. For example, you may have a number of deferred giving plans, such as unitrusts, annuity trusts, or pooled-income funds. Your development officer should be familiar with these methods.
- Goals. You need to define realistic targets for long-range planning.

There are many ways to encourage people to give to charitable, tax-exempt health care firms. Many large firms employ full-time development staff. These individuals can do much to increase charitable giving.

One of the most promising areas of philanthropic giving is in deferred gift arrangements. In a deferred giving plan, a taxpayer donor may get an immediate tax benefit in return for a gift to be given to the tax-exempt firm later. An interesting recent example of deferred giving is the case of a hospital in California that initiated a provocative new fundraising effort, called

Table 20–2 Sources of Giving (Dollars in Billions)

	1995 (inflation adj.)	%	*2000 (inflation adj.)*	%	*2004*	%
Individuals	$118.2	77	$191.4	76	$187.9	76
Bequests	12.9	8	21.8	9	19.8	8
Foundations	13.1	9	27.0	11	28.8	12
Corporations	9.1	6	11.8	5	12.0	5
Total	$153.3	100	$252.0	100	$248.5	100

Source: Giving USA 2005, Giving USA Foundation™, AAFRC Trust for Philanthropy.

Table 20-3 Distribution of Giving (Dollars in Billions)

	1995		2000		2004	
	Giving (inflation adj.)	%	Giving (inflation adj.)	%	Giving	%
Religion	$58.1	47	$77.0	34	$88.3	36
Education	17.6	14	31.7	14	33.8	14
Health	12.6	10	18.8	8	22.0	9
Human services	11.7	9	18.0	8	19.2	8
Arts and culture	10.0	8	11.5	5	14.0	6
Other	13.7	11	72.7	32	71.2	29
Total	$123.7	100	$229.7	100	$248.5	100

Source: Giving USA 2005, Giving USA Foundation™, AAFRC Trust for Philanthropy.

the home value program (HVP). HVP is designed for senior citizens, aged 70 or older, who own mortgage-free homes. The homeowners sign a revocable agreement that, upon their deaths, transfers the title to their homes to the hospital. In return, they receive a monthly payment that is based on a loan from the hospital. In concept, HVP is similar to the reverse annuity mortgages that are being used in some banking circles. An HVP program is also being used to finance long-term care for individual patients in nursing homes and home health agencies. It is especially useful for the elderly who have no means of supporting themselves other than the equity built up in their homes.

The following case illustrates the mechanics of an HVP. Assume that Mrs. Jones, aged 70, has a mortgage-free home with a market value of $100,000. The hospital, or its foundation, executes a loan of $50,000 at 12 percent interest that will pay Mrs. Jones $717 per month for 10 years. Mrs. Jones signs a revocable agreement.

How does the hospital benefit? First, for a $50,000 loan, the hospital receives title to property that is valued at $100,000. Second, the hospital benefits from any appreciation on the property. In 10 years, if the annual appreciation rate is five percent, Mrs. Jones' $100,000 home will be worth $163,000. Third, the hospital establishes a relationship with Mrs. Jones that may lead to other donations.

How does Mrs. Jones benefit? First, the monthly payment is considered tax-free income. Second, there is no risk to Mrs. Jones because the agreement is revocable and can be rescinded with payment of the loan plus a penalty. Third, the HVP provides Mrs. Jones

with a tangible way of supporting the hospital. The last factor is the key to the ultimate success of the program.

An HVP, or some adaptation of it, can provide a significant return to a hospital. However, some forethought is required. For one thing, working capital obviously is necessary. Payments to homeowners will precede any financial recovery through sale of the donated homes. Also, a significant amount of legal, accounting, and actuarial consulting is essential. Finally, such a program should not be perceived as a pure donation program. It is intended to be a method of investment diversification, albeit one with unusually high returns. Thus, a program such as an HVP can provide an excellent vehicle for long-term equity capital growth.

Both taxable and tax-exempt health care providers have shown great interest in the issuance of equity to investors. For taxable health care firms, this interest is not new; for most such firms, the issuance of equity has been a major source of financing over the years. Most taxable health care firms began with a small amount of venture capital. They were able to use that original funding to develop a successful track record of operations. Based on that record of success, an initial public offering (IPO) of stock was made. The resulting funds were then used to expand operations, part of which was fueled by leveraging funds acquired during the initial public offering.

The technique of expanding operations quickly through the issuance of equity and then leveraging that equity through the issuance of debt has been used extensively in the taxable sector. Table 20–4 illustrates the growth potential of a taxable entity.

Table 20–4 Capital Growth in Alternative Organizations

Organizational Type	Historical Net Income	Equity Issue (Stock)	Debt Addition	Possible Total Capital
Tax-exempt	$1.0	$0.0	$2.0	$3.0
Taxable	$0.7	$14.0	$28.0	$42.7

These data indicate that a taxable entity could raise approximately 14 times the amount of total capital that a tax-exempt entity could. Let us examine these data and their related assumptions more closely to clearly understand the underlying process behind capital formation. It is assumed that some business unit or firm has generated $1 million in before-tax income. If the firm was a taxable entity, it would be required to pay approximately 30 percent of this income as tax. However, the taxable firm could issue stock, limited partnership units, or some other type of equity security. Furthermore, it is assumed that a price earnings multiple of 20 is in effect. This means that the taxable firm could raise $14 million in equity based on its net income of $700,000. Both the tax-exempt and the taxable firms could issue debt based on their equity positions. We have assumed that a leverage ratio of 2 to 1 exists; that is, the firms could borrow $2 for every $1 of equity. The taxable firm could issue $28 million in debt, whereas the tax-exempt firm would be limited to $2 million in debt. Total capital, both debt and equity, would be $3 million for the tax-exempt firm and $42.7 million for the taxable firm.

In the preceding example, some of the assumptions might be changed, but the relative growth potential would remain the same. In this situation, is there any way that a tax-exempt firm can take advantage of this growth potential? The answer is yes: a tax-exempt firm could change its status to taxable. This is not an easy thing to do, but it is not impossible. Several large health maintenance organizations (HMOs) started out as tax-exempt firms, but changed their ownership status to maximize their growth potential.

An easier alternative method is to restructure the firm. Figure 20–1 presents a generic structure that is used by many tax-exempt health care firms to create an equity capital formation alternative. This structure involves the creation of taxable entities that can issue equity securities directly to investors. In the parent

holding company model in Figure 20–1, there are several taxable entities that could issue equity to investors and help generate capital for the entire consolidated structure.

An actual case example may help to illustrate the potential for capital formation created by restructuring a tax-exempt health care firm. ABC Hospital needed to replace its computed tomography (CT) scanner with a new one. The estimated cost of the new scanner was $1,160,000. The hospital did not wish to use any of its debt capacity in this project. The solution was to create a limited partnership and joint venture with its physicians. A new entity was created, called ABC Scanner, which was a limited partnership. The ABC Properties Company, which was a subsidiary of the hospital's parent holding company, was the general partner. A bank loan of $1,180,000 was obtained; the loan was guaranteed by the limited partners (30 limited partners) and the general partner. The source and use-of-funds statement for the new structure is presented in Table 20–5.

Table 20–5 documents the capability of the new structure to enhance ABC Hospital's capital position with little funding commitment from the hospital. The general partner, a member of the restructured health care entity, has contributed only $50,000 of cash and guaranteed $295,000 in loans. For this relatively modest level of commitment, total funding of $1,380,000 was made available. However, while the level of required capital was reduced, the expected future returns from the investment will also be reduced because of the presence of physician limited partners.

LEARNING OBJECTIVE 2

Explain the factors that influence the desirability of alternative sources of financing.

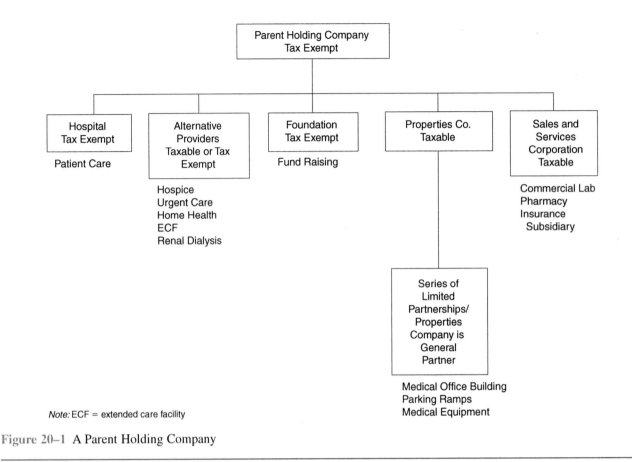

Note: ECF = extended care facility

Figure 20–1   A Parent Holding Company

LONG-TERM DEBT FINANCING

An examination of the specific sources of long-term debt financing in the health care industry can be a complex and confusing process. Part of the problem stems from the use of jargon by those involved. Unless one is familiar with this jargon, meaningful communication with financing people may be difficult. Before describing the alternatives for long-term debt financing in the health care industry, we should note five key characteristics of financing that greatly affect the relative desirability of alternative sources of financing. As we describe these characteristics, we will introduce some new terminology that will facilitate later discussion.

The five key characteristics are:

1. Cost
2. Control
3. Risk
4. Availability
5. Adequacy

Cost

Interest rates are the most important characteristic that affects the cost of alternative debt financing. The fixed return of a long-term debt instrument is often called the coupon rate. For example, a 9.8 percent revenue bond indicates that the issuer will pay the investor $98 annually for every $1,000 of principal. Sometimes the term "basis point" is used to describe differences in coupon rates. A basis point is 1/100 of 1 percent. For example, the difference between a coupon rate of 9.80 percent and 9.65 percent is 15 basis points.

Although interest is the primary measure of financing cost, it is not the only aspect of cost that should be considered. Issuance costs can be sizable in some types of financing. Issuance costs are simply those expenditures that are essential to consummate the financing. There is a great difference in the amount of issuance costs for publicly-placed and privately-placed issues. A privately-placed issue is not sold to the general market, but rather is purchased directly by only a few major buyers. In a publicly-placed issue,

Table 20–5 Source and Use of Funds for CT Scanner

Sources of Funds		
Bank loan		$1,180,000
Guaranteed by:		
General partner	$295,000	
Limited partners (@ $29,500)	885,000	
General partner's cash contribution		50,000
Limited partner's cash contribution (@ $5,000)		150,000
Total sources		$1,380,000
Uses of Funds		
Purchase and installation of CT scanner		$1,160,000
Leasehold (suite) improvements		95,000
Loan placement fee		35,400
Legal and other organizational expenses		15,000
Reserve for working capital		74,600
Total uses		$1,380,000

there are a number of costs that must be incurred to legally sell the securities to the general public. Printing costs are associated with producing the official statements that will be sent to prospective clients. There are costs for attorneys and accountants who must certify various aspects of the issue, such as its financial feasibility and its tax-exempt status. Finally, there is the underwriter's spread that is charged by the investment banking firm that arranges the sale of the securities. The underwriter's spread represents the difference between the face value of the bonds and the price the underwriter or investment banker pays to purchase the bonds. When aggregated, issuance costs can sometimes amount to as much as five percent of the total issue. This means that an issuer must borrow $100 to get $95.

Another large cost of financing is reserve requirements. Some types of financing require the creation of fund balances in escrow accounts under the custody of the bond trustee. The bond trustee is designated by the issuer to represent the interests of the bondholders. The obligations of the trustee are defined in the Trust Indenture Act of 1939, which is administered by the Securities and Exchange Commission. There are two primary categories of reserve requirements. The first is the debt service reserve. This fund represents a cushion for the investors if the issuer gets into some type of fiscal crisis. It is usually set equal to one year's worth of principal and interest payments. The second category of reserve requirement is the depreciation reserve. This fund is sometimes set up to equal the cumulative dif-

ference between debt principal repayment and depreciation expense on the depreciable assets financed with debt. Usually, the amount of depreciation expense is greatest during the immediate years after a major construction program has been completed, when debt principal may be at its lowest level. Because depreciation may represent the primary source of debt principal payment, there is a need to accumulate these funds to ensure their availability in later years, when the amount of debt principal payment exceeds depreciation. Figure 20–2 presents a graphic display of this relationship.

Control

Ideally, when issuing debt financing, the issuer would like to have little or no interference in management by the investors. It is usually not possible to avoid such interference, however. The investors often will specify some conditions or restrictions that they would like included in the bond contract. Such conditions or restrictions are often known as covenants. These are explained in great detail in the indenture, which is the written contract between the investors and the issuing company.

One category of restrictive covenants concerns specific financial performance indicators. For example, most indentures define values for the firm's debt service coverage ratio and its current ratio. If actual values for these indicators are below the defined values, the bond trustee may take certain actions. The trustee may assume a position on the board of trustees, replace

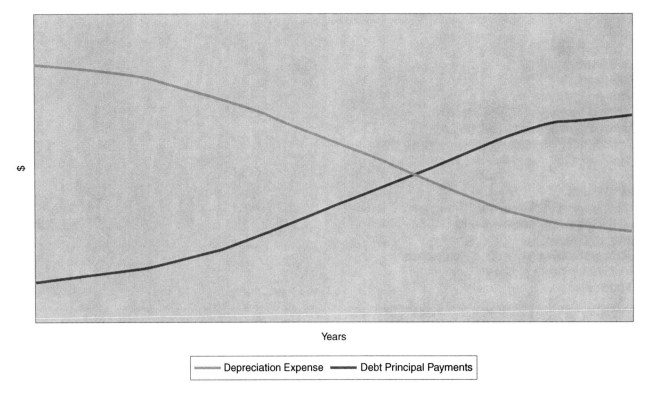

Years

Depreciation Expense ▬▬ Debt Principal Payments

Figure 20–2 Depreciation Reserve Requirement: Relationship between Depreciation Expense and Debt Principal Payments

current management, or require the entire outstanding principal to be paid immediately.

Another category of covenants concerns future financing. A section in the indenture referred to as additional parity financing defines the conditions that must be satisfied before the firm can issue any additional debt. The most important condition is usually prior and projected debt service coverage.

There is a trend developing in the issuance of tax-exempt bonds to replace the projected debt service coverage provision with a stated level of debt to equity. For example, the initial bond placement may specify that new financing can be issued if long-term debt does not equal a multiple of 1.5 times present equity or net assets. This would permit large health care systems more flexibility when issuing future debt and is more closely akin to provisions that exist in the corporate taxable debt markets.

Risk

From the issuer's perspective, flexibility of repayment terms is highly desirable. An issuer with flexible

repayment terms can alter payments to meet the issuer's current cash flow. The investor, however, wants some guarantee that the principal will be repaid in accordance with some pre-established plan.

One of the most important indenture elements is the prepayment provision. This provision specifies the point in time at which the debt can be retired, and the penalty that will be imposed for an early retirement. For example, the indenture may prohibit the issuer from prepaying the debt for the first ten years of issue life. Thereafter, the debt may be repaid, but only if there is a call premium. The call premium is some percentage of the par or face value of the bonds. Thus, a call premium of five percent would mean that a $50 premium would be paid for each $1,000 of bonds. The issuer would like to have the option of retiring outstanding debt at any point with no call premium. However, investors do not usually permit this for debt that has a fixed interest rate.

Another aspect of risk relates to the debt principal amortization pattern. Most debt retirement plans can be categorized as level-debt service or level-debt principal. In a level-debt service plan, the amount of interest and principal that is repaid each year remains fairly constant. This is the type of repayment that is usually associated with home mortgages. In the early years, the amount of interest is much greater than the debt principal. Over time, this pattern changes and the amount of principal repaid each year begins to exceed the interest payment. Figure 20–3 presents a graphic view of a level-debt service plan.

Level-debt principal means that equal amount of debt principal is repaid each year. In this pattern of debt retirement, the total debt service payment decreases over time. Figure 20–4 shows this relationship.

Many financing plans approximate a level-debt service plan. This pattern of debt amortization extends the debt retirement life and may benefit the issuer. The benefit is predicated on three factors:

1. The ability of the issuer to earn a return greater than the interest rate on the debt
2. The presence of reimbursement for capital costs
3. The availability of tax-exempt financing

To illustrate the desirability of principal repayment delay, we will examine a simple case. Let us assume that we have two alternative financing plans. One plan will permit us to borrow $10 million for five years with no payment of principal until the fifth year. We will be required to pay ten percent per year as our interest payment for each of the five years. The second financing plan will permit us to borrow the same $10 million for five years; however, there will be an annual payment of principal equal to $2 million per year. The interest rate on this financing plan will be eight percent per year, which is below the interest rate in the first plan. Let us further assume that 80 percent of our interest expense will be repaid by our third-party payers, who still pay us for the actual costs of capital incurred because this is a critical access designated hospital. Finally, let us assume that any differences in cash flow between the two plans could be invested at ten percent. Table 20–6 provides a comparison of the net present values for these two financing plans. The values indicate that the higher-interest balloon payment plan is the lower cost source of financing. This is a direct result of the large percentage (80 percent) of capital cost payment. An 80 percent capital cost payment means that the effective interest rate is $(1 - .80)$ times the

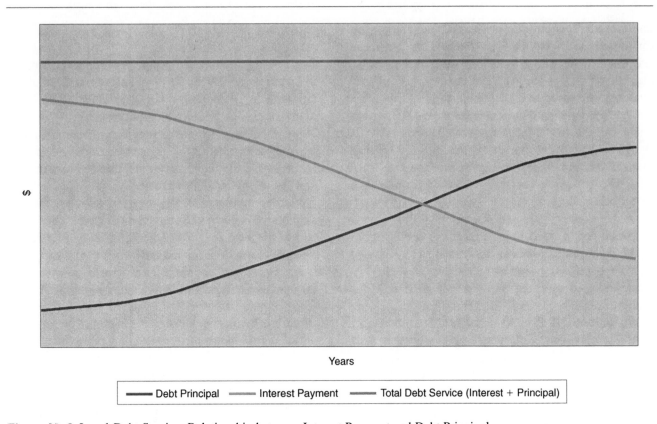

Years

Debt Principal ——— Interest Payment ——— Total Debt Service (Interest + Principal)

Figure 20–3 Level-Debt Service: Relationship between Interest Payment and Debt Principal

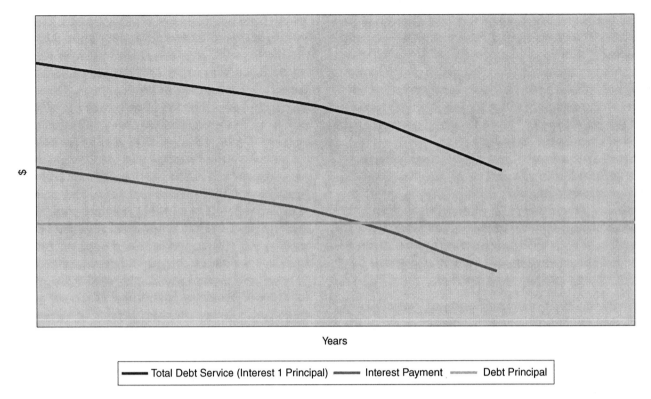

Years

Total Debt Service (Interest 1 Principal)   Interest Payment   Debt Principal

Figure 20–4 Level-Debt Principal: Relationship between Interest Payment and Total Debt Service

interest rate. This means that the effective interest rate for the balloon repayment plan would be 2 percent, and the corresponding value for the equal principal plan would be 1.6 percent. The difference in interest rates has decreased from 2 percent to .4 of 1 percent. An investment yield of two percent means that we can make money from delaying principal payment. In short, our cost is less than our return. It is only natural to want to retain money as long as possible.

Availability

Once a health care firm decides that it needs debt financing, it usually wants to obtain the funds as quickly as possible. A delay can result in severe consequences and postpone the start of a construction program. This might increase the cost of the total program because of normal inflation in construction costs. A delay also could result in an unexpected increase in interest rates. Although privately-placed issues usually can be arranged more quickly than publicly-placed issues, there is usually a higher interest rate associated with privately-placed issues. However, the difference in interest rates may more than offset the costs of delay.

Adequacy

A key requirement of any proposed plan of financing is that it covers all the associated costs. One of the key areas of adequacy is that of refinancing costs. In many situations, a new construction program that requires financing may not be possible unless existing financing can be retired or refinanced. Not all types of financing permit the issuer to include the costs of refinancing in the amount borrowed.

Funding during construction is another important area of financing. Some types of financing do not permit the issuer to borrow during the construction period. A loan will be issued only after the construction has been completed and the new assets are available for operations. In this situation, the issuer must arrange for a separate source of funding to finance the construction. Permanent financing then must be arranged upon completion of the construction program.

Interest incurred during construction can be sizable. For example, a $50 million construction program might incur $5 to $10 million in interest during the construction period. Thus it is important to have a source of financing that also permits the issuer to borrow to cover interest costs.

Table 20–6 Cost of Alternative Debt Amortization Plans

Item	Amount before Reimbursement Effect	Amount after Reimbursement Effect	Years	Present Value Factor (10%)	Present Value
Equal Principal Payment—8%					
Principal	$2,000,000	$2,000,000		3.791	$7,582,000
Interest	800,000	160,000		0.909	145,440
Interest	640,000	128,000		0.826	105,728
Interest	480,000	96,000		0.751	72,096
Interest	320,000	64,000		0.683	43,712
Interest	160,000	32,000		0.621	19,872
Net present value cost					$7,968,848
Balloon Principal—10%					
Interest	$1,000,000	$200,000	1–5	3.791	$758,200
Principal	10,000,000	10,000,000	5	0.621	6,210,000
Net present value					$6,968,200

The percentage of financing available varies across financing plans and is another key area of adequacy. Some plans permit up to 100 percent of the cost, whereas others may limit the amount to 70 or 80 percent. Depending on the availability of other funds, these limitations may pose real problems in some situations.

ALTERNATIVE DEBT FINANCING SOURCES

Sources

Presently, the following four major alternative sources of long-term debt are available to health care facilities:

1. Tax-exempt revenue bonds
2. Federal Housing Administration (FHA)-insured mortgages
3. Public taxable bonds
4. Conventional mortgage financing

Table 20–7 compares these four sources of financing regarding the factors that affect capital financing desirability.

Tax-Exempt Revenue Bonds

Tax-exempt revenue bonds permit the interest earned on them to be exempt from federal income taxation. The primary security for such loans is usually a pledge of the revenues of the facility seeking the loan, plus a first mortgage on the facility's assets. If the tax

revenue of a government entity is also pledged, the bonds are referred to as "general obligation bonds." Because of the income tax exemption, the interest rates on a tax-exempt bond are usually 1.5 to 2 percent lower than other sources of financing.

Most tax-exempt revenue bonds are issued by a state or local authority. The health care facility then enters into a lease arrangement with the authority. Title to the assets remains with the authority until the indebtedness is repaid.

Congress has issued legislation that has begun to limit both the total amount of tax-exempt revenue bonds that can be issued and the purpose for which the financing can be used. For example, a hospital can no longer issue tax-exempt revenue bonds to finance the construction of a medical office building because the medical office building is not perceived as a central element of the non-profit hospital's mission.

FHA-Insured Mortgages

FHA-insured mortgages are sponsored by the Federal Housing Administration, but initial processing begins in the Department of Health and Human Services. Through the FHA program, the government provides mortgage insurance for both proprietary and nonproprietary hospitals. This guarantee reduces the risk of a loan to investors and thus lowers the interest rate that a hospital must pay. However, obtaining the appropriate approvals often can be a time-consuming process.

Table 20–7 Comparative Analysis: Long-Term Debt Alternatives for Hospitals

Program Characteristics	Conventional Mortgage	Taxable Bonds	Tax-Exempt Bonds	FHA-Insured Mortgage (GNMA Guarantee)
Security	First mortgage given to lender; pledge of gross revenues (substantially all hospital assets pledged)	First mortgage given to trustee bank for benefit of bondholder; pledge of gross revenue (substantially all assets pledged)	First mortgage or negative pledge if A rated or higher, given to trustee bank for benefit of bondholders; pledge of gross revenue (substantially all assets pledged)	First mortgage given to FHA-approved mortgage for benefits of HUD; pledge of gross revenue (substantially all assets pledged)
Timing for alternative	2–6 months	4–6 months	3–6 months	6–12 months
Percentage financing available	Usually 70%–80% of eligible assets available to be pledged (as determined by appraisal)	Up to 100%, limited by available cash flow and available assets in some cases	Up to 100%, subject to available cash flow	90% of value; up to 100% of cost.
Construction financing	Normally required	Optional	Not required	Required because a minimum of 20% of the mortgage must be used for renovation or equipment.
Financing costs	Covers all costs of assets, excluding some movable equipment	Covers all cost	Covers all cost	Covers all cost, including startup costs
Term of financing	5–15 fixed balloon 20–25 amortization	10–20 years (occasionally with balloon payment based on longer amortization)	30 years	25 years fully amortizing starting after completion of construction, plus construction period.
Front-end fees	1%–2% commitment fee subject to amount financed; other fees $5–$25,000	1% underwriting (private placement) or 2%–4% underwriting (public offering); other expenses approximately 1/2 of 1% plus feasibility study	Fees directly related to a published bond rating; size; and financing structure (variable vs. fixed).	.80% filing fee, 0.5% insurance (FHA) fee, plus a maximum of 2.0% Financing and 1.5% Placement Fees. Another 2.0% may be used to cover tax-exempt bond costs
Continuing annual fee	1/8 of 1% servicing if multiple lenders	Trustee fees (nominal)	Trustee fees (nominal)	0.5% FHA insurance fee; 0.25% GNMA fee
Prepayment provisions	Make whole provision with lender	Normally 5 year and prepayment; no penalty unless refinancing	10 year, no prepayment; 1% penalty descending thereafter	Taxably, 2 year lockout, then 8% declining 1.0% per year. Tax-exempt, no call for 10 years, then 3% declining 1% per year
Required reserves	Usually none; depreciation reserve optional	None	Debt service reserve equal to 1 year's principal and interest (P & I); depreciation reserve equal to defeciency amount	A "Mortgage Reserve Fund" is required, to equal 1 year's debt service after 5 years and 2 year's debt service after 10 years
Restriction on leasing	Yes; subject to cash-flow levels by convenant	None	None	None
Additional parity financing	Yes; normally subject to lender approval	Yes; subject to approval of underwriter or to provisions of financing agreement; normally required coverage of 110%–150%	Yes; subject to meeting coverage requirement of 110%–120% on both historical and pro forma basis	Generally, none allowed because the FHA mortgage requires a 1st lien. A very "soft" second mortgage is allowed. FHA has the Section 241 program to finance renovations secured by 2nd mortgage liens.
Payment	Monthly	Semiannually	Quarterly/semiannualy	Monthly debt service payments to HUD approved lender.
Reporting	Lender(s) only	Lender(s) or bond trustee and underwriter as appropriate, and rating agencies	Bond trustee, underwriter, and rating agencies as appropriate	Annual financial statement reporting requirement.

Source: Ziegler Capital Markets Group, Chicago, Illinois.

Public Taxable Bonds

Public taxable bonds are issued in much the same way as tax-exempt revenue bonds, except that there is no issuing authority and no interest income tax exemption. An investment banking firm usually underwrites the loan and markets the issue to individual investors. Interest rates are thus higher on this type of financing than they are on a tax-exempt issue.

Conventional Mortgage Financing

Conventional mortgage financing is usually privately-placed with a bank, pension fund, savings and loan institution, life insurance company, or real estate investment trust. This source of financing can be arranged quickly, but, compared with other alternatives, does not provide as large a percentage of the total financing requirements for large projects. Thus, greater amounts of equity must be contributed.

Parties Involved

Figure 20–5 is a schematic representation of the parties involved and their relationships when issuing a public tax-exempt revenue bond. This schematic also could be used to illustrate the process of issuing a public taxable bond. The only change would be the deletion of the issuing authority and addition of a line showing the direct issuance of the bonds by the health care facility. The specific parties involved in financing a bond include the following:

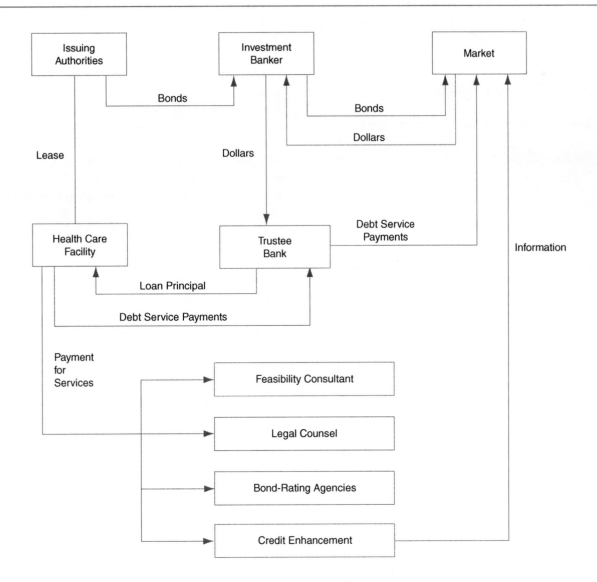

Figure 20–5 Parties Involved in a Public, Tax-Exempt, Revenue Bond Issue

* Issuing authority
* Investment banker
* Health care facility
* Market
* Trustee bank
* Feasibility consultant
* Legal counsel
* Bond-rating agency

Issuing Authority

The issuing authority is involved only in tax-exempt financing. In most cases, the issuing authority is some state or local governmental authority, which may be specially created for the sole purpose of issuing revenue bonds. The issuing authority serves as a conduit between the health care facility and the investment banker. In a public taxable issue or in a situation in which tax-exempt revenue bonds are issued directly by the health care facility, the role of the issuing authority may be eliminated.

LEARNING OBJECTIVE 3

Explain what an investment banker does.

Investment Banker

In public or private issues, investment bankers have a dual role. First, they serve as advisors to the health care facility that is issuing the bonds. In many circumstances, they are the focal point for coordinating the services of the feasibility consultant, the legal counsel, and the bond-rating agencies. Their advice can be extremely important in obtaining timely funding under favorable conditions. Second, investment bankers serve as brokers between the market and the issuer of the bond. If investment bankers underwrite the issue, it means that they technically buy the entire issue and are at risk for the sale of the bonds to individual investors. If investment bankers place the issue on a best-efforts basis, they do not purchase the issue, and any unsold bonds become the property of the issuer.

Health Care Facility

The health care facility is the ultimate beneficiary of the bond issue. The health care facility is also responsible for repayment of the loan principal. The health care facility's financial condition and its ability to repay the indebtedness are thus the central concerns of the investor. To provide evidence of its financial condition and the risk of the investment to the market, the health care facility usually employs independent consultants who assess various aspects of the facility. Such consultants include the feasibility consultant, the legal counsel, and the bond-rating agencies.

Market

For any given bond issue, the market may consist of a large number of individual investors or it may consist of a small number of large institutional investors. In any case, the market purchases the bonds of the issuer with the expectation of some stated rate of return. The market also wants assurances that the bonds will be repaid on a timely basis and that there is not an unreasonable amount of risk.

Trustee Bank

A trustee bank serves as the market's agent once the bonds are sold. Typically, the trustee bank is a commercial bank—in some cases, the same bank at which the health care facility has its accounts. The trustee bank may receive the proceeds from the sale of the bond issue and deliver the monies directly to the hospital or to the contractor, as required. The trustee bank also receives the debt service payments from the health care facility and distributes these to the market or investors. It may retire outstanding bonds according to a prearranged schedule of retirement, and hold additional reserve requirements deposited by the health care facility. Finally, the trustee bank ensures that the health care facility is adhering to the provisions of the bond contract or indenture, such as those concerning adequate debt service coverage and working capital positions.

Feasibility Consultant

The feasibility consultant is usually an independent, certified public accountant, who may or may not be the health care facility's outside auditor. The feasibility consultant's primary function is to assess the financial feasibility of the project and the ability of the health care facility to meet the associated indebtedness. Financial projections are usually made for a five-year period. These projections provide a basis for the investor and the bond-rating agency to assess the risk of default.

Legal Counsel

Legal counsel is needed for several reasons. First, in a tax-exempt revenue bond issue, the market is concerned with the legality of the tax exemption. If the interest payments are not determined to be tax-exempt by the Internal Revenue Service, the investors will suffer a significant loss. Second, legal opinion is necessary to ensure that the security pledged by the health care facility, whether it be revenue or assets, is legal and enforceable.

LEARNING OBJECTIVE 4

List the major bond-rating agencies and explain their role in the debt market.

Bond-Rating Agencies

Moody's and Standard & Poor's are the two primary bond-rating agencies, although other smaller ones exist. Their function is to assess the relative risk associated with a given bond issue. The two agencies have developed detailed coding systems to assess risk (Table 20–8). The resulting bond rating has important implications. First, there is a definite correlation between the interest rate that an issuer must pay and the bond rating associated with the issue. Generally speaking, the higher the bond rating, the lower the interest rate. Thus, a bond rated AAA by Standard & Poor's would be likely to have a much lower rate of interest than one rated BBB. Second, issues rated below BBB by Standard & Poor's or Baa by Moody's are not classified as investment grade. Many institutional investors are prohibited from investing in bonds that carry a rating lower than investment grade. Thus, the market for such issues is likely to be small.

Credit Enhancement

Credit enhancement is a term that has come into use in the health care financing field only recently. A credit enhancement device is simply a mechanism by which the risk of default can be shifted from the issuer to a third party. Thus, the FHA-insured mortgage program provides a form of credit enhancement.

Aside from the FHA program, two basic types of credit enhancement are commonly used. The first type is municipal bond insurance. Municipal bond insurance is a surety bond that ensures that the debt service will be repaid. When municipal bond insurance is used, the credit rating for the issue becomes the credit rating of the insurance firm that is writing the insurance. In most cases, this means that the bond rating would be AAA or Aaa. Table 20–9 presents a summary of the major firms that currently provide municipal bond insurance and gives some idea of the relative cost of such insurance.

The second form of credit enhancement is a letter of credit. A letter of credit, usually issued by a commercial bank, provides a formal assurance that a specified sum of money will be available during some defined period. Usually, the period matches the maturity of the debt, and the amount provided in the letter of credit corresponds to the amount of indebtedness. As with bond insurance, the credit rating of the bank would be substituted for the credit rating of the issuer. In most situations, this would mean an automatic AAA or Aaa rating. The bank requires a fee for providing the letter of credit, and the issuer must determine whether the cost of the letter of credit exceeds any possible savings in reduced interest expense that would result from an improved bond rating.

MORE RECENT DEVELOPMENTS

The following four more recent modifications of the traditional sources of long-term debt should be noted at this juncture:

Table 20–8 Bond Ratings

Classification	Moody's	Standard & Poor's
Investment grade	Aaa	AAA
	Aa	AA
	A	A
	Baa	BBB
Not investment grade	Ba	BB
	B	B
	Caa	CCC
	Ca	CC
	C	C

Moody's assigns sub-category ratings of 1, 2, and 3 that are designated with superscripts. A Baa[1] rating woud be at the higher end of the rating and the modifier 3 would be at the lower end. Standard and Poor's uses plus and minus modifiers for their rating catgories.

Table 20–9 Municipal bond Insurers

Insurer	Types of issues	Rating	Premiums	Principal and Interest Insured (Billions)	
				All Types	Health Care
AMBAC Indemnity (212-248-3307)	New-issue general obligation bonds (GOs), tax and revenue anticipation note	AAA Aaa	.33–.94%	$86.2	$12.9
MBIA (914-765-3893)	New-issue GOs, utility issues, commercial paper, hospital goods	AAA Aaa	.30–.90%	$157.7	$32.1
FGIC (212-607-3009)	New issues, Gos, revenue bonds, and unit investment trusts	AAA Aaa	NA	$92.5	NA
Capital Guarantee (415-995-8012)	New issues, Gos, and revenue bonds	AAA NR	.20–2.00%	$9.0	$0.6
FSA (212-826-0100)	New issues, Gos, revenue bonds, and municipal utilities	AAA Aaa	NA	$21.6	$0.7

Source: Prepared by Ziegler Securities, Chicago, Illinois.

1. Variable rate financing
2. Pooled or shared financing
3. Zero-coupon and original issue discount bonds
4. Interest rate swaps

Variable Rate Financing

Recently in the health care sector, as well as in other industries, there has been a shift to the use of variable rate financing. In variable rate financing, the outstanding debt principal is fixed, but the interest rate on the principal is variable. This contrasts with the traditional situation in which the interest rate is fixed for the life of the bonds. Variable rate financing requires that the interest rate be adjusted periodically—in some cases, weekly—to a current market index.

A feature that is often associated with variable rate financing is the use of a tender option or put. A tender option or put permits investors to redeem their bonds at some predetermined interval—perhaps daily—at the face value. In reality, this type of financing is short-term, not long-term. As a result, the interest rate may be significantly below a comparable long-term rate at the initiation of the financing. Many firms—not just health care

firms—have opted to use variable rate financing to achieve a lower cost of financing. Sometimes this strategy is referred to as "moving down the yield curve." Figure 20–6 shows a typical upward-sloping yield curve.

Pooled Financing

In the health care sector, there has been increasing interest in developing financing packages that encompass more than one entity. The major rationale for this interest lies in the relationship between size and cost of debt; larger organizations are better able to obtain debt capital and to realize lower costs of financing.

In general, there are three ways in which pooled or shared arrangements have been created in the health care sector. The first is through the use of master indenture financing by health care systems. In such cases, master indenture financing means that the debt is guaranteed by all the members who are a part of the master indenture. For example, a system of ten hospitals could finance through some master indenture arrangement in which all ten hospitals, or some subset of the ten hospitals, would be involved in the financing. The subset of hospitals involved in the financing is referred to as the "obligated group."

The Yield Curve

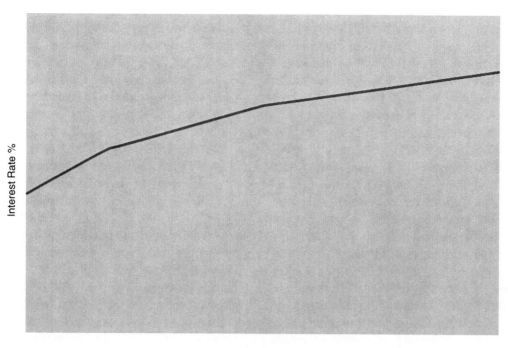

Figure 20–6 The Yield Curve

A second alternative is the use of pooled equipment financing programs. These programs are often sponsored by the state hospital association or some regional association. Individual hospitals are involved in the financing and can obtain funds from the pool. The interest rate is usually much lower because the risk is spread across several hospitals.

The third alternative is an arrangement similar to the previous, except that the sponsor is different. Here, the pooled approach is used either for equipment needs, or in some cases, for major building programs. The issuer and sponsor of the pool is not the state or regional association, however, but some voluntary association of health care entities. The Voluntary Hospitals of America have created such pooled financing for their members, and other associations are developing similar financing programs.

Zero-Coupon and Original Issue Discount Bonds

Bonds that are issued at a great discount have a coupon rate of interest that is below the rate required by the market for that type of security. In a zero-coupon

situation, there is no interest paid, thus the term "zero coupon." Certain investors think advantages accompany the purchase of zero-coupon bonds and these advantages help investors meet their portfolio needs. For example, pension plans may have a schedule of future pension payments by year, Purchase of zero coupon bonds could meet the required payments due in future years. There also may be advantages for the issuer, such as the delay of interest payments. This can conserve needed cash flow and may match the cash needs of the issuer. There is also the possibility that the after-reimbursement cost of the debt will be below the investment yield. It is important to note that, in most zero-coupon situations, there is a periodic payment to a sinking fund. The sinking fund is an account under the control of the bond trustee, and the proceeds of the fund are used to retire the bonds at maturity.

The mechanics of a zero-coupon situation may be illustrated in the following case example. Assume that General Hospital issues $100,000,000 in zero-coupon, five-year bonds. General Hospital would receive $62,100,000 from the market if the current market rate of interest is ten percent. Although no interest is paid, each year an amount is recorded for interest expense. This amount is an amortization of the difference between the face value of the bonds ($100,000,000) and the actual cash received ($62,100,000). Thus, during the five-year period, $37,900,000 will be recognized as interest expense. General also will be required to make semiannual payments of $7,586,793 to a sinking fund. This fund is assumed to earn interest at 12 percent annually or 6 percent semiannually. Assume also that equal amounts of the total discount will be recognized as interest expense each year. This would amount to $7,580,000 ($37,900,000/5). The calculation in Table 20–10 shows the net present value cost of this financing, assuming that 50 percent of capital costs are reimbursed and that the appropriate discount rate for the hospital is its investment yield of 12 percent.

The net present value cost of General Hospital's financing is $46,174,086, which is significantly less than the $62,100,000 that the hospital will receive. The sinking fund is not recognized as a capital expense item, which explains why the before and after reimbursement amounts are the same. The annual amortization of the discount, which is recognized by third-party payers as a reimbursable capital item, reduces the cost of the financing significantly. In some cases, this pattern of amortization may not be permitted by the payers. Instead, the payer may require a type of amortization called effective yield. This type of amortization requires that the same total amount of interest expense be recorded over the five years ($37,900,000), but the amounts in the earlier years would be less. This would reduce the present value of the benefit somewhat.

Interest Rate Swaps

Many hospitals and other health care providers have begun to use interest rate swaps. Interest rate swaps may enable firms to deal with the volatility in the financial markets and obtain lower-cost financing that better meets their needs. To understand an interest rate swap, three questions must be answered:

1. What is an interest rate swap?
2. Why are interest rate swaps beneficial? For every winner, won't there be a loser?
3. How can a swap arrangement be analyzed?

An interest rate swap is merely an exchange of interest rate payments between two firms, with a bank usually acting as a broker. For example, a firm that has issued fixed-rate debt may wish to make floating-rate payments. If a firm that makes floating-rate payments can be found that would like to substitute this type of payment with fixed-rate payments, a swap may be arranged. It is also possible to swap two different types of floating-rate debt. In a swap, only the coupon payments are exchanged, not the principal.

The basic nature of the swap is easy to understand. The aspect that is often puzzling is, how could both parties benefit from the swap? Many people believe that the only party that truly benefits is the broker.

The rationale for swaps is purely and simply a function of a supposed market imperfection. This means that one borrower has a better relative position in one maturity market than another. This difference is often ascribed to differential information and institutional restrictions that lead to differences in transaction costs.

Table 20–10 Net Present Value of Zero-Coupon Financing

Item	Amount before Reimbursement	Amount after Reimbursement	Years (Periods)	Present Value Factor (12%)	Present Value
Sinking fund	$7,586,793	$7,586,793	1–10*	7.8869	$59,836,278
Interest expense (amortization)	(7,580,000)	(3,790,000)	1–5	3.6048	(13,662,192)
Net present value cost					$46,174,086

*Ten semiannual payments; the present value factor is for ten periods at 6%.

Table 20–11 Interest Rates for Two Hospitals

Type of Debt	Hospital A	Hospital B	Rate Differential
Fixed	7.15%	8.10%	95 bps
Floating	Variable + 25 bps*	Variable + 40 bps	15 bps

*bps = Basis point (1/100 of 1 percent).

Because of these imperfections, the opportunity for financial arbitrage occurs.

To understand this concept more fully, let us assume that Hospital A and Hospital B encounter the interest rates in Table 20–11.

In the example in Table 20–11, Hospital A has a better relative position in both markets, fixed and floating. The differential, however, is much larger in the fixed-rate market [95 basis points (bps)] than in the floating-rate market (15 bps). The net differential is 80 (95 − 15). This difference implies that there is a swap opportunity present and that the total advantage is 80 bps. It is this 80 bps differential that will be split among Hospital A, Hospital B, and the broker.

Assume now that both hospitals issue $50 million of debt. Hospital A issues fixed-rate debt and Hospital B issues floating-rate debt. A broker could put these two hospitals together, and the set of payments in Table 20–12 might result. These data show that all parties have realized some financial advantage as a result of the swap.

Hospital A has reduced its floating rate to variable minus 10 basis points from variable plus 25 basis points. This is a savings of 35 basis points from its initial position. Hospital B also has gained. It now has fixed-rate debt at 7.80 percent, which is 30 basis points under its projected rate of 8.10 percent. Of course, the

broker has kept 15 basis points for the time and effort required to bring the parties together.

This is the way in which a swap is supposed to work. Everyone has benefited. It is not always true, however, that every party will benefit, and each swap opportunity must be carefully analyzed to ensure that benefits will be realized. The information following describes the use and valuation of interest rate swaps in Hospital Corporation of America's (HCA) 2005 financial statement:

LEARNING OBJECTIVE 5

List some of the pros and cons of retiring debt early.

EARLY RETIREMENT OF DEBT

In many cases, an issuer prefers to retire an existing debt issue before its maturity. There are a variety of reasons for wanting to do this. One important reason is that it permits the issuer to take advantage of a reduction in interest rates. An issue may have been marketed several years ago when interest rates were ten percent, and rates may now have decreased to seven percent. If

Table 20–12 Interest Rate Swap Payments

Payments	Hospital A	Hospital B	Broker
To bondholders	715 bps	Variable + 40 bps	0
To broker	Variable + 15 bps	750 bps	Variable + 765 bps
From broker to A	740 bps	0	740 bps
From broker to B	0	Variable + 10 bps	Variable + 10 bps
Net payment	Variable − 10 bps	780 bps	15 bps
Advantage	35 bps	30 bps	15 bps

HCA has entered into interest rate swap agreements to manage its exposure to fluctuations in interest rates. These swap agreements involve the exchange of fixed- and variable-rate interest payments between two parties based on common notional principal amounts and maturity dates. Pay-floating swaps effectively convert fixed-rate obligations to LIBOR indexed variable-rate instruments. The notional amounts and timing of interest payments in these agreements match the related liabilities. The notional amounts of the swap agreements represent amounts used to calculate the exchange of cash flows and are not assets or liabilities of HCA. Any market risk or opportunity associated with these swap agreements is offset by the opposite market impact on the related debt. HCA's credit risk related to these agreements is considered low because the swap agreements are with creditworthy financial institutions. The interest payments under these agreements are settled on a net basis.

The following table sets forth HCA's interest rate swap agreements at December 31, 2005 (dollars in millions):

	Notional Amount	Transaction Date	Fair Value
Pay-floating interest rate swap	$500	June 2006	0
Pay-floating interest rate swap	350	November 2008	(11)
Pay-floating interest rate swap	500	December 2009	14)

The fair value of the interest rate swaps at December 31, 2005 represents the estimated amounts HCA would have paid upon termination of these agreements. The fair values were based on valuations obtained from the financial institutions with which HCA has the interest rate swap agreements.

At December 31, 2005 and 2004, the fair values of cash and cash equivalents, accounts receivable, and accounts payable approximated carrying values due to the short-term nature of these instruments. The estimated fair values of other financial instruments subject to fair value disclosures are generally determined based on quoted market prices. The estimated fair values and the related carrying amounts are as follows (dollars in millions):

	2005		2004	
	Carrying Amount	Fair Value	Carrying Amount	Fair Value
Assets:				
Investments	$2,384	$2,284	$2,322	$2,322
Interest Rate Swaps			10	10
Liabilities				
Long Term Debt	$10,475	$10,733	$10,530	$10,789
Interest Rate Swaps	25	25	—	—

the present lower interest rate could be substituted for the original rate, a major improvement in net income could result. Other reasons for wishing to retire an existing indebtedness early might be:

1. to avoid onerous covenants in the existing indenture.
2. to take advantage of changes in bond ratings.
3. to take advantage of changes in policy regarding tax-exempt financing.

Whatever the reason, most health care issues, in fact, do not remain outstanding for their full life cycles; most are retired early.

The following are two common ways of retiring an issue early: (1) refinancing and (2) refunding. In a refinancing situation, the issuer buys back the outstanding bonds from the investors. This can be accomplished in one of two ways. First, the issuer may have the option of an early call. If the outstanding bonds are callable, the issuer would notify the present bondholders that the bonds are being called and should be ten-

dered for payment. The principal or face value would then be paid, along with any call premium plus accrued interest. A second way to effect a refinancing would be for the issuer to buy back the bonds in open-market transactions or to send a letter to existing bondholders, offering to buy the bonds at some stated dollar amount.

Early retirement of existing bonds also can be accomplished through refunding. In a refunding situation, the outstanding bonds are not acquired by the issuer, and the present bondholders continue to maintain their investment. Although the refunding does not actually retire the bonds, the bonds are not shown on the issuer's financial statements, and the covenants present in the indenture are now voided. The process of voiding existing indenture covenants and removing the bonds from the issuer's financial statements is called defeasance. In effect, defeasance in a refunding situation involves the deposit of a sum of money with the bond trustee, which is then used to buy specially-designated securities of the federal government. With these securities, there is a guarantee that all future interest and principal payments can be met from the proceeds controlled by the bond trustee.

The following is a simple example to illustrate the refunding process: On January 1, 2008, $1 million of 15-percent, level-debt service bonds are issued. The bonds have a five year life. The earliest call date is January 1, 2010. No call premium is involved. On January 1, 2009, interest rates have decreased to seven percent, and management advance-refunds the January 1, 2008 issue. In this example, the original issue would have the debt service schedule included in Table 20–13.

To retire or advance-refund the issue on January 1, 2009, management must place on deposit with a trustee a sum of money that will guarantee payment of the following amounts on January 1, 2010 (the earliest call date):

Interest due Jan. 1, 2010	$127,750
Debt principal due Jan. 1, 2010	170,570
Ending debt principal on Jan. 1, 2010	681,110
	$979,430

If management borrows all the funds necessary to meet the $979,430 payment on January 1, 2010, how much must it borrow on January 1, 2009? Ignoring placement fees and other debt issuance costs, the hospital would borrow $915,360. Why $915,360? It is assumed that the hospital will be able to invest the proceeds at seven percent, the effective interest rate on January 1, 2009 (1.07 × $915,360 = $979,430). In tax-exempt issues, an arbitrage restriction limits investment yields for all practical purposes to the interest rate of the refunding issue.

Are there any real savings in debt service costs? Yes; the new issue schedule in Table 20–14 shows an-

nual savings of $28,080 ($298,320 − $270,240) for the next four years.

Thus far, the refinancing looks good. However, there is an accounting loss that must be recorded. At the end of the first year (January 1, 2009), the value for the old debt, $851,680, will be removed from the balance sheet. But the defeased debt will be replaced by $915,360 of new debt, and this will reduce income in that year by $63,680 ($915,360 − $851,680). This will be treated as an extraordinary loss during the period in which refunding takes place.

A "real-world" case may make the magnitude of these numbers more apparent. A hospital recently refunded $65 million of two-year-old debt with $79 million of new debt at a lower effective interest rate. Estimated savings in debt service over the life of the issue were $22 million, but there was an accounting loss of approximately $13 million during the initial year. More important, this loss reduced the hospital's ratio of equity to assets from 26 percent to 16 percent. This is a sizable reduction that could have some impact on future credit availability. Many lenders establish target equity-to-debt ratios beyond which they will not lend funds at reasonable interest rates.

In summary, refunding to take advantage of reduced interest rates usually makes a lot of economic sense. But the presence of an accounting loss should be considered, especially its potential impact on future credit availability.

SUMMARY

The major sources of capital financing available to health care firms may be categorized as (1) equity and (2) debt. Equity has become an important source of

Table 20–13 Debt Service Schedule of January 2008 Issue

Date	Interest	Principal	Total Debt Service	Ending Debt Principal
Jan. 1, 2009	$150,000	$148,320	$298,320	$851,680
Jan. 1, 2010	127,750	170,570	298,320	681,110
Jan. 1, 2011	102,170	196,150	298,320	484,960
Jan. 1, 2012	72,740	225,580	298,320	259,380
Jan. 1, 2013	38,940	259,380	298,320	0

Table 20–14 Debt Service Schedule of January 2009 Issue

Date	Interest	Principal	Total Debt Service	Ending Debt	Savings in Debt Service
Jan. 1, 2010	$64,080	$206,160	$270,240	$709,200	$28,080
Jan. 1, 2011	49,640	220,600	270,240	488,600	28,080
Jan. 1, 2012	34,200	236,040	270,240	252,560	28,080
Jan. 1, 2013	17,680	252,560	270,240	0	28,080

capital, even for traditional tax-exempt health care firms. Corporate restructuring can greatly facilitate the process of accessing equity capital. However, long-term debt probably will continue to represent the major source of capital for most health care firms. Evaluation of alternative sources of long-term debt requires more than a simple comparison of interest rates. The impact of other factors also should be carefully reviewed to determine the overall attractiveness of alternative financing packages.

ASSIGNMENTS

1. Explain the term defeasance. What does it mean?

2. Assuming a normal or typical yield curve (that is, upward sloping), discuss the advantages and disadvantages of borrowing money for a major construction program with three-year term financing.

3. When is a master trust indenture used, and what is its value?

4. Under what circumstances might your firm be interested in issuing zero-coupon bonds?

5. In an advance refunding of debt, accounting gains or losses usually occur. Under what conditions could there be an accounting gain?

6. United Hospital has received a leasing proposal from Leasing, Inc., for a Siemens cardiac catheterization unit. The terms are:

   - Five-year lease
   - Annual payments of $200,000 payable one year in advance
   - Payment of property tax estimated to be $23,000 annually
   - Renewal at end of year 5 at fair market value

   Alternatively, United Hospital can buy the catheterization unit for $725,000. This purchase would require United Hospital to debt-finance this equipment. It anticipates a bank loan with an initial down payment of $125,000 and a three-year term loan at 16 percent with equal principal payments. The residual value of the equipment at year 5 is estimated to be $225,000. The lease is treated as an operating lease. Depreciation is calculated on a straight-line basis. Assuming a discount rate of 14 percent, what financing option should United Hospital select? Assume that there is no reimbursement of capital costs.

7. Nutty Hospital wishes to advance-refund its existing 15-percent long-term debt. The present $30,000,000 is not callable until five years from today. The payout on the issue over the next five years is as presented in Table 20–15.

Table 20–15 Nutty Hospital Debt Service Schedule

	Interest	Principal	Total
End of year 1	$4,500,000	$1,000,000	$5,500,000
End of year 2	4,350,000	1,000,000	5,350,000
End of year 3	4,200,000	1,000,000	5,200,000
End of year 4	4,050,000	1,000,000	5,050,000
End of year 5	3,900,000	1,000,000	4,900,000

At the end of the fifth year, the debt ($25,000,000 outstanding balance at that time) may be called with a ten percent penalty. If present interest rates are ten percent and the investment rate on the funds to be received from the new issue cannot exceed ten percent, what amount must Nutty Hospital borrow today? Assume that underwriting fees and other issuance costs will be five percent of the issue and that all debt service on the old issue must be met from the proceeds of the refunding issue and related investment income.

8. You have the option of leasing an asset for $100,000 per year, with payments to be made at the end of each year of use. This lease cannot be cancelled. Alternatively, you may buy the asset for $248,700. For reimbursement purposes, the lease must be capitalized. If the asset is purchased, it will be debt-financed with $210,000 of three-year serial notes (that is, $70,000 of principal will be repaid each year). The effective interest rate on this loan will be eight percent. Assume that the asset has an allowable useful life of three years with no estimated salvage value.

   - Determine the amount of expense that would be reported during each of the three years under the two financing plans.
   - Assuming that 80 percent of all reported capital expenses are reimbursed and that the discount rate is six percent, determine the present value of the asset in these two methods of financing.

9. Happy Valley is considering moving from its present location into a new 200-bed facility. The estimated construction cost for the new facility is $40 million. The hospital has no internal funds and is considering a 20-year mortgage with interest scheduled to be eight percent. The issue will be repaid over 20 years with equal annual principal payments of $2 million. Interest expense would decline each year by $160,000.

   The cost of the plant and fixed equipment would be 80 percent of the total cost or $32 million, and the movable equipment would be $8 million. The movable equipment would need to be replaced in ten years, and it is estimated that the replacement cost would be $17,271,200 (inflation is assumed to be eight percent per year). The plant and fixed equipment would need to be replaced in 30 years at a cost of $322,006,400 (inflation again assumed to be eight percent per year). All costs reflect only the investment required to provide inpatient services. A separate analysis will be done for outpatient services.

   Happy Valley anticipates that its operation will generate about 9700 discharges per year. The hospital anticipates that its operating costs, excluding capital costs, will be $4,000 per discharge, or $38,800,000 in the first full year of operation.

   The payer mix at Happy Valley is expected to be 60 percent Medicare and Medicaid on the inpatient side. These payers will pay approximately $4,400 per discharge. This payment reflects both operating and capital cost payments. Approximately ten percent of Happy Valley's operating and capital costs will be paid by payers who reimburse the hospital on a cost-related basis for both capital and operating costs. The remaining 30 percent of Happy Valley's business will be charge-based, but it is expected that discounts to commercial insurers and bad debt and charity write-offs will average 30 percent.

   Assuming that Happy Valley wishes to break even on a cash-flow basis during the first year of operation, what charge per discharge must be set? If the hospital wanted to include an element in its rate structure to reflect replacement cost of the building and movable equipment, what additional amount would that be? Assume that 50 percent of the movable equipment cost would be debt financed and 80 percent of the building and fixed equipment would be debt financed. Also assume that the hospital can earn ten percent on any invested money, so use ten percent as your discount rate.

10. Mayberry Hospital is considering a joint venture relationship with your physicians to acquire a full-body CT scanner. Projected revenues and expenses for the scanner are presented in Table 20–16.

Table 20–16 CT Scanner Financial Forecast

	Year 1	Year 2	Year 3	Year 4	Year 5
Revenues	$521,000	$531,000	$542,000	$533,000	$564,000
Less bad debts and discounts	52,100	53,100	54,200	53,300	56,400
Net revenues	468,900	477,900	487,800	479,700	507,600
Expenses					
Wages and employee benefits	$60,000	$63,000	$66,150	$69,459	$72,930
Maintenance	55,000	57,750	60,638	63,669	66,853
Supplies	20,000	21,000	22,050	23,153	24,310
Rent	18,000	18,900	19,845	20,837	21,879
Administrative	10,000	10,500	11,025	11,576	12,155
Utilities	5,000	5,250	5,513	5,788	6,078
insurance	5,000	5,250	5,513	5,788	6,078
Taxes	10,000	10,000	10,000	10,000	10,000
Depreciation	94,050	137,940	131,670	131,670	131,670
Other	40,620	33,384	25,271	16,176	5,977
Total expenses	317,670	362,974	357,675	358,116	357,930
Net income before tax or interest	$151,230	$114,926	$130,125	$121,585	$149,670

The scanner is expected to cost $627,000 and have a useful life of five years. Two possible financing plans have been proposed. The first plan would be a limited partnership arrangement. There would be 34 shares; 33 would be sold to investors for $19,000 apiece (total funds generated would be $627,000). The 34th would be retained by the hospital for its development effort. In the second financing plan, a $380,000 level-debt service plan with a five-year maturity and interest at ten percent would be arranged. The remainder of the funding would be generated through the sale of 33 limited partnership shares at $7,485 per share ($247,000). Again, a 34th share would be issued to the hospital for its development efforts. Assuming that a 30 percent marginal tax rate will exist, project cash flow per partnership unit under each financing alternative for each of the five years.

SOLUTIONS AND ANSWERS

1. Defeasance means that upon final payment of all interest and principal, the rights of the bond trustee cease to exist; that is, they are defeased. The security covenants in an indenture also may be satisfied through the creation of a trust (escrow) in which sufficient monies are held to guarantee payment at some future date. Defeasance means that the issue defeased is no longer an obligation of the issuer and can be removed from the issuer's books.

2. The typical upward-sloping yield curve implies that a three-year interest rate probably will be much lower than a twenty- to twenty-five-year rate. Therefore, cost will be lower with a three-year construction loan. At the end of the third year, however, permanent financing must be sought; also, there is no guarantee that interest rates will not have increased during the period or that financing will be available at the end of the third year.

3. A master trust indenture usually pledges the assets and revenues of several firms in a combined financing package. It is often used by health care systems to gain better access to capital and lower interest rates.

4. Zero-coupon bonds are especially desirable if the issuer's effective interest rate on the bonds is well below the issuer's cost of capital. In a zero coupon bond issue, the postponement of interest payment maximizes the possibility for additional arbitrage, that is, for investing at a yield greater than the cost of funds.

5. Accounting gains usually take place when the advance-refunding issue has a higher rate of interest than the refunded issue. Accounting losses often occur when the reverse is true, or the refunding interest rate is less than the initial borrowing rate.

6. United Hospital's financing options for the cardiac catheterization unit are detailed in Table 20–17. From the data in Table 20–17, it can be seen that purchase of the catheterization unit would produce a higher net present value cost, compared with a lease.

Table 20–17 Lease/Purchase Analysis

Item	Amount before Reimbursement	Amount after Reimbursement	Years	Present Value Factor (14%)	Present Value
Lease					
Rent	$200,000	$200,000	0	1.000	$200,000
Rent	200,000	200,000	1–4	2.914	582,800
Property tax*	23,000	23,000	1–5	3.433	78,959
			Net present value cost of lease		$861,759
Purchase					
Down payment	$125,000	$125,000	0	1.000	$125,000
Principal	200,000	200,000	1-3	2.322	464,400
Interest	96,000	96,000	1	0.877	84,192
Interest	64,000	64,000	2	0.769	49,216
Interest	32,000	32,000	3	0.675	21,600
Salvage	(225,000)	(225,000)	5	0.519	(116,775)
			Net present value of purchase		$627,633

*Property tax would be passed on to the lessee or hospital. There is no property tax on the purchase because the hospital is a tax-exempt firm.

7. Nutty Hospital's present borrowing needs are detailed in Table 20–18.

Table 20–18 Nutty Hospital Refunding Requirements

Item	Amount Required	Years	Present Value Factor (10%)	Present Value
Debt service-year 1	$5,500,000	1	0.909	$4,999,500
Debt service-year 2	5,350,000	2	0.826	4,419,100
Debt service-year 3	5,200,000	3	0.751	3,905,200
Debt service-year 4	5,050,000	4	0.683	3,449,150
Debt service-year 5	4,900,000	5	0.621	3,042,900
Principal at year 5	25,000,000	5	0.621	15,525,500
Call premium	2,500,000	5	0.621	1,552,500
				$36,893,850

Net present value

Amount borrowed = $36,893,850/.95 = $38,835,631

8. The data in Tables 20-19 and 20-20 show the comparative expense and present values for leasing versus debt financing the asset during the three-year period.

Table 20–19 Leasing Versus Purchase Analysis

Leasing Expenses

	Year 1	Year 2	Year 3
Lease payment per year(3 Yr. @ 10%)	$100,000	$100,000	$100,000
Interest @10%	$24,870	$17,357	$9,073
Principal payment	$75,130	$82,643	$90,927
Ending principal	$173,570	$90,927	$0
Depreciation expense	$82,900	$82,900	$82,900
Total expenses (Interest and Depreciation)	**$107,770**	**$100,257**	**$91,973**
Debt financing expenses			
Interest @8%	$16,800	$11,200	$5,600
Principal payment	$70,000	$70,000	$70,000
Ending principal	$140,000	$70,000	$0
Depreciation expense	$82,900	$82,900	$82,900
Expenses (Interest and Deprec.)	**$99,700**	**$94,100**	**$88,500**
Expense difference			
Leasing less debt	$8,070	$6,157	$3,473

Table 20–20 Leasing Versus Debt Finance-Present Value Analysis

Item	Amount Before Reimbursement	Amount After Reimbursement	Years	PV Factor	Present Value
Lease financing					
Depreciation	−$82,900	−$66,320	1 to 3	2.673	−$177,273
Interest	$24,870	$4,974	1	0.943	$4,690
Interest	$17,357	$3,471	2	0.890	$3,090
Interest	$9,073	$1,815	3	0.840	$1,524
Principal	$75,130	$75,130	1	0.943	$70,848
Principal	$82,643	$82,643	2	0.890	$73,552
Principal	$90,927	$90,927	3	0.840	$76,379
Net present value cost of lease					$52,809
Debt financing					
Depreciation	−$82,900	−$66,320	1 to 3	2.673	−$177,273
Down payment	$38,700	$38,700	Present	1.000	$38,700
Principal payment	$70,000	$70,000	1 to 3	2.673	$187,110
Interest	$16,800	$3,360	1	0.943	$3,168
Interest	$11,200	$2,240	2	0.890	$1,994
Interest	$5,600	$1,120	3	0.840	$941
Net present value cost of purchase					$54,640

9. Table 20-21 reflects the required charge that Happy Valley must set to break even on a cash-flow basis and the additional charge required to cover the funded depreciation requirement necessary for eventual replacement.

Table 20–21 Happy Valley Required Rate Structure

Cash Expenditures

Principal amount	$2,000,000
Interest payment	$3,200,000
Operating costs	$38,800,000
Total cash costs	$44,000,000

Reimbursement

Medicare & Medicaid ($4,400 × .6 × 9,700)	$25,608,000
Reimbursed interest (.10 × $3,200,000)	$320,000
Reimbursed operating costs (.10 × $38,800,000)	$3,880,000
Reimbursed equip. depreciation (.10 × $800,000)	$80,000
Reimbursed build. depreciation (.10 × $1,066,667)	$106,667
Total payments	$29,994,667

Required charge to cover cash expenditures

Remaining cash costs to be covered	$14,005,333
Number of charge paying discharges (.3 × 9,700)	2,910
Required charge without discount	$4,812.83
Required charge with discount (30%)	$6,875.47

Additional requirements for replacement

Equipment (.5 × $17,271,200/ F(10%,10 Years)	$541,838
Plant (.2 × $322,006,400/F(10%,30Years)	$391,506
Total annual deposit	$933,344
Number of charge-paying discharges	2,910
Required charge without discount	$320.74
Required charge with discount	$458.20

10. The data in Table 20–22 show the projected cash flow per partnership unit under the two financing alternatives.

Table 20–22 CT Scanner Cash Flow Per Share

	Years				
	1	2	3	4	5
Alternative 1—no debt					
Income before tax and interest	$151,230	$114,926	$130,125	$121,585	$149,670
Less income tax	45,369	34,478	39,038	36,476	44,901
Income after tax	$105,861	$80,448	$91,088	$85,110	$104,769
Add depreciation	94,050	137,940	131,670	131,670	131,670
Cash flow	199,911	218,388	222,758	216,780	236,439
Cash flow per share (34 shares)	5,880	6,423	6,552	6,376	6,954
Percentage return	30.9%	33.8%	34.5%	33.6%	36.6%
Alternative #2—debt financing					
Income before tax and interest	$151,230	$114,926	$130,125	$121,585	$149,670
Less interest	38,000	31,776	24,929	17,398	9,111
Taxable income	113,230	83,150	105,196	104,187	140,559
Less income tax	33,969	24,945	31,559	31,256	42,168
Income after tax	79,261	58,205	73,637	72,931	98,391
Add depreciation	94,050	137,940	131,670	131,670	131,670
Less principal	62,243	68,467	75,314	82,845	91,132
Cash flow	$111,068	$127,678	$129,994	$121,756	$138,930
Cash flow per share (34 shares)	$3,267	$3,755	$3,823	$3,581	$4,086
Percentage return	43.6%	50.2%	51.1%	47.8%	54.6%
Debt Service for $380,000 Loan					
Total debt service (5 Yr. @ 10%)	$100,243	$100,243	$100,243	$100,243	$100,243
Interest @ 10%	$38,000	$31,776	$24,929	$17,398	$9,111
Prinicpal payment	$62,243	$68,467	$75,314	$82,845	$91,132
Ending principal	$317,757	$249,290	$173,977	$91,132	$0

Working Capital and Cash Management

After studying this chapter, you should be able to do the following:

1. Explain why cash management is especially crucial in most sectors of the health care industry.
2. Explain what working capital is and why it is needed.
3. Describe the activities covered in the cash budget that affect working capital.
4. Describe the tools that an organization manager can use to manage receivables.
5. List the external resources available to an organization for its short-term financing needs.
6. List and explain the criteria that should be used when investing an organization's cash in the short term.

Dr. Noah Johnson is the chair of the Ear, Nose and Throat (ENT) Department in a hospital. As the end of the month approached, he decided that the revenues for the current month already were above budget. Therefore, he decided to hedge his bets for the following month by delaying some of the end-of-month revenues until the following month. This was not difficult to accomplish. The charges simply were not submitted for a few days. The few days were followed by a weekend and before charges were actually posted to the account, seven days had passed without posting any charges.

The loss of revenues became evident in accounting. An inquiry into the situation found that there were no problems with the charging system, but rather that the delay was intentional. Soon, everyone was angry. The ENT Department had not followed the hospital's charging policy. Accounting was angry because the delay distorted the monthly revenues.

Accrual accounting matches the revenue and expenses in the month they actually occur. The chair of the ENT Department had bypassed the process and moved charges into the wrong month. This distorted reporting of the results of operations for the period. Also, this information is used for forward planning. Therefore, the cyclical nature of revenues may be distorted going forward.

Finally, billing was upset. They collect charges four days after discharge, and on the fifth day they create and send the bill. In this case they had some charges not posted until the bill had been sent. Some minor charges would never be billed, because it costs more to bill them than the cash received. Other charges would be rebilled, but the additional cost was unnecessary.

In the end, the most significant financial result was the lost reimbursement on some of the late charges. Organizationally, relations were strained, and information was distorted. This situation highlights the principle that the collection of financial information should not be manipulated, but rather analyzed.

Few topics in finance are more important than cash and investment management. Cash is the lifeblood of a business operation. A firm that controls its access to cash and the generation of cash usually will survive and thrive. A firm that ignores or manages its cash position poorly may fail. Experience has shown that more firms fail because of a lack of ready cash than for any other reason—even firms with sound profitability. It is important, therefore, to recognize and appreciate that profit and cash management are not the same thing.

It would seem logical to expect that great volumes of literature would be devoted to such an important topic as cash and investment management. Unfortunately, this is not the case. Although a major portion of a financial manager's time is devoted to working capital problems, relatively little space is devoted to them in most financial management textbooks. A typical text often contains only several chapters that deal with working capital management and perhaps a single chapter that discusses cash management.

Cash management is probably more important in the health care industry than in many other industries, but often it is less understood. Health care financial executives frequently advance through the accounting route.. Many health care financial executives traditionally think of cash management in terms of receivables control. They often believe that better cash management will result if accounts receivable can be reduced or the collection cycle shortened. Although accounts receivable management in health care organizations is clearly important, limiting attention to this one area is myopic. Good cash management should focus not only on the acceleration of receivables, but also on the complete cash conversion cycle. Reduction of the cash conversion cycle, along with the related investment of surplus funds, should be a critical objective of financial managers.

Many hospitals and health care firms often are willing to allow their banks to handle most of their cash management decisions. Although this strategy is acceptable in some situations, it may produce a result that is less than optimal. Risks are sometimes unnecessarily increased or yields on investments are sacrificed. Real or perceived conflicts of interest also exist if the bank is represented on the health care firm's governing board.

LEARNING OBJECTIVE 1

Explain why cash management is especially crucial in most sectors of the health care industry.

Why is cash and investment management important to health care executives? Hospitals have large sums of investment eligible funds compared with firms of similar size in other industries. Hospitals and other health care firms are also more likely to have greater investment management needs than other industries for several reasons:

* Many health care firms are voluntary, not-for-profit firms, and must set aside funds for replacement of plants and equipment. Investor-owned firms can rely on the issuance of new stockholders' equity to finance some of their replacement needs.
* Health care firms are increasingly beginning to self-insure all or a portion of their professional liability risk. This requires that sizable investment pools be available to meet estimated actuarial needs.
* Many health care firms receive gifts and endowments. Although these sums may not be large for

individual firms, they can provide additional sources of investment.

* Many health care firms also have sizable funding requirements for defined-benefit pension plans and debt service requirements associated with the issuance of bonds. These funds are usually held by a trustee.

With greater investments, one should expect to find greater levels of investment income. For the average acute care hospital in 2004, approximately 25 percent of total net income was derived from non-operating revenue sources, such as donations and investment income. Ninteen percent of total net income was investment income (State of the Hospital Industry 2006 Edition, Cleverley and Associates).

CASH AND INVESTMENT MANAGEMENT STRUCTURE

Effective cash management is often related to the cash conversion cycle, as depicted in Figure 21–1. In its simplest form, the cash conversion cycle represents the time that it takes a firm to go from an outlay of cash to purchase the needed factors of production, such as labor and supplies, to the actual collection of cash for the produced product or service, such as a completed treatment for a given patient. Usually, the objectives in cash management are to minimize the collection period and to maximize the payment period. Tradeoffs often exist; for example, accelerating collection of re-

ceivables may result in lost sales, and delaying payments to vendors could result in increased prices.

LEARNING OBJECTIVE 2

Explain what working capital is and why it is needed.

The primary tool used in cash planning is the cash budget. (Cash budgeting is discussed more fully in Chapter 22.) Cash balances are affected by changes in working capital over time. Working capital may be defined as the difference between current assets and current liabilities. The following items are usually included in these two categories:

1. Current assets
   * cash and investments
   * accounts receivable
   * inventories
   * other current assets
2. Current liabilities
   * accounts payable
   * accrued salaries and wages
   * accrued expenses
   * notes payable
   * current position of long-term debt

LEARNING OBJECTIVE 3

Describe the activities covered in the cash budget that affect working capital.

The cash budget focuses on four major activities that affect working capital:

1. Purchase of resources
2. Production/sale of service
3. Billing
4. Collection

These activities represent intervals in the cash conversion cycle. The purchase of resources relates to the acquisition of supplies and labor, such as the level of inventory necessary to maintain realistic production schedules and the staff required to ensure adequate provision of services. Production and sale are virtually

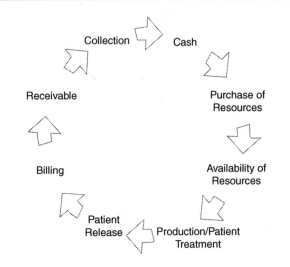

Figure 21–1 Cash Conversion Cycle

the same in the health care industry; there is no inventory of products or services. However, there is a delay between the production of service and final delivery. A patient may be in the hospital for ten to fifteen days or in a skilled nursing facility for two months, which could be regarded as the final point of sale. Billing represents the interval between the release or discharge of a patient and the generation of a bill. Collection represents the interval between the generation of a bill and the actual collection of the cash from the patient or the patient's third-party payer.

Estimating these four intervals is critical to cash budgeting, and therefore, cash planning. For example, the average collection period will dramatically influence the need for cash assets. During periods when sales are expected to increase, a long collection period will require the hospital to finance a larger amount of working capital in the form of increased receivables. The hospital must pay for its factors of production (that is, supplies and labor) at the beginning of the cycle and wait to receive payment from its customers at the end of the cycle.

The previous example also illustrates why a focus on a static measure of liquidity, such as a current ratio, sometimes can be deceiving. A rapid buildup in sales results in a large increase in accounts receivable, which increases the current ratio. Liquidity position, however, might not be improved in this case. The speed with which these receivables can be turned into cash is also an extremely important measure of liquidity.

The major purpose of a cash budget, an example of which is shown in Table 21–1, is to prepare an accurate estimate of future cash flows. With this estimate, the firm can arrange for short-term financing from a bank through a line of credit if it projects a period of

Table 21–1 Sample Cash Budget

| | First Quarter | | | | | |
	January	February	March	Second Quarter	Third Quarter	Fourth Quarter
Receipts from operations	$300,000	$310,000	$320,000	$1,000,000	$1,100,000	$1,100,000
Less disbursements from operations	280,000	280,000	300,000	940,000	1,000,000	1,000,000
Cash available from operations	$20,000	$30,000	$20,000	$60,000	$100,000	$100,000
Other receipts						
Increase in mortgage payable				500,000		
Sale of fixed assets		20,000				
Unrestricted income—endowed		_____	40,000	40,000	40,000	40,000
Total other receipts	0	$20,000	$40,000	$540,000	$40,000	$40,000
Other disbursements						
Mortgage payments			150,000		150,000	
Fixed-asset purchase				480,000		
Funded depreciation			30,000	130,000	30,000	30,000
Total other disbursements	0	0	180,000	610,000	180,000	30,000
Net cash gain (loss)	$20,000	$50,000	($120,000)	($10,000)	($40,000)	$110,000
Beginning cash balance	100,000	120,000	170,000	50,000	40,000	0
Ending cash	$120,000	$170,000	$50,000	$40,000	$0	$110,000
Desired level of cash	100,000	100,000	100,000	100,000	100,000	100,000
Cash above minimum needs (financing needs)	$20,000	$70,000	($50,000)	($60,000)	($100,000)	$10,000

Management of Working Capital 475

cash deficiency, or it can invest surplus funds. Because yields are usually higher on longer-term investments, an investment for a six-month term is likely to result in greater income than an investment broken down into two three-month cycles. The cash budget, then, is the key document in terms of providing information regarding short-term investment and short-term financing decisions. A key factor in these projections is the desired level of cash balances that the firm would like to maintain. Firms that set low cash requirement levels are assuming more risks. The entire cash management process can be broken down into five sequential steps.

1. Understand and manage the cash conversion cycle. In most situations, the objective is to minimize the required investment in working capital, when working capital is defined as current assets less current liabilities.
2. Develop a sound cash budget that accurately projects cash inflows and cash outflows during the planning horizon.

3. Establish the firm's minimum required cash balance. This level should be set in a manner consistent with the firm's overall risk assumption posture.
4. Arrange for working capital loans during those periods when the cash budget indicates that short-term financing will be needed.
5. Invest cash surpluses in a way that will maximize the expected yield to the firm, subject to a prudent assumption of risk.

MANAGEMENT OF WORKING CAPITAL

The management of working capital items is related to short-term bank financing and investment of cash surpluses, which are discussed in subsequent sections of this chapter. The balance sheet for ABC Medical Center in Table 21–2 presents a useful way to examine the relevant items of working capital management. As examples, the following two categories are discussed: (1) receivables and (2) accounts payable and accrued salaries and wages.

Table 21–2 ABC Medical Center, Consolidated Balance Sheets, June 30, 2008 and 2007

	Assets	
	2008	2007
Current assets		
Cash	$1,216,980	$362,422
Investments	4,042,407	4,597,806
Patient accounts receivable (2008, $7,356,120; 2007, $6,253,629), less allowance for uncollectables	5,892,339	5,143,471
Other receivables		
Medicare	2,672,612	2,113,655
Miscellaneous	213,726	164,631
Inventories	1,302,598	1,174,295
Prepaid expenses	1,021,972	249,455
Current portion of deferred receivables from Medicare	454,404	502,904
Assets held by trustee	180,000	247,181
Total current assets	$16,997,038	$14,555,820
Other assets		
Investments	$10,642,621	$10,983,125
Accounts receivables—affiliated companies	4,510,105	2,036,436
Notes receivable—affiliated company	700,000	700,000

continues

Table 21–2 *continued*

	Assets	
	2008	*2007*
Assets held by trustee		
Temporary cash account		
Construction fund	2,717,846	59,643
Sinking fund	6,751,942	4,018,948
Interest receivable	118,142	6,112,530
Self-insurance funds	10,942,749	94,231
Unamortized debt issuance expenses	934,535	7,875,602
Investment in ABC Insurance, Ltd.	209,655	954,078
Deferred receivables for Medicare	2,620,162	–
Prepaid pension cost	840,449	3,074,567
Unamortized past service cost	1,784,160	–
Total other assets	$42,772,366	$35,909,160
Property, plant, and equipment		
Land	$1,654,394	$1,649,912
Buildings	36,505,277	34,504,398
Improvements to land and leaseholds	1,272,205	1,263,959
Fixed equipment	8,812,615	8,713,615
Movable equipment	20,290,037	15,461,276
Capitalized leases	2,998,295	3,293,693
Total property, plant, and equipment	$71,532,823	$64,886,853
Less allowance for depreciation	27,763,195	22,037,503
	43,769,628	42,849,350
Construction and other work in progress	$4,396,463	$3,869,866
Total property, plant, and equipment	$48,166,091	$46,719,216
Total assets	$107,935,495	$97,184,196

	Liabilities fund balances	
	2008	*2007*
Current liabilities	$2,297,672	$2,531,257
Accounts payable trade	1,366,777	1,035,496
Accrued salaries and wages	1,232,586	1,119,800
Accrued Medicare liability	317,302	1,881,895
Accrued indigent care assesment	1,170,001	1,061,742
Other accrued liabilities	611,230	444,916
Current portion of long-term debt	1,528,910	1,442,420
Total current liabilities	$8,524,478	$9,517,526
Other liabilities		
Accounts payable—affiliated companies	$1,993,815	—
Self-insurance liabilities	8,904,000	$7,048,000
Total other liabilities	$10,897,815	$7,048,000
Long-term, less current maturities		
Series B bonds, less unamortized discount		
(2000, $1, 144, 348; 1995, $1, 186, 425)	$45,745,652	$46,063,575
Notes payable	3,902,113	1,888,504
Capital leases payable	127,535	595,407
Total long-term debt	$49,775,300	$48,547,486
Net assets	$38,737,952	$32,071,204
Total liabilities and net assets	$107,935,545	$97,184,216

LEARNING OBJECTIVE 4

Describe the tools that an organization manager can use to manage receivables.

Receivables

Industry experience suggests that receivables constitute the most critical, but not exclusive, area of importance in cash management. In general, accounts receivable usually represent about 60 to 70 percent of a hospital's total investment in current assets. ABC Medical Center has $8,778,677 ($5,892,339 + $2,672,612 + $213,726) of receivables, or 51.6 percent of its total current assets, in 2008. This value is below the range cited previously, largely because ABC Medical Center has a relatively low value for days in accounts receivable (50.3 days). This situation, of course, is favorable and is an objective of most financial managers. In general, the following three objectives are usually associated with accounts receivable management:

1. Minimize lost charges
2. Minimize write-offs for uncollectable accounts
3. Minimize the accounts receivable collection cycle

All three objectives are important, but our attention will be directed at the third—minimizing the collection cycle. Figure 21–2 provides a schematic that predicts intervals involved in the entire accounts receivable cycle. The following intervals usually exist in the hospital inpatient accounts receivable collection cycle:

- Admission to discharge
- Discharge to bill completion
- Bill completion to receipt by payer
- Receipt by payer to mailing of payment
- Mailing of payment to receipt by hospital
- Receipt by hospital to deposit in bank

Figure 21–2 also provides the estimated time that could be involved in each interval, but these numbers vary widely among hospitals and payer categories within hospitals. They are intended only to show the relative importance of each interval in the overall accounts receivable collection cycle. The total number of days represented in Figure 21–2 is 64, which is reasonably close to the national average of 62 days during 2003.

Admission to Discharge (5 Days)

Shortening this interval is not the critical objective from an accounts receivable perspective. This does not imply, however, that a reduction in length of stay is not an objective, because clearly it is. With fixed prices per case, reduced length of stay is particularly desirable from a cost management viewpoint.

In terms of managing the accounts receivable cycle, the real solution appears to be what occurs during this interval to expedite later collection. The following specific suggestions are provided:

- Determine whether interim billings are possible for patients with a long length of stay. Some third-party payers permit interim billings if the length of stay exceeds a specified interval. Often, this is 21 days. Although there may be relatively few patients in this category, it is important to recognize that the absolute value of accounts receivable represented by these patients can be large.
- Use advance deposits for nonemergent admissions. If insurance coverage can be verified, estimates of the total deductible and copayment amounts can be made. These amounts can be requested from the patient before or during admission. In situations when this is not possible, a financing plan should be developed jointly between the hospital and the patient. Many patients appreciate being told beforehand what their insurance will pay and what their individual liability is likely to be.

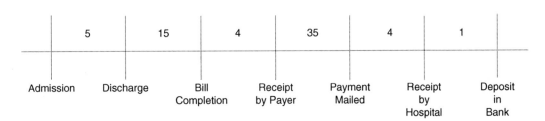

Figure 21–2 Accounts Receivable Collection Cycle in Days

- Obtain required insurance and eligibility information before admission for nonemergent patients. For emergency admissions, obtain the same data during the hospital stay. This will permit the preparation of a bill during, or shortly after, discharge.
- For patients with Health Savings Account (HSA) coverage, arrange for the deductible payment portion during patient registration.

Discharge to Bill Completion (15 Days)

Ideally, this interval should be reduced as much as possible. Although this may be an objective, there are clearly some cost/benefit tradeoffs to be evaluated. For example, speeding up the processing of bills is desirable only if the cost involved does not exceed the benefits of more rapid bill preparation. An acceleration of the billing process can also create a reduction in final payments if the acceleration results in some late charges not being posted to the final bill. Inaccurate coding could also result from an acceleration of billing that could cause later delays in payment or inaccurate payment amounts. Basic suggestions include the following:

- Implement more timely billing and remove "bottlenecks." Usually, bills are not prepared during discharge so that late charges can be posted. If certain ancillary departments experience constant delays, corrective steps should be taken to improve posting. A holding period longer than two to three days is probably not reasonable.
- Develop educational programs to show the effects of physicians delaying completing medical charts. Often, an incomplete medical chart is the reason for delay in billing. Physicians must be informed of the effect these delays have on the hospital. Some hospitals have suspended admitting privileges of physicians who are constantly delinquent. Although this strategy may not be useful in many hospitals, it is worth considering in some situations.

Bill Completion to Receipt by Payer (4 Days)

The estimated four-day length of this interval may be grossly overstated where electronic claim submission is utilized. Several steps may be useful in shortening this interval including the following:

- Consider electronic invoicing for large payers when this alternative is available. This decreases mail time to zero, and it may reduce the account

receivable cycle for these payers by as much as four days.
- Try to settle all outpatient accounts at the point of discharge or departure. Each outpatient should be presented with a bill at the point of departure, and payment should be requested at this time.
- Submit a bill for any deductible and copayment amounts for hospital inpatients at the point of discharge. Settlement should take place at this point if the patient has been advised previously of the total amount due.

Receipt by Payer to Mailing of Payment (35 Days)

This interval varies greatly by type of payer. Some self-pay patients may have outstanding accounts for more than a year. Insurance companies may take an inordinate amount of time to settle bills because of disputes over coverage or reasonableness. Steps to be considered include the following:

- Sell some accounts receivable. Until recently, hospitals could not legally sell Medicare accounts, but this is no longer true. More and more hospitals are considering selling accounts receivable because the rates of interest charged for these loans are relatively low. On a taxable basis, the interest rate will be slightly below prime for these asset-backed transactions.
- Use discounts for prompt payment. Many businesses have long provided discounts as financial incentives for early payment. This strategy may be used for self-pay portions of hospital bills and also for insurance payers. Sufficiently large discounts also can greatly reduce collection costs and write-offs. How large an inducement should be offered? This decision, of course, is firm-specific, but a five-percent reduction for payment during discharge does not seem excessive.
- Create a system to respond quickly to third-party requests for additional data. Third-party payers often delay payment until requested information has been received and reviewed. At a minimum, a log should be maintained that shows dates of requests and responses.
- Claim all bad debts on the Medicare deductible and copayment portion of hospital bills. Medicare is liable for payment of bad debts experienced on their patients. It is important, however, to document reasonable collection efforts on the part of

the hospital before Medicare liability for payment can be ensured.

- Make frequent follow-up telephone calls to detect problems or concerns with bills. In many situations, self-pay hospital bills are not paid because there is a disagreement over the amount of the bill. This type of dispute can be avoided by a non-threatening hospital employee promptly contacting the patient and inquiring about the patient's health and the amount of the bill. Sometimes this may be better handled by an independent party. When this approach has been used, reductions in bad debt write-offs have been large.

Payment Mailed to Receipt by Hospital (4 Days)

Mail time is the cause for this four-day interval. These delays cannot be prevented for most small, personal accounts. In the case of a government or large insurance payer, a courier service can be used. Checks are picked up as they become available. For large, out-of-town payers, a special courier arrangement can be used or direct deposits to an area bank can be initiated. Relatively large sums of money must be involved for these strategies to be cost effective. In addition, direct wire transfer of funds between payer and the health care provider's bank is also an alternative that makes great sense, if available. Many major commercial payers and public programs, such as Medicare and Medicaid, arrange for wire transfer of payments.

Receipt by Hospital to Deposit in Bank (1+ Days)

Perhaps the only effective way this interval can be shortened is through the use of a lockbox arrangement in which payments go directly to a post office box that is cleared at least once a day by bank employees. Bank employees deposit all payments, usually photocopy the checks, and send the copies—along with any enclosures—to the hospital for proper crediting. There is usually a cost for this service. The hospital must determine whether improvement in the cash flow, plus potential reduction in clerical costs, are worth the fee charged.

Accounts Payable and Accrued Salaries and Wages

Accounts payable and accrued salaries and wages represent spontaneous sources of financing. This means that these amounts are not usually negotiated, but vary directly with the level of operations. Table 21–2 shows that ABC Medical Center had $2,297,672 in accounts payable trade and $1,366,777 in accrued salaries and wages in 2008. In addition, $1,993,815 of accounts payable from affiliated companies also existed. These amounts are not small and represent a sizable proportion of ABC's total financing.

Managing accounts payable and accrued salaries is similar to the management of accounts receivable, except in a reverse direction. Instead of acceleration, most financial managers would like to slow payment to these accounts. A number of approaches, as discussed in the literature, attempt to do this. Several relevant approaches for a free-standing hospital are as follows:

- Delay payment of an account payable until the actual due date. Many hospitals often process invoices upon receipt and initiate payment even when the invoices are not due for several weeks or months. For example, many invoices for subscriptions to journals are sent out three to five months before their due dates. There is no reason to pay these invoices until they are actually due.
- Stretch accounts payable. This technique has been described frequently in the literature and is familiar to most individuals. Stretching accounts payable simply means delaying payment until some point after the due date. Although this technique is often used, the ethics of the method are clearly debatable. In addition, delays may cause a hospital's credit rating to deteriorate. Vendors eventually will be unwilling to grant credit, or they may alter payment terms.
- Change the frequency of payroll. Although not a popular decision with employees, lengthening the payroll period can provide a significant amount of additional financing that is virtually free. For example, ABC Medical Center has an estimated weekly payroll of approximately $1,150,000. If ABC changes its payroll period from a weekly to a biweekly basis, it can create an additional source of financing equal to one week's payroll, or $1,150,000. Investing that money at eight percent provides $92,000 in annual investment income. Fewer payroll periods may also reduce bookkeeping costs.
- Use banks in distant cities to pay vendors and employees. This method may delay check clearing and create a day or two of "float." Float is defined

as the difference between the bank balance and the checkbook balance. It also may be a questionable practice, depending on applicable state laws. With the advent of direct deposit for most employees, float is no longer a possibility.

- Schedule deposits to checking accounts to match expected disbursements on a daily basis. A daily cash report can be prepared for each account, using information obtained daily by calling the bank or accessing the account electronically. The report can thus reconcile data on beginning cash balances and disbursements expected to be made that day. Separate accounts for payroll are often maintained to recognize the predictability of check clearing. For example, payroll checks issued on a Friday may have a highly predictable pattern of check clearing. Knowledge of this distribution enables the treasurer to minimize the amount of funds needed in the account on any given day to meet actual disbursements and thus maximize the amount of invested funds.

LEARNING OBJECTIVE 5

List the external resources available to an organization for its short-term financing needs.

SHORT-TERM BANK FINANCING

Many health care firms may experience a short-term need for funds during their operating cycles. The need for funds may have resulted from a predictable seasonality in the receipt and disbursement of cash or it may represent an unexpected business event, such as a strike. Commercial banks are the predominant sources of short-term loans, but other sources are also available. Several common arrangements used by health care firms to arrange for short-term loans include those discussed below.

Single-Payment Loan

The single-payment loan is the simplest credit arrangement and is usually given for a specific purpose, such as the purchase of inventory. The note can be either on a discount or an add-on basis. In the discount arrangement, the interest is computed and deducted

from the face value of the note. The actual proceeds of the loan, then, would be in an amount less than the face value of the note. In an add-on note, the interest is added to the final payment of the loan. In this arrangement, the borrower receives the full value of the loan when the loan is originated.

Line of Credit

A line of credit is an agreement that permits a firm to borrow up to a specified limit during a defined loan period. For example, a commercial bank may grant a $2 million line of credit to a hospital during a specific year. In that year, the hospital could borrow up to $2 million from the bank with presumably little or no additional paper work required. Lines of credit are either committed or uncommitted. In an uncommitted line, there is no formal or binding agreement on the part of the bank to loan money. If conditions change, the bank could decide not to loan any funds at all. In a committed line of credit, there is a written agreement that conveys the terms and conditions of the line of credit. The bank is legally required to lend money under the line as long as the terms and conditions have been met by the borrower. To cover the costs and risks incurred by the commercial bank in a committed line of credit, the bank charges a commitment fee. The fee is usually based on either the total credit line or the unused portion of the line.

Revolving Credit Agreements

A revolving credit is similar to a line of credit except that it is usually for a period longer than one year. Revolving credit agreements may be in effect for two to three years. Most revolving credit agreements are renegotiated before maturity. If the renegotiation occurs more than one year before maturity, a revolving credit agreement loan may be stated as a long-term debt and never appear as a current liability on a firm's balance sheet. Terms of revolving credit agreements are similar to those of lines of credit. Interest rates are usually variable and based on the prime rate or other money-market rates.

Term Loans

Term loans are made for a specific period, usually ranging between two and seven years. The loans usually require periodic installment payments of the principal. This type of loan is frequently used to finance a tangible asset that will produce income in future periods, such as a computed tomography scanner. The asset acquired with the loan proceeds may be pledged as collateral for the loan.

Letters of Credit

Some hospitals use letters of credit as a method of bond insurance. A letter of credit is simply a letter from a bank stating that a loan will be made if certain conditions are met. In hospital bond financing, a letter of credit from a bank guarantees payment of the loan if the hospital defaults.

LEARNING OBJECTIVE 6

List and explain the criteria that should be used when investing an organization's cash in the short term.

INVESTMENT OF CASH SURPLUSES

The term surplus is confusing, even among financial executives. For the purpose of this discussion, cash surplus is defined as money exceeding a minimum balance that the firm prefers to maintain to meet immediate operating expenses and minor contingencies, plus any compensating balance required at its banks.

The balance sheet for ABC Medical Center shown in Table 21–2 lists a cash balance of $1,216,980 plus $4,042,407 in short-term investments as of June 30, 2008. These are the funds that are most often referred to as surplus cash when discussing short-term investment strategy. It is important to note that ABC Medical Center has significant investments in other areas. Most hospitals follow this procedure. For example, ABC Medical Center, as of June 30, 2008, has $10,642,621 in an investments account under the "other assets" section of the balance sheet. These funds probably are designated for the eventual replacement of the hospital plant. In addition, sizable balances of funds are maintained with a trustee. For example, there is $2,717,846 in the construction fund account, $6,751,942 in the sinking fund account, $118,142 in the interest receivable account, and $10,942,749 in the self-insurance

fund account. Most hospitals and health care firms maintain similar fund balances. It is critical for management to make investments that will meet the objectives of each specific fund and maximize the potential yield to the firm.

Often, a portion of a firm's investment funds is restricted to money-market investments. The term money market refers to the market for short-term securities, including U.S. Treasury bills, negotiable certificates of deposit, bankers' acceptances, commercial paper, and repurchase agreements. Maturities for money-market investments can range from one day to one year. Funds invested in money-market securities usually serve two roles. They represent (1) a liquidity reserve that can be used if the firm experiences a need for these funds, and (2) a temporary investment of surplus funds that can result in the earning of a return.

If the funds are invested for periods longer than one year (for example, the investment of a replacement reserve fund), higher yields often result. These longer-term maturity investments may not be referred to as money-market securities.

When evaluating alternative investment strategies, there are usually five basic criteria that should be reviewed:

1. Price stability
2. Safety of principal
3. Marketability
4. Maturity
5. Yield

Price Stability

The importance of price stability, especially for money-market investments, cannot be overemphasized. If a firm has a sudden need for cash, most major money-market investments can be sold without any serious capital losses. Generally, U.S. Treasury bills are the most credit-worthy money-market investments, followed closely by other U.S. Treasury obligations and federal agency issues. Investment in securities with long-term maturities are subject to risk if interest rates increase. This explains why money-market investments are usually restricted to maturities of less than one year.

Safety of Principal

Financial managers expect that the principal of their investment is generally not at risk. Treasury and federal agency obligations have little risk of principal loss through default. Bank securities (such as negotiable certificates of deposit and bankers' acceptances) and corporate obligations (such as commercial paper) are different matters. There may be a loss of principal through default, and care should be exercised when choosing these instruments. Information on banks is available in Polk's World Bank Directory and Moody's Bank and Finance Manual. There is no reason why a firm should not review the creditworthiness of its banks as carefully as banks review the financial position of loan applicants. It should be noted, however, that erosion of principal can occur through increases in money-market interest rates, and these increases subsequently will have an impact on fixed-rate securities.

Marketability

Marketability varies among money-market instruments. The term refers to the ability to sell a security quickly and with little price concession before maturity. In general, an active secondary trading market must exist to ensure the presence of marketability. Most major money-market instruments do have active secondary markets, especially obligations of the U.S. Treasury. Some commercial paper, especially that of industrial firms, may be difficult to redeem before maturity.

Maturity

There is a clear relationship between the yield of a security and its maturity that can be summarized in a yield curve. Table 21–3 shows a set of values for U.S. Treasury securities on March 21, 2006. Some firms use a strategy of investment described as "riding the yield curve." This strategy relies on the existence of an upward-sloping yield curve. Investments are made in longer-term securities that are sold before maturity.

Table 21–3 Yield to Maturity for US Treasuries, March 21, 2006

Maturity	Yield%
30 day	4.56
90 day	4.66
180 day	4.79
One Year	4.74
Two Years	4.65
Three Years	4.62
Five Years	4.61
Seven Years	4.62
Ten Years	4.66
Twenty Years	4.87
Thirty Years	4.70

Yield

Yield is a measure of the investment's return and is an important consideration. Yield is usually affected by maturity, expected default risk of principal, marketability, and price stability. In addition, taxability is often an issue. A tax-exempt health care firm has no incentive to invest in securities that are exempt from federal income taxes.

SUMMARY

Working capital management involves decisions that have an impact on operating cash flows of the firm. Ideally, the objective of most working capital management systems is to accelerate the collection of cash from customers and to slow down the payment to suppliers and employees. Investment management is important in many health care firms because of the relative size of their investment portfolios. Hospitals, for example, generate about 40 percent of their total net income from nonoperating sources, largely investment income. With so much at stake, health care firms need to improve performance in the cash and investment management area.

ASSIGNMENTS

1. Data from Table 21–2 indicate that $8,778,677 of accounts receivable were present at the end of 2008. If this value represented 50 days of average net patient revenue, and the hospital believed that this value could be reduced to 40 days, what dollar amount of new cash flow would be generated? If these funds were invested at 8.5 percent, how much additional investment income would result per year?

2. Alpha Home Health Inc. has received an invoice for medical supplies for $5,000 with terms of a two-percent discount if paid within ten days. The invoice is due on the thirtieth day. What is the annual effective cost of interest on this invoice?

3. Pauly Hospital has been thinking about changing its payroll period from biweekly to monthly. Pauly currently has 600 employees with an annual payroll of $18,000,000. If Pauly could earn 9.5 percent on invested funds, what amount of new investment income could be generated on an annual basis? If the cost of writing a payroll check is $1.50, what additional amount could be saved on an annual basis from switching to a monthly payroll period?

4. Your firm has negotiated a $1,000,000 line of credit with your local bank. The terms of the line of credit call for an interest rate of two percent above prime on any borrowing plus 0.5 percent on any unused balance. If the line is not used during the year, what cost will your firm incur?

5. ABC Medical Center (Table 21–2) expects its revenues to increase by ten percent next year. If the firm can increase its current liabilities by 12 percent through payment extensions and limit its increase in current assets, excluding cash and investments, to eight percent, what additional cash will be required to finance working capital?

SOLUTIONS AND ANSWERS

1. The amount of new cash flow would be $1,755,735:

$$[(\$8,778,677)/50] \times [50 - 40]$$

   The amount of additional investment income per year would be $149,238 (.085 × $1,755,735).

2. The two-percent discount would be realized for making payment 20 days before required. The annual interest cost would be approximately 36 percent:

$$2\% \times [360 \text{ days}/20\text{days}] = 36\%$$

3. There are two ways to estimate the annual savings. The easiest method would be to multiply the difference in average wages payable by 9.5 percent:

$$\left[\frac{(18,000,000 \div 12)}{2} - \frac{(18,000,000 \div 26)}{2} \right] \times .095 = \$38,365$$

   Alternatively, the difference in average payable amount per day can be calculated and multiplied times the average daily interest rate (.095/360), which is shown in Table 21–4.

   Assuming that the pattern presented in Table 21–4 holds, the annual return would be $39,353 (12 × $3,279.42). The savings from reduced checks would be $12,600 = [600 (26 − 12) × $1.50].

4. The firm must pay 0.5 percent on the entire $1,000,000, or $5,000 (.005 × $1,000,000).

5. The schedule presented in Table 21–5 shows the increase in net working capital.

Table 21–4 Investment Payable Income from Longer Payroll Cycle

Day	Average Payable Balance*		Incremental Amount Invested	Investment Income**	
	Monthly	*Biweekly*			
1		$49,315	$49,315	$ —	$
2		98,630	98,630	—	—
3		147,945	147,945	—	—
4		197,260	197,260	—	—
5		246,575	246,575	—	—
6		295,890	295,890	—	—
7		345,205	345,205	—	—
8		394,521	394,521	—	—
9		443,836	443,836	—	—
10		493,151	493,151	—	—
11		542,466	542,466	—	—
12		591,781	591,781	—	—
13		641,096	641,096	—	—
14		690,411	690,411	—	—
15		739,726	49,315	690,411	182.19
16		789,041	98,630	690,411	182.19
17		838,356	147,945	690,411	182.19
18		887,671	197,260	690,411	182.19
19		936,986	246,575	690,411	182.19
20		986,301	295,890	690,411	182.19
21		1,035,616	345,205	690,411	182.19
22		1,084,932	394,521	690,411	182.19
23		1,232,877	443,836	690,411	182.19
24		1,183,562	493,151	690,411	182.19
25		1,232,877	542,466	690,411	182.19
26		1,282,192	591,781	690,411	182.19
27		1,331,507	641,096	690,411	182.19
28		1,380,822	690,411	690,411	182.19
29		1,430,137	49,315	1,380,822	364.38
30		1,479,452	98,630	1,380,822	364.38

Monthly Total $3,279.42

* Average Payable Balance = $18,000,000/365 Days
** ($690,411 × .095) / 360

Table 21–5 Net Increase in Working Capital

Present current assets	$16,997,038
—Cash	1,216,980
—Investments	4,042,407
Noncash current assets	$11,737,651
8% Increase	0.08
Increase in noncash current assets	$939,012
Present current liabilities	$8,524,478
× 12% increase	0.12
Increase in current liabilities	$1,022.937
Net increase in working capital	($83,925)

Chapter 22

Developing the Cash Budget

LEARNING OBJECTIVES

After studying this chapter, you should be able to do the following:

1. Explain the importance of a cash budget.
2. Explain why an organization needs to carry cash balances.
3. List and describe how cash is generated by an organization and how an organization uses its cash.
4. Understand how to prepare a cash budget.

REAL-WORLD SCENARIO

Ainsley Campbell, the CEO of Mikaela Grace Medical Center, was briefed by her CFO, Joshua Douglas. regarding the current liquidity crisis at the medical center, which is the largest hospital in the market area. Joshua informed Ainsley that their cash balances have eroded by about $25 million in the last six months. The primary cause for this erosion is the removal of the medical center from the network of the largest commercial payer in the region. The loss of contract means that all beneficiaries of this plan are now considered out-of-network if they receive care at the hospital. A large number of physicians, especially the cardiovascular surgeons, have begun to perform procedures at Mikaela Grace's primary competitor in the market. Major elective procedures are being shifted to this competitor, and as a result revenues are down almost five percent from budget in the first six months.

Ainsley questioned Joshua regarding their financial ability to withstand another six months of reduced volume if a new contract cannot be negotiated. Joshua said their large existing reserves of capital funds will protect them from any default on existing obligations, but they will be forced to use their present line of credit from the local bank. Joshua wanted to give special credit to Riley Ilene, the controller, who had anticipated the current crisis when developing the hospital's cash budget last year. Her forecast was almost perfect; and as a result Mikaela Grace Medical Center negotiated a new expanded line of credit with the bank. Ainsley instructed Joshua to try to finalize negotiations with the health plan as quickly as possible to avoid a permanent reduction in their service lines, especially cardiology, which is the hospital's most profitable line.

Explain the importance of a cash budget.

Chapter 21 stressed the importance of developing a sound cash budget that accurately projects cash inflows and cash outflows in the cash-management process. Cash budgets embody the key source of information that permits management to determine the firm's short-term needs for cash. When a cash budget is modified to include the effects of alternative outcomes, financial executives can better assess the issue of liquidity risk and make decisions that will reduce the probability of a liquidity crisis. One of the following three courses of action can be taken:

1. Increase the level of cash and investment reserves
2. Restructure the maturity of existing debt
3. Arrange a line of credit with a bank

Explain why an organization needs to carry cash balances.

DETERMINING REQUIRED CASH AND INVESTMENT RESERVES

Businesses maintain cash and investments for four primary purposes:

1. Short-term working capital needs
2. Capital investment needs
3. Contingencies
4. To supplement operating earnings

Short Term Working Capital Needs

The area of need most easily projected is usually short-term working capital transactions. In 2004, the average nonprofit U.S. hospital held between 15 and 20 days of short-term cash and investments to meet short-term working capital needs. This represents less than one month of cash transactions, and standards do not vary much across different industry sectors. It is safe to assume that most health care firms should carry approximately 20 days of expected cash transactions at any point in time to meet normal short-term working capital needs for cash. However, it is not safe to say that a nonprofit health care firm would need only 20 days of cash. Twenty days of cash meets current operating short-term needs, such as payroll and supplies. It would not cover the larger long-term needs for capital replacement and contingencies.

Capital Investment Needs

Nonprofit health care providers must retain cash to finance replacement and renovation of existing capital assets, as well as investment in new product and service line areas. Their position is very different from that of taxable firms, whose access to capital for both replacement and new capital assets can and should be directed back to equity investors. Shareholders decide whether they wish to supply more capital to the firm based upon their expected return. Nonprofit entities, in general, and nonprofit health care firms, in particular, must routinely set aside funds for replacement. Unlike investor-owned health care firms, nonprofit entities have no access to the equity capital markets.

The amount of money that a nonprofit health care firm should reserve for capital assets is dependent upon two factors:

1. Percentage of debt financing to be used
2. Projected future levels of capital expenditures

Health care firms that choose or are forced to limit their debt financing of capital assets must clearly set aside larger sums of money for capital replacement and expansion. The absence of debt in a firm's capital structure should permit a greater accumulation of capital reserves because there is no interest being paid to decrease earnings and lower cash reinvestment potential. The absence of debt in a health care firm's capital structure also reduces the financial risk and lowers the probability of failure.

It is the responsibility of the board of directors to establish appropriate levels of debt financing. Boards usually make trade-offs between the risk that is associated with debt financing and the firm's needs for capital to meet mission-related goals. Access to debt capital is usually related to both historical and projected financial performance. Nonprofit health care firms that maintain high levels of cash and reserves will usually have greater access to debt financing with lower interest rates.

Projecting future levels of capital expenditures over a long period of time is very difficult. Capital expenditure decisions result from both routine replacement factors, as well as strategic considerations regarding the future direction of the firm. Most health care firms also experience years when capital expenditures are especially large due to major replacement needs. In general, however, most firms spend more on new capital expenditures than they depreciate in any given year.

One method that is commonly used to estimate future capital expenditures is based upon present levels of allowances for depreciation. If all of a firm's existing assets were to be replaced, if no inflation in replacement cost occurred, and if no new capital assets other than replacement items were purchased, the present allowance-for-depreciation balance would be an accurate estimate of future capital expenditures. A simple example may help to illustrate this concept. If a digital mammography unit were acquired today for $500,000 and had a five-year estimated life, it would be depreciated at a rate of $100,000 per year. At the end of the first year, the allowance for depreciation would be $100,000 and would increase each year by $100,000. For example, at the end of year three, the allowance for depreciation would be $300,000. Nonprofit hospitals without access to equity capital often adopt a program called "funding depreciation." If this practice were adopted, the hospital would place $100,000 in a fund each year. At the end of the five-year useful life, it would have $500,000 available for replacement, assuming no pricing increase. However, new capital assets not presently in the firm's capital asset pool are purchased, and replacement capital assets do typically increase in price. While it is true that some capital assets are not replaced, in most situations, projected capital expenditures exceed present allowance-for-depreciation balances. To adjust this forecast of capital expenditures, an inflation factor is usually applied in the following way. The present allowance-for-depreciation balance is increased at some projected inflation rate compounded at the average age of the firm's present capital assets. The formula can be stated as follows:

$$\text{Estimated Capital Expenditures} =$$
$$[\text{Allowance for Depreciation}] \times$$
$$[1 + \text{Inflation Rate}]^{\text{Average Age of Plant}}$$

As a general rule of thumb, most voluntary health care firms should try to have the following amount of cash available for replacement needs:

$$(100\% - \text{Desired debt policy \%}) \times$$
$$\text{Estimated Capital Expenditures}$$

Contingencies

Many firms try to sequester some funding to meet unexpected demands for cash flow. The amount they reserve reflects their tolerance for risk, as well as their estimates of unexpected cash demands upon the firm. Values for underfunded pension or professional liability claims should be considered contingency funds. Payment of these liabilities will require funding at some future date. This investment is over and above short-term working capital needs.

Supplementing Operating Earnings

A number of nonproft health care firms in the United States have established "operating endowments." The purpose of these funds is to provide a dependable flow of investment earnings that can be used to supplement expected weaknesses in operating earnings. While this practice is not widespread, it is worthy of consideration if a significant deterioration in operating earnings is expected, or if current operating margins have been weak with no expectation of future improvement.

CASE EXAMPLE—DEFINING REQUIRED CASH BALANCES

Table 22–1 identifies the sources of cash and investments available at our case example firm, Saint Alexus Health System, as of December 31, 2008. Cash and investments are limited to those balances that are not restricted by a third party.

Based upon the 2008 income statement, Saint Alexus Health System should carry $114,860,000 to maintain a 20-day cash-on-hand position. The estimated days of

Table 22–1 Saint Alexus Health System Cash & Investment Position

	(000)
Current Asset Cash & Short-Term Investments	$201,013
Assets Limited as to Use— Board Designation	540,211
Total	**$741,224**

cash expenses are defined by taking 2008 total operating expenses ($2,186,536,000) and subtracting depreciation ($90,339,000) to derive annual cash expenses ($2,096,197,000). This value is then divided by 365 to yield daily cash expenses ($5,743,005). Multiplying that number by 20 days, which is the short term working capital need, produces the $114,860,000 requirement.

A desirable cash and investment position for capital asset needs can be estimated using the methodology described earlier. To estimate projected future capital asset expenditures based upon the December 31, 2008, allowance-for-depreciation balance of $1,203,185,000; we assumed a range of possible inflation factors ranging from four percent to eight percent.

Inflation factors were compounded at the present average age of plant at Saint Alexus Health System (13.3 years). Finally, we assumed that the percentage of debt financing to be used would be 40%, 50%, 60%, or 70%. For example, the replacement cost of the plant and equipment assuming a six percent inflation rate would be $2,611,562,000 ($1,203,185,000 × $1.06^{13.3}$). If it was determined that a 40 percent debt and 60 percent equity financing mix was to be used, the required level of funding would $1,566,937,000 (.60 × $2,611,562,000).

Table 22–2 presents the required cash and investment position under these scenarios.

Contingency Needs

There is no really good methodology for establishing a desired contingency reserve. To a large extent, the desired balance is a reflection of the firm's propensity to tolerate risk. Specifically, we identified two areas where funds must be set aside. First, Saint Alexus Health System reported a negative funded status for its defined benefit retirement plan of $111,552,000 in 2008. This is a sizable deficit and has been increasing. The comparable 2007 value was $87,381,000. Second,

Saint Alexus Health System reported $90,194,000 of accrued liability for medical malpractice in 2008 that was not currently funded. This value is also increasing dramatically; the comparable 2007 value was $63,496,000. While it is unclear at what future point actual funds will be utilized, the deficits are very large and indicate that funding for these liabilities must be established.

No supplement to operating earnings was established because prior operating earnings are assumed to be adequate. Table 22–3 summarizes the determination of required cash balances at Saint Alexus Health System.

LEARNING OBJECTIVE 3

List and describe how cash is generated by an organization and how an organization uses its cash.

SOURCES AND USES OF CASH

In its most basic form, a cash budget is a statement that projects how the firm's cash balance position will change between two points in time. Changes to cash position are categorized as either sources of cash flow (sometimes called receipts) or uses of cash flow (sometimes called disbursements). Sources of cash include:

* Collection of accounts receivable
* Cash sales
* Investment income
* Sale of assets
* Financings
* Capital contributions

Table 22–2 Required Capital Fund (000s)

| Debt | Inflation Rate | | |
	4%	6%	8%
40%	$1,216,266	$1,566,937	$2,009,184
50%	1,013,552	1,305,781	1,674,320
60%	810,841	1,044,625	1,339,456
70%	608,131	783,469	1,004,592

Table 22–3 Required Cash and Investment Position (000s)

Investment Need	Desired Balance	Days Cash
Working Capital	$114,860	20
Capital Asset	783,469	136
Contingency	201,746	35
Supplement Operating Earnings	0	0
Total Required	$1,100,075	191
less Present Available Funds	741,224	129
Surplus (Deficit)	**($358,851)**	**62**

Uses of cash include:

* Payments to employees
* Payments to suppliers
* Payments to lenders for interest and principal
* Purchase of fixed assets
* Investments

It is important to note that the definition of income and the definition of cash flows are not the same. This means that the amount reported for revenues in any given period most likely will not equal the actual amount of cash realized. The only exception would be a case in which all revenues were produced by cash sales. In most health care settings, there is a lag between the recording of revenue and the collection of the resulting account receivable. In the same manner, expenses reported for wages and salaries and supplies may not actually equal the amount of cash expended within the period. As the period expands, for example, from a month to a year, the differences between revenues and expenses and receipts and disbursements begin to narrow. If one expanded the period from one year to twenty years, the difference between cash flows and income would be minimal. Unfortunately, most financial managers are interested in cash flows over much shorter periods. Many firms have cash budgets defined on at least a monthly basis, and some have biweekly or weekly cash budgets.

When cash flows are extremely volatile but reasonably forecastable, cash budgets for shorter terms are desirable. If cash flows are reasonably stable, a cash budget defined on a quarterly basis may be appropriate. Although most firms develop cash budgets on a monthly basis, it is common for these budgets to be revised periodically because original budget assumptions often prove to be inaccurate.

The primary factor affecting the validity of the cash budget is the accuracy of the forecasts for individual cash flow categories. The greater the degree of possible variation between actual and forecasted cash flow, the higher the liquidity need of the firm. Firms that cannot predict cash flow with much certainty should increase their cash balances or negotiate lines of credit to escape the possibility of severe cash insolvency problems.

LEARNING OBJECTIVE 4

Understand how to prepare a cash budget.

PREPARING THE CASH BUDGET

The most important area in cash budgeting is the revenue forecast. The revenue for health care providers will be a function of the following two factors: (1) volumes by product line and (2) expected prices by payer category.

Most firms use a variety of methods to estimate volumes of services during the cash budget period. As discussed in Chapter 15 and shown in Figure 22–1, the revenue budget is critically related to the statistics budget. In general, the following two major categories of methods are used to develop estimates of volumes: (1) subjective forecasts and (2) statistical forecasts.

In reality, most forecasts probably combine elements of both subjective and statistical methods. Subjective forecasts are often referred to as "seat-of-the-pants" methods and other less flattering names. Subjective forecasts do, however, have a place in the estimation of product line volumes. The critical factors in the reliability of a subjective forecast are the wisdom and understanding of the forecaster. In cases when future volumes are likely to deviate from historical patterns, subjective forecasts may be the most reliable method of forecasting. Surveying medical staff members regarding their expected utilization during the next year is a form of subjective forecasting, but one that may be extremely reliable.

Statistical forecasts run the gamut from major econometric studies to simple time series techniques. Whatever the method, an underlying assumption surrounds a statistical forecast that states the future can be predicted based on some mathematical model extrapolated from the past. If the relationships or models on

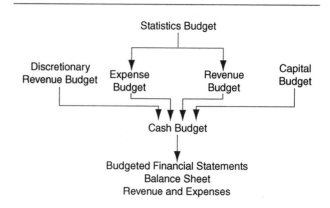

Figure 22–1 Integration of the Budgetary Process

which the forecasts are based have changed, future forecasts can be misleading.

In some cases, predicting prices for the firm's products and services may be almost as difficult as projecting volumes. Health care firms are price takers in most situations. This means that they rely on someone else to establish prices for their services. Medicare and Medicaid are two organizations that set prices and exert tremendous influence on a major portion of the total revenue budget. One would think that these payers would establish prices far enough in advance so that forecasting prices would be a simple matter. Unfortunately, sometimes interim prices stay interim for longer than expected, and promised increases never materialize. Although the differences between expected and actual prices may be relatively small, the volume of the Medicare and Medicaid business is so large that small changes in prices have a major impact on net cash flows. Most health care providers operate with relatively small margins—somewhere between one and five percent. When Medicare and Medicaid account for 50 percent or more of a firm's total business, a small forecast error of one or two percent in the final prices to be paid by Medicare and Medicaid can have a disastrous impact on final operating margins.

Health care firms also increasingly are being asked to discount more and more of their business to other major groups, such as health maintenance organizations (HMOs), preferred provider organizations, commercial insurers, and self-insured employers. This makes projecting actual realized net prices more and more difficult.

Projecting revenues does not equate to projecting cash flows. Collections will lag the actual booking of revenues for some period. One common way to develop forecasts of patient receipts is through the use of "decay curves." These curves relate future collections to past billings. Figure 22–2 depicts a decay curve with the following pattern of collections:

1. The first 15 percent of any month's revenue is collected in the first month.
2. The next 30 percent of any month's revenue is collected in the second month.
3. The next 25 percent of any month's revenue is collected in the third month.
4. The next 20 percent of any month's revenue is collected in the fourth month.
5. The next 5 percent of any month's revenue is collected in the fifth month.

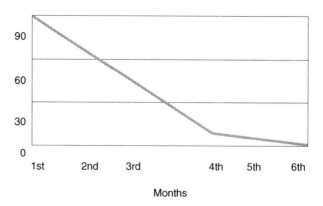

Figure 22–2 Decay Curve Analysis: Percentage Uncollected by Month after Billing

6. The remaining 5 percent of any month's revenue is written off and not collected.

Table 22–4 presents a cash receipts summary for the first six months of the year. The collection pattern reflected in the decay curve of Figure 22–2 can be seen in Table 22–4. For example, of the $2,000,000 of January revenue, 15 percent ($300,000) is collected in January, 30 percent ($600,000) is collected in February, 25 percent ($500,000) is collected in March, 20 percent ($400,000) is collected in April, 5 percent ($100,000) is collected in May, and the remaining 5 percent ($100,000) is written off and not collected. The revenues in the following months reflect the same collection pattern. Although cash receipts and revenues are most often correlated, it is not always true that the months producing the highest revenue will be the months with the highest cash collection. For many health care firms, the highest cash collection month is often one to two months after the highest revenue month.

Changes in collection patterns of major third-party payers can have a significant effect on cash flows and should be reflected immediately in revised cash budgets. For example, if Medicaid decides to delay the payment of patient bills by sixty days to conserve cash, the cash budget must be revised to reflect this new payment pattern. Increasing values for deductibles and copayments under many health care insurance plans also may delay collection patterns and increase eventual write-offs because the self-pay portion of the total health care bill may not be paid by the patient.

Additional cash receipts may come from sources other than revenue collection. Investment income and sale of assets are identified as the only other sources in

Table 22–4 Cash Receipts Summary (in Thousands)

		January	February	March	April	May	June
Beginning accounts receivable revenue	$3,600	$1,600	$1,000	$500	$100		
January sales	2,000	300	600	500	400	$100	$ 0
February sales	2,100	0	315	630	525	420	105
March sales	2,000	0	0	300	600	500	400
April sales	1,900	0	0	0	285	570	475
May sales	1,800	0	0	0	0	270	540
June sales	1,800	0	0	0	0	0	270
Subtotal		$1,900	$1,915	$1,930	$1,910	$1,860	$1,790
Other cash receipts							
Investment income		561	420	496	420	406	432
Sale of assets		0	0	25	0	0	0
Subtotal		$561	$420	$521	$420	$406	$432
Estimated cash receipts		$2,461	$2,335	$2,451	$2,330	$2,266	$2,222

Table 22–4, but other sources also may exist. Contributions, sale of stock, and the issuance of new debt are also possibilities.

After forecasting cash receipts, a schedule of expected cash disbursements is necessary before the cash budget is complete. The two largest categories in most health care firms are labor and supplies. Labor costs or payroll most often represent about 60 percent or more of a health care firm's total expenses. The expense budget will identify expected labor or payroll expenses by month, but payroll expenses do not translate into cash disbursements. Most health care firms meet the majority of their payroll obligations on a biweekly basis, which necessitates some accruals. For example, labor expense in January might be $1,200,000, but actual payroll might be $1,731,000 because there were three biweekly payroll periods. (There are 26 biweekly payroll periods in a year. Every month will have at least two payroll periods, but two months will have three.) Conversely, in other months during which only two biweekly pay periods were present, actual payroll disbursements might be less than labor expense.

Payroll expense also must be adjusted for withholding and other deductions. For example, the January payroll of $1,731,000 might be broken down as presented in Table 22–5. In Table 22–5, the figure for net payroll—$1,190,000—does not include additional payroll

taxes, such as workers' compensation, unemployment, and the employer's share of social security. Other fringe benefits, such as pension and health insurance, also are not included. The employee deductions, such as income tax and social security, will involve a cash outlay, but the payment will go the federal government.

As with payroll, the expense budget will include a value for supplies expense, but that value will not equal the actual disbursement for supplies. Table 22–6 presents a schedule of expected cash disbursements. The only remaining task is to combine the cash receipts summary and the cash disbursements summary to create the cash budget. Before doing so, a desired level of cash balances must be defined. For this example, it will be assumed that a short-term cash balance of $1,350,000 is required to meet the firm's short-term working capital needs. If the firm cannot maintain this balance, it must

Table 22–5 Payroll Disbursements

Total payroll	$1,731,000
Less:	
Income taxes	330,000
Social Security	126,000
Other deductions	85,000
Net payroll disbursed to employees	$1,190,000

Table 22–6 Cash Disbursements Summary (in Thousands)

	January	February	March	April	May	June
Salary and wages	$1,190	$900	$980	$880	$850	$840
Payroll deductions	541	400	446	400	386	382
Fringe benefits	155	130	135	125	115	110
Purchases	315	385	405	390	385	385
Other disbursements	185	205	225	190	210	250
Capital expenditures	25	15	100	350	45	60
Debt service	0	0	300	0	0	300
Estimated disbursement	$2,411	$2,035	$2,591	$2,335	$1,991	$2,327

make a decision whether it will transfer funds from its replacement reserves or whether it will borrow short term through a line-of-credit arrangement.

Table 22–7 combines the cash receipt and cash disbursement summaries to produce the cash budget. The cash budget shows that the firm will experience negative cash flows in some months. However, in this initial six-month forecast, no month will show a balance less than the required cash balance of $1,350,000. If the forecast proves to be accurate, the firm will not need to arrange any short-term financing, nor will it need to transfer any replacement reserves. In fact, it could transfer some of the short-term cash balances that are more than the required minimal balance of $1,350,000 to replacement reserves. The firm could transfer all of the $50,000 in cash flow that occurs in January to replacement reserves, but only $160,000 of the $300,000 net cash flow in February could be transferred because the March cash flow will be a negative $140,000.

By examining the pattern of expected cash flows, the treasurer of the firm can better decide the duration

and maturity of possible investments. Usually, longer-term securities will yield higher returns. Therefore, if the funds are not expected to be needed for six months, the firm would be better off investing in a six-month Treasury bill than a 30-day Treasury bill.

SUMMARY

Cash budgets are critical pieces of information that financial executives in all health care firms need to prepare and monitor closely. The forecast of cash flows should help management determine whether additional financing will be needed, in what amounts, and for what duration. The information also will permit the short-term investment of surplus funds so that yields on those investments might be improved.

Cash budgets are forecasts, and there is no guarantee that the forecasted results will be achieved. It is important for management to test the sensitivity of the forecasts regarding alternative scenarios, such as slowdowns in collections or declines in revenues.

Table 22–7 Cash Budget Summary (in Thousands)

	January	February	March	April	May	June
Beginning cash balance	$1,350	$1,400	$1,700	$1,560	$1,555	$1,830
Add receipts	2,461	2,335	2,451	2,330	2,266	2,222
Less disbursements	2,411	2,035	2,591	2,335	1,991	2,327
Cash flow	50	300	(140)	(5)	275	(105)
Ending cash balance	$1,400	$1,700	$1,560	$1,555	$1,830	$1,725

ASSIGNMENTS

1. Morgan Village is a voluntary, nonprofit, continuing care retirement center. Presently it has $1,200,000 set aside for replacement and renovation. Its current accumulated depreciation is $1,800,000 and the average age of the plant is ten years. If it can be assumed that capital assets for Morgan Village are inflating at six percent per year, what balance would Morgan Village need to have set aside today to meet their replacement needs if they will not be using any debt financing?

2. Huntley Hospital must maintain $3.3 million in a debt service reserve fund maintained by the bond trustee. The board members would like to count this balance when determining the amount of cash that they should carry for meeting normal transaction needs. Is this reasonable?

3. Dean Nursing Home has a payer mix of approximately 60 percent Medicaid and 40 percent private pay. The state Medicaid program recently has experienced major funding problems, and the frequency of payment for Medicaid beneficiaries is unclear for the next year. How might this information affect Dean's cash management?

4. Prepare a cash budget for Aztec Home Health Agency for the months of May, June, and July. The firm wishes to maintain a $200,000 minimum cash balance during the period, and it presently has a $220,000 balance as of April 30. Revenues are presented in the following:

January	$ 500,000
February	500,000
March	600,000
April	600,000
May	700,000
June	800,000
July	1,000,000
August	1,000,000

The firm collects 30 percent of its revenue in the month billing occurred, 30 percent in the next month, and 25 percent in the following month. The firm fails to collect 15 percent of its revenue because of either bad debt or contractual allowances. Expense budget relationships are presented in the following:

Payroll = $50,000 per month plus .50 × revenues
Supplies = .10 × revenues
Rent = $50,000 per month
Debt service = $150,000 in July
Capital expenditures = $75,000 in June

Eighty percent of payroll expense is paid in the month this expense was incurred, and 20 percent is paid in the following month. Supplies expense is paid in the following month. All other items are paid in the month reported. Determine during which months Aztec will be able to invest surplus funds and during which months it might need to borrow.

SOLUTIONS AND ANSWERS

1. The total amount of required replacement reserves should be:

   $1,800,000 \times (1.06)^{10}$, or $3,223,525

2. No. The debt service reserve fund is not under the control of Huntley Hospital management and could not be used to meet normal transactional needs for cash such as payroll and purchases.

3. Because cash flows are likely to be more volatile next year, Dean should consider enhancing its liquidity position. This might be accomplished by increasing the amount of short-term cash reserves or negotiating a line of credit.

4. Surplus funds will be available during May and June, but a loan will need to be obtained during July, as the cash budget in Table 22–8 shows.

Table 22–8 Cash Budget for Aztec Home Health Agency

	May	June	July
Receipts			
March revenue	$150,000	$0	$0
April revenue	180,000	150,000	0
May revenue	210,000	210,000	175,000
June revenue	0	240,000	240,000
July revenue	0	0	300,000
Total receipts	$540,000	$600,000	$715,000
Disbursements			
Payroll			
April	$70,000	$0	$0
May	320,000	80,000	0
June	0	360,000	90,000
July	0	0	440,000
Total payroll disbursed	$390,000	$440,000	$530,000
Supplies	60,000	70,000	80,000
Rent	50,000	50,000	50,000
Debt service	0	0	150,000
Capital expenditures	0	75,000	0
Total disbursements	$500,000	$635,000	$810,000
Net cash flow	$40,000	($35,000)	($95,000)
Beginning balance	$220,000	$260,000	$225,000
Ending cash	260,000	225,000	130,000
Less required minimum	200,000	200,000	200,000
Net investment (borrowing)	$60,000	$25,000	($70,000)

Glossary

Accountability—Being subject to sanctions with respect to carrying out responsibilities.

Accounting period—The elapsed time between financial statements. Common accounting periods include a month, a quarter, and a year.

Accounts payable—Amounts the organization is obligated to pay others, including suppliers and creditors.

Accounts receivable—Amounts due to the organization from patients, third parties, and others.

Accrual basis of accounting—The system of accounting that recognizes revenues when earned and expenses when resources are used. This method is used by most nongovernmental health care organizations. *See also* Cash basis of accounting.

Accrued expenses—Expenses that have been incurred, but not yet paid.

Accumulated depreciation—The cumulative amount of depreciation recognized on an asset since its purchase. An asset's book value is equal to its purchase price less the amount of accumulated depreciation.

Acid test ratio [(cash + marketable securities)/ current liabilities]—A liquidity ratio that measures how much *cash* and *marketable securities* are available to pay off all *current liabilities*.

Activity-based costing (ABC)—A method to determine the costs of a service, product, or customer by tracing the resources consumed. ABC focuses on: 1) controlling, as well as calculating costs, 2) tracing as opposed to allocating costs, and 3) the importance of indirect costs. *See also* Step-down method.

Activity ratios—Ratios that measure how efficiently an organization is using its assets to produce revenues.

Administrative cost centers—Organizational units responsible for their own costs that provide administrative support to other organizational units or the organization as a whole.

Administrative profit centers—Organizational units responsible for providing administrative support at a profit to other organizational units or to the organization as a whole and/or raising funds externally.

Admitting diagnosis—The initial diagnosis made upon admission to a hospital.

Age of plant ratio (accumulated depreciation/ depreciation expense)—This ratio indicates the average number of years an organization has owned its plant and equipment.

Aggressive strategy—An attempt to maximize returns by investing funds in higher-earning (i.e., more risky) nonliquid investments at the expense of higher liquidity.

Aging schedule—A method of classifying accounts receivable by the amount of time that has passed since they were recognized.

Allocation base—A statistic used to allocate costs from a cost center based on a cause-and-effect relationship. For example, a common allocation base to allocate the costs of maintaining medical records is number of visits. *See also* Cost driver.

Allowance for uncollectibles—A balance sheet account that estimates the total amount of patient accounts receivable that will not be collected. It is also called allowance for bad debts and allowance for doubtful accounts.

Allowed charge—The Medicare-approved payment amount reported on a line item on the physician/supplier claim.

Amortization of a loan—The gradual process of paying off debt through a long series of equal periodic payments. Each payment covers a portion of the principal plus current interest. The periodic payments are equal over the lifetime of the loan, but the proportion going towards principal gradually increases.

Annuity—A series of equal cash flows made or received at regular time intervals. *"Ordinary annuities"* occur at the end of each period whereas *"annuities due"* occur at the beginning of each period.

Appropriations—Monies provided by governmental agencies to organizations.

Approximate percentage cost {[Discount percent/(1 − discount percent)] × [365/net period]}—An estimate of the annualized interest rate incurred by not taking a discount.

Asset mix—The percentage of each asset relative to total assets.

Assets—The resources owned by the organization. It is one of the three major categories on the balance sheet.

Assets limited as to use—Funds, excluding those restricted by donors, that have been set aside for specific purposes and are not available for general use. The balance sheet presentation of *assets limited as to use* must differentiate both between current and noncurrent assets limited as to use and separate internally-designated amounts from externally-designated amounts either on the balance sheet or in the notes to the financial statements.

Assignment—Under Part B, if a physician chooses to accept assignment on a claim, the physician bills Medicare and is paid an amount equal to 80 percent of the fee schedule amount (less any unmet deductible). The physician is not permitted to charge the beneficiary more than the applicable deductible and coinsurance amounts. If the physician does not accept assignment, the physician still bills Medicare; but the Medicare payment is made to the beneficiary. In addition to the coinsurance and deductible amounts, the beneficiary is liable for the difference between the fee schedule amount and the physician's actual charge, subject to certain limits.

Authoritarian approach—An approach to carrying out organizational tasks that relies heavily on higher management decision making with little employee input. It is also called the top-down approach.

Authority—The power to carry out a given responsibility. Authority may be formal or informal.

Average payment period {current liabilities/[(total expenses − depreciation expense)/365]}—This ratio measures how long, on average, it takes an organization to pay its bills.

Avoidable fixed cost—A fixed cost that is avoided if a particular service is no longer offered.

B

Bad debt—An amount owed to the organization that will not be paid. Charity care is not considered a bad debt since nothing is owed to the organization for services provided.

Balance sheet—One of the four major financial statements of a health care organization. It presents a summary of the organization's assets, liabilities, and net assets as of a certain date.

Basic accounting equation (Assets = Liabilities + Owners' Equity)—In nonprofit, business-oriented health care organizations, the analogous equation is (Assets = Liabilities + Net Assets).

Basis points (bps)—A method to describe the change in a bond's interest rate where a 1 percent change equals 100 basis points. One basis point is one hundredth of one percent in the yield of an investment.

Beginning inventory—The amount of inventory on hand at the beginning of an accounting period. *See also* Ending inventory.

Benefit period (spell of illness), Medicare—The unit of time for measuring use of Part A benefits. The period begins upon the beneficiary's admission to a hospital or other facility, and ends after 60 consecutive days during which the individual was not an inpatient of any hospital, skilled nursing facility, or rehabilitative facility. Although there are limits to covered benefits per benefit period, there is no limit to the number of benefit periods a beneficiary can have. The beneficiary must pay the Part A deductible for each new benefit period.

Billing, collections, and disbursement policies and procedures—Tools used to increase the amount of cash available to the organization. The objective of billing, credit, and collection policies is to accelerate cash receipts; the objective of cash disbursement policies is to slow down cash outflows.

Billing float—The delay between providing the service and getting the bill to the patient or third party. There are two aspects of billing float: assembling the bill, and delivering the bill to the patient or third-party payor.

Bond rating—An assignment or grading of the likelihood that an organization will not default on a bond.

Bond-rating agency—Agencies that assess the "credit worthiness" of an organization. The three major rating agencies are Moody's, Standard & Poor's, and Fitch.

Bonds—A form of long-term financing whereby the issuer receives cash and in return issues a note called a bond. By issuing the bond, the issuer agrees to make principal and/or interest payments on specific dates to the holders of the bond.

Book value—The cost of a capital asset minus accumulated depreciation.

bps—*See* basis points.

Break-even analysis—An approach to analyzing the relationship among revenues, costs, and volume. It is also called Cost-Volume-Profit or CVP analysis.

Break-even point—The point at which total revenues equal total costs. It is described by the equation: (price × volume) = fixed costs + (variable cost per unit × volume).

Budget—The central document of the planning/control cycle. It identifies revenues and resources that will be needed by an organization to achieve its goals and objectives.

Budget variance—The difference between what was planned (budgeted) and what was achieved (actual).

Bundling—The pricing mechanism that combines services that are charged for separately into a single package with a single price.

C

Callable bonds—Bonds that may be redeemed by the issuer before they mature. Callable bonds have a higher interest rate than do noncallable bonds.

Cannibalization—A situation that occurs when a new service decreases the revenues or cash flows from existing services.

Capital—The sources of funds to finance the non-current assets of the organization. It is also considered the debt and equity of the organization.

Capital appreciation—The increase in the value of an investment from the time it is purchased until the time it is sold.

Capital assets—Assets that have a useful life greater than one year, such as plant, property, and equipment. Plant and equipment are depreciated over time; land (property) is not.

Capital budget—The budget used to forecast, and in some cases justify, the expenditures (and in some cases the sources of financing) for noncurrent assets.

Capital financing—Financing used expressly for the purchase of noncurrent assets.

Capital investment decisions—Decisions regarding the acquisition of capital assets. The capital investment decision should be separate from the decision on how to finance capital assets.

Capital lease—A lease in which the lessor aims to lease an asset for virtually all of its economic life. In return, the lessee is committed to lease payments for the entire lease period. Also called a financial lease.

Capital structure decisions—Decisions regarding the relative amount of debt and equity used to finance the organization's noncurrent assets.

Capital structure ratios—Ratios that measure how the organization's assets are financed and/or whether the organization can take on new debt.

Capitated profit centers—Organizational units responsible for making a profit. They agree to take care of specific health care needs of a population over a given time period for a specific fixed amount paid in advance.

Capitation—A payment system in which providers receive a specific amount in advance to care for specific health care needs of a defined population over a specific period. Providers are usually paid on a per member per month (PMPM) basis. A capitated provider assumes the risk of caring for the covered population for the PMPM amount. The capitation dollars are derived from premiums paid by enrollees. Typically, administrative fees for claims payment, case management, profit, and other costs are taken out of the premium before any payment is made to providers.

Care maps—Guidelines that detail suggested regimens of treatment for patients in a given category. Also called critical pathways.

Carrier—A Medicare contractor that processes and pays Medicare physician and supplier claims.

Case management—The coordination of services provided to a patient by a specific entity. Case management is often provided by a primary physician or by clinical experts who have the responsibility to approve, monitor, and/or evaluate the care given to a patient.

Case mix—The mix of patients served by a provider classified by one or more salient characteristics (age, sex, diagnosis, acuity, etc.).

Case rates—A fixed reimbursement amount depending on the type of case (hip replacement, normal newborn delivery, cardiac catheterization, etc.). This payment type typically includes both physician and hospital charges, limits the liability of the payor, and shifts some of the financial risk to the provider.

Cash—Coin and currency and cash equivalents, such as interest-bearing savings and checking accounts.

Cash and cash equivalents—The balance sheet category that includes actual money on hand, as well as money equivalents, such as savings and checking accounts. It excludes cash restricted for something other than current operations.

Cash basis of accounting—The system of accounting that recognizes revenues when cash is received and expenses when cash is paid out. *See also* Accrual basis of accounting.

Cash budget—The budget that projects the organization's cash inflows and outflows. The bottom line in the cash budget is the amount of cash available at the end of the period.

Cash flows from financing activities—Cash inflows and outflows resulting from financing activities, such as obtaining grants or endowments, or from borrowing or paying back long-term debt.

Cash flows from investing activities—Cash inflows and outflows for the organization resulting from investing activities, such as purchasing and selling investments or investing in itself by purchasing or selling noncurrent assets. It also includes transfers to and from the parent corporation.

Cash flows from operating activities—The changes in cash resulting from the normal operating activities of the organization.

Centralization—1) The degree to which power and authority is concentrated in an organization. 2) The degree to which a variety of services are offered at a single location. *See also* Decentralization.

Certainty—The absence of risk in an investment.

Certificate of need (CON)—The process by which a provider justifies the necessity for capital expenditures in order to obtain approval from an independent agency, such as the government. If approved, a CON is issued.

Charge-based system—A system in which providers set the rates for services. Reimbursement is based upon the charge rather than being predetermined by the payor.

Charity care—Free care provided to those who cannot pay for their services. Also called indigent care. Each organization must have rules to determine when care is charity care as opposed to bad debt. Some health care institutions may receive appropriations from the government to help offset the costs of charity care.

Claim—A request by a provider for payment for services provided to a beneficiary.

Clinical cost centers—Organizational units responsible for providing health care related services to clients, patients, or enrollees, and the related costs thereof.

Coinsurance (Medicare)—Coinsurance is that portion of covered hospital and medical expenses, after subtraction of any deductible, for which the beneficiary is responsible. Under Part A, there is no coinsurance for the first 60 days of inpatient hospital care; from the 61st through the 90th day of inpatient care, the daily coinsurance amount is equal to one-fourth of the inpatient hospital deductible. For each of the 60 lifetime reserve days used, the daily coinsurance amount is equal to one-half of the inpatient hospital deductible. There is no coinsurance for the first 20 days of skilled nursing facility (SNF) care; from the 21st through the 100th day of SNF care, the daily coinsurance amount is equal to one-eighth of the inpatient hospital deductible. Under Part B, after the annual deductible has been met the beneficiary must generally pay 20 percent of the approved amount (plus any charges above the approved amount).

Collateral—A borrower's assets on which a lender has legal claim if a borrower defaults on a loan.

Collection float—The time between the issuance of the bill and the time funds are available for use by the health care organization. It has two components: mail float and processing float.

Collections policies and procedures—Policies and procedures that address when and how to collect revenues, such as paying at time of service, sending accounts to collection agencies, and writing off accounts as bad debt.

Commercial paper (CP or C.P.)—A negotiable promissory note (essentially an IOU) issued at a discount by large corporations.

Commitment fee—A percentage of the unused portion of a credit line charged to the potential borrower. The annual fee is a function of the credit risk of the borrower and the reason for the line of credit.

Common costs—Costs (such as rent, administration, insurance, etc.) that are shared by a number of services or departments and cannot easily be broken down to the services attributable to each (surgery, emergency medicine, etc.). Also called joint costs.

Common stocks—Stock that entitles its holders to ownership rights in the corporation and to dividends only after the rights of preferred stockholders have been satisfied.

Comparative approach—The method of capital budgeting that compares the cash flows resulting from continuing with the existing alternative to those that would result if the equipment were replaced.

Compensating balance—The amount required to be maintained on deposit with the bank for such things as maintaining a credit line and fee-free checking.

Compound interest method—The method of determining the future value of money in which interest is calculated on the cumulative principal and interest earned up to that point. *See also* Simple interest method.

Compounding—1) Calculating interest using the compound interest method. 2) Adjusting for the time value of money forward in time to a future value. *See also* Compound interest method *and* Discounting.

Concurrent review—Monitoring the continued medical necessity of hospital treatment and assessing discharge needs to determine the appropriateness of payment.

Conservative strategy—An attempt to maximize liquidity by foregoing returns that could be earned by investing funds in higher-earning non-liquid assets.

Contingencies—Uncontrollable changes in the environment that may affect the financial condition of the organization (changes in the payment system, labor shortages, and catastrophic events).

Contra asset—An asset that, when increased, decreases the value of a related asset. Two primary examples are accumulated depreciation, which is the contra asset to properties and equipment, and the allowance for doubtful accounts, which is the contra asset to accounts receivable.

Contribution margin—The amount remaining after subtracting variable costs from revenues. When the organization is not at capacity, it is the "profit" the organization makes on providing each new unit that is available to cover all other costs. Contribution margin may be determined on a total or per unit basis.

Controlling activities—Activities that provide guidance and feedback to keep the organization within its budget, such as staff meetings, regular reports, and bonuses.

Conversion factor—A dollar multiplier used to convert the geographically-adjusted relative value for a

physician service to a Medicare payment amount for the service.

Copayments—Requiring the patient to pay part of his/her health care bill. These payments are used to prevent overutilization of services.

Cost—1) The resources used to produce a good or service. 2) The amount of cash given up in a transaction. 3) Price. The first definition is based on accrual accounting and the second on cash accounting.

Cost + approach—The method of determining prices that adds a margin to the cost of an item for profit. It is most often used with ancillary services such as radiology, pharmacy, and laboratory services.

Cost avoidance—The ability of an organization to find new ways to operate that obviate the need for certain classes of costs, such as doing procedures on an outpatient rather than inpatient basis.

Cost-based systems—A payment system that uses provider cost, as opposed to charges, as the starting point to determine the amount of payment.

Cost centers—Organizational units responsible for providing services and controlling their costs. There are two major types: clinical cost centers and administrative cost centers.

Cost containment—1) Actions that control or reduce the total amount of costs incurred. 2) The act of not spending more than is budgeted.

Cost driver—1) An activity or event that causes activities to occur and thus, resources to be used and costs to be incurred. 2) A statistic correlated to why a cost occurred. *See also* Allocation base.

Cost object—Anything for which a cost is found (a test, a visit, a patient day).

Cost of capital—The rate of return required to undertake a project. *See also* Discount rate *and* Hurdle rate.

Cost of goods used—The amount of supplies used to provide a service. It can be calculated by multiplying the number of RVUs provided by the cost per RVU.

Coupon—A certificate attached to a bond representing the amount of interest to be paid to the holder.

Coupon payment (CP or C.P.)—The amount the holder of the coupon receives periodically, usually semiannually. Over the year, it equals the coupon rate times the face value of the bond.

Coupon rate—Stated interest rate on a bond, as promised by the issuer.

Covenant—Legal provisions in a bond that must be followed by the issuer. Also called a loan covenant.

Coverage approach—A method of setting charges to cover costs.

CP or C.P.—*See* coupon payment on a bond; or commercial paper.

Creditor—An entity that is owed money for lending funds or supplying goods or services on credit.

Critical pathways—*See* Care maps.

Current assets—Generally, assets that will be used or consumed within one year. Some organizations use a period of less than one year.

Current liabilities—An organization's financial obligations that are to be paid within one year.

Current procedural terminology (CPT) codes—CPT codes are codes for reporting medical services and procedures performed by physicians. *See also* Healthcare Common Procedure Coding System (HCPCS).

Current ratio (current assets/current liabilities)—This liquidity ratio measures the proportion of all current assets to all current liabilities to determine how easily current debt can be paid off. It is one of the most commonly used ratios.

D

Daily operations—The usual and common activities of an organization.

Days' cash-on-hand {[cash + marketable securities]/[(operating expenses – depreciation)/ 365]}—A ratio that indicates the number of days' worth of expenses an organization can cover with its most liquid assets (cash and marketable securities).

Days in accounts receivable [net accounts receivable/(net patient revenues/ 365)]—This ratio indicates how quickly a hospital is converting its receivables into cash. It provides an estimate of how many days' revenues are yet to be collected.

Debenture—An unsecured bond—one that is not backed by any specific lien on the property. *See also* Subordinated debenture.

Debt financing—Borrowing money from others at a cost in the form of interest. It is an alternative to equity financing. *See also* Equity financing.

Debt service coverage [(excess of revenues over expenses + interest expense + depreciation expense)/ (interest expense + principal payments)]—A ratio that measures an organization's ability to pay back a loan. In for-profit organizations, it is calculated as: (net income + interest expense + depreciation expense)/(interest expense + principal payments).

Decentralization—The degree of dispersion of responsibility within an organization. *See also* Centralization.

Decentralized collection centers/concentration banking—Locations near a payor designed to reduce mail and processing float.

Deductible—A set amount the patient is responsible for paying before third-party coverage begins. These are used to prevent overutilization of services.

Deferred revenues—Monies received that have not yet been earned. One of the most common types of deferred revenues is the receipt of capitation on the basis of per member per month (PMPM).

Depreciation—An estimate/measure of how much a tangible asset (such as plant or equipment) has been "used up" during an accounting period. It is an expense that does not require any cash outflow under the accrual basis of accounting. *See also* Accumulated depreciation.

Depreciation tax shield—An inflow of funds that provides a reduction in the amount of taxes that have to be paid.

Diagnosis related groups (DRGs)—DRGs are a patient classification system that categorizes patients into groups that are clinically coherent and homogeneous with respect to resource use. The Prospective Payment System (PPS) uses approximately 550 DRGs as the basis for payment to hospitals.

Direct costs—Costs that are traced to a cost object. *See also* Indirect costs *and* Cost object.

Disbursement float—The amount of time between when an organization receives a service and pays for it.

Discount—1) A reduction in the charge for services. 2) When the market rate is higher than the coupon rate, a bond is said to be selling at a discount from its par value. *See also* Premium.

Discount rate—1) The returns that must be generated on a project to compensate the organization for its risk. 2) The returns the organization is foregoing by investing its money in one project as opposed to an alternative of similar risk. *See also* Cost of capital *and* Hurdle rate.

Discounted cash flows—Cash flows that have been adjusted to their present value to account for the cost of capital (over time) and the time value of money.

Discounting—The process of adjusting for the time value of money backward in time to present value. *See also* Compounding.

Disproportionate share hospital—A hospital that serves a relatively large volume of low-income patients.

Dividends—Portion of profit an organization distributes to investors. By law, only investor-owned health care organizations can distribute dividends outside the organization.

Donation—Funds provided by a private entity or individual without the requirement of repayment. Donations can either be restricted or unrestricted.

Donor—Private entity or individual who makes a donation.

DRGs—*See* Diagnosis related groups.

Dual entitlement—Indicates that an individual is entitled for both Medicare and Medicaid coverage.

Durable medical equipment (DME)—Under Medicare, DME includes certain medical supplies and such items as hospital beds and wheelchairs used in a patient's home.

E

Effectiveness—The degree to which standards are met.

Efficiency—1) Measuring inputs against outputs. 2) The cost of service per unit rendered.

Electronic billing—A process whereby bills are sent electronically to third parties through electronic data interfacing (EDI).

Ending inventory—The amount of inventory on hand at the end of an accounting period. *See also* Beginning inventory.

Equity financing—The purchase of assets with contributed and internally generated funds. *See also* Debt financing.

Estimated third-party payor settlements—Amounts due to (or from) third-party payors for advances or overpayments (or underpayments) from third parties.

Excess of revenues over expenses—Operating income plus other income. This is analogous to net income before taxes in for-profit entities.

Expansion decisions—Capital investment decisions designed to increase the operational capability of a health care organization.

Expense budget—The budget used to forecast operating expenses.

Expense cost variance [(actual cost per unit – budgeted cost per unit) × actual volume]—The difference between the variable expenses that would have been expected at the actual volume and those actually incurred.

Expense volume variance [(actual volume – budgeted volume) × budgeted cost per unit]—The portion of total variance that is due to actual volume being either higher or lower than budgeted volume. It is the difference between the expenses forecast in the original budget and what would have been expected at the actual volume.

Expenses—A measure of the resources used to generate revenue and/or provide a service. Often used synonymously with costs. *See also* Costs.

Extraordinary item—An extremely unusual and infrequent occurrence.

F

Factoring—The selling of accounts receivable at a discount, usually to a bank, in order to obtain cash.

Favorable variance—1) When actual revenues are higher than budgeted revenues. 2) When actual expenses are lower than budgeted expenses. *See also* Unfavorable variance.

Feasibility study—A study that looks at factors affecting an issue's ability to generate the necessary cash flows to meet principal and interest requirements.

Fee-for-service arrangement (FFS)—Arrangements in which providers receive "reasonable charges" for "necessary" services as the services are provided.

Federal Housing Administration (FHA) program loans—Mortgage insurance provided by the Federal Housing Administration that guarantees the principal and interest on a loan for a health care provider.

Financing activities—A section of the statement of cash flows used to report such activities as borrowing and paying back loans.

Financing mix—How an organization chooses to finance its working capital needs.

Fiscal intermediary (FI)—A Medicare contractor that processes and pays Medicare institutional claims.

Fixed asset turnover [total revenues/net plant & equipment]—This ratio measures the number of dollars generated for each dollar invested in an organization's plant and equipment.

Fixed assets—Literally nonmovable assets. Generally used to refer to buildings and equipment.

Fixed costs—Costs that stay the same in total over the relevant range as volume increases, but that change inversely on a per unit basis.

Fixed income securities—Securities that pay a fixed amount of interest periodically, usually semiannually, over the lifetime of the bond.

Fixed labor budget—The section of the expense budget that forecasts salary and benefits.

Fixed (interest) rate debt—A security with an interest rate that does not change during the lifetime of the bond.

Fixed supplies budget—The section of the expense budget that forecasts the cost of those supplies that will not vary as a direct result of changes in the amount of services provided (such as administrative office supplies).

Flat fee systems—Flat fee systems pay a predefined amount for a unit of service. By paying a flat fee, the payor limits its liabilities. By accepting a flat fee, the provider accepts the risk that the cost to offer the service may exceed the payment. An example is the DRG system.

Flexible budget—A budget that estimates the revenues and/or expenses over a range of service volume.

Float—Time delays in the billing and collection process. There are four categories of float: billing, collection, transit, and disbursement. An organization's goal is to optimize float for incoming revenues and outgoing bills.

Footnotes—The bottom area of the financial statements that contains key information not available in the body of the statements, such as how charity is determined, the position of investments, which assets are restricted, and the depreciation method used.

For-profit—A type of organization whose profits can be distributed outside the organization and must pay taxes. Also called investor-owned organizations.

FTE—Full-time equivalent employees. Two half-time employees equal one FTE.

Fully allocated costs—The costs of a service after taking into account its direct and fair share of allocated costs.

Future value (FV)—What an amount invested today (or a series of payments made over time) will be worth at a given time in the future using the compound interest method. This accounts for the time value of money. *See also* Present value.

Future value factor (FVF)—A factor that, when multiplied by a present amount, yields the future value of that amount. It is calculated using the formula $(1 + i)^n$, where i is the interest rate and n is the number of periods. *See also* Present value factor.

Future value factor of an annuity (FVFA)—A factor that when multiplied by a stream of equal payments equals the future value of that stream. *See also* Present value factor of an annuity.

Future value of an annuity—What a series of equal payments will be worth at some future date using compound interest. *See also* Future value factor of an annuity *and* Present value of an annuity.

Future value table—The table that contains factors to determine the future value of an amount.

G

Gain or loss—1) The difference between the amount received in selling a capital asset and its book value. 2) The difference between the purchase price of a stock and its sale price.

Gatekeepers—Persons who must preapprove the care received by a patient, such as a primary care physician who must approve a patient visiting a specialist. Gatekeepers are utilized in most point-of-service and HMO plans.

General and administrative (G & A) expenses—Operating expenses that are not contained in the labor or supplies budgets.

Geographic adjustment factor (GAF)—A measure of the effect of geographic location on the cost of a service—used in calculating Medicare physician payment.

Geographic practice cost index (GPCI)—A measure of the differences in resource costs among physician fee schedule areas. There are three GPCIs, one for each relative value unit (RVU) component: a work GPCI, an overhead GPCI, and a malpractice GPCI.

Global payments—Payments in which the fees for all providers and suppliers (hospitals, physicians, nurses, home health care agencies, drugs, etc.) are included in a single negotiated amount. Often called bundling of services.

Grants—Funds given to a health care organization for special purposes, usually for only a limited time.

Gross patient service revenues—The total amount the health care organization earns at full retail price for its services (i.e., before discounts and allowances).

GROUPER—Computer software that translates variables such as age, diagnosis, and surgical codes into the diagnosis related group (DRG) under which Medicare payment amount is determined.

H

Health care common procedure coding system (HCPCS)—The HCPCS is a coding system for all services performed by a physician or supplier. It is based on the American Medical Association Physicians' Current Procedural Terminology (CPT) codes and is augmented with codes for physician and nonphysician services (such as ambulance and durable medical equipment [DME]), which are not included in CPTs.

Health maintenance organization (HMO)—Entities that receive premium payments (fixed periodic prepayment) from enrollees with the understanding that the HMO will be financially responsible for all predefined health care required by its enrollees for a specified period of time. The health care is provided through the HMO's provider network.

Hedge—A transaction that reduces the risk of an investment.

Historical/market/payor approach—Setting charges based on a combination of: 1) charging what the organization has traditionally charged; 2) what similar organizations charge; and 3) what payors will pay. Sometimes called the UCR (usual, customary, and reasonable) system.

Home health agency (HHA)—A public agency or private organization that is primarily engaged in providing skilled nursing services and other therapeutic services in the patient's home. Service examples are physical, occupational, or speech therapy; medical social services; and home health aid services.

Horizontal analysis—Looks at the percentage change in a line item's value from one year to the next using the formula: [(subsequent year − base year)/base year] × 100. *See also* Vertical analysis.

Hospice—Hospice care is palliative care, such as medical relief of pain, provided to patients who are certified to be terminally ill.

Hospital insurance (HI, Medicare)—Medicare HI, also referred to as Part A, covers expenses of inpatient, hospice, skilled nursing facility (SNF), or home health agency (HHA) services for individuals who are age 65 or older and are eligible for retirement benefits under the Social Security or Railroad Retirement systems. Coverage is also provided for individuals under age 65 who have been entitled for not less than 24 months to benefits under the Social Security or Railroad Retirement systems on the basis of disability, and for certain other individuals who are medically determined to have end stage renal disease (ESRD) and are covered by the Social Security or Railroad Retirement systems.

Hurdle rate—*See* Cost of capital *and* Discount rate.

I

Income from investments—A category of income that includes unrestricted interest, dividends, and gains from the sale of unrestricted investments.

Increase in unrestricted net assets—The bottom line in the statement of operations. It includes such items as operating and nonoperating income, contributions of long-lived assets, transfers to parent company, and extraordinary items.

Incremental cash flows—Cash flows that occur solely as a result of undertaking a project. Basically the marginal difference between alternatives.

Incremental/decremental approach—An approach to budgeting that begins with what exists and either gives a slight increase, no change, or a slight decrease to various line items, programs, or departments. *See also* Zero-based budgeting.

Indenture—Legal document that states the conditions and terms of a bond.

Indirect costs—Costs not traced to a cost object, but that must eventually be allocated across cost objects. *See also* Direct costs.

Individual practice associations (IPA) model HMO—Loose affiliation of providers who agree to cover the health care needs of a covered population on a capitated basis, usually through a per member per month payment arrangement.

Inflation—The rise in an economy's general level of prices.

Institutional services—Services provided by hospitals (outpatient and inpatient), home health agencies (HHAs), hospices, comprehensive outpatient rehabilitation facilities, end stage renal disease (ESRD) facilities, rural health clinics, and skilled nursing facilities (SNFs).

Interest—1) The cost to borrow money. It can be expressed in dollars or as a percentage. 2) Payment to creditors for the use of money on credit.

Interim claim—A request for payment that does not cover a complete stay in a hospital or skilled nursing facility (SNF). It is submitted by a provider when a beneficiary is still receiving services (i.e., has not yet been discharged).

Internal claims processing—Reviewing claims sent to payors in order to assure that care has appropriately described and decrease the chances that the claims will be denied. This process usually includes utilization review.

Internal rate of return (IRR)—The percentage return on an investment. It is the rate of return at which the net present value equals zero. Often used as a comparison to cost of capital.

International Classification of Diseases-9th Revision-Clinical Modification (ICD-9-CM)—The ICD-9-CM is a diagnosis and procedure classification system. ICD-9-CM codes are the basis for grouping patients into diagnosis related groups (DRGs).

Investment banker—One who advises corporate clients on their financial strategy and/or is primarily involved in the distribution of securities from the issuing organization to the public.

Investment centers—Responsibility centers responsible for making a certain return on investments.

Investment grade—Bonds that have received a rating ranging from AAA to BBB (at S&P), or Aaa to Bbb (Moody's), of which the highest are called quality ratings.

Investor—An entity that gives capital to another entity in expectation of a financial or nonfinancial return.

Issuer—An entity that sells bonds in order to raise money.

J

Joint costs—*See* Common costs.

Junk bonds—Bonds rated BB and below by S&P or Ba and below by Moody's. They usually have a high default rate.

L

Labor budget—That part of the expense budget that forecasts the cost of fixed and variable labor.

Lease—A contract in which the lessee (user) agrees to pay the lessor (owner) a specific amount over a period of time for the use of an asset.

Lender—An entity that temporarily grants the use of money or an asset to another in return for compensation, usually in the form of interest.

Liabilities—The organization's legal obligations to pay its creditors. Liabilities are classified as current and noncurrent. Liabilities are one of the three major categories on the balance sheet and are part of the fundamental accounting equation.

Lien—A security interest in one or more assets granted to lenders in a secured loan.

Lifetime reserve days, Medicare—A beneficiary is entitled to 60 lifetime reserve days for inpatient hospital care. When more than 90 days of inpatient care are required in a benefit period, a patient may choose to draw upon the reserve days. Patients are required to pay a daily coinsurance amount equal to one half of the inpatient hospital deductible for each reserve day.

Line of credit—A contract between a lender and a potential borrower preauthorizing the potential borrower's right to borrow up to a specific amount on request as long as they fulfill the terms and conditions of the contract. Also called a letter of credit.

Line-item budget—The budget format that lists revenues and expenses by category, such as labor, travel, and supplies. Categories are sometimes broken down into subcategories. *See also* Performance budget *and* Program budget.

Liquidity—The ease and speed with which an asset can be turned into cash.

Liquidity ratios—Ratios that answer the question: How well is the organization positioned to meet its short-term obligations?

Loan amortization schedule—A schedule detailing the principal and interest payments required to repay a loan. Typically, the periodic payments remain unchanged, but the proportion used to pay off the principal increases over time.

Lockboxes—A mailbox directly accessible by a bank that deposits receipts directly into the health care provider's account.

Longitudinal data—Information that covers multiple periods. Used in horizontal and ratio analysis.

Long-term debt to net assets ratio (long-term debt/net assets)—A measure of the proportion of an organization's assets that are financed by debt as opposed to equity. In for-profit organizations, it is called the *long-term debt to equity ratio* and is calculated using the formula (long-term debt/owners' equity).

Long-term debt, net of current portion—The total amount of multiyear debt due in future years.

Long-term financing—Debt to be paid off in a period longer than one year.

Long-term investments—A category of noncurrent assets not intended to be used for operations, but only for capital appreciation and dividends, and that will be held for a period longer than one year.

M

Mail float—The elapsed time between when the patient or third-party payor sends the payment and the time the health care provider receives the payment.

Managed care—Any of a number of arrangements designed to control health care costs through monitoring, prescribing, or proscribing the provision of health care to a patient or population. *See also* Health maintenance organizations (HMOs).

Managed care organization (MCO)—A prepaid or capitated health plan that is a State-licensed legal entity which provides health care directly or under arrangements for its members, and does participate under agreement or contract in a Federal Medicare managed care program.

Management information system—A system designed to gather, store, manipulate, and analyze data in order to provide information for management decision making.

Management service organization (MSO)—Organizations whose main purpose is to provide administrative services (claims management, utilization review, etc.) to or for health care organizations.

Mandatory services—Those services that each State Medicaid program is required to cover, including hospital, physician, and skilled nursing facility services.

Market rate of interest—The current traded rate for similar risk securities.

Market value (MV)—The price at which something, such as bonds and stocks, could be bought or sold today on the open market.

Marketable securities—Short-term claims that can be bought and sold through a capital market. Examples are treasury bills, commercial paper, and certificates of deposit.

Maturity—The end of a bond's life.

Medicaid—A joint, Federal-State entitlement program intended to provide basic medical services for certain groups of low-income persons.

Medicare beneficiary—An individual who is enrolled for coverage under the Medicare program.

Medicare eligibility—Medicare eligibility is determined by whether an individual meets the legal requirements for Medicare coverage (age 65 or older, disabled, or requiring kidney transplant or renal dialysis due to chronic kidney disease).

Medicare provider—A facility, supplier, or physician who furnishes Medicare services.

Mission statement—A statement intended to guide the organization into the future by identifying the unique attributes of the organization, why it exists, and what it hopes to achieve.

Money market mutual funds—Pooling of investors' funds for the purchase of a diversified portfolio of short-term financial instruments, such as treasury bills and certificates of deposit. This pooling of funds allows small investors, such as small health care facilities, to earn short-term money market rates on their investments.

Mortgage—A note payable that has as collateral real assets and that requires periodic payments.

Mortgage bonds—Bonds that hold the health care provider's real property and equipment as security or collateral in case of default.

Multiyear budget—Budgets that typically cover two to five years.

Mutually exclusive projects—A situation in which if one project is implemented the other(s) will not be.

N

Negative pledge—A bond covenant that restricts the health care provider from giving a lien (claim) on its real estate to any other creditor.

Negotiable certificates of deposit (CDs)—Certificates of deposit an investor may sell before maturity.

Net accounts receivable—The amount expected to be collected from payors. It is calculated as: (gross accounts receivable—discounts and allowances—allowance for uncollectibles).

Net assets—Assets minus liabilities. One of the three major categories on the balance sheet. Traditionally known as *stockholders' equity* in investor-owned organizations and *fund balance* in not-for-profit organizations. In not-for-profit health care organizations, net assets must be categorized into three categories: unrestricted, temporarily restricted, and permanently restricted.

Net assets released from restriction—Previously restricted assets no longer restricted because the terms of the restriction have been met.

Net assets released from restrictions used for purchase of property and equipment—Previously-restricted assets that must be used to purchase property and equipment. Since they are for the purchase of long-lived assets, they are not considered revenue.

Net assets to total assets (net assets/total assets)—This ratio reflects the proportion of total assets financed by equity. In for-profit organizations it is called the *equity to total asset ratio* and is calculated using the formula (owners' equity/total assets).

Net increase (decrease) in cash and cash equivalents—The section of the statement of cash flows that reports the total change in cash and cash equivalents over the accounting period.

Net patient service revenue—The revenue that the organization has a right to collect. It is computed as: gross patient service revenues—contractual allowance and charity care.

Net present value—The difference between the initial amount paid for an investment and the related future cash inflows after they have been adjusted (discounted) by the cost of capital.

Net proceeds from a bond issuance—Gross proceeds less the underwriter's fee and other issuance fees.

Net working capital—The difference between current assets and current liabilities.

Non-current assets—Assets that provide service for a period exceeding one year. Sometimes referred to as long-term assets.

Non-current liabilities—Financial obligations that will be paid off over a time period longer than one year.

Nonoperating expenses—Expenses of the organization incurred in non-health-care related activities.

Nonoperating income—The income (operating revenues – operating expenses) earned in non-health care-related activities.

Nonoperating ratio (nonoperating revenues/total operating revenues)—A ratio that reflects how dependent the organization is on nonpatient care related net income.

Nonoperating revenues—Revenues of the organization earned in non-healthcare-related activities.

Nonregular cash flows—Irregular cash flows, typically occurring at the end of the life of a project.

Notes payable—A legal obligation to pay the holder of the note or lien.

Not-for-profit—1) Organizations that have a special designation because they provide goods or services that result in needed community benefit. In turn, such organizations are not required to pay most taxes. 2) The designation of an organization as one that is not generally required to pay taxes and may not distribute its profits.

O

Offering memorandum—A document that outlines the terms of the offering of a private placement security.

Opening inventory—The cost of the supplies on hand at the beginning of the year.

Operating activities—The activities of an organization directly related to its main line of business.

Operating budget—The revenue and expense budgets of an organization.

Operating cash flows—The cash flows derived from an organization's operating activities.

Operating expenses—The expenses incurred from an organization's operating activities.

Operating income—A measure of the income earned from operating activities. It is calculated as: (unrestricted revenues, gains, and other support – expenses and losses).

Operating lease—A lease for a period shorter than the equipment's economic life, usually cancelable.

Operating margin (operating income/total operating revenues)—The proportion of profit remaining after subtracting total operating expenses from operating revenues.

Operating revenues—Revenues generated from an organization's operating activities.

Opportunity cost—Proceeds lost by foregoing other opportunities.

Ordinary annuity—A series of payments made or received at the end of each period.

Other expenses—A catch-all category for miscellaneous expenses and losses not included in other categories (telephone, travel, meals, etc.).

Other income—Nonoperating income.

Other revenues—Operating income not reported elsewhere under revenues, gains, and other support.

Other support—Amounts given to the organization for operating purposes, such as governmental appropriations and unrestricted donations.

Outlier—An outlier is an extremely long or unusually high cost inpatient hospital stay when compared to most stays classified in the same diagnosis related group (DRG).

P

Par value—Amount that a bondholder is paid at the time of the bond's maturity. Also called face value.

Parent organization—An entity that owns other companies.

Part A—See Hospital insurance (HI).

Part B—See Supplementary medical insurance (SMI).

Participatory approach—An approach to carrying out organizational tasks in which the roles and responsibilities are diffused throughout the organization. This approach is opposite of the authoritarian approach.

Passthrough payment—Payments to hospitals for costs that are excluded from the Prospective Payment System (PPS), including bad debt, kidney acquisition costs, and direct costs of medical education.

Payback—A method to evaluate the feasibility of an investment by determining how long it would take until the initial investment is recovered. As it is usually applied, this method does not account for the time value of money.

Penalties (out-of-network)—Charging patients a penalty for seeking care from out-of-network providers.

Per diem rates—A set reimbursement per inpatient day based on the type of case.

Per member per month (PMPM)—The most common way in which providers receive captitated payments.

Performance budget—A budget which presents not only line items and programs, but also the performance goals that each program can be expected to attain. *See also* Line-item budget *and* Program budget.

Performance measure—Financial and nonfinancial standards against which organizational performance is measured.

Periodic payments—Series of payments over time, such as interest paid to bondholders.

Permanently restricted net assets—Donated assets that have restrictions on their use which will never be removed.

Perpetuity—An investment that generates an annuity for an indefinite period of time, basically forever.

Planning/control cycle—A classification of the activities of the organization into four major components, with budgeting being the focus: strategic planning, planning, implementing, and controlling.

PMPM—*See* Per member per month.

Point-of-service (POS) arrangement—A hybrid between an HMO and a PPO in which patients are given the incentive to see providers participating in a defined network, but may see non-network providers, though usually at some additional cost.

Preadmission certification and second opinions—A requirement that prior approval or review of service take place before care is delivered.

Precautionary purposes—Setting aside cash to meet unexpected demands, such as unexpected maintenance of a facility or piece of equipment.

Preferred provider organization (PPO)—An independent provider or provider network preselected by the payor to provide a specific service or range of services at predetermined (usually discounted) rates to the payor's covered members.

Premium—1) An amount paid by an employee or employer to pay for health care insurance. 2) When the market rate is lower than the coupon rate, a bond is said to be selling at a premium.

Premium revenues—Revenues earned from capitated contracts.

Prepaid asset—A benefit paid for in advance (rent, insurance, etc.). Also called prepaid expense.

Present value (PV)—The value today of a payment (or series of payments) to be received in the future taking into account the cost of capital. It is calculated using the formula: future value × present value factor [$PV = FV \times PVF$ *or* $PV = FV \times 1/(1 + i)^n$]. *See also* Future value.

Present value factor (PVF)—A factor used to discount future cash flows. It is the reciprocal of the future value factor and is calculated by the formula: $1/(1 + i)^n$. *See also* Future value factor.

Present value of an annuity—What a series of equal payments in the future is worth today taking into account the time value of money. *See also* Present value factor of an annuity *and* Future value of an annuity.

Present value of an annuity table—The table that contains factors to determine the present value of an annuity.

Present value factor of an annuity (PVFA)—A factor that when multiplied by a stream of equal payments equals the present value of that stream. *See also* Future value factor of an annuity.

Present value table—The table that contains factors to determine the present value of an amount to be received in the future.

Prevention—A set of activities designed to decrease morbidity and mortality in a population.

Principal—Amount invested.

Principal diagnosis—The medical condition that is chiefly responsible for the admission of a patient to a hospital or for services provided by a physician or other provider. It is determined after the patient has been examined.

Private placement—The sale of securities directly to investors without a public offering.

Processing float—The elapsed time between processing a payment once received and depositing it in the bank.

Product margin (Total contribution margin – Avoidable fixed costs)—It represents the amount that a service contributes to cover all other costs after it has covered those costs which are there solely because the service is offered (its total variable cost and avoidable fixed costs) and would not be there if the service were dropped.

Product margin rule—If a service's product margin is positive, the organization will be better off financially if it continues with the service, all other things equal. Conversely, if a service's product margin is negative, the organization will be better off financially if it discontinues the service, all else being equal.

Professional fees—Fees paid to contract clinicians such as physicians, social workers, and physical therapists. Nursing expenses are usually reported under a category such as Labor Expenses.

Profit centers—Organizational units responsible for controlling their costs and earning revenues. There are three types of profit centers: traditional profit centers, capitated profit centers, and administrative profit centers.

Profitability ratios—Ratios designed to answer the question: How profitable is the organization?

Pro-forma financial statements—These are customized financial statements that do not necessarily conform to generally-accepted accounting principles (GAAP). When they are prepared before the accounting period, they present what the organization's financial statements will look like if all budgets are met exactly as planned. Pro-forma financial statements also can be prepared for historical statements. In that case, the financial statements are remade to illustrate the effect of a proposed transaction, such as a business combination, acquisition, or proposed issue of securities. The role of a pro-forma balance sheet is to present underlying assumptions and events that permit investors to understand the potential effect of that proposed transaction.

Program budget—A budget in which line items are presented by program. *See also* Line-item Budget *and* Performance budget.

Properties, plant, and equipment—The category of assets summarizing the amount of the major capital investments of the facility in plant, property, and equipment. *Plant* means buildings, *property* is land, and *equipment* includes a wide variety of durable items from beds to CAT scanners. Property, plant, and equipment are recorded on the organization's books at cost, and over time, plant and equipment (but not land) are subject to depreciation.

Properties, plant, and equipment, net—Properties, buildings, and equipment less accumulated depreciation.

Prospective payment system (PPS)—The system used by Medicare to reimburse providers a set amount based on the patient's DRG. This system is commonly referred to as the PPS or DRG payment system.

Provider networks—A preselected list of providers from which a patient can choose without being liable for additional costs beyond any deductibles and copayments.

Provision for bad debt—A statement of operations account which estimates the portion of receivables that are not likely to be collected. The provision for bad debt is the cost recognized in a particular period only. The related allowance for uncollectibles on the balance sheet is a cumulative account.

Public offering—A bond sold to the investing public through an underwriter (sometimes called an investment banker).

Q

Qui tam—*Qui tam* is an abbreviation of a Latin phrase which has the meaning "he who as well for the king as for himself sues in this matter." Qui tam is the technical legal term for the mechanism in the Federal False Claims Act that allows persons and entities with evidence of fraud against federal programs or contracts to sue the wrongdoer on behalf of the government.

Quick ratio [(cash + marketable securities + net accounts receivable)/current liabilities]—A measure of the organization's liquidity.

R

Ratio analysis—An approach to analyzing the financial condition of an organization based on ratios calculated from line items found in the financial statements. There are four major categories of ratios: liquidity, profitability, capitalization, and activity.

RBRVS—*See* Resource-based relative value system. *See also* RVUs.

Realized gains and losses—The increases or decreases in the value of a stock from the time it was purchased until the time it is sold.

Red herring—A preliminary prospectus offered by the underwriters to prospective buyers of bonds to determine a fair price for which they will be sold.

Relative value unit (RVU)—A standard for measuring the value of a medical service provided by physicians relative to other medical services provided by physicians. The RVU for each service has three components: the physician work component (reflecting physician time and intensity), the overhead component (reflecting all categories of practice expenses, exclusive of malpractice insurance costs), and the malpractice expense component (reflecting the cost of obtaining malpractice insurance).

Relevant range—The range over which fixed costs in total and variable costs per unit do not change.

Replacement decisions—Capital investment decisions designed to replace older assets with newer ones, using a net present value approach.

Resource-based relative value scale (RBRVS)—A system for measuring physician input to medical services for the purpose of calculating a physician fee schedule. The relative value of each service is the sum of relative value units (RVUs) representing physician work, practice expenses, and the cost of malpractice insurance.

Responsibility—Duties and obligations of a responsibility center.

Responsibility center—Organizational unit given the responsibility to carry out one or more tasks and/or achieve one or more outcomes.

Restricted donation—A donation that has conditions which must be satisfied. *See also* Temporarily restricted net assets.

Retained earnings—Portion of the profits the organization keeps in-house to use in support of its mission.

Retrospective review—Reviewing all services after they have been performed, and only reimbursing for those services deemed medically necessary by the payor.

Return on investment (ROI)—The percentage gain or loss experienced from an investment.

Return on net assets (excess of revenues over expenses/net assets)—In not-for-profit health care organizations, it measures the rate of return for each dollar in net assets. In for-profit organizations, it measures the rate of return for each dollar in owners' equity; called *return on equity* and has the formula: (net income/owners' equity).

Return on total assets (excess of revenues over expenses/total assets)—A measure of how much profit is earned for each dollar invested in assets. In for-profit organizations it is called *return on assets* and is calculated as: (net income/assets).

Revenue—Amounts earned by the organization from the provision of service or sale of goods.

Revenue attainment—Earning the amount of revenue budgeted.

Revenue budget—The budget that forecasts the operating, and in some cases, the nonoperating revenues that will be earned during the budget period.

Revenue center—A facility cost center for which a separate charge is billed on an institutional claim.

Revenue enhancement—Supplementing traditional sources of revenue with new sources.

Revenue rate variance—The amount of the total revenue variance that occurs because the actual average rate charged varies from that originally budgeted. It can be calculated using the formula: [(actual rate – budgeted rate) × actual volume].

Revenue volume variance—The portion of total variance in revenues due to the actual volume being either higher or lower than the budgeted volume. It can be computed using the formula: [(actual volume – budgeted volume) × budgeted rate].

Revolving line of credit—A contract that requires a lender to fulfill the borrower's credit request up to the prenegotiated limit.

Rolling budgets—Budgets updated on an ongoing basis, continually forecasting a given time frame, e.g., 3 years in advance.

RVUs—See Relative value units.

S

Salvage value—The amount an organization would receive by selling a fixed asset, usually either at the end of a project or at the end of its useful life.

Secondary diagnosis—A medical condition other than the principal diagnosis that affected the treatment received or length of stay in a hospital, or services rendered by a physician or other provider.

Secondary market—Markets that deal in the buying and selling of bonds that have already been issued.

Secured loan—A loan in which specific assets are pledged as collateral.

Securities and Exchange Commission (SEC)—This governmental agency ensures that market trading is fair, among other things.

Security—A (contractual) claim on future cash flows.

Seller—An organization selling an asset.

Serial bonds—Bonds issued at various maturities and coupon rates.

Service centers—Organizational units primarily responsible for ensuring that services are provided to a population in a manner that meets the volume and quality requirements of the organization. Service centers are the most basic type of responsibility centers.

Service mix—1) The range of services offered by a provider. 2) Issues focusing on the appropriateness of care.

Short-term financing—Financing that will be paid back in less than one year.

Short-term investments—Investments that will be liquidated within one year, such as certificates of deposit, commercial paper, and treasury bills.

Simple interest method—Financing in which only the interest on the principal is calculated each period. *See also* Compound interest method.

Sinking fund—As part of the bond contract, a covenant may establish that part of the principal be paid each year, earmarked for the orderly retirement or the redemption of bonds before maturity. These funds are paid periodically to the trustee who maintains the fund for the health care provider. They are analogous to the principal repayment of a mortgage.

Skilled nursing facility (SNF)—An institution that meets specified regulatory certification requirements and is engaged primarily in providing inpatient skilled nursing care and rehabilitative services.

Speculative bonds—Relatively high-return, high-risk bonds. Sometimes called junk bonds.

Speculative purposes—Setting aside cash that can be used to take advantage of unexpected opportunities.

Spillover cash flows—If a project is undertaken, these cash flows are the indirect increases or decreases in cash flows that will occur elsewhere in the organization.

Spread—The difference between the price paid for a security by an investment banker and its sale price. Usually quoted in terms of basis points.

Staff mix—1) The amount of staff in various categories. 2) Issues pertaining to the appropriateness of who provides service (RN vs. LPN, etc.).

Staff model HMO—An HMO in which the providers are employees of the HMO.

Statement of cash flows—One of the four major financial statements. It answers the questions: Where did our cash come from and where did it go during the accounting period?

Statement of changes in net assets—One of the four major financial statements. It explains the changes in net assets from one period to the next on the balance sheet. Also called *statement of changes in owners' equity* in a for-profit business.

Statement of operations—One of the four major financial statements. It summarizes the organization's revenues and expenses during an accounting period, as well as other items that affect its unrestricted net assets. It is analogous to, but different from, an *income statement* in a for-profit organization.

Static budgets—Budgets that forecast for a single level of activity.

Statistics budget—The budget that identifies the amount of services that will be provided, usually by payor type.

Stay record—A record that summarizes all services rendered to a beneficiary from admission to an institution through discharge from that same institution.

Steerage discounts—Agreements by which payors agree to send patients to selected providers in return for discounts.

Step-down method—A method of allocating costs that are not directly paid for (utilities, rent, administration) into those products or services to which payment is attached (day of care, a brief visit). *See also* Activity-based costing.

Step-fixed costs—Fixed costs which increase in total at certain points as the level of activity increases. For instance, labor is often a step-fixed cost that increases when new employees are added after certain volumes of service are reached.

Stop-loss limit—A method used by providers to limit the risk in cases where costs incurred are significantly greater than standard reimbursements for those services.

Strategic decisions—Capital investment decisions designed to increase a health care organization's strategic position.

Strategic financial planning—A method by which the organization develops its strategies and budgets to meet future financial targets.

Strategic planning—The planning process that identifies the organization's mission and strategy in order to position itself for the future.

Subordinated debenture—Unsecured bond junior to debenture bonds. In the case of default, debenture bondholders are paid first.

Subsidiary—An organization owned and/or managed by another organization.

Substandard bonds—Very risky "junk bonds."

Sunk cost—Costs already incurred. They should not be included in cost analyses of future projects.

Supplementary medical insurance (SMI)—Medicare SMI, also referred as Part B, is a voluntary insurance program that covers physician services (in or outside of the hospital), outpatient hospital services, ambulatory services, and certain medical supplies and other services, for all persons age 65 or older and persons eligible for Part A due to disability or chronic renal disease.

Supplies budget—The expense budget that forecasts fixed and variable supplies.

SWOT analysis—A technique to evaluate an organization's *s*trengths, *w*eaknesses, *o*pportunities, and *t*hreats. This technique often is used as part of the strategic planning process.

T

Tangible assets—Assets that have a physical presence.

Target costing—An approach to designing products and services so that their cost is below a certain level, rather than the traditional method of producing a product and then setting a price based on its cost.

Tax-exempt bonds (tax-exempt revenue bonds)—Bonds in which the interest payments to the investor are exempt from IRS taxation. These bonds must be issued by an organization that has received tax exemption from the IRS and be used to fund projects that qualify as "exempt uses." Tax-exempt revenue bonds are backed by the organization's revenues. They offer lower interest rates than do taxable bonds.

Tax shield—An investment that reduces the amount of income tax to be paid, often because interest and depreciation expenses are tax deductible.

Temporarily restricted net assets—Assets that have restrictions on their use which will be removed either with the passage of time or the occurrence of some event. *See also* Restricted donation.

Term—A specified amount of time.

Term loans—A form of long-term financing that typically must be paid off within ten years. They require the borrower to pay off or amortize the principal value of the loan over its life.

Terminal value—The value of a bond at maturity.

Third-party payor—An agent that agrees to pay on behalf of a patient or group of patients. Examples include: Medicare, Medicaid, indemnity insurance companies, and HMOs.

Time value of money—The idea that a dollar today is worth more than a dollar in the future.

Times interest earned [(excess of revenues over expenses + interest expense)/interest expense]—This ratio enables creditors and lenders to evaluate an organization's ability to generate earnings necessary to meet interest expense requirements. In for-profit organizations the ratio is calculated using the formula: [(net income + interest expense)/interest expense]. The ratio answers the question: For every dollar in interest expense, how many dollars are there in profit before interest?

Top-down/bottom-up approach—Opposite of the authoritarian approach. The roles and responsibilities of the budgeting process are diffused throughout the organization. Often called the participatory approach.

Top-down budgeting—That process of budgeting where the environmental assessment and planning of future activities are largely decided upon by a few individuals, and the budget is essentially dictated to the rest of the organization. Often called authoritarian approach.

Total asset turnover (total revenues/total assets)—This ratio measures the overall efficiency of the organization's assets to produce revenue. It answers the question: For every dollar in assets, how many dollars of revenue are being generated?

Total revenue—Price times total quantity.

Trade credit—Credit granted by a firm to another firm for the purchase of services or products.

Traditional profit centers—Organizational units primarily responsible for providing services and earning a profit based on the health care services provided.

Transaction—A good or service provided in return for some type of compensation.

Transaction notes—A short-term, unsecured loan made for some specific purpose, such as the financing of inventory purchases. Transaction notes have compensating balance requirements.

Transfer to parent—Transfer of assets from a subsidiary to its parent company.

Transit float—The time elapsed between the time a check is deposited in the banking system and when the funds are available.

Treasury bills (T-bills)—Financial instruments that can be purchased from the government and are considered default-free. They are among the most liquid short-term investments available. Rather than earning interest directly, T-bills are purchased at a discount rate and redeemed at face value when they mature.

Trend analysis—A type of horizontal analysis that looks at changes in line items compared to a base year. It is calculated: [(any subsequent year − base year)/base year] × 100.

Trustee—An agent for bondholders who performs two primary functions: the trustee makes the principal and interest payments to the bondholders and the trustee ensures that the healthcare provider complies with the legal covenants of the bond.

U

Underwriter—A firm that brings out new securities issues, agreeing to purchase and resell them. Often a lead underwriter and several other underwriters will work together on a given issue. Underwriters help healthcare facilities issue bonds and advise management on the terms of the structure of the bonds. Sometimes underwriters guarantee the proceeds to the firm from a future security sale, in effect taking ownership of the securities.

Unfavorable variances—1) When actual revenues are lower than budgeted revenues. 2) When actual expenses are lower than budgeted expenses. *See also* Favorable variance.

Uniform Bill 92 (UB92)—The UB92 is a Medicare claim form used by institutional providers.

Unit of service—1) A unit of measure of the amount of service delivered. 2) A system of paying for services based on the number of units delivered (per procedure, per inpatient day, per admission, per discharge, per diagnosis).

Unrealized gains and losses—The change, since the last balance sheet, in the market value of stocks held for investment. The gains and losses are recognized as realized gains and losses only when the stocks are sold.

Unrestricted net assets—All net assets (including those that have been restricted by management, the governing board, contractual agreements, or other legal documents) not restricted by donors.

Unrestricted revenues, gains, and other support—The income of the organization derived from providing patient service, the sale of assets for more than their book value, contributions, appropriations, and assets released from restriction (except those used to purchase property and equipment).

Unsecured bank loan—A short-term loan not backed by collateral.

V

Variable costs—Costs that stay the same per unit, but change directly in total with a change in activity over the relevant range. (Total variable cost = Variable cost per unit × Number of units of activity).

Variable labor budget—The expense budget that forecasts labor costs that vary as additional personnel or overtime hours are needed.

Variable (interest) rate debt—A security whose rate changes are based on market conditions.

Variable supplies budget—The expense budget that forecasts the costs of supplies that vary with the number of patients seen, such as disposable syringes, disposable gloves, and x-ray films. Also called the nonfixed supply budget.

Vertical analysis—A method to analyze financial statements which answers the general question: What percentage of one line item is another line item? Also called common-size analysis because it converts every line item to a percentage, thus allowing comparisons among the financial statements of different organizations. *See also* Horizontal analysis.

Virtual corporations—Corporations that save cash and limit their financial risk by hiring a limited number of employees, owning few physical assets, and contracting out for most services.

W

Weighted-average approach—An approach to setting charges as a function of the number and type of procedures and the financial requirements of the organization.

Wire transfer—An approach used to eliminate mail and transit float by electronically depositing payments in the bank. Related techniques are zero-balance accounts and sweep accounts, where the bank automatically removes any excess from subsidiaries and places it in the account of the parent corporation.

Working capital—Current assets. (Net working capital = current assets − current liabilities).

Working capital cycle—The activities of the organization that encompass: 1) obtaining cash; 2) turning cash into resources, such as inventories and labor, and paying bills; 3) using the resources to provide services; and 4) billing patients for the services, and collecting revenues so that the cycle can be continued.

Working capital strategy—The degree of risk the organization is willing to take in financing and investing its working capital.

Y

Yield to maturity (YTM)—(market interest rate of a bond). The rate at which the market value of a bond is equal to the bond's present value of future coupon payments plus par value.

Z

Zero-coupon bonds—Bonds issued with a very low coupon value or with no coupon at all.

Zero-based budgeting (ZBB)—An approach to budgeting that regularly questions both the need for existing programs and their level of funding and the need for new programs. *See also* Incremental/decremental approach.

Common Health Care Financial Management Acronyms

A

A&D—admission and discharge

A/P—accounts payable

AAAHC—Accreditation Association for Ambulatory Health Care

AAE—affirmative action employer

AAHAM—American Association of Healthcare Administrative Management

AAHP—American Association of Health Plans

AAMA—American Academy of Medical Administration

AAMC—Association of American Medical Colleges

AAPA—American Academy of Physician Assistants

AAPCC—adjusted average per capita cost

AAR—after-hours activity report

ABA—American Bar Association

ABC—activity-based costing

ABM—activity-based management

ABN—advance beneficiary notice

ACC—ambulatory care center

ACI—average cost of illness

ACHE—American College of Healthcare Executives

ACPE—American College of Physician Executives

ACPPD—average cost per patient day

ACR—adjusted community rate

ACRS—accelerated cost recovery system

ACS—ambulatory care services

AD—admitting diagnosis

ADA—American Dietetic Association; American Dental Association

ADC—average daily census

ADFS—alternative delivery and financing systems

ADP—automatic data processing

ADPL—average daily patient load

ADRG—adjacent diagnosis-related group, alternative diagnosis-related group

ADS—alternative delivery system

ADSC—average daily service charge

ADT—admission/discharge/transfer

AEP—appropriate evaluation protocol

AFDC—Aid to Families with Dependent Children

AFDS—alternative financing and delivery systems

AFS—alternative financing systems

AG—affiliated group

AHA—American Hospital Association

AHCA—American Health Care Association (long-term care)

AHIMA—American Health Information Management Association

AHIP—assisted health insurance plan

AICPA—American Institute of Certified Public Accountants

ALC—alternate level of care

ALOH—average length of hospitalization

ALOS—average length of stay

AMA—American Medical Association

AMGA—American Medical Group Association

ANSI—American National Standards Institute

APA—American Psychiatric Association; American Psychological Association

APC—ambulatory payment classification

APG—ambulatory patient group

APHA—American Public Health Association

APHP—acute partial hospitalization program

APPAM—Association for Public Policy Analysis and Management

APR—annual percentage rate

AR—accounts receivable

AS—admissions scheduling

AS-SCORE—age of patient; systems involved; state of disease; complications; response to therapy

ASC—administrative services contract; ambulatory surgical/surgery center

ASCII—American Standard Code for Information Interchange

ASCS—admission scheduling and control system

ASF—ambulatory surgical facility

ASO—administrative services only

AVG—ambulatory visit group

AWI—area wage index

AWP—average wholesale price

B

BA—budget authority

BBA—Balanced Budget Act of 1997

BBRA—Balanced Budget Refinement Act (1999)

BCD—binary code decimal

BHU—basic health unit

BLS—Bureau of Labor Statistics

BOL—bill of lading

BQA—Bureau of Quality Assurance

BSR—bill summary record

C

C&E—consultation and examination

CAP—capitated ambulatory plan

CAH—critical access hospital

CBA—cost-benefit analysis

CBO—Congressional Budget Office

CC—complications and/or comorbidities

CCH—Commerce Clearing House

CCI—correct coding initiative

CCMU—critical care medical unit

CCR—cost-to-charge ratio

CCRC—continuing care retirement community

CD—chemical dependency

CDC—Centers for Disease Control (and Prevention)

CE—continuing education

CEA—cost-effectiveness analysis

CEO—chief executive officer

CER—capital expenditure review

CEU—continuing education unit

CFO—chief financial officer

CFR—Code of Federal Regulations

CHAMPUS—Civilian Health and Medical Program of the Uniformed Services

CHAMPVA—Civilian Health and Medical Program of the Veterans Affairs

CHC—community health center

CHFP—Certified Healthcare Financial Professional

CHI—consumer health information

CHIP—comprehensive health insurance plan, Children's Health Insurance Program; Consumer Health Information Program

CHMSA—critical health manpower shortage area

CHP—comprehensive health planning

CHRIS—computerized human resources information system

CIC—captive insurance company

CIO—chief information officer

CIS—computer information system

CM—case mix

CME—continuing medical education

CMHC—community mental health center

CMI—case-mix index; chronic mental illness

CMN—certificate of medical necessity

CMP—competitive medical plan

CMS—Centers for Medicare & Medicaid Services (formerly known as the Health Care Financing Administration)

CNH—community nursing home

CNHI—Committee for National Health Insurance

CNS—clinical nurse specialist

CO—coinsurance

COB—coordination of benefits; close of business

COI—cost of illness

COLA—cost-of-living adjustment

CON—certificate of need

COO—chief operating officer

CORF—comprehensive outpatient rehabilitation facility

CPA—certified public accountant

CPD—central processing department

CPEHS—Consumer Protection and Environmental Health Service

CPEP—Carrier Performance Evaluation Program

CPI—consumer price index

CPR—customary, prevailing, and reasonable

CPT-4™—Current Procedural Terminology, Fourth Edition

CPU—central processing unit

CQI—continuous quality improvement

CS—complexity-severity; consumer satisfaction
CSPS—corporate strategic planning system
CWF—common working file
CY—calendar year

D

D/A—date of admission
DA—disability assistance
DAW—dispense as written
DBMS—database management system
DC—diagnostic code
DDR—discharge during referral
DEFRA—Deficit Reduction Act
DHHS—Department of Health and Human Services
DI—disability insurance
DIB—disability insurance benefit
DISA—Data Interchange Standards Association
DJIA—Dow Jones Industrial Average
DME—durable medical equipment
DMEPOS—durable medical equipment, prosthetics, orthotics, and supplies
DMS *see* DBMS
DNR—do not resuscitate
DOA—date of admission; dead on arrival
DOD—Department of Defense
DOE—Department of Energy; Department of Education
DOH—Department of Health
DOJ—Department of Justice
DOL—Department of Labor
DOS—date of service
DOT—Department of Transportation
DP—data processing
DPH—Department of Public Health
DRA—Deficit Reduction Act
DRC—diagnosis-related category
DRG—diagnosis-related group
DRS—data retrieval system
DSH—disproportionate share hospital
DSM-IV—Diagnostic and Statistical Manual of Mental Disorders, Fourth Edition
DSO—debt service obligation

E

E&A—evaluate and advise
E&M—evaluation and management
EA—environmental assessment
EAC—estimated acquisition cost

EACH—essential access community hospital
EBCDIC—extended binary coded decimal information code
EBRI—Employee Benefit Research Institute
EC—emergency center
ECF—extended care facility
ECHO—electronic computing, health-oriented
ECI—employment cost index
ECD—electronic data processing
EDI—electronic data interchange
EDIFACT—EDI for administration, commerce, and trade
EDP—electronic data processing
EEO—equal employment opportunity
EEOC—Equal Employment Opportunity Commission
EFT—electronic funds transfer
EGHP—employer group health plan
EHIP—employee health insurance plan
EMTALA—The Emergency Medical Treatment and Active Labor Act
EO—executive order
EOB—explanation of benefits
EOC—episode of care
EOMB—explanation of medical benefits; Executive Office of Management and Budget; explanation of Medicare benefits
EOQ—economic order quantity
EPA—Environmental Protection Agency
EPEA—expense per equivalent admission
EPFT—electronic payment funds transfer
EPO—exclusive provider organization
ER—emergency room
ERISA—Employment Retirement Income Security Act
ERTA—Economic Recovery and Taxation Act
ES—emergency service
ESA—Employment Standards Administration
ESRD—end-stage renal disease
ET—expenditure target
EV—expected value
EVA—Economic Value Added

F

F&A—fraud and abuse
FAC—freestanding ambulatory care
FAHS—Federation of American Health Systems
FASB—Financial Accounting Standards Board
FDA—Food and Drug Administration
FDO—formula driven overpayment

FEC—freestanding emergency center
FFC—federal funding criteria
FFP—federal financial participation
FFS—fee for service
FFSS—fee-for-service system
FFY—federal fiscal year
FHA—Federal Housing Administration
FHFMA—Fellow of Healthcare Financial Management Association
FI—financial institution; fiscal intermediary
FICA—Federal Insurance Contributions Act
FIFO—first in, first out
FIG—fiscal intermediary group
FOIA—Freedom of Information Act
FPR—Federal Procurement Regulations
FQHC—federally qualified health center
FR—Federal Register
FSI—financial strength index
FTC—Federal Trade Commission
FTE—full-time equivalent
FWHF—Federation of World Health Foundations
FY—fiscal year

G

GAAP—generally accepted accounting principles
GAF—geographic adjustment factor
GAO—General Accounting Office
GDP—gross domestic product
GME—graduate medical education
GNP—gross national product
GOCO—government-owned, contract operated
GOGO—government-owned, government operated
GPCI—geographic practice cost index
GPM—gross profit margin
GPO—Government Printing Office; group purchasing organization

H

H-B—Hill-Burton Act
HAP—hospital accreditation program
HAR—hospital associated representatives
HAS—hospital administration services
HAT—hospital arrival time
HB—hospital based
HBCS—Hospital Billing and Collection Service
HBO—hospital benefits organization
HBP—hospital-based physician
HC—health care; home care

HCC—health care corporation
HCCA—health care commuting area
HCD—health care delivery
HCFA—Health Care Financing Administration, previous name for CMS. *See* CMS.
HCFAR—Health Care Financing Administration ruling
HCPCS—HCFA Common Procedure Coding System
HCRIS——Hospital Cost Reporting Information System
HCTA—health care trust account
HCUP—hospital cost and utilization project
HDS—health delivery system
HEAL—Health Education Assistance Loan
HEDIS— Health Plan Employer Data and Information Set
HEF—Health Education Foundation
HFMA—Healthcare Financial Management Association
HFPA—health facilities planning area
HFSG—health care financing study group
HH—hold harmless
HHO—home health organization
HHRG—home health resource groups
HHS—Health and Human Services (Department of)
HI—Hospital Insurance (refers to Medicare Part A)
HIAA—Health Insurance Association of America
HIBAC—Health Insurance Benefits Advisory Council
HIBCC—Health Insurance Business Communications Council
HIC—health information center; health insurance claim; health insurance company
HINN—hospital-issued notice of noncoverage
HIP—health insurance plan
HIPAA—Health Insurance Portability and Accountability Act of 1996
HIS —hospital information system
HITF—health insurance trust fund
HMO—health maintenance organization
HMO/CMP—health maintenance organization/competitive medical plan
HMPSA—health manpower shortage area
HOPD—hospital outpatient department
HPAC—Health Policy Advisory Center
HPB—historic payment basis
HPC—Health Policy Council
HPR—hospital peer review
HR—hospital record; hospital report; House of Representatives; House Resolution
HRET—Hospital Research and Education Trust
HRSA—Health Resources and Services Administration

HSA—Health Services Administration
HSQB—Health Standards and Quality Bureau
HSR—health services research
HSRC—Health Services Research Center
HUD—Housing and Urban Development (Department of)
HURA—Health Underserved Rural Area
HURT—hospital utilization review team
HV—hospital visit

I

IBNR—incurred but not reported
ICD—International Classification of Diseases
ICD-9—International Classification of Diseases, Ninth Revision
ICD-9-CM—International Classification of Diseases, Ninth Revision, Clinical Modification
ICD-10—International Classification of Diseases and Related Health Problems, Tenth Revision
ICD-10-CM—International Classification of Diseases and Related Health Problems, Tenth Revision, Clinical Modification
ICF—intermediate care facility
IDS—integrated delivery system
IG—Inspector General
IHS—Indian Health Service
IME—indirect medical education
IMS—information management system
I/O—input/output
IO—investor owned
IOL—intraocular lens
IOV—initial office visit
IP—inpatient
IPA—individual practice association
IPS—interim payment system
IRS—Internal Revenue Service
ITC—investment tax credit

J

JCAHO—Joint Commission on Accreditation of Healthcare Organizations
JIT—just in time
JUA—Joint Underwriting Association

L

LBO—leveraged buyout
LIFO—last in, first out

LOS—length of stay
LPN—licensed practical nurse
LTC—long-term care
LTCF—long-term care facility
LTCG—long-term capital gain
LTCU—long-term care unit
LTD—long-term debt
LVN—licensed vocational nurse

M

M&A—merger and acquisition
M+C—Medicare+Choice
MAC—major ambulatory category; maximum allowable charge
MADC—mean average daily census
MADRS—Medicare Automated Data Retrieval System
MB—market basket; Medicare Bureau
MCO—managed care organization
MDC—major diagnostic category
MDDRG—physician (MD) diagnosis-related group
MDG—major diagnostic group
MDH—Medicare dependent hospital
MDS—minimum data set
MEDISGRPS—Medical Illness Severity Grouping System
MEDLARS—Medical Literature Analysis and Retrieval System
MedPAC—Medicare Payment Advisory Commission
MedPAR—Medicare Provider Analysis and Review file
MEI—Medicare economic index
MET—multiple employer trust
MHB—maximum hospital benefit
MIA—medically indigent adult; multi-institutional arrangement
MIS—management information system
MLP—mid-level practitioner
MPFS—Medicare physician fee schedule
MR—management review
MRA—medical record administrator
MRD—medical record department
MRDF—machine-readable data file
MRI—magnetic resonance imaging; mortality risk index
MRP—maximum reimbursement point
MSA—metropolitan statistical area
MSO—medical service organization
MSP—Medicare secondary payer
MUA—medically underserved area
MVPS—Medicare volume performance standard

N

NACHA—National Automated Clearing House Association

NAHC—National Association for Home Care

NAIC—National Association of Insurance Commissioners

NAPH—National Association of Public Hospitals

NAR—net accounts receivable

NAS—National Academy of Sciences

NBS—National Bureau of Standards

NCAHC—National Council on Alternative Health Care

NCCBH—National Council for Community Behavior Healthcare

NCHS—National Center for Health Services

NCI—National Cancer Institute

NCQA—National Committee for Quality Assurance

NF—nursing facility

NFA—net fixed assets

NFP—not-for-profit

NFPC—not-for-profit corporation

NH—nursing home

NHC—National Health Council

NHCT—National Health Care Trust

NHF—National Health Federation

NHI—national health insurance

NHIP—national health insurance plan

NIH—National Institutes of Health

NOA—notice of admission

NOI—net operating income

NOL—net operating loss

NonPAR—nonparticipating physician

NOR—net operating revenue

NP—nurse practitioner

NPI—national provider identifier

NPO—nonprofit organization

NPPR—notice of proposed rulemaking

NPR—notice of program reimbursement

NPSR—net patient service revenue

NRHA—National Rural Health Association

NSF—not sufficient funds

NTIS—National Technical Information Services

NUBC—National Uniform Billing Committee

O

OASDHI—Old Age Survivors, Disability, and Health Insurance Program

OASIS—Outcome and Assessment Information Set

OBRA—Omnibus Budget Reconciliation Act

OD—organizational development

ODR—Office of Direct Reimbursement

OHTA—Office of Health Technology Assessment

OIG—Office of Inspector General

OJT—on-the-job training

OMB—Office of Management and Budget

OOP—out of pocket

OP—outpatient

OPD—outpatient department

OPL—operational policy letter; other party liability

OPM—Office of Personnel Management

OR—occupancy rate; operating room

OSG—Office of the Surgeon General

OSHA—Occupational Safety and Health Act; Occupational Safety and Health Administration

OTA—Office of Technology Assessment

OTC—over the counter

OWCP—Officer of Workers' Compensation Programs

P

PA—physician assistant

PAAF—preadmission assessment form

PAC—preadmission certification

PACE—performance and cost efficiency

PAM—patient accounts manager

PAR—participating (provider or supplier)

PATH—Physicians at Teaching Hospitals (fraud audit)

PCP—primary care physician

PE—practice expense; physician extender

PH—partial hospitalization

PHO—partial hospitalization organization

PHP—partial hospitalization program

PL—Public Law

PM—program memorandum

PMPM—per member per month

PO—physician organization

POS—place of service; point of service

PPA—preferred provider arrangement

PPD—per patient day; prepaid

PPM—physician practice management

PPO—preferred provider organization

PPR—patient-physician relationship; physician payment reform

PPS—prospective payment system; prospective pricing system

PR—peer review

PRO—peer review organization
ProPAC—Prospective Payment Assessment Commission
PRP—prospective reimbursement plan
PRRB—Provider Reimbursement Review Board
PRS—prospective reimbursement system
PSO—provider-sponsored organization
PTA—prior to admission
PUFF—proposed use of federal funds
PVH—private voluntary hospital

Q

QA—quality assurance
QAM—quality assurance monitor/monitoring
QAP—quality assurance program
QAS—quality assurance standards
QA/RM—quality assurance/risk management
QA/UR—quality assurance/utilization review
QM—quality management
QMB—Qualified Medicare Beneficiary
QPC—quality of patient care

R

RADT—registration, admission, discharge, and transfer
RB—rating board
RBRVS—resource-based relative value scale
RCC—ratio of cost to charges
R&D—research and development
REIT—real estate investment trust
RFI—request for information
RFP—request for proposal
RFQ—request for quotation
RHA—regional health administrator
RHC—rural health clinic
RHP—regional health planning
RIF—reduction in force
RM—risk management
RMIS—risk management information systems
ROE—return on equity
ROI—return on investment
RPCH—rural primary care hospital
RR—rate review
RRC—rural referral center
RTU—relative time unit
RUG—resource utilization groups
RVS—relative value scale/schedule/study
RVU—relative value unit

S

SB—Senate Bill (National)
SBC—school-based clinic
SBU—strategic business unit
SCH—sole community hospital
SCP—sole community provider
SD—standard derivation
SDC—secondary diagnostic category
SDI—selective dissemination of information
SE—standard error
SEC—Securities and Exchange Commission
SG—Surgeon General
SGO—Surgeon General's Office
SGR—sustainable growth rate
SHA—state health agency
SHC—state health commissioner
SI—severity index
SMI—Supplementary Medical Insurance (refers to Medicare Part B)
SNF—skilled nursing facility
SOB—statement of benefits
SOC—standard of care
SOI—severity of illness
SOP—standard operating procedures
SP—standard of performance
S&P—Standard and Poor's
SPA—state planning agency
SPD—supply, processing, and distribution
SPP—select provider program
SPR—system performance review
SR—Senate Resolution
SSA—Social Security Administration
SSDI—Social Security Disability Insurance
SSI—Supplemental Security Income
SSOP—Second Surgical Opinion Program
ST—standard treatment
STD—short-term disability
SUBC—State Uniform Billing Committee

T

TAAC—Technology Assessment Advisory Council
TAR—technology assessment report
TDA—tax-deferred annuity
T&E—travel and expense; trial and error
TEFRA—Tax Equity and Fiscal Responsibility Act
TPA—third-party administrator
TQM—total quality management

TR—turnover rate
TRO—temporary restraining order
TSA—tax-sheltered annuity
TT—transferred to; turnover time

U

UB—uniform billing
UB-92—Uniform Billing–Form 92
UBI—unrelated business income
UCAS—Uniform Cost Accounting Standards
UCR—usual, customary, and reasonable
UCR/PACE—usual, customary, and reasonable/performance and cost efficiency
UCRS—utilization control reporting system
UHCIA—Uniform Health Care Information Act
UHDDS—Uniform Hospital Discharge Data Set
UL—unauthorized leave
UM—utilization management
UPC—Uniform Product Code
UR—utilization review
USDA—United States Department of Agriculture
USDT—United States Department of Transportation
USFMG—United States foreign medical graduate
USFMSS—United States foreign medical school student
USMG—United States medical graduate
USPCC—United States per capita cost
USPHS—United States Public Health Service
USSG—United States Surgeon General

V

VA—Veterans' Affairs
VAH—Veterans' Affairs Hospital
VC—voluntary closing
VIP—voucher insurance plan

W

WC—Workers' Compensation
WCB—Workers' Compensation Board
WHF-USA—World Health Foundation, United States of America
WHO—World Health Organization
WIC—Women, Infants, Children
WL—waiting list

X

XR—x-ray

Y

YTD—year-to-date

Z

ZBB—zero-base budgeting
ZPG—zero population growth
ZPHMO—zero premium health maintenance organization

Index

S

U

V

LaVergne, TN USA
16 September 2010
197231LV00002B/19/P